D0166230

Communication and Cognition in Normal Aging and Dementia

COMMUNICATION AND COGNITION IN NORMAL AGING AND DEMENTIA

Kathryn A. Bayles, Ph.D.
Associate Research Scientist
Department of Speech and Hearing Sciences

Alfred W. Kaszniak, Ph.D.
Associate Professor of Psychology
Adjunct Associate Professor of Psychiatry

With the Assistance of
Cheryl K. Tomoeda, M.S.
Research Assistant
Department of Speech and Hearing Sciences
University of Arizona

pro·ed
8700 Shoal Creek Boulevard
Austin, Texas 78757

©1987 by PRO-ED, Inc.

All rights reserved. No part of this book may be reproduced in any form or by any means without the prior written permission of the publisher.

Printed in the United States of America

Library of Congress Cataloging-in-Publication Data

Bayles, Kathryn A., 1942–
Communictaion and cognition in normal aging and dementia / Kathryn A. Bayles, Alfred W. Kaszniak ; with assistance of Cheryl K. Tomoeda.
p. cm.
Reprint. Originally published: Boston : Little, Brown, ©1987.
Includes bibliographical references and indexes.
ISBN 0-89079-330-1
1. Communicative disorders in old age. 2. Language disorders in old age. 3. Cognition disorders in old age. 4. Dementia. 5. Aged–Communication. I. Kaszniak, Alfred W., 1949– . II. Tomoeda, Cheryl K. III. Title.
[RC423.B35 1991]
618.97'68—dc20 90-21692
CIP

pro·ed

8700 Shoal Creek Boulevard
Austin, Texas 78757

5 6 7 8 9 10

To Ed, Sara, and Tyler

K.A.B.

Mary Ellen, Jesse, and Ellie

A.W.K.

My parents and Barry

C.K.T.

CONTENTS

PREFACE

Our goal in writing this book was to describe the effects of normal aging and dementing diseases on communication and cognition. The purpose of the description is to provide health professionals and graduate students with an appreciation of aging and dementia that will guide them in their clinical responsibilities of diagnosis, evaluation, therapy, counseling, education, and research. To write about communication in dementia necessarily involves writing about cognition, and this book is unique in that it is a collaboration between brain-language scientists and a neuropsychologist. It is the first of its kind on this topic. It is intended to be useful to professionals in the fields of speech-language pathology, psychology, gerontology, and neurology. It may also be of interest to linguists, particularly neurolinguists. Professors in speech and hearing sciences may find it appropriate for classes in neurogenic communication disorders, aphasia, and aging and communication. Psychology professors may find it appropriate for classes in the psychology of aging, human neuropsychology, cognitive neuroscience, and clinical psychology. Additionally, the book may be a useful resource for students in nursing, medicine, and other health professions.

To assist the reader in understanding the multidisciplinary literature in dementia, and gleaning from it practical suggestions, the clinical implications of the material in each chapter have been specified. A glossary has been included after the last chapter.

Many of the data in the book are from the study of Alzheimer's patients. It is important for the reader to understand that the diagnosis of Alzheimer's disease is presumptive until autopsy confirmation (or brain biopsy in life, an uncommon practice in the United States). Thus, when reference is made in the text to the diagnosis of Alzheimer's disease, it is recognized that the diagnosis is presumptive.

ACKNOWLEDGMENTS

We wish to acknowledge the fine work of our colleagues, on which most of this book is based. For our own contributions, we are indebted to the National Institute of Aging, the National Institute of Mental Health, the National Institutes of Health Biomedical Research Program, the AARP Andrus Foundation, the Robert Wood Johnson Foundation, the University of Arizona Foundation, and Dr. Stanley Glickstein.

A colleague who was thinking about dementia and communication long before us, and who has provided inspiration for much of our work, is Dan Boone—a mentor and a friend.

Larry Stern, our colleague in neurology and our co-investigator, has challenged us always to do more and shown us how to do it better.

We are deeply indebted to Tom Slauson, our talented and tireless research assistant, who has innovated, edited, helped in the preparation of the manuscript, and managed the office. The fact that he forgot he had a home, other than the office, for the past year immeasurably contributed to the book's production. Thank you, Tom.

Who says research is no fun? Not Jill Caffrey! For the past decade her enthusiasm has made doing research fun for us, and her suggestions have improved the quality of our projects. She, too, read the manuscript and made suggestions. Special mention must be made of the contributions that Jill and Tom Slauson made in the development of Chapter 15, Management of Dementia.

The support of a friend who believes in you makes burning the midnight oil easier. Ray Bayles is such a friend. His moral support, wit, and technical advice made this writing adventure more enjoyable.

We would like to thank Jim Allender for many hours of consultation, discussion, and collaboration in research endeavors over the past several years.

Jay Rosenbek and Tom Hixon, our respected colleagues and awesome editors, shared their talents in editing the manuscript. We are grateful to them.

Thanks are in order for several other individuals: to Dick Demers, a distinguished linguist and friend who helped us better understand phonology.——To Karen Bressler, a cheerful, capable, and willing assistant, our thanks for helping in the office.——And to Marilyn Cauthon, a home-care provider to Alzheimer's patients, whose respect for research and cooperative spirit made the conduct of many of our studies easier.

As anyone who has conducted behavioral research with dementia patients knows, the data collection is challenging. Many graduate students have helped. Thanks to Fang Ling Lu, Elliot Smith, Cindy Spier, Lynne Jacobsen, Bob Boies, Tom Marks, Barbara Rende, Sherry Semrad, Alissa Berkin, Karen Eagans, Nancy Gibb, Glenn Stebbins, Mary Fox, Rex Swanda, Diane Pitz, and Paul Guest.

Finally, we want to thank the Tucson nursing home personnel, who have been so cooperative over the years. And most of all we thank the patients and their families. There is, of course, no way to thank our families for their sacrifices.

ACKNOWLEDGMENTS

INTRODUCTION

Sample #1

E: Tell me about this (marble).

S: Well, it's about half and half. It's a marble and its half and half. Uhm, that uhm, I'm trying to think what the and ya know and I've been doing all this color work and uhm. I'm trying to think. There's a white and there's a black and there's a, uhm, uhm, I'm trying to think, uh, it, it's, like uhm, oh, what is that called? Ym, more of a, oh damn, in the colors that I have in my book is uh more vivid, and this is a little darker, and I'm trying to think, what's it called, purple, more on the purple order this is.

Sample #2

E: Why are you here?

S: I'm not sure. I think I just started getting trouble with colds and they found out I was tied up with some virus affair that the Army had and uh used me as a means to cure that or . . . to put out a spread to it.

E: And, what's the name of the hospital?

S: Uh patients or etymology, one of the two, I'm not sure. I've been in part where you have the majority of them on the floor and some of them were not.

One of these language samples was produced by a dementia patient, the other by an aphasia patient. Which is which? Notice that both contain instances of perseveration, paraphasia, and dysnomia. The fact that these samples are hard to differentiate is a reminder that two very different neurologic disorders can produce similar results.* To differentiate between the neurologic conditions associated with these two samples, the clinician must consider something other than linguistic discourse. Most clinicians have a theory of aphasia that accounts for the discourse produced by aphasia patients, but lack a theory to account for the discourse of dementia.

Speech-language pathologists, neuropsychologists, and other professionals interested in communication disorders are educated in aphasia theory and recognize it as the consequence of focal damage in the area of the brain subserving language function, usually the left cerebral hemisphere. Aphasia theory is related to a more general theory of brain localization which enables clinicians to understand other nonlinguistic problems common in aphasia patients, such as hemiplegia and hemianopsia.

*Although not all discourse samples of dementia and aphasia patients are indistinguishable, some are.

CLINICIANS NEED A THEORY OF DEMENTIA

Few clinicians have a theory that accounts for the discourse of the patient with dementia. Stated differently, they lack a set of organizing principles that enables them to interpret the patient's behavior. Not only is a theory helpful for understanding the patient's behavioral changes; it can also guide the clinician in developing an evaluation plan and in predicting the course of the disease. One purpose of this book is to present a theory of dementia that accounts for the dissolution of cognition and communication.

The authors could recite the facts about behavioral change in dementing illness without suggesting a theory. However, the theory is the adhesive that binds together, in a meaningful way, the behavioral facts about dementia patients. To have a theory, albeit a good theory, is more helpful than memorizing facts about behavior, because a theory gives clinicians a context in which to interpret previously unlearned behavioral facts. Thus, in the course of this book, behavioral facts about communication and cognition in dementia will be specified, whenever possible, in relation to a theory.

ISN'T APHASIA THEORY THE SAME AS THE THEORY OF DEMENTIA?

No, they are very different. The commonly accepted theory of aphasia is that individuals suffer impairment in the comprehension and/or production of language, in one or more modalities, as a result of focal brain damage in the language dominant cerebral hemisphere. Further, the degree of language/communicative impairment is greater than that of cognitive impairment. This theory is inappropriate for dementia patients because they always suffer impairment in both language comprehension and production but retain (in the early and moderate stages) the ability to speak, read, and write. Additionally, they have brain damage in many regions of both cerebral hemispheres. Finally, in dementia, the degree of communicative impairment is generally proportional to the degree of cognitive impairment.

A critical difference between aphasia and dementia patients is that dementia patients have greater difficulty with the concepts underlying intentional communication and their manipulation. Grammatical and phonological rules, and the mechanics of linguistic expression, are not as vulnerable in dementia patients as in aphasia patients.

A THEORY ABOUT COMMUNICATION AND COGNITION IN DEMENTIA

Simply stated, the theory to be presented in this book is that dementia patients have particular impairment of semantic memory and a subsystem of semantic memory known as episodic memory. This term, *semantic memory*, will be confusing for most speech-language pathology readers. It sounds like a synonym for word memory, and the theory seems to be saying that word memory is broken. Quite the opposite. We will argue that word memory, or lexical representation, is intact in most persons with dementia, whereas conceptual memory is impaired. Semantic memory is a term commonly used by cognitive psychologists and linguists to refer to the central conceptual system in which information from the various sensory modalities is ultimately processed and represented. It is in this system that thinking occurs. We appreciate that the term is something of a misnomer, but we have elected to use it because it is so firmly rooted in the psychological and linguistic literature. Occasionally, however, synonyms such as the *central system*, the *conceptual system*, or the *central conceptual system* will be substituted.

The nature of semantic memory and the perceptual input systems that feed it are widely debated in numerous disciplines. One volatile issue about the nature of the mind's perceptual and central systems is the degree to which they are "modular," or uniquely organized to process a certain kind of information. Modularity is of interest to scholars who seek to characterize the structure of the mind and how the brain works to produce language.

Because it is the case that the performance of dementia patients raises some interesting points about the criteria used to define whether a system is modular, we will attempt to relate the data from dementia to the modularity debate.

HOW THE BOOK IS ORGANIZED

In the last two decades, an explosion of information about dementia and healthy aging has occurred. The study of both has become a priority in the scientific community. In relation to dementia, guidelines have been developed for defining, evaluating, and diagnosing primary degenerative dementing illnesses. Dementia severity rating scales have been validated. Cognitive and communicative changes have been documented. Tests have been validated for use with dementia patients. Patient management approaches have been suggested and caregiver counseling techniques evaluated. A primary purpose of this book is to share the research about dementia with clinicians and researchers.

Another purpose is to share recent research and theories about healthy aging. In order to differentiate a patient with dementing pathology from healthy individuals, considerable research has been conducted on the effects of healthy aging on cognition and communication. We have attempted to include enough of this research to build within the reader appropriate expectations about the cognitive and communicative abilities of the normal elderly.

To understand the dementia syndrome, most scholars will find themselves exploring new disciplines, mastering new research paradigms and terminology. The process of understanding is likely to be a time of personal intellectual growth, and the reader will make forays into neurology, cognitive psychology, speech and hearing sciences, neuropsychology, linguistics, and philosophy. This book is a collaborative effort between a speech-language pathologist and a neuropsychologist because in dementia, cognition affects communication and communication affects cognition.

In Chapter 1, The Brain and Age-Related Dementing Diseases, the reader is introduced to the dementia syndrome and the major dementing disorders, their epidemiology, neuropathology, and neurochemistry. Mastery of Chapter 1 will enable the clinician to anticipate and better understand the behavioral manifestations of the primary degenerative diseases discussed in subsequent chapters.

In Chapter 2, Linguistic Communication, Cognition, and the Conceptual System, a theoretical framework is constructed for interpreting the data from the study of communication and cognition in dementia. Considerable attention is given to delineating the putative contents and processes of semantic memory because the aforestated thesis of the book is that dementia patients suffer impairment of the conceptual and inferential system, where ideas are born and processed.

In Chapter 3, The Effects of Dementing Illness on Linguistic Communication, the reader is introduced to the recent literature concerning communication deficits of persons with dementia. The evidence of communicative impairment is classified according to whether it represents deterioration of the contents of semantic memory or its processes.

The effect of dementia etiology on the nature of communicative impairment is one of two topics discussed in Chapter 4: Linguistic Communication: Interetiologic and Longitudinal Considerations. The second topic is the nature of communicative dissolution over time, the principal points of which have been summarized in a series of charts at the chapter's end.

The effects of aging on linguistic communication are considered in Chapter 5. The information in this chapter is designed to help clinicians define what portion of a diminished performance may be due to the effect(s) of aging and what is due to pathology.

Changes in linguistic theory over the past two decades have influenced the way in which language is defined and evaluated, changes which are discussed in Chapter 6: Linguistic Theory and Knowledge, and Dementia. Among language scholars, a shift of emphasis has occurred from the study of language structure to the study of its meaning and use. The implications of this paradigmatic shift for the evaluation of dementia patients is specified.

In Chapter 7, Differentiating Dementia and Aphasia, the clinician is introduced to a testing approach for differential diagnosis. Specific tests are described and performance data of dementia and aphasia patients, as well as the normal elderly, are provided.

Chapter 8, Case Histories, is a natural sequel to the previous two chapters. It is unique in that the reader has been given the descriptive histories of several different types of dementia patients in addition to their performance scores on a communication test battery. It is in the reading of these case histories that the clinician can come to appreciate the relation of clinical performance to performance in real-life situations.

Chapter 9 is a reference chapter in which methodologic issues in aging and dementia research are discussed. Readers unsophisticated in the research issues related to measuring behavioral change in a progressively deteriorating population will be introduced to the pitfalls of dementia research. Further, they will receive guidance in how to evaluate published research findings.

Chapters 10 and 11 are concerned with intelligence and information processing speed as well as perception and attention, in normal aging and dementia. Together with Chapter 12, Memory in Normal Aging, and Chapter 13, Memory in Dementia, they provide a scholarly comprehensive account of the nature of cognitive change in both the normal elderly and dementia victims. Because the topic of memory has been the most popular in gerontologic psychology, the data related to memory and normal aging and memory and dementia are so substantial that each warrants its own chapter. In Chapter 13, considerable effort has been spent explicating episodic memory because of its value in differentiating dementia patients from other amnesic individuals and the normal elderly.

Evaluation of cognitive functions is the subject of Chapter 14, Neuropsychological Assessment of the Dementia Patient. The topics emphasized are the role of neuropsychological assessment in the diagnosis of dementing disease and the validity and reliability of commonly used neuropsychological tests.

The final chapter is entitled Management of Dementia. Because dementia patients and their caregivers are likely to be elderly, a profile of the average elderly person is developed. This profile forms a backdrop for considering the imposition of dementing illness on both the patient and caregiver. The most difficult problems of caregiving are reviewed, and an approach for management of the caregiver is suggested. The roles of the speech-language pathologist and neuropsychologist are detailed, and specific suggestions are provided for management of communicative and cognitive deficits.

Incidentally, the first language discourse sample is from a dementia patient, the second from an aphasic stroke patient.

His tundra'd mind sprouts leaflets
here and there
and causes me to stare
in new awareness of the man
he must have been.
Where he now
                    struggles
                                        to retain
such meagre lichen to his brain
he must have raised
rare orchids
years ago.

PAT FOLK, 1979*

---

*From Folk, P. (1979). Senile. In P.B. Janeczko (Ed.), *Postcard poems: A collection of poetry for sharing* (pg. 89). Scarsdale, NY: Bradbury Press.

Chapter 1

The Brain and Age-Related Dementing Diseases

This chapter is presented as an introduction to the most common causes of irreversible dementia, including Alzheimer's, Parkinson's, and Huntington's diseases, and vascular disease resulting in multiple infarctions. The information contained herein will provide a foundation for the interpretation of data obtained in behavioral studies of persons with dementia. The reader is referred to the sources listed in the bibliography for more comprehensive descriptions of the neuropathology and neurochemistry of specific dementing diseases. Also, the authors would like to draw the reader's attention to Figures 1-20 and 1-21 at the end of this chapter. These drawings of neuroanatomic structures and brain regions will assist the reader in identifying the important structures affected by the pathologic processes discussed in this chapter.

WHAT IS DEMENTIA?

Dementia is a syndrome and not a consequence of the normal process of aging. In medical terms, a syndrome is a constellation of signs and symptoms associated with a morbid process. Dementia refers to a condition of chronic progressive deterioration in intellect, personality, and communicative functioning (Table 1-1) and can be associated with numerous causes, among them infection, anoxia, tumor, trauma, toxicity, nutritional disturbances, and Alzheimer's and other diseases. In fact, Haase (1977) has identified more than 50 causes of dementia.

It is important to realize that when the term "dementia" is applied to a patient, the condition is not necessarily irreversible, for many of the causes of dementia are treatable. Lishman (1978) notes that the term has been used in two different ways. One refers to degenerative brain diseases such as Alzheimer's and Pick's disease, which are irreversible, and the other refers to a clinical syndrome of mental status impairments associated with a variety of conditions and illnesses.

American psychiatrists have adopted the term "primary degenerative dementia" (American Psychiatric Association, 1980) to refer to the clinical syndrome of progressive insidious intellectual deterioration commonly seen in elderly individuals, the defining characteristics of which are presented in Table 1-2. Although the syndrome of primary degenerative dementia is most frequently caused by Alzheimer's disease, the term does not imply causative factors or specific physiopathic concomitants. Not all patients with primary degenerative dementia are found to have the neuropathologic changes characteristic of Alzheimer's disease.

TABLE 1-1. Diagnostic Criteria for Dementia

A. Deterioration of intellect of sufficient magnitude to interfere with social or occupational functioning
B. Impairment of memory
C. At least one of the following:
   (1) impairment of abstract thinking
   (2) impairment of judgment
   (3) impairment of other higher cortical functions as evidenced by presence of: (a) aphasia, (b) apraxia, (c) agnosia, (d) constructional difficulty
   (4) personality change
D. Unclouded state of consciousness (does not meet the criteria for delirium or intoxication; however, these conditions may be superimposed)
E. One of the following:
   (1) a specific organic factor judged to be etiologically related to the disturbance through evidence from the history, physical examination, and laboratory tests
   (2) in the absence of such evidence, an organic factor can be presumed if: (a) conditions other than organic mental disorders have been excluded, and (b) cognitive impairment is apparent in many areas

Modified from DSM-III, 1980.

However, the term and the criteria established for its use have been criticized. Cummings and Benson (1983) argue that the term "primary degenerative dementia" contributes to confusion between the diagnosis of a specific type of dementia and the identification of a syndrome that has many causes. To avoid confusion, in recent years researchers have referred to the "dementia" associated with Alzheimer's disease as either Alzheimer's dementia or dementia of the Alzheimer's type (DAT), or even as senile dementia of the Alzheimer's type (SDAT).

TABLE 1-2. Diagnostic Criteria for Primary Degenerative Dementia

A. Dementia (see Table 1-1)
B. Insidious onset with steady, progressive deteriorating course
C. Exclusion of all other specific causes of dementia determined through evidence from medical history, physical examination, and laboratory tests

Modified from DSM-III, 1980.

Like the term "dementia," the term "Alzheimer's disease" has been applied to more than one population. Until recently, "Alzheimer's disease" was a diagnostic label used to refer to presenile patients, patients younger than 65 years of age; "senile dementia," and "senile brain disease," were the terms used with patients over age 65. As a result of several studies in which no difference was found in the histopathology of Alzheimer's patients and those with senile brain disease (Blessed, Tomlinson, and Roth, 1968; Terry and Wisniewski, 1972), the two conditions were reconceptualized as the same disease entity. Thus, the term "Alzheimer's disease" is used regardless of age of onset. If a specification of early onset is desired, patients can be described as having presenile dementia of the Alzheimer's type; to specify late onset, the term senile dementia of the Alzheimer's type can be used.

CAUSES OF DEMENTIA

Although the dementia syndrome has many causes, Alzheimer's disease is the most common. The data from postmortem studies reveal that between 50 and 60 percent of all dementia patients have Alzheimer's disease (Jellinger, 1976; Sourander and Sjögren, 1970; Tomlinson, Blessed, and Roth, 1970). Other causes of dementia range from hypothyroidism to chemical intoxication to sensory deprivation. Early identification of potentially treatable causes of the dementia is of particular importance, for, if untreated, the dementia can become fixed and irreversible (Besdine, 1982).

Reversible Causes of Dementia

Reports from six neurologic and neuropsychiatric studies indicate that in 10 to 33 percent of adults with the characteristics of dementia, the condition has a reversible cause (Fox, Topel, and Huckman, 1975; Freemon, 1976; Harrison and Marsden, 1977; Marsden and Harrison, 1972; Rabins, 1981;

Smith and Kiloh, 1981). One feature distinguishing many reversible from irreversible causes is whether the cognitive deterioration has a structural basis. For example, AD patients have structural changes in their brains, whereas those with dementia due to systemic infection do not. When the disease process lies outside the central nervous system and structural changes are not associated, some physicians use the term "secondary dementia" to emphasize that the disease exerts a secondary detrimental effect on the brain (Besdine, 1982).

Delirium or Acute Confusional State. True dementia must often be distinguished from delirium. Delirium, or acute confusional state, is common in the elderly and suggests systemic illness. The essential feature of delirium, according to the DSM-III (1980), is a clouded state of consciousness (Table 1-3). In aged individuals, brain homeostasis is easily disrupted because of its greater sensitivity to pathophysiologic changes caused by physical illness (Engel and Romano, 1959; Libow, 1973). Unlike dementia, in which confusion insidiously occurs, delirium develops abruptly, being provoked most frequently by reversible disease (Besdine, 1982). The primary behavioral manifestation is impaired attention (Cummings and Benson, 1983). Other features include impaired memory, incoherence of thought and conversation, hallucinations, disturbances of the sleep-wakefulness cycle, an abnormal electroencephalogram, and evidence of systemic illness (Chedru and Geschwind, 1972; Engel and Romano, 1959; Lipowski, 1980; Wolff and Curran, 1935).

TABLE 1-3. Diagnostic Criteria for Delirium

A. Clouded state of consciousness or reduced awareness of the environment
B. At least two of the following: (1) perceptual impairment (e.g., hallucinations), (2) incoherent speech or language, (3) sleep disturbance, or (4) change in psychomotor activity
C. Disorientation
D. Memory impairment
E. Abrupt onset and fluctuating course
F. A specific organic factor judged to be etiologically related to the disturbance through evidence from medical history, physical examination, and laboratory tests

Modified from DSM-III, 1980.

Pseudodementia. The term "pseudodementia" is often used to refer to the cognitive impairment seen in association with a number of psychiatric disorders. The dementia is presumed not to be structurally based. Approximately 10 percent of patients evaluated for progressive cognitive decline have been found to have pseudodementia (Marsden and Harrison, 1972; Seltzer and Sherwin, 1978). Tyler and Tyler (1984) report that cognitive impairment related to severe depression is commonly mistaken for dementia and may account for 50 percent of the cases of pseudodementia. It is important to emphasize that in cases of pseudodementia, the primary cause of intellectual impairment is a psychiatric disorder, and if treatment is successfully implemented, the intellectual disturbance may be reversible.

Normal Pressure Hydrocephalus. Normal pressure hydrocephalus (NPH) is a condition in which enlargement of the ventricular system is observed in the presence of normal cerebrospinal fluid pressure (Katzman, 1978). Researchers have suggested that there are two forms of NPH. One form occurs secondary to bleeding from an arteriovenous malformation or trauma (Katzman, 1978). In the other form, idiopathic NPH (Adams, Fisher, Hakim, Ojemann, and Sweet, 1965), the cause is not apparent. The incidence of NPH is estimated at 5 percent among patients younger than 65 who exhibit dementia symptoms (Jellinger, 1976; Marsden and Harrison, 1972) and 0.2 percent in patients older than 65 (Jellinger, 1976). It is a well-recognized cause of reversible dementia and was the most common potentially treatable cause in studies conducted by Marsden and Harrison (1972) and Freemon (1976). The symptom constellation that makes this a clinically distinct condition is urinary incontinence, ataxia of gait, and mental status change.

Mental and Sensory Deprivation. Finally, it should be mentioned that mental deprivation and sensory impairment may alter the behavior of affected individuals to the degree that they appear demented. People undergoing voluntary visual, auditory, and tactile deprivation have been found to develop anxiety, tension, impaired comprehension, somatic complaints, intense emotions, and vivid sensory imagery akin to hallucinations (Solomon, 1961). In his chapter on mental deprivation and the development of dementia-like characteristics, Charatan (1984) reminds readers that older individuals typically experience reduction in visual and auditory acuity, tactile and olfactory sensitivity, and restricted mobility (Figure 1-1).

Although the aforementioned diseases and conditions are those most commonly associated with reversible dementia, many other causes, too numerous to discuss, also exist. The point to be emphasized is that because so many conditions are associated with dementia, cognitive decline and mental status change must not be presumed to be irreversible.

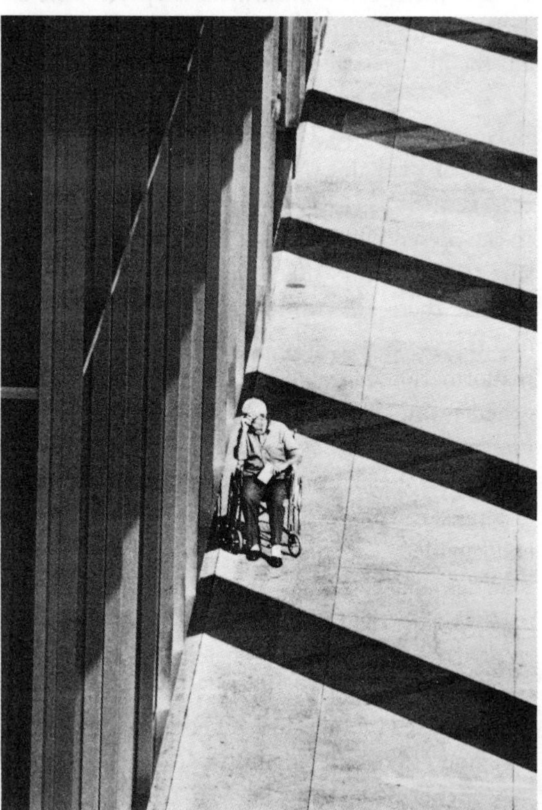

Figure 1-1. *Mental deprivation and sensory impairment may cause elderly individuals to appear demented.*

EPIDEMIOLOGY OF DEMENTIA

Declining birth rates, reduced mortality, and rising life expectancy have resulted in the aging of the world's population. In 1970, approximately 307 million people in the world were over the age of 60. This figure is expected to rise to 600 million by the year 2000, with the very elderly subgroup accounting for the greatest increase (Lauter, 1985). Indeed, most Asian countries are predicted to experience an increase in excess of 80 percent (Table 1-4). Indonesia is expected to experience the largest increase, an increase of 134 percent!

The projections are further dramatized by the fact that the estimated percentage increases in the period between the years 2000 and 2025 are expected to be twice as great as in the years 1975 to 2000 (Figure 1-2). By the year 2025, the proportion of Americans over 65 years of age will rise from 11 to 20 percent, and their numbers will more than double from 26 million to more than 58.5 million (Brody, 1984).

With such phenomenal growth expected in the elderly population, scientists and health planners predict a rapid increase in the number of individuals affected by Alzheimer's disease. By the year 2000, over 2 million people in the United States will be affected (Finch, 1985). It is also predicted that by the twenty-first century, more than 11 million elderly people in Asia will suffer moderate to severe dementing disease; of existing health services on that continent, those for the geriatric patient are the least developed.

In their chapter on aging and dementia in the developing world, Andrews and Davidson (1984) write that history will judge the health planners of today severely if they fail to acknowledge that caring for dementia patients is one of the most significant problems associated with the growing elderly population. Although health planners in developed nations are beginning to respond to the challenge of caring for dementia patients, little

TABLE 1-4. Examples of Projected Percentage Increases in Populations in Selected Asian Countries

	Projected Percent Increase of the Total Population 1980 to 2000	Percentage of the Population ≥ 60 years		Projected Percent Increase of Population ≥ 60 years 1980 to 2000
		1980	2000	
China (People's Republic)	24.3	8.6	10.6	54.7
Japan	10.8	12.6	19.8	73.8
Korea (Republic)	33.7	6.2	9.3	100.0
Philippines	63.6	4.8	5.6	89.2
Malaysia	48.0	5.4	6.6	80.1
Indonesia	45.9	4.3	6.8	134.4

From the United Nations Centre for Social Development and Humanitarian Affairs (UNCSDHA 1981), *Demographic aspects of the aging population in the Asian and Pacific region.* Report of the Technical Meeting on Aging. Bangkok, ESP/P/WP.65. Reprinted with permission.

attention is being given by underdeveloped nations, geographic areas in which the impact of population aging will be greatest (Myers, 1982; Schade, 1982; United Nations, 1982).

Prevalence and Incidence of Dementia

Dementia is most commonly caused by Alzheimer's disease which affects between 1.2 and 4 million Americans (U.S. Office of Technology Assessment, 1985). The prevalence of AD is hard to specify precisely because of variations in regional and historical methods of diagnosing and reporting. Reliable prevalence estimates come from population studies conducted in northern Europe. Severe Alzheimer's dementia was reported to affect between 1.1 and 6.2 percent of those over age 65, with mild and moderate dementia affecting another 2.6 to 15.4 percent (Bollerup, 1975; Broe et al., 1976; Essen-Moller, Larsson, Uddenberg, and White, 1956; Kay, Beamish, and Roth, 1964; Kay, Bergmann, Foster, McKechnie, and Roth, 1970; Nielsen, 1962). Recently an investigation was conducted in the United States of the prevalence of severe dementia in a Mississippi county (Schoenberg, Anderson, and Haerer, 1985). Severe dementia was reported in approximately 1 percent

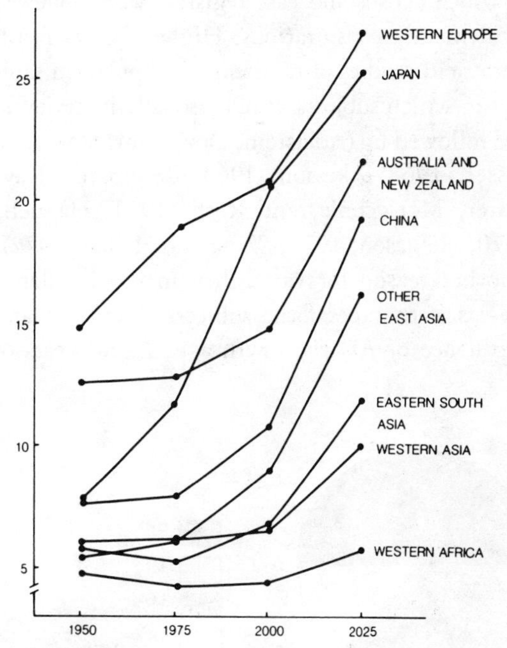

Figure 1-2. *Proportion of the total population that is 60 years and over, by selected subregions, for 1950, 1975, 2000, 2025. (From the United Nations World Assembly on Aging (1982).* Introductory document: Demographic considerations. *A/Conf.113/4. Reprinted with permission.)*

of individuals over 40 years of age. This prevalence figure rose to 7 percent for those 80 years of age or older.

The incidence (frequency of occurrence of new cases) of Alzheimer's disease approximates 1 percent of the elderly population per year (Mortimer, 1983). Incidence studies require follow-up of a population over time with careful medical review to detect new cases. Few such investigations have been conducted. Mortimer (1983) analyzed the incidence studies and reported that with the exception of the study by Jarvik, Ruth, and Matsuyama (1980), in which the population studied was older, investigators reported an incidence of approximately 1 percent per year.

Incidence rates may vary, depending upon whether the investigator is considering only mild dementia or moderate and severe dementia as well. Lauter (1985) reports that moderate and severe dementia in the over-60 population varies between 4 and 5 per 1,000 and 15 per 1,000. The lower incidence figures are associated with investigations in which census and case registers were reviewed for dementia consultations. Higher figures result from field studies of randomized population samples in which subjects were personally interviewed and followed up (Adelstein, Downham, Stein, and Susser, 1968; Åkesson, 1969; Bergmann, Kay, Foster, McKechnie, and Roth, 1971; Hagnell, 1970; Helgason, 1977; Wing and Hailey, 1972). Another reason for variability in the incidence reports is the age of the subjects. Incidence and prevalence of AD rises with age. At 80 years of age, the incidence is 3 to 4 percent, and prevalence approaches 20 percent. These figures are especially significant because the 85-plus age group is the fastest growing segment of the United States population.

Dementia is the most common nursing home diagnosis (U.S. Office of Technology Assessment, 1985) given to approximately two thirds of all nursing home residents. Yet, one third to one half of dementia patients are cared for at home (Terry and Katzman, 1983).

For dementia, prevalence figures (percentage of people afflicted at given time) are likely to be conservative because few epidemiologists have recognized the frequency of dementia in Parkinson's patients. Although not all Parkinson's patients develop dementia, a significant percentage do: on the average, 30 percent (Boller, Mizutani, Roessmann, and Gambetti, 1980; Lieberman et al., 1979; Loranger, Goodell, McDowell, Lee, and Sweet, 1972; Pollock and Hornabrook, 1966).

Accounting for approximately 15 to 20 percent of the dementia patient population is vascular disease (Tomlinson, Blessed, and Roth, 1970). Vascular or multi-infarct dementia (MID) is the cumulative worsening of cognitive function due to repeated strokes. It can and does co-occur with Alzheimer's disease in another 15 percent of cases (Figure 1-3). The burgeoning population of dementia patients will challenge the emotional resources of a large portion of the population and the financial resources of the nation.

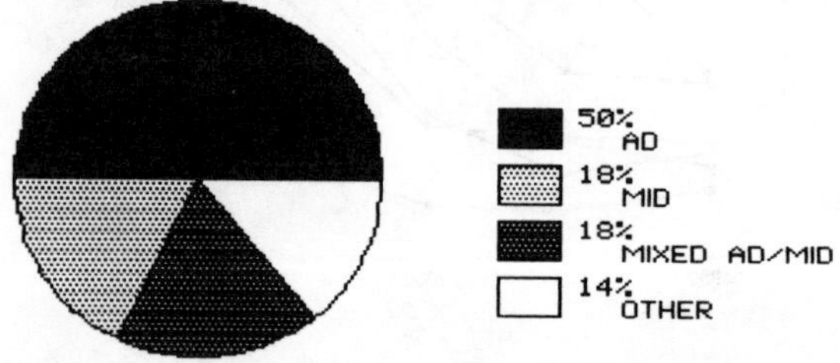

Figure 1-3. *Prevalence of dementia according to type. AD = Alzheimer's disease; MID = multi-infarct dementia. (Based on data from Tomlinson, Blessed, and Roth, 1970)*

Cost of Caring for Dementia Patients

The Health Care Financing Administration has estimated that the United States government spends over 6 billion dollars annually in nursing home costs on Alzheimer's patients alone. This figure represents 30 percent of the total Federal health care budget. Furthermore, an additional 2 to 4 billion dollars in Federal funds are spent on acute-hospital, home, and rehabilitative care for these patients.

Under present arrangements, federal funds for long-term care will escalate to $43 billion by 1990, and Alzheimer's disease will account for 30 to 50 percent of this outlay.

ALZHEIMER'S DISEASE

Whereas a decade ago the majority of Americans were unfamiliar with our fastest growing and most expensive clinical population, today most know about Alzheimer's disease and its consequences. Americans have begun to realize the dramatic rate at which the older segment of the population is growing. Increasing numbers of people have had to cope with the economic exigencies of caring for an AD patient, an undertaking that depletes their financial and emotional resources. The social and economic realities of caring for AD patients have motivated government leaders to provide support for scientists studying the disease, its cause, and its behavioral manifestations. In 1984 the National Institute on Aging encumbered 3.5 million dollars to establish as many as five national centers for the study of AD. Additionally, the National Institute of Neurological, Communicative Disorders and Stroke and the National Institute of Mental Health have increased the numbers of research dollars destined for AD research. Indeed, AD has become a top research priority of both governmental and private research organizations.

The disease is named for the German neurologist, Alois Alzheimer, who in 1906 first described the relation between neurofibrillary tangles and the symptomatology of dementia (Alexander and Selesnick, 1966). Using newly developed silver impregnation histologic staining techniques, Alzheimer was able to observe neurofibrillary tangle formations in the brain of a demented 55 year old woman. The age of the woman and her lack of vascular disease convinced Alzheimer to attribute the woman's dementia to the presence of tangle formations in the brain.

At the turn of the century, Alzheimer's assertion of a relationship between dementia symptomatology and neuronal changes in the brain was notable because of the disagreement within the academic community as to the cause of mental disease. Alzheimer's organic concept of his patient's dementia contradicted the Freudian concept of mental disease as a conflict between the conscious and subconscious minds. However, within 5 years of Alzheimer's paper, 11 additional cases with similar clinical and pathologic characteristics were reported, and the concept of Alzheimer's disease as an organically caused presenile dementia gained credibility. However, the same silver staining techniques used by Alzheimer were soon employed in studying the neuropathology of other illnesses, and it became apparent that AD was not the only disease in which the tangle formations occurred. In fact, tangle formations were noted in the brains of healthy individuals. These findings caused much confusion about the nature of Alzheimer's disease—confusion that persists today. As yet, brain scientists are unable to explain why the morphologic changes typical of AD occur in the brains of normal individuals.

Clinical Presentation

Alzheimer's disease begins subtly; in fact, in most individuals, identification of the precise onset is a matter of speculation. Often, it is only after the disease is diagnosed that families of AD victims begin to remember seemingly isolated instances of unusual behavior that occurred during the previous 2 or 3 years. In a survey of 284 caregivers of AD patients, the question was asked, "How did you first become aware something was wrong?" (Chenoweth and Spencer, 1986). Sixty-two percent reported memory problems, 20 percent indicated work-related problems, and 19 percent observed personality changes. These same respondents also were asked, "What was the main symptom that first caused you, your relative with Alzheimer's, or someone else to look for help?" Again, memory loss and disorientation were the most common distressing symptoms occurring in 52 percent of the cases, followed by personality change in 16 percent and physical changes in 16 percent. Other symptoms included inability to function, work-related and driving problems, difficulty managing money, and drinking.

These reports by caregivers are in accord with clinical observations. In the first phase of the disease (Table 1-5), changes in memory, personality, problem-solving ability, visuospatial skills, and communicative functioning are apparent to family members, and detectable with formal testing, but may go unnoticed in casual encounters. In the second phase, these defects are more prominent, appearing even in casual encounters. Motor problems, particularly restlessness, may now be present. By the third phase, intellectual functioning is globally deteriorated and persons need continuous supervision. Patients become incontinent of bowel and bladder and require assistance with all aspects of personal hygiene and daily living. Because of disease effects on the motor system, patients may exhibit limb rigidity and flexion posture. (For case descriptions of AD patients, see Chapter 8.)

TABLE 1-5. Clinical Presentation of Alzheimer's Disease

FIRST PHASE

Memory: Recent and remote recall impaired

Personality: Irritability, hostility, apathy, suspiciousness, frustration

Communication: Content of language disordered, dysnomia, linguistic reasoning defects

Problem-solving: Inferential ability impaired

Visuospatial ability: Defective constructions, topographic disorientation

Motor system: Generally normal, subset with extrapyramidal signs

SECOND PHASE

Memory: Prominent impairment in all memory and learning

Personality: Indifference, hostility, poor social judgment, flattening of affect

Communication: Content disordered and some structural defects, dysnomia

Problem-solving: Needs assistance to solve very simple problems

Visuospatial ability: Spatial disorientation, poor constructions, misperception

Motor system: Restlessness

THIRD PHASE

Intellectual functions: Globally deteriorated

Personality: Disorganized

Communication: Globally deteriorated, mutism, echolalia, palilalia, perseveration

Motor system: Limb rigidity and flexion posture

Adapted from Cummings and Benson (1983).

Neuropathy of Alzheimer's Disease

The brains of AD patients atrophy and undergo microscopic changes, notably the development of neurofibrillary tangles (NFTs), neuritic plaques (NPs), and areas of granulovacuolar degeneration (GVD). Total cortical and white matter volume is diminished. Large neurons are lost, primarily in the frontal and temporal regions (Figure 1-4) and the substantia innominata, an area deep within the brain. Other regions are affected as well. Brody (1955, 1970) and Shefer (1972) studied the four lobes of the brain and noted the most severe cell loss in the frontal lobe. Their data suggested a trend of increasing neuronal cell loss from primary cortices to association cortices. The atrophic process can be seen in the dilation of the lateral ventricles and the sunken gyri and widened sulci (Figure 1-5). Indeed, there is a decrease in the absolute volume of neuron-bearing cortex. While the weight of an aged normal brain is 7 to 8 percent less than that of an average adult brain, in AD patient brains, weight is reduced by approximately 10 percent from that of healthy age-mates (Terry and Davies, 1983).

The fact that large neurons are lost may be important, because the loss of the larger neurons may distinguish abnormal from normal aging. Brody (1955) has reported that the major cell loss in normal aging is among small neurons. Then too, Brody describes the greatest neuronal loss among normal persons to be in the superior temporal cortex, whereas the greatest loss in AD patients is in the midfrontal area, superior temporal gyrus (Terry, 1981), and anterior temporal lobes (Lauter, 1985).

Not only are neurons lost in the brains of AD patients, but the number of dendritic branches decreases. Dendrites are cell body projections by which neurons receive impulses from other neu-

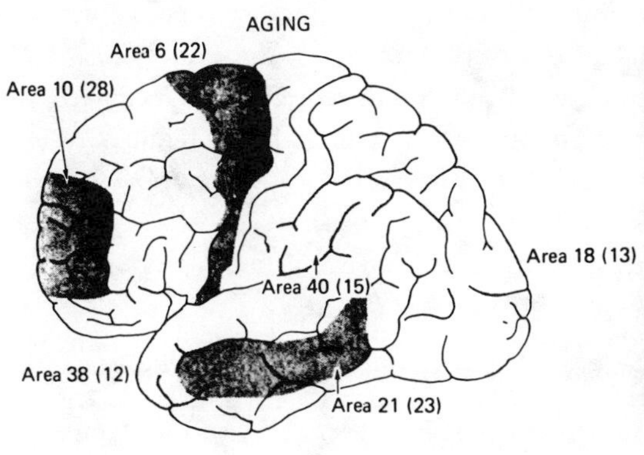

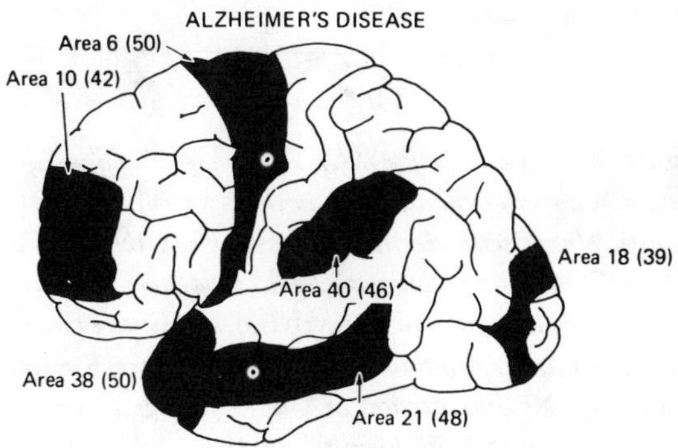

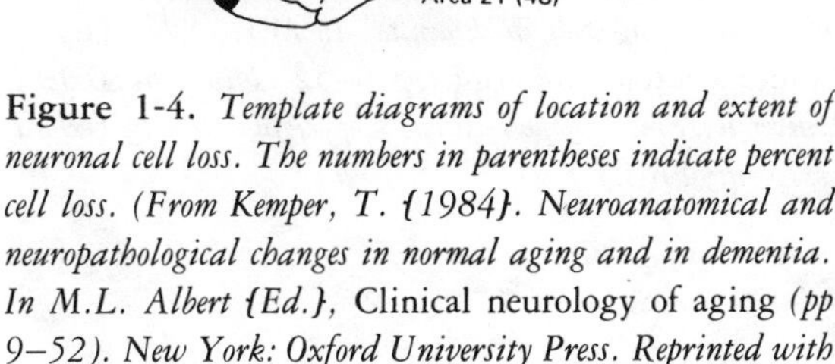

Figure 1-4. *Template diagrams of location and extent of neuronal cell loss. The numbers in parentheses indicate percent cell loss. (From Kemper, T. {1984}. Neuroanatomical and neuropathological changes in normal aging and in dementia. In M.L. Albert {Ed.},* Clinical neurology of aging *(pp 9–52). New York: Oxford University Press. Reprinted with permission.)*

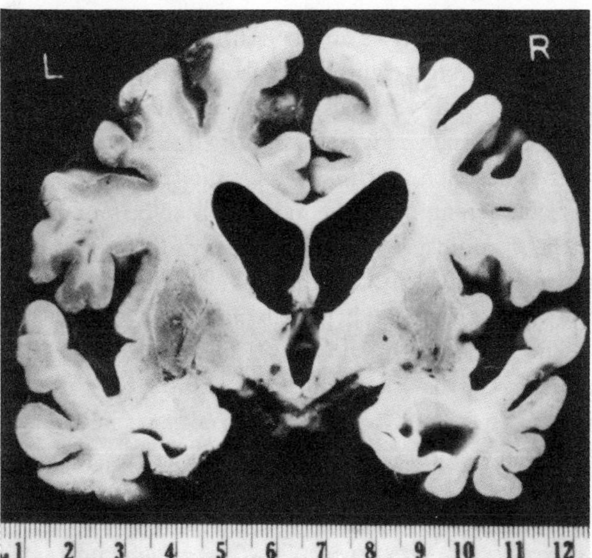

Figure 1-5. *Alzheimer's disease, showing general shrinkage of the brain in a coronal cut. (From Adams, J.H., Corsellis, J.A.N., and Duchen, L.W. {1984}.* Greenfield's neuroanatomy. *New York: John Wiley and Sons, by permission. Copyright 1984 by Edward Arnold (Publishers) Ltd.)*

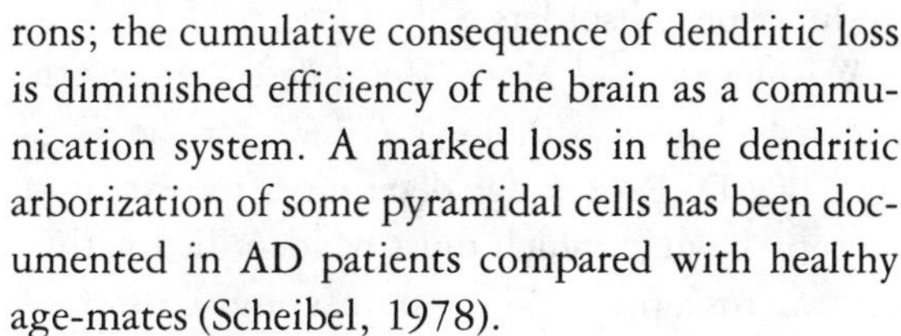

rons; the cumulative consequence of dendritic loss is diminished efficiency of the brain as a communication system. A marked loss in the dendritic arborization of some pyramidal cells has been documented in AD patients compared with healthy age-mates (Scheibel, 1978).

Neurofibrillary Tangles. The most characteristic morphologic change is the formation of neurofibrillary tangles (NFTs), (Figure 1-6). NFTs are filaments within the cell body that pair together in a helical fashion (Kidd, 1963; Wisniewski, Narang, and Terry, 1976) and course throughout

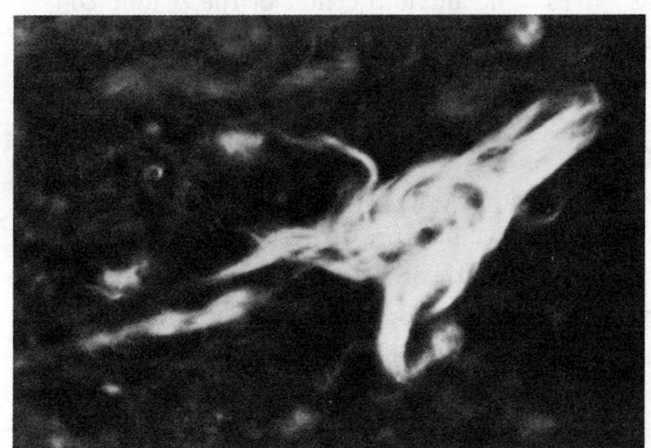

Figure 1-6. *A thioflavine S–stained neuron with a well-formed neurofibrillary tangle. The paired helical filaments glow bright yellow in ultraviolet illumination. (From Terry, R., and Katzman, R. {1983}. Senile dementia of the Alzheimer type: Defining a disease. In R. Katzman and R. Terry {Ed.},* The neurology of aging *(pp. 51–84). Philadelphia, PA: F.A. Davis Company, by permission. Copyright 1983 by the F.A. Davis Company.)*

the cytoplasm. NFTs are thought to result from abnormal protein synthesis (Iqbal, Wisniewski, Grundke-Iqbal, Korthals, and Terry, 1975), but yet to be discounted is the possibility that they represent a reaction to damage in another part of the nervous system. NFTs are most likely to be found in the pyramidal cells of the hippocampus and the amygdaloid nucleus, but they can occur throughout the neocortex and hypothalamus.

The hippocampus and amygdaloid nucleus, for which NFTs have a predilection, are part of the limbic system, a network of nuclei and tracts influential in emotion and memory. NFTs are not unique to AD and may represent a common cellular sequela after physical or chemical trauma. Their presence in older people may account for the difficulty many elders have with memory.

Neuritic Plaques. Neuritic plaques (NPs), also called senile plaques, are clumps of degenerating neurons surrounding an amyloid core (Figure 1-7). The degenerative neuronal processes consist primarily of axonal terminals or preterminals (Reisberg, 1981). They are found in the same brain regions as NFTs. The amyloid center of the plaque consists of either protein material or a complex of immunoglobulin chains. Amyloid is deposited in tissues when a condition of altered immunity exists (Behan and Behan, 1979). Reisberg (1981) described immunoglobulins as protein antibodies that organisms manufacture in response to antigenic material. It is theorized that plaques are formed when antigen-antibody complexes are ingested by white blood cells (Glenner, Ein, and Terry, 1972).

In AD patients, the plaques are found in large numbers primarily in the outer half of the cortex, where the number of neuronal connections is greatest (Sholl, 1956). In intellectually normal individuals, plaques are seen in smaller numbers in the inner half of the cortex (Gibson, 1983).

Tomlinson et al. (1970) observed that 14 plaques per microscopic field was a valid threshold value for differentiating the demented elderly from normal persons. Whereas plaques were common in the normal elderly in their study, large numbers of them were uncommon. Roth (1971) reported that the cutoff point of an average of 12 plaques or more per visual field correctly classified 85 percent of patients with senile dementia, whereas a plaque count of less than 12 classified 90 to 100 percent of mentally normal subjects and those with different functional disorders.

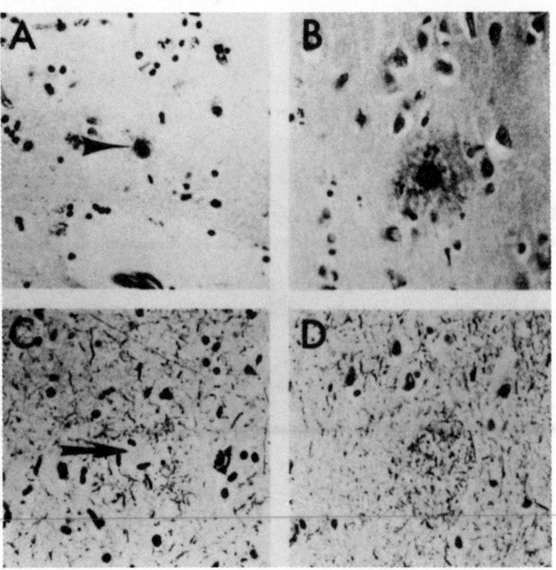

Figure 1-7. *Senile plaques.* **(A)**, *a "burned-out" plaque represented by a small focal deposit of amyloid* (arrowhead); **(B)**, *a classic plaque with reactive cells surrounding the amyloid deposit;* **(C)**, *a classic plaque with degenerating axons surrounding focal deposit of amyloid* (arrow); **(D)**, *a primitive plaque with degenerating axons throughout the plaque. (From Kemper, T. {1984}. Neuroanatomical and neuropathological changes in normal aging and in dementia. In M.L. Albert {Ed.},* Clinical neurology of aging *(pp. 9–52). New York: Oxford University Press, by permission. Copyright 1984 by Oxford University Press.)*

Wisniewski and Merz (1985) describe recently established neuropathologic criteria for the diagnosis of AD. Patient age determines the extent of neuropathology, which must be identified within any microscopic field encompassing 1 mm^2 of brain tissue.

1. In any patient *less than 50 years of age,* the number of neuritic plaques and neurofibrillary tangles seen anywhere in the neocortex should be greater than two to five per field. This enables the anatomical pathologist to

establish a very firm diagnosis, even in mediocolegal cases and in the absence of any helpful clinical history.

2. In any patient *between age 50 and 65 years,* there will be some number of tangles, but the number of plaques must be eight or greater per field. This will again permit a diagnosis with a very high degree of confidence (±95 percent).
3. In any patient *between 66 and 75 years of age,* some tangles will still be present, but the number of neuritic plaques must be greater than ten per field.
4. In any patient *older than 75 years,* tangles may sometimes not be found in the neocortex, but the number of plaques should exceed 15 per microscopic field. (pp. 232-233)

Granulovacuolar Degeneration. Granulovacuolar degeneration (GVD) is a descriptive term that refers to the presence of fluid-filled spaces and granular debris within the cell (Figure 1-8). Like NFTs and NPs, areas of GVD occur in the brains of normal individuals and have a predilection for the hippocampal formation. The degree of GVD is significantly related to the presence of dementia. Tomlinson and Henderson (1976) reported that 90 percent of persons with more than 9 percent of hippocampal cells affected exhibit dementia.

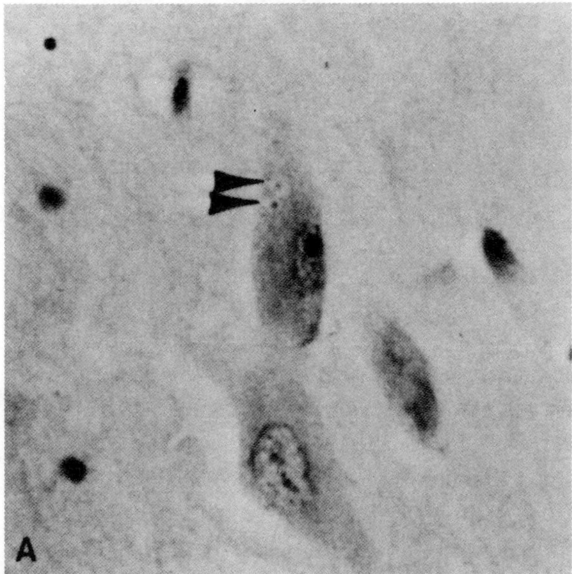

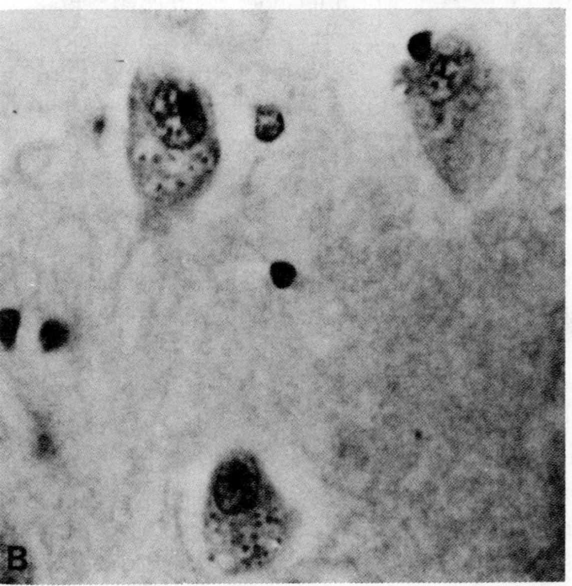

Figure 1-8. *Granulovacuolar degeneration in hippocampal pyramidal cells.* **(A)**, *two granules, indicated by arrowheads;* **(B)**, *three neurons with multiple granules. (From Kemper, T. {1984}, Neuroanatomical and neuropathological changes in normal aging and in dementia. In M.L. Albert {Ed.},* Clinical neurology of aging *(pp. 9–52). New York: Oxford University Press, by permission. Copyright 1984 by Oxford University Press.)*

Neurochemical Changes

Cholinergic System. Neurochemical deficiencies in the brains of AD patients are now well documented. The best known is the cholinergic deficit. The first clue that central cholinergic neurons were impaired in AD patients came from a published report of significant reduction in the activity of a marker enzyme for choline, acetylcholinesterase (AChE) (Pope, Hess, and Lewin, 1964). At first, the report received little attention because AChE is not specific to cholinergic neurons, but by 1976, several reports were published of reductions in the level of choline acetyltransferase (ChAT), an enzyme thought to be unique to cholinergic neurons (Bowen, Smith, White, and Davison, 1976; Carlsson,

Adolfsson, and Aquilonius, 1980; Davies and Maloney, 1976; Kuhar, 1976; Perry, Gibson, Blessed, and Tomlinson, 1977; Perry, Perry, Blessed, and Tomlinson, 1977; Reisine, Yamamura, Bird, Spokes, and Enna, 1978; White et al., 1977). The deficiency in choline acetyltransferase was beyond that typical of normal aging (Davies, 1979; McGeer and McGeer, 1975) and was most apparent in the neocortex and hippocampus, where the losses ranged from 50 to 97 percent (Davies and Maloney, 1976; Perry, Perry et al., 1977; White et al., 1977). Reduction in cholinergic neurotransmission has been associated with degree of cognitive impairment (Perry et al., 1978) and may account, at least partially, for degree of overall dementia severity (Perry and Perry, 1985).

Simultaneously with the investigations of ChAT levels, neuroscientists worked to trace the cholinergic innervation of the cortex. As a result of these investigations, scientists learned that the medial basal forebrain, which includes the medial septal nucleus, the nucleus of the diagonal band of Broca, and the nucleus basalis of Meynert (nbM) (Figure 1-9), is composed of a sheet of giant cholinergic cells (Divac, 1975; Kievit and Kuypers, 1975; Mesulam and van Hoesen, 1976; Nagai, Pearson, Peng, McGeer, and McGeer, 1983). These cells innervate the hippocampus, amygdala, and neocortical areas. The first report of a large loss of these cholinergic cells in AD came from Price and colleagues (1982), a finding that is now well substantiated (Nagai, McGeer, Peng, McGeer, and Dolman, 1983; Perry et al., 1982; Rossor et al., 1982). Subsequently, the giant cells of the medial basal forebrain were shown to be a single population of cholinergic cells, thereby enabling researchers to assess the relationship between AD and the cholinergic cell population in the medial basal forebrain (McGeer, 1984).

Most cortical cholinergic inputs originate in the nbM. This nucleus lies beneath the lentiform nuclei, near the anterior commissure, and contains large cholinergic neurons that project diffusely to the cortex (Figure 1-10). Coyle, Price, and DeLong (1983) have reviewed the evidence for marked and widespread degeneration of these cells in AD patients.

More recently Rogers, Brogan, and Mirra (1985) compared degeneration in the nbM in the brains of patients with a broad variety of neurologic disorders, some associated with dementia. Rogers and colleagues found the most striking degeneration to be among the AD patients, though degeneration was apparent in Parkinson's disease, Creutzfeldt-Jakob disease, and progressive supranuclear palsy.

Currently, research is underway to discover why the cholinergic neurons in the nbM are selectively affected. An important point to be emphasized is that within the cortex, the postsynaptic elements of the cholinergic system are well preserved (Davies and Verth, 1977; Perry, Perry et al., 1977; Reisine et al., 1978), suggesting that the problem in cortical cholinergic neurotransmission is due to a dysfunction of presynaptic cholinergic neurons. Because of this finding, neuropharmacologists have considered ways to bring choline to the intact cortical receptors.

Noradrenergic System. In addition to a cholinergic deficit, evidence has accumulated of abnormalities in the noradrenergic system in AD patients (Adolfsson, Gottfries, Roos, and Winblad, 1979; Berger, Tassin, Rancurel, and Blanc, 1980). The marker enzyme for the noradrenergic transmission system is dopamine-β-hydroxylase, which is known to be reduced in AD (Cross et al., 1981), though not as prominently as ChAT, nor in all patients. Noradrenergic cell bodies are located in the nucleus locus coeruleus, found within the dorsal brainstem (Figure 1-11). Interestingly, the loss of dopamine-β-hydroxylase has been found to be more severe in younger AD patients (Bondareff, Mountjoy, and Roth, 1981).

The locus coeruleus is believed to influence higher-order mental functions, including learning and memory (van Dongen, 1981). Nerve cells in this nucleus form an extensive network of fibers, which terminate on capillary walls within the brain (Swanson, Connelly, and Hartman, 1976). Electrical stimulation of the locus coeruleus is associated with a reduction in cerebral blood flow and an increase in water permeability (Raichle, Hartman, Eichling, and Sharpe, 1975), findings interpreted to mean that the nucleus locus coeruleus is influential in maintaining central nervous system homeostasis.

Neuropeptides. Additionally, reductions have been reported in certain other brain chemicals, among them the neuropeptides, somatostatin, and substance P (Davies, Katz, and Crystal, 1982; Davies, Katzman, and Terry, 1980; Davies and Terry, 1981; Rossor, Emson, Mountjoy, Roth, and Iverson, 1980). Neuropeptides are small proteins that play important roles in brain function as neurotransmitters, neuromodulators or neurohormones (Barchas, Akil, Elliott, Holman, and Watson, 1978). Reductions in somatostatin as great as 75 percent have been reported in several brain regions, while substance P has been reported diminished by 30 to 50 percent. Davies (1983) suggested that these reductions may occur only in the late stages of AD.

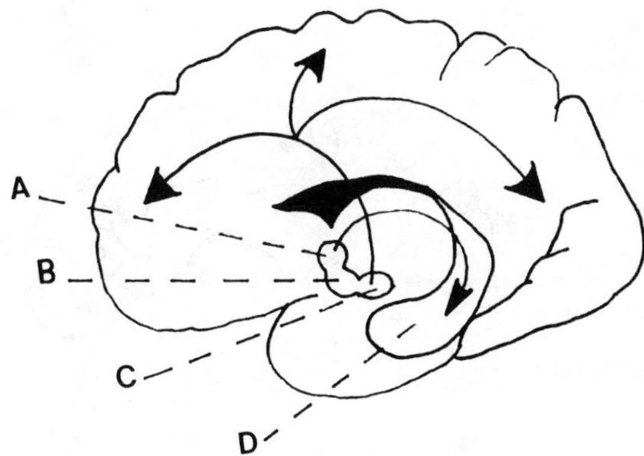

Figure 1-9. *Cholinergic pathways innervating cortex. (A) Medial septal nucleus. (B) Diagonal band of Broca. (C) Nucleus basalis of Meynert. (D) Hippocampal formation.*

Evidence of Alzheimer's Disease Subgroups

As research data from various disciplines have accumulated, the question has been raised whether dementia of the Alzheimer's type is a homogeneous clinical entity (Albert, 1968; Chui, Teng, Henderson, and Moy, 1985; Lauter and Meyer, 1968; Mayeux, Stern, and Spanton, 1985; Rossor, Iversen, Reynolds, Mountjoy and Roth, 1984; Seltzer and Sherwin, 1983; Sulkava and Amberla, 1982). So provocative have been the research findings that in July 1984, the National Institute of Neurological, Communicative Disorders and Stroke—Alzheimer's Disease and Related Disorders Association (NINCDS-ADRDA) sponsored work group, under the auspices of the Department of Health and Human Services Task Force on Alzheimer's disease (McKhann et al., 1984) recommended that researchers classify AD patients according to the following criteria: age of onset (before or after age 65), familial occurrence and presence of trisomy-21 (Down syndrome), and coexistence of other relevant conditions such as Parkinson's disease.

Then too, several researchers have reported an association between the aforementioned classification variables and certain communication disorders (Chui et al., 1985; Folstein and Breitner, 1981; Seltzer and Sherwin, 1983; Sulkava and Amberla, 1982). Chui and colleagues (1985) reported more prominent and prevalent aphasia in patients with early onset of AD. No relationship was observed between family history of dementia and either aphasia or age at onset. Independently of duration of illness, myoclonus and noniatrogenic extrapyramidal disorder were associated with greater severity of dementia.

Recently, data have been reported emphasizing the frequency of extrapyramidal signs in AD patients (Leverenz and Sumi, 1984; Mayeux et al., 1985; Turnbull and Aitken, 1983). Leverenz and Sumi (1984) documented the occurrence of Parkin-

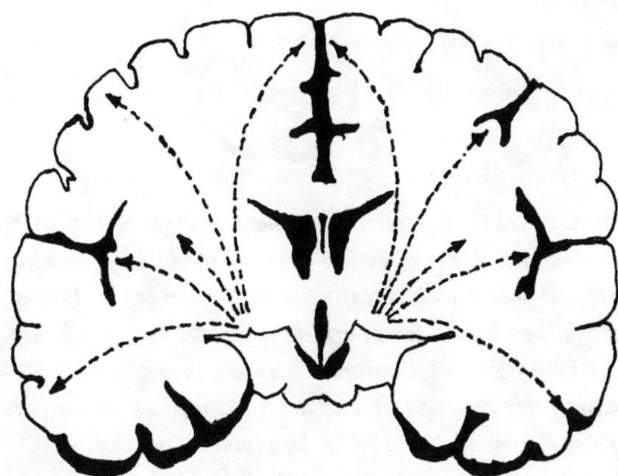

Figure 1-10. *Projections of cholinergic neurons from nucleus basalis of Meynert to cortical grey matter.*

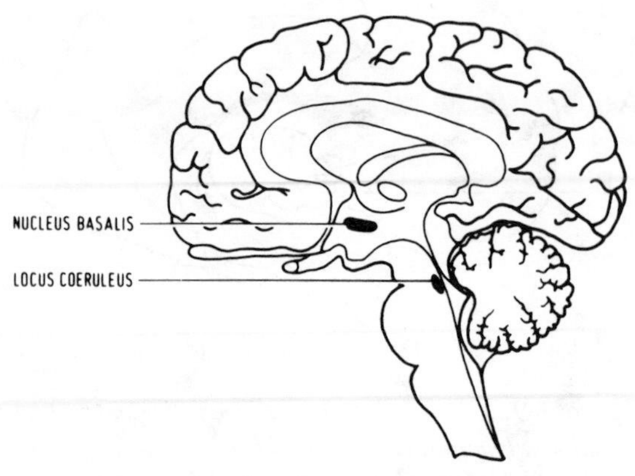

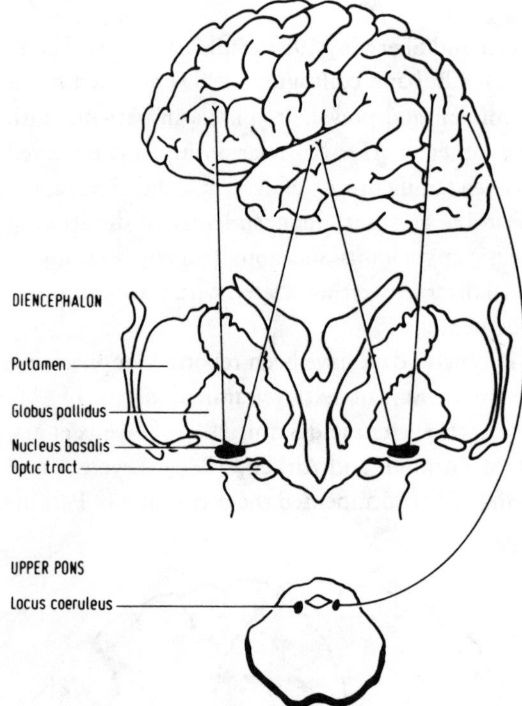

Figure 1-11. *Cholinergic and noradrenergic projections to the neocortex.* Upper; *nucleus basalis and the locus coeruleus projected onto a midsagittal section of human brain.* Lower; *nucleus basalis and locus coeruleus in coronal section. The diffuse projections to the cerebral cortex are shown in diagrammatic form, as the detailed anatomy has not been established. (From Rossor, M.N. {1982}. Dementia.* Lancet, *2, 1200–1204, by permission. Copyright 1982 by The Lancet, Ltd.)*

son-like signs in 18 of 40 patients with histopathologically confirmed AD. Mayeux and colleagues (1985) reported extrapyramidal signs in approximately 30 percent of their sample of 121 AD patients. The group with extrapyramidal signs performed significantly worse on mental status examination, exhibited greater impairment of functional activities, and was more likely to have organic psychosis and a family history of dementia.

Although the NINCDS-ADRDA work group (McKhann et al., 1984) did not recommend rate of disease progression as a criterion for classification, it is thought by many to distinguish AD patients (Seltzer and Sherwin, 1983; Sulkava and Amberla, 1982). Whereas death typically occurs 6 to 12 years after the onset of disease (Goodman, 1953), individuals with the more fulminating form die within a year of diagnosis (Ehle and Johnson, 1977; Watson, 1979).

Theories of Causation

The cause of the neuropathologic and neurochemical changes associated with AD is unknown. The principal theories relate to infectious agents, exposure to toxic substances, and genetic factors.

Infectious Agent Theory. To date, the credibility of the infectious agent theory is wanting from a lack of evidence of the transmissibility of AD. Because two other dementia-related conditions, kuru and Creutzfeldt-Jakob disease, are transmissible infectious disorders, scientists have speculated that AD is caused by an unconventional virus (Gajdusek, 1977). Transmission of Creutzfeldt-Jakob spongiform encephalopathy from humans to nonhuman primates (Gajdusek, 1977; Gibbs and Gajdusek, 1978) and other humans (Duffy et al., 1974) has been documented. However, attempts at infecting primates using material from patients with either the familial or the sporadic (nonfamilial) form of AD have all proved unsuccessful (Goudsmit et al., 1980).

Alzheimer's disease is considered as the possible human analog of scrapie, a neurodegenerative disease affecting sheep. When the scrapie agent was extracted and injected into brains of mice, AD-like changes were reported (Wisniewski, Moretz, and Lossinsky, 1981). Brain tissue from scrapie-infected animals show the same ChAT enzyme deficit found in AD and morphologic changes like the neuritic plaque, which has an amyloid deposit. Notable pathologic similarities have been reported in AD, Creutzfeldt-Jakob, kuru, and scrapie, specifically neuronal loss, gliosis, and amyloid plaques (Chou and Martin, 1971; Masters, Gajdusek, and Gibbs, 1981; Pro, Smith, and Sumi, 1980). The overlap in clinical and pathologic features suggests an etiologic relationship between these diseases.

Investigators continue to search for a link between AD and prions, the smallest known infectious agent. A prion or *pro*teinaceous *in*fectious particle (Prusiner, 1982), is approximately 1/100 the size of the smallest virus and cannot be viewed under an electron microscope. Prusiner (1984) has detected many similarities in the physical and chemical properties between prions and amyloid, the material found in the core of neuritic plaques. It is hypothesized that amyloid is composed of aggregates of prions (Prusiner, 1984). However, before entertaining the theory that prions cause Alzheimer's disease, scientists must account for the apparent lack of evidence of the transmissibility of Alzheimer's disease.

Toxic Substance Theory. Another possible cause of AD is aluminum toxicity in the brain. Several investigators have reported elevated aluminum in the brains of AD patients at postmortem examination (Crapper, Krishnan, and Dalton, 1973; Crapper, Krishnan, and Quittkat, 1976). The aluminum was aggregated in neurons having neurofibrillary tangles (Perl and Brody, 1980). However, the likelihood of elevated aluminum seems related to geographic area. For example, higher than normal aluminum deposits were found in the brains of AD patients from the Toronto area (Crapper et al., 1973) and Vermont. Because the water in both Toronto and Vermont has high levels of aluminum, it was conjectured that the aluminum was absorbed from the water.

Other investigators in different geographic regions, specifically Kentucky and New York (areas with low levels of aluminum in water), have not found significantly elevated brain aluminum levels in AD patients (Markesbery, Ehmann, Hossain, Alauddin, and Goodin, 1981; McDermott et al., 1977, 1979). Further, Markesbery and colleagues (1981) examined the brains of histologically verified Alzheimer's disease patients and adult control subjects and found that density of aluminum content did not correlate with density of neurofibrillary tangles and neuritic plaques; rather, the level of brain aluminum significantly increased as a function of age. Klatzo, Wisniewski, and Streicher (1965) reported that the injection of aluminum salts into rabbit cerebrospinal fluid produces neurofibrillary tangles, although the tangles are not identical to those seen in AD patients. Instead, these argyrophylic tangles are composed of straight rather than helical filaments.

The mixed results from the studies of aluminum and AD have lead to the general consensus that aluminum alone is not the cause. Another factor appears to be required. For example, high intake of aluminum may need to be coupled with long-term low intake of vital minerals, such as calcium and magnesium, for a breakdown to occur in the normal mechanisms that metabolize minerals (Garruto, Yanagihara, and Gajdusek, 1985).

Genetic Transmission Theory. The question most commonly asked by relatives of AD patients is whether the disorder can be inherited. Although a genetic marker for the disease is nonexistent, the members of some families clearly have a greater risk of developing the disease (Bucci, 1963; Feldman, Chandler, Levy, and Glaser, 1963; Heston, Lowther, and Leventhal, 1966; Lowenberg and Waggoner, 1934; Nee et al., 1983, Wheelan, 1959). The pedigrees of such families reveal that the ratio of affected males to females is equal, and approximately one half of the children are affected, a pattern associated with an autosomal dominant mode of inheritance (Powell and Folstein, 1984; Slater and Cowie, 1971).

Heston and Mastri (1977) investigated the medical history of 30 families in which there was a well-documented case of AD and found much higher morbidity risks for parents and siblings. Parents had an associated morbidity risk of 23 ± 7 percent and siblings 10 ± 3.6 percent.

Other evidence confirming a genetic factor in the development of AD comes from the studies of Kallmann (1950, 1955). He calculated the morbidity risk of AD parents to be 3.4 percent, siblings 6.5 percent, dizygotic twins 8.0 percent, and monozygotic twins 42.8 percent. Larsson, Sjögren, and Jacobson (1963) studied the relatives of Swedish patients with AD and determined the risk for primary relatives of AD patients to be 4.3 times that for the general population. The aggregate risk for the general Swedish population was 0.4 percent at age 70, increasing to 3.8 percent at age 85. The aggregate morbidity risk for parents and siblings of AD victims was 1.7 percent until the age of 70 and 16.3 percent at 85. However, because the methodology used in this study may have resulted in an underestimate of the morbidity risk for the general population (Mortimer, Schuman, and French, 1981), the increased risk in relatives is likely to be smaller than was reported. Heston, Mastri, Anderson, and White (1981) avoided the methodologic difficulties of the Larsson study and concluded that the risk of AD in the relatives of early-onset probands, individuals developing the disease before age 70, is significantly increased, whereas that for late onset probands is small.

Wright and Whalley (1984) partitioned the data from the Swedish studies of Sjögren, Sjögren, and Lindgren (1952) and Larsson and colleagues according to age of onset and estimated the heritabilities associated with early- and late-onset AD. The highest heritability estimates (0.89 to 1.03 percent) were found for early-onset disease in the relatives of early-onset probands. In fact, the heritability for all types of AD was higher for the relatives of early-onset probands. Carter (1969) associated the early-onset illness with a more extreme deviation and greater genetic risk.

Breitner and Folstein (1984) investigated the hypothesis that the clinical features of apraxia, agnosia, and aphasia would characterize the familial form of AD. They identified 16 AD patients with a family history of the disease and 23 without, and obtained clinical and family histories from multiple informants. The AD patients participating in the study were asked to write a sentence. By analysis of the sentence each subject wrote and the answers to a few questions about a history of speaking difficulty, word-finding, reading, and writing, judgments were made as to the presence of aphasia, agraphia, and apraxia. Breitner and Folstein concluded that language-disordered AD is a dominant genetic disorder with age-dependent penetrance; that is, the incidence rises with age. They reported that the relatives of language-disordered probands bear a 50 percent or greater risk of developing the disease by the age of 90.

Because of the very limited data on which these judgments about aphasia, agraphia, and apraxia were made and the lack of definition of the term "language-disordered," this conclusion seems premature. A thesis of this book is that all AD patients are disordered in their ability to communicate, a disorder that is likely to take more than one form. Perhaps the AD patients in the Breitner and Folstein study, without a family history of the disease, had communication problems that were unidentified.

Down Syndrome Patients: More Evidence for a Genetic Factor

Evidence for a genetic factor comes from another source, the study of Down syndrome patients. Several investigators report AD-like morphologic changes to be an almost inevitable consequence in Down syndrome patients surviving into their 40s (Burger and Vogel, 1973; Olson and Shaw, 1969; Owens, Dawson and Lowsin, 1971) (Figure 1-12). Although only a small proportion of Down syndrome patients survive to the fourth and fifth decades of life (Smith and Bergg, 1976), those who do survive develop the neuritic plaques and neurofibrillary tangles characteristic of AD and in addition suffer a decrease in ChAT (Malamud, 1972; Yates, Simpson, Maloney, Gordon, and Reid, 1980).

Attempts to identify chromosomal abnormalities in AD patients have not produced any evidence of an abnormality in chromosome 21, although some degree of aneuploidy (state of having an abnormal number of chromosomes) is often noted in the chromosomes of cultured white blood cells from AD patients (Brun, Gustafson, and Mittleman, 1978; Cook, Ward, and Austin, 1979; Jarvik, Altshuler, Kato, and Blummer, 1971; Sourander and Sjögren, 1970).

The question of whether the development of AD-like changes in the brains of Down syndrome patients is associated with cognitive decline is harder to answer. Some clinicians report decline (Jervis, 1970; Lott, 1982); others do not accept cognitive decline as an invariable consequence (Ropper and Williams, 1980). Most studies of Down syndrome patients have been retrospective, such as the one by Wisniewski, Howe, Williams, and Wisniewski (1978), who compared the neuropsychiatric features of 50 Down syndrome patients older and younger than 35 and reported evidence of greater change in cognition and personality in the older group. However, in this study there is no assurance that the older patients were not more psychologically impaired than the younger when they were the same age as the younger patients. In a prospective study, Dalton, Crapper, and Schlotterer (1974) observed progressive deterioration in learning ability in Down syndrome patients who were later examined at autopsy. Dalton and colleagues reported a positive correlation between the severity of morphologic changes and the extent of cognitive deterioration (Crapper, Dalton, Skopitz, Scott, and Hachinski, 1975). Thase, Liss, Smeltzer, and Maloon (1982) conducted a cross-sectional study in which they compared the neuropsychiatric status of Down syndrome patients in the following age classes: 25 to 34, 35 to 44, 45 to 54, and 55 to 64. With advancing age, a decline in performance was seen; however, less than half of the older Down patients met the diagnostic criteria for dementia, and one 59-year-old individual had no evidence of dementia. They concluded that clinically significant dementia does not invariably develop in Down syndrome patients after age 35.

A possible chemical relationship between AD and Down syndrome has been suggested by Glenner and Wong (1984), who analyzed the cerebrovascular amyloid protein from a patient with Down syndrome and found it to be homologous to that of the protein of Alzheimer's disease. These researchers are hopeful that a protein sequence homology between the two diseases will yield evidence that establishes Down syndrome as a predictable model for Alzheimer's disease.

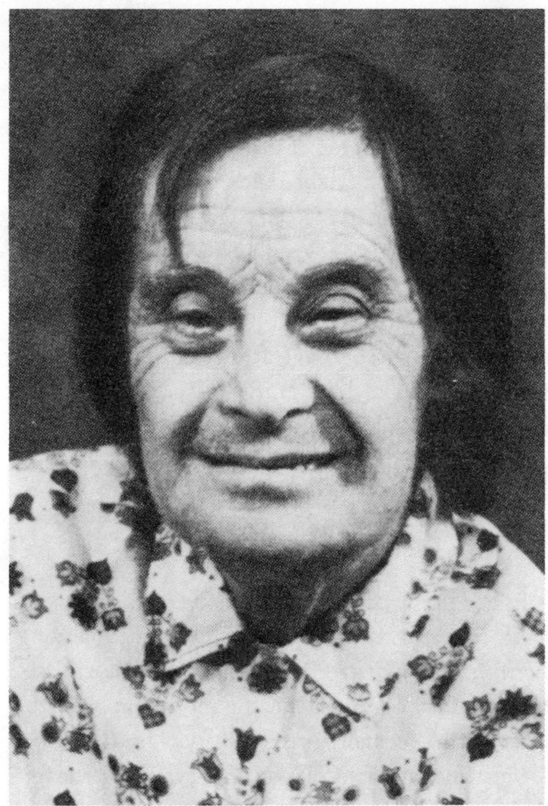

Figure 1-12. *Down syndrome and Alzheimer's disease. A photograph of a 55-year-old woman who regressed from a 6- or 7-year mental level to a state in which she cannot speak or comprehend language, is disoriented, and is incontinent. (From Kolata, G. {1985}. Down syndrome–Alzheimer's linked.* Science, 230, *1152–1153, by permission. Copyright 1985 by the American Association for the Advancement of Science. {Photo by Krystyna Wisniewski, chief of the Neuropathology Laboratory at New York State's Institute for Basic Research in Developmental Disabilities on Staten Island.})*

Another possible association between Down syndrome and AD patients may be the advanced age of their mothers. Advanced maternal age is a well-known risk factor for Down syndrome (Creasy,

1974; Erickson, 1978; Hook and Lindsjo, 1978; Penrose, 1933), and some evidence has been published that AD patients have older mothers. Cohen, Eisdorfer, and Leverenz (1982) studied the parental age data for 80 Alzheimer's patients and found a marked difference between the age of the patient's mothers, (median 35.5, SD 1.4) and the median age of the mothers of persons born in Washington state in 1907 (median 27.0). However, neither maternal nor parental age at birth of persons with AD was found to be significantly different from that of control subjects in a recent study by Heyman and colleagues (1983).

Risk Factors for Alzheimer's Disease

In the previous discussion of the possible causes of AD, certain risk factors were mentioned, among them, having a first-order relative with the disease. Another may be the age of the mother at the subject's birth. Yet another is a history of head injury.

Mortimer and associates (1985) evaluated the frequency of prior head injury in 78 patients with presumptive AD and 124 control subjects matched for age, sex, and race. A history of head injury in adulthood with loss of consciousness was reported in 25.6 percent of the AD patients and only 5.3 and 14.6 percent of the hospital and neighborhood control subjects, respectively. These data become more compelling with the realization that neither the interviewers nor the respondents knew that the purpose of the study was to identify risk factors in AD.

The report by Mortimer and colleagues corroborated a similar earlier report by Heyman and colleagues (1984), who observed that 15 percent of 40 AD patients had head injury history, compared with 3.8 percent of matched control subjects. Rudelli, Strom, Welch, and Ambler (1982) detailed the case history of a 38-year-old man who died of AD 16 years after severe head trauma. Postmortem examination of his brain revealed the morphologic changes typical of AD. Rudelli and colleagues argued that head injury may have provided a "permissive role in the development of the pathologic Alzheimer's disease changes" (p. 574). If head trauma is a true risk factor for the development of AD, the pathogenetic mechanism is not well understood. Some scientists have suggested that damage to the blood-brain barrier permits access of serum proteins to the brain parenchyma, which may sensitize the immune system. Any alterations in the blood brain barrier later may provide the impetus for a secondary response (Ishii, 1969; Rapoport, 1976).

Physiologic Markers of Alzheimer's Disease

Electrophysiological Measures. One of the most consistent correlates of progressive degenerative change in AD brains is symmetric, usually diffuse slowing of the electroencephalogram (EEG) (Terry and Katzman, 1983). Among healthy individuals, a dominant frequency of 8 to 12 Hz (alpha rhythm) is typically observed. Only a small percentage of healthy elderly have diffuse EEG slowing into the theta range (5 to 7 Hz), and no normal elderly have been found with slowing in the delta range of 4 or less Hz (Wang and Busse, 1969). Frequently observed is a slowing or absence of alpha rhythm with replacement by theta- and eventually delta-slow activities (Duffy, Albert, and McAnulty, 1984; Lauter, 1985). The degree of slow wave activity has been found to correlate significantly with the degree of cognitive deficit (Johannesson, Hagberg, Gustafson, and Ingvar, 1979; Kaszniak, Garron, Fox, Bergen, and Huckman, 1979; Kidd, 1963; Müller and Schwartz, 1978; Obrist and Henry, 1958; O'Connor, Shaw, and Ongley, 1979; Roberts, McGeorge, and Caird, 1978; Stefoski et al., 1976). Kaszniak and colleagues (1978, 1979) found the EEG to be a better correlate of dementia than the computerized tomographic scan.

Evoked potentials (EP) are brain waves associated with sensory events. In patients with moderate to severe dementia, the late components of the EP show increased latency and reduced amplitude, especially the P300 event-related component (Duffy et al., 1984). Prolonged latency of P300 potentials occurs in 50 to 80 percent of Alzheimer patients and may be clinically useful in differentiating AD patients from depressed patients, the P300 wave being normal in the latter group (McKhann et al., 1984).

Cerebral Blood Flow. The technique of measuring cerebral blood flow (CBF) has been used to help neuroscientists understand which areas of the brain are involved in particular activities. In the normal brain, CBF is proportional to cerebral oxidative metabolism. Cerebral blood flow and metabolism can be measured through the 133Xe inhalation technique in which the xenon isotope is inhaled, and gamma emissions given off by the isotope are measured in multiple brain regions.

The resting pattern of cerebral blood flow is sufficiently stable and reproducible to enable comparisons to be made between resting flow and flow uptake in specific brain regions during various activities. The CBF measurement technique reveals those areas of the cortex active in a particular task, thus allowing researchers to study brain-behavior relationships.

In AD patients, cerebral blood flow and cerebral metabolic rate have been found to be consistently reduced (Freyhan, Woodford, and Kety, 1951; Lassen, Munck, and Tottey, 1957), and the degree of flow reduction correlates with the severity of dementia (Grubb, Raichle, Gado, Eichling, and Hughes, 1977; Obrist, Chivian, Cronquist, and Ingvar, 1970; Yamaguchi, Meyer, Yamamoto, Sakai, and Shaw, 1980). Additionally, regional cerebral blood flow (rCBF) rates closely correspond to the distribution of neuropathologic changes in AD brains (Lauter, 1985). Accentuated blood flow reductions in the parieto-temporo-occipital area are typically observed (Gustafson and Risberg, 1974; Hagberg and Ingvar, 1976).

Regional cerebral blood flow measurements have been shown to have diagnostic utility in differentiating subgroups of dementia patients from each other (Gustafson, Brun, and Ingvar, 1977; Risberg and Gustafson, 1983) and from patients with depression (Gustafson and Risberg, 1979; Risberg, 1985). The results of a large study conducted in Sweden of rCBF in four clinical subgroups of dementia patients indicate that marked and significant rCBF differences among groups can be delineated (Risberg, 1985). Included in the study were patients with presenile AD, senile dementia of the Alzheimer type (SDAT), Pick's disease, and multi-infarct dementia (MID). Compared with patients with Pick's disease, AD patients had significant flow reductions in the parietal, parieto-occipital, and parieto-temporal regions bilaterally. The pattern in Pick's disease was diminished flow in premotor, supplemental motor, and prefrontal regions bilaterally. Although the senile and presenile AD groups showed similar flow patterns, presenile AD patients had a greater localized postcentral flow deficiency whereas late-onset AD patients had greater widespread disturbance and greater involvement of the frontal lobes. Because of the heterogeneity of flow disturbances, averaging the flow values of MID patients resulted in a flat mean rCBF pattern. Patients with more advanced MID tended to have right-left asymmetries in hemispheric mean flow. Thus, irregular and asymmetric flow patterns distinguished MID patients from the other clinical subgroups in this study. No significant difference in values between depressed patients and normal control subjects was observed.

Computerized Tomography. Computerized tomography (CT) allows for the non-invasive examination of intracranial contents and the exclusion of other causes of dementia such as subdural hematoma, brain tumor, hydrocephalus, cerebral infarction, and abscesses (Cummings and Benson, 1983). Enlarged ventricles and widened cortical sulci have been documented in AD patients through CT scanning (Jacoby and Levy, 1980); however, these neuroanatomic changes also occur with normal aging. Even more of a problem in interpreting CT data is that the brains of some AD patients show no evidence of cortical atrophy (Fox et al., 1975). Thus, the diagnostic utility of CT scanning in reliably identifying AD patients has been questioned (Kaszniak et al., 1978, 1979; Jacoby and Levy, 1980; Yerby, Sundsten, Larson, Wu, and Sumi, 1985). However, other investigators (Bondareff, Baldy, and Levy, 1981; Damasio et al., 1983; Naeser, Albert, and Kleefield, 1982) continue to develop new quantitative techniques and suggest that refinement of the CT technique may yield data useful for the identification of AD and quantification of the severity of dementia.

Positron Emission Tomography. Positron emission tomography (PET) is a noninvasive neuroscanning technique in which the amount of glucose uptake is measured in brain tissue. Subjects inhale or are injected with a positron-emitting radioactive substance, and the brain's use of that substance is monitored by positron detectors to provide a cross-sectional image of brain radioactivity (Kuhl and Edwards, 1963; Kuhl, Edwards, Ricci, and Reivich, 1973; Phelps, 1977). The underlying assumption of PET is that reduction in glucose utilization by some area of the brain indicates a pathologic condition. Indeed, AD patients have been found to have markedly reduced overall cortical glucose utilization (Foster et al., 1984).

Although PET studies have shown patients with AD to have decreased metabolism in all brain areas, reductions are most prominent in association cortices, both frontal and temporoparietal, and least common in primary motor and sensory cortex (Benson et al., 1983; Foster et al., 1984). Benson and colleagues found these results to be consistent with the retention of normal primary neurologic functions until the most advanced stages of AD.

Friedland, Prusiner, Jagust, Budinger, and Davis (1984) have reported regionally diminished glucose utilization in patients with AD and Creutzfeldt-Jakob disease. Markedly diminished flows in the temporal lobes and temporoparietal areas with hemispheric asymmetry were apparent in both types of patients.

The lateral asymmetries in hypometabolism, found in the inferior temporoparietal area, have been associated with differences in degree of cognitive deficits and age of disease onset (Koss, Friedland, Ober, and Jagust, 1985). Patients with greater right than left hemispheric impairment in cortical glucose metabolism were younger than 65, and the hemispheric asymmetry was associated with poor visuospatial performance. These authors concluded that PET study data do not support the concept that regardless of age, AD patients are a homogeneous population; rather, they suggest the existence of two separate populations with different patterns and severity of neuropathology.

Other investigators have reported disproportionate language impairment in patients with marked reductions in glucose metabolism in the left frontal, temporal, and parietal regions (Foster et al., 1983). Patients with predominantly visuoconstructive problems had greater right than left hypometabolism in the parietal area. No consistent asymmetry was observed in patients with predominant memory failure.

Magnetic Resonance Imaging. Another technique, magnetic resonance imaging (MRI), also known as nuclear magnetic resonance (NMR), is a noninvasive technique that allows for high-resolution imaging of brain structure without ionizing radiation. The technique permits measurement of brain and cerebrospinal fluid volume and can distinguish gray from white matter (Bryan, 1985). It can provide evidence of abnormal morphologic changes such as intracranial tumors (Brant-Zawadzki, Badami, Mills, Norman, and Newton, 1984), infarction, regional or global brain atrophy, and arteriovenous malformations (Brant-Zawadzki, Mills, and Davis, 1983).

Magnetic resonance imaging studies of AD patients have revealed enlarged ventricles and widened sulci (Alavi et al., 1986) A benefit of MRI is the visibility of infarcted tissue and tumor, enabling the diagnostician to rule out tumor and vascular disease as the cause of dementia (Bryan, 1985).

Treatment Approaches

As yet, a treatment for altering the course of AD is unknown. Progress in recent years in recognizing the cholinergic deficit has prompted several treatment strategies: raising brain concentration of choline and therefore, it is hoped, acetylcholine through diet; inhibition of normal hydrolysis of acetylcholine; use of an analog of acetylcholine as a substitute for the natural transmitter; and increasing the sensitivity of the central muscarinic receptors to acetylcholine. Though minimal transient memory improvement has been reported in 10 AD patients (Davis and Mohs, 1982) with the use of intravenous physostigmine, an anticholinesterase drug that readily crosses the blood-brain barrier (Smith, Swash, and Hart, 1985), sustained improvement in cognitive/communicative functioning has not been found when other drugs known to increase levels of acetylcholine or stimulate cholinergic receptors have been used. The lack of success thus far may be due to incorrect pharmacologic approaches, involvement of other noncholinergic systems, or the need for a possible cotransmitter that exists together with acetylcholine in cortical cholinergic projection systems (Perry and Perry, 1985).

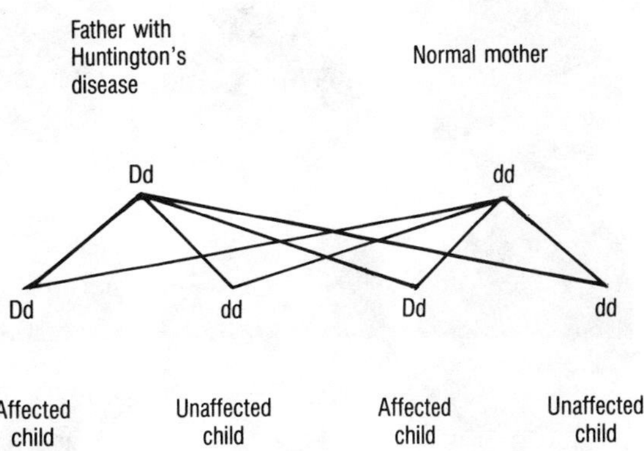

Figure 1-13. *Genetic transmission of Huntington's disease. D = defective gene; d = normal gene.*

HUNTINGTON'S DISEASE

Huntington's disease (HD), also known as Huntington's chorea, is an inherited degenerative disease of the nervous system characterized by dementia and bizarre uncontrollable dancelike movements or chorea. The Huntington's gene is autosomal dominant (Figure 1-13). "Autosomal" means that the gene is located on a chromosome other than the sex chromosome, and therefore the disease is not sex-linked; male and female patients are equally likely to be affected. "Dominant" means that the defective gene dominates its normal partner gene from the unaffected parent. Each child of an affected parent has a 50 percent chance of inheritance. If a child has not received the Huntington's gene from a parent, the child and his or her children will be free of the disease. Children who inherit the gene will develop the disease if they live long enough.

The reports of average age of onset of HD have ranged from 35 to 42 years (Bolt, 1970; Myers, Madden, Teague, and Falek, 1982; Myers and Martin, 1982; Negrette, 1958). In approximately 3 percent of cases, however, the signs and symptoms begin in childhood (Martin, 1984). When onset is in childhood, the disease is more likely to have been inherited from the father (Hayden, MacGregor, Saffer, and Beighton, 1982; Myers et al., 1982; Newcombe, Walker, and Harper, 1981). Irrespective of when the disease occurs, the onset is insidious, and many patients try to hide or ignore early signs.

The first signs can be changes in personality, motor function, or cognition. Deterioration ultimately occurs in all of these areas. When the first manifestation of the disease is psychologic, depression is the most common feature (Folstein, Abbott, Chase, Jensen, and Folstein, 1983; Folstein, Franz, Jensen, Chase, and Folstein, 1983). Early changes include irritability, untidiness, apathy, and impulsive behavior. Families of HD patients report that impulsive behavior may eventuate in social problems such as substance abuse and sexual promiscuity. The physical and mental signs may appear simultaneously or individually. The duration of the disease is approximately 10 to 15 years, although some individuals live longer. Death does not result from the disease per se, but from secondary complications such as heart failure, aspiration, or pneumonia (Bruyn, 1968).

The tragedy of the disease is the realization by affected individuals of their prognosis, and suicide is high among those recently diagnosed. It accounts for the deaths of 7.8 percent of male and 6.4 percent of female patients with HD (Reed and Chandler, 1958). Unsuccessful suicide attempts are common (Dewhurst, Oliver, and McKnight, 1970).

The choreic movements are jerky, irregular, and stretching and first appear in the extremities as "pia-

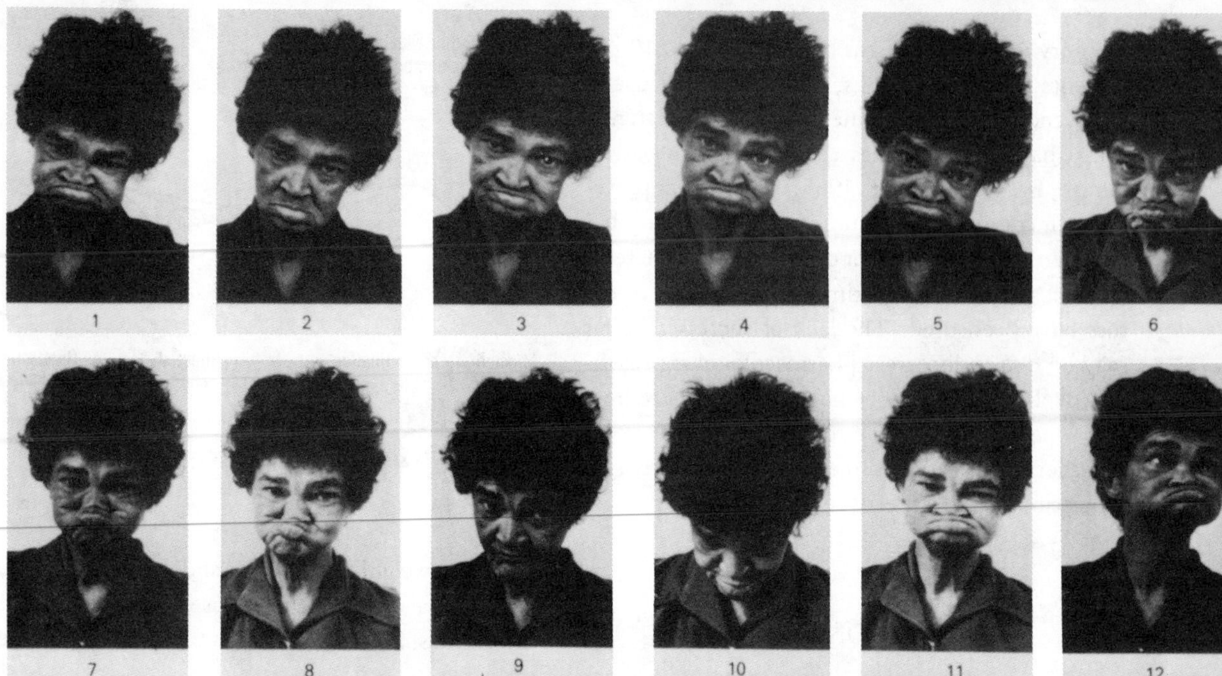

Figure 1-14. *Sequential photographs taken at one-second intervals showing gross choreiform movements of face and neck. (From Hayden, M.R. {1981}.* Huntington's chorea. *New York: Springer-Verlag, by permission. Copyright 1981 by Springer-Verlag, Berlin, Heidelberg.)*

no playing" movements of the fingers. The face, neck (Figure 1-14), and arms (Brown, 1973) also are affected early and are associated with noticeable changes in speech. As the disease progresses, dysarthria worsens, and ultimately the patient becomes hard to understand. Dysphagia is a common sign in the late stages (Young et al., 1986). HD patients are described as having a shuffling, jerky gait with the upper body seeming to move ahead of the hips and legs.

The Neuropathy and Neurochemistry of HD

The signs and symptoms of HD result from brain atrophy and neurochemical deficiencies. Atrophy occurs in the caudate nucleus and putamen of the basal nuclei (Figure 1-15), (brain areas that help control motor movement), the cortex, and the substantia nigra. Initially, small Golgi type II neurons located in the caudate and putamen are lost. These cells serve to inhibit movement. Later, larger neurons in these areas are affected (Lange, 1981; Lange, Thorner, Hopf, and Schroder, 1976).

PET studies of deoxyglucose uptake in early cases of HD reveal a significant decrease in metabolism in the basal ganglia (Kuhl et al., 1982). In the cortex, diffuse neuronal loss occurs, particularly in the occipital lobes and frontobasal cortex (Lange, 1981). These neuropathic abnormalities are accompanied by neurochemical deficits; that is, the caudate nucleus is deficient in the neurotransmitters gamma-aminobutyric acid (GABA) and acetylcholine (Bird and Iversen, 1974; Stahl and Swanson, 1974) and their respective synthesizing enzymes, glutamic acid decarboxylase and choline acetyltransferase (Bird and Iversen, 1974; McGeer and McGeer, 1975; Perry, Hansen, and Kloster, 1973).

To understand the movement disorder of HD, it is necessary to appreciate that the components of the basal nuclei are influenced by a set of reverberating neuron networks, each reliant upon specific neurotransmitters. Through interconnections with the thalamic nuclei, cerebral hemispheres, and cerebellum, movements of the body are controlled. In HD an imbalance occurs between the neurochemicals needed to control movement. The amount of dopamine is excessive in relation to acetylcholine and GABA within the caudate nucleus. When the balance between these three neurotransmitters is restored, choreiform movements are reduced (Stipe, White, and Van Arsdale, 1979).

Clinical ratings of the functional abilities of HD patients show a strong linear relationship to the extent of caudate atrophy, as assessed by CT (Shoulson, Plassche, and Odoroff, 1982; Stober, Mussow, and Schimrigk, 1984), and caudate hypometabolism, as measured by PET (Penney et al., 1984).

In 1983, a breakthrough occurred when Gusella and colleagues (1983) identified a polymorphic DNA marker genetically linked to Huntington's disease. Once the linkage to HD was established by Gusella and colleagues, other studies were undertaken to assign the marker to the correct chromosome. Subsequent investigations have shown its location to be on the short arm of chromosome 4. This research is essential to the development of a test for persons at risk for Huntington's disease.

Treatment of HD

As yet no treatment alters the course of HD, but progress has been made in recent years in developing a test to determine which individuals carry the defective gene. At present, medical treatment consists of attempting to ameliorate the signs. To reduce the bizarre writhing movements associated with the disease, tranquilizers frequently are given. A report recently published by Young and colleagues (1986), of a longitudinal study involving 65 diagnosed HD patients and 225 at risk individuals in Venezuela, revealed that untreated HD patients demonstrated a rate of decline similar to that of medicated patients in the United States who received neuroleptic drugs. The authors of this report recommended that neuroleptic drugs be used sparingly to treat hyperkinetic and psychiatric signs. A similar recommendation has been made by other researchers (Shoulson, 1984).

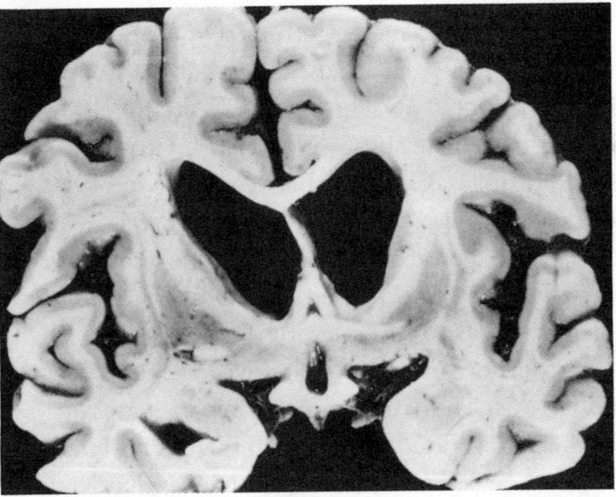

Figure 1-15. *Huntington's chorea. There is bilateral symmetrical dilatation of the frontal horns. (From Hirano, A., Iwata, M., Llena, J.F., and Matsui, T. {1980}.* Color atlas of pathology of the nervous system. *New York: Igaku-Shoin Medical Publishers, Inc., by permission. Copyright, first edition, 1980 by Igaku-Shoin, Ltd., Tokyo.)*

PARKINSON'S DISEASE

Parkinson's disease (PD) is a cluster of signs resulting from a variety of causes. Four variants of the parkinsonian syndrome account for the majority of cases: idiopathic, drug-induced, postencephalitic, and arteriosclerotic. The most common variant is idiopathic. In a recent epidemiologic study of PD (Rajput, Offord, Beard, and Kurland, 1984), the idiopathic form was found to account for 86 percent of cases.

The reported frequency of occurrence of other forms of PD has been somewhat variable. With the increased general use of neuroleptic drugs, or drugs that act on the nervous system, a noticeable increase in the number of cases of drug-induced Parkinsonism has been recorded (Ayd, 1961; Korczyn and Goldberg, 1976). In the study by Rajput and colleagues (1984), drug-induced PD was found to be the second most common type, representing 7.2 percent of their cases.

Postencephalitic PD patients have a history of encephalitis or influenza with acute febrile illness in which they were drowsy, delirious, or comatose or all three for days or weeks (Pollock and Hornabrook, 1966). According to results of studies conducted in the Rochester, Minnesota, region, the number of postencephalitic cases has dropped steadily from 20 percent in 1955 (Kurland, 1958) to 6.6 percent in 1965 (Nobrega, Glattre, Kurland, and Okazaki, 1967). Between 1967 and 1979, no new cases were seen (Rajput et al., 1984).

As with postencephalitic PD, the number of patients with arteriosclerotic PD appears to be decreasing. In arteriosclerotic Parkinsonism, the symptoms occur in association with cerebral arteriosclerosis. The patient typically reports onset during an acute episode after which there is a steplike progression of the illness. In early reports (Kurland, 1958; Nobrega et al., 1967), arteriosclerotic PD accounted for 20 to 30 percent of the cases of parkinsonism. More recently, arteriosclerotic parkinsonism accounted for only 1.4 percent of the cases in a study by Rajput and colleagues (1984).

The prevalence rate of PD is approximately 106 per 100,000 individuals, but it increases with age (Pollock and Hornabrook, 1966), reaching 1 in 100 over the age of 50 years (Pearce, 1978). It is the most common age-related disease of the basal ganglia. The overall annual incidence of parkinsonism per 100,000 population is approximately 20.5 (Rajput et al., 1984), with the peak incidence occurring between 75 and 84 years.

In the majority of PD patients, the age at onset is between 50 and 69 years for both men and women (Hoehn and Yahr, 1967). The presence of the disease is reported to shorten longevity (Hoehn and Yahr, 1967; Kurland, 1958; Nobrega et al., 1967). Hoehn and Yahr (1967) reported mortality to be three times that of the general population of the same age, sex, and color, and Nobrega and coworkers (1967) observed mortality to be 1.6 times higher than expected.

Symptomatology of PD

Considerable variation exists in the symptomatology of PD. Some patients show only motor signs, whereas others have cognitive deficits and some a full dementia. The classic motor signs are tremor, rigidity, and bradykinesia, or slowness in movement and in the ability to initiate movement.

Of these motor manifestations, the most obvious is tremor, "an involuntary oscillatory movement produced by contractions of reciprocally innervated antagonistic muscles" (Jankovic and Fahn, 1980, p. 460). The typical resting tremor is seen in the fingers and thumb and is often likened to pill rolling. Hoehn and Yahr (1967) reported tremor to be the most common initial sign; they observed that patients with tremor as the initial sign exhibited a slower rate of progression during the first 10 years of the disease. Similarly, Zetusky, Jankovic, and Pirozzolo (1985) noted that tremor was associated with earlier age at onset, family history of PD, less severe oropharyngeal disorder, preserved mental and functional status, and more favorable prognosis.

Rigidity is an increase in the resting tone of muscle or resistance to passive stretch and is present throughout the muscle's range of motion (Newman and Calne, 1984). When a resting tremor is superimposed on increased resting tone, the resistance may be jerky, a type of response referred to as cogwheel rigidity.

The bradykinesia of PD patients makes it difficult for them to start a movement such as walking or writing. Once a movement is in progress, they have difficulty stopping it.

Other signs of PD are stooped posture, shuffling gait, and micrographia (Figure 1-16), or the tendency for the handwriting to become small. Facial expressions are diminished, giving the person a masklike immobile face (Figure 1-17), and the voice may be monotonous with low volume. Depression is common.

The cardinal features of PD, tremor, rigidity, and bradykinesia, often affect the body asymmetrically in the early and middle stages. Direnfeld and colleagues (1984) reported that PD patients with greater involvement of the left side demonstrated greater neuropsychologic deficits than those with greater involvement of the right side and more closely resembled AD patients in neuropsychologic performance.

Neuropathology and Neurochemistry of PD

The aforementioned signs result from neuronal and degenerative changes in the basal nuclei, cortex, nucleus basalis of Meynert (nbM), and nucle-

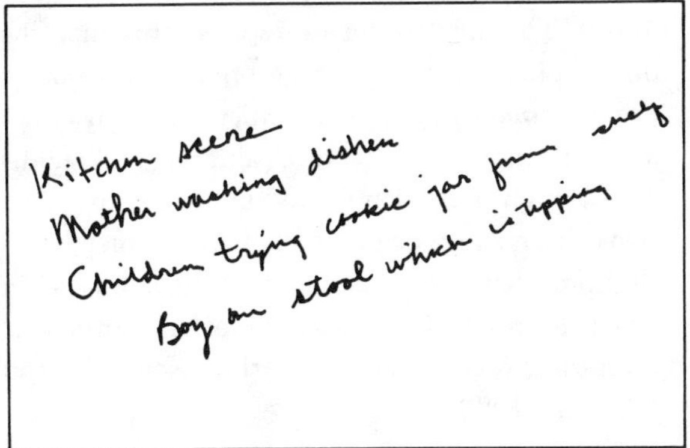

Figure 1-16. *Micrographia is evident in the written description of the Cookie Theft Picture provided by a mildly demented Parkinson's patient.*

us locus coeruleus (nLC) (Figures 1-9, 1-10, and 1-11). The most conspicuous neuropathologic change is depigmentation of the substantia nigra in the basal ganglia and loss of the neurotransmitter dopamine. The dopamine deficiency in the brain (Bernheimer, Birkmayer, Hornykiewicz, Jellinger, and Seitelberger, 1974) is manifested as a low level of homovanillic acid in the cerebrospinal fluid (Johansson and Roos, 1967).

Because of the discovery of cholinergic cell loss in the nucleus basalis of Meynert in AD patients, researchers have attempted to define other diseases with basal nucleus pathology. Tagliavini, Pilleri, Bouras, and Constantinidis (1984) studied the basal nucleus in PD patients and found neuronal losses ranging from 29.9 to 68.3 percent, a finding similar to that reported by several other investigators (Arendt, Bigl, Arendt, and Tennstedt, 1983; Whitehouse, Price, Clark, Coyle, and DeLong, 1981; Wilcock, Esiri, Bowen, and Smith, 1983). This loss is less severe than that observed in AD patients but significantly greater than that in normal age-matched subjects.

The involvement of both the nucleus basalis of Meynert and the nucleus locus coeruleus raises a question about the relation of PD to AD, and rightly so, for it appears that idiopathic PD shares several symptomatologic, neurochemical, and neuropathologic features with AD (Nakano and Hirano, 1984). For example, Alzheimer's-like morphologic changes have been found in many PD patients with dementia (Hakim and Mathieson, 1979; Hirano and Zimmerman, 1962), but it is unclear whether all PD patients with dementia have such changes. Also, researchers using PET have demonstrated abnormal metabolic processes throughout the parkinsonian brain (Kuhl, Metter, and Riege, 1984), a metabolic pattern similar to that seen in AD patients. Finally, choline acetyltransferase activity in the cortices of PD patients is reduced in apparent proportion to the severity of dementia (Ruberg, Ploska, and Javoy-Agid, 1982).

Evidence of PD Subgroups

Several investigators suggest the existence of two forms of PD (Boller et al., 1979; Garron, Klawans, and Narin, 1972; Lieberman et al., 1979): a motor disorder without dementia in which changes are limited to subcortical structures, and a second form in which dementia is associated with motor dysfunction and both cortical and subcortical changes.

Mortimer, Pirozzolo, Hansch, and Webster (1982) studied the relation of motor signs to intel-

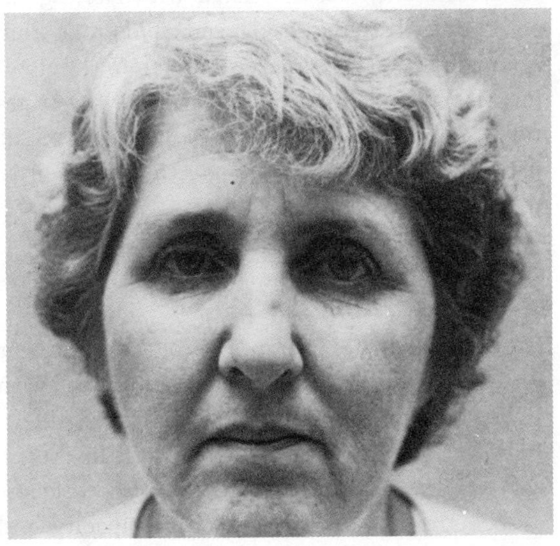

Figure 1-17. *Typical masked facies in a patient with Parkinson's disease. (From Weiner, W.J. (1981). Parkinson's disease. In W.J. Weiner and C.G. Goetz (Eds.),* Neurology for the non-neurologist. *Philadelphia: Harper and Row Publishers, Inc., by permission. Copyright 1981 by Harper and Row Publishers, Inc.)*

lectual deficits, reasoning that a strong positive correlation would suggest that the subcortical damage responsible for motor problems was also responsible for dementia. The results were mixed; that is, although bradykinesia was associated with psychologic impairment, other motor signs, such as tremor and rigidity, were not. This finding was corroborated by Agnoli and colleagues (1984). In a study by Mayeux and Stern (1983), both bradykinesia and rigidity were found to be the strongest predictors of overall intellectual performance. Mortimer and colleagues (1982) further reported an inverse relation between tremor severity and visuospatial function, a finding earlier reported by Lieberman (1974).

However, Martilla and Rinne (1976) found severity of tremor to be related to severity of dementia. Recently, Zetusky et al., (1985) examined tremor, bradykinesia, rigidity, postural instability, and gait difficulty in relation to mental status in 334 patients with idiopathic PD. Rather than tremor severity, postural instability and gait disturbance were found, to correlate strongest with mental status, followed by bradykinesia. Additionally, postural instability was associated with later age at onset, dysarthria, dysphagia, and rapid progression of the disease. These mixed results from the aforementioned studies indicate that further investigations are necessary to resolve the question of the nature of cognitive deficits and their relation to motor symptoms in PD.

Treatment of PD

Levodopa Drug Therapy. Levodopa treatment greatly ameliorates the motor signs associated with PD and decreases the mortality rate (Rinne, 1983). However, long-term administration of the drug is associated with serious problems, most notably loss of benefit, declining intellectual capacity and dementia, low threshold for certain side effects, and fluctuations in disability. After an average of 5 to 8 years of treatment, individuals are found to experience fluctuations in response (McDowell and Sweet, 1976) and a gradual return to pretreatment level (Rinne, Sonninen, Siirtola, and Martilla, 1980). The fluctuations in response are called the on-off phenomenon. The on-off phenomenon is characterized by rapid, "unpredictable swings from a hyperkinetic state to one of akinesia and rigidity" (Clough, Bergmann, and Yahr, 1984, p. 131) It has been suggested that PD patients may benefit from medically supervised "drug holidays" in order to reset the sensitivity of dopaminergic receptors (Weiner, Koller, Perlik, Nausieda, and Klawans, 1980).

Others have studied the long-term effects of levodopa treatment on cognitive function, among them Portin, Raininko, and Rinne (1984). Analysis of their longitudinal data revealed that even before treatment, the PD patients differed significantly in cognitive and emotional functions from normal age-matched control subjects. After the initiation of levodopa treatment, most patients showed significant improvement in cognitive function but did not reach the level of normal subjects. After 2 to 3 years of drug treatment, some cognitive processes began to decline, a finding reported by other investigators (Halgin, Riklan, and Misiak, 1977; Loranger et al., 1973). With 8 to 10 years of drug treatment, highly significant deterioration occurred in motor, visuospatial, memory, and verbal skills.

Anticholinergic Drug Therapy. If PD patients are unable to tolerate levodopa, anticholinergic compounds sometimes are administered to alleviate the parkinsonian signs. These drugs result in modest improvement in severity of tremor and ridigity, but little or no benefit for bradykinesia (Adams and Victor, 1977; McDowell, Lee, and Sweet, 1978). Side effects include dry mouth, urinary retention, constipation, blurred vision, delirium, agitation, and hallucinations (Cummings and Benson, 1983). Use of anticholinergic medications in PD patients with intellectual impairment is questionable because these patients have been shown to be particularly sensitive to the mental side effects of anticholinergics (Klawans, 1982). Memory function in both animal and human studies is in some way dependent upon cholinergic neurotransmission; thus, anticholinergics disrupt memory (Koller, 1984). DeSmet and associates (1982) reported confusional states in 93 percent of PD patients in their study who were taking anticholinergics but in only 46 percent of those not receiving anticholinergic medication. Further, while cholinergic neurotransmission is known to be disrupted in AD, it is considered to be an integral feature in PD patients with dementia (Ruberg et al., 1982).

VASCULAR DEMENTIA

In the not distant past, the gradual loss of mental faculties in the elderly was commonly ascribed to "hardening of the arteries," and patients were treated with vasodilators (Ditch, Kelly, and Fesnick, 1971; Rao and Norris, 1972). The NFTs and neuritic plaques seen in the brains of demented patients were theorized to result from cerebral ischemia and tissue hypoxia. Now it is recognized that it is not the existence of vascular disease per se that causes the dementia, but the repeated occurrence of stroke. As a result of well-controlled pathologic studies, repeated strokes as the sole cause of dementia are recognized to account for approximately 17 percent of dementia cases (Tomlinson and Henderson, 1976). Tomlinson et al., (1970) reported that the characteristics of dementia are influenced by the location and total amount of infarcted tissue. Changes in the perception of what causes vascular dementia was reflected in the term used by the American Psychiatric Association (1980), "multi-infarct dementia" (MID); this phrase was introduced by Hachinski, Lassen, and Marshall, (1974).

Signs of Vascular Dementia

The distinguishing clinical features of MID are hypertension, abrupt onset, stepwise deterioration, fluctuating course, relative preservation of the personality, focal neurologic signs and symptoms, history of strokes, emotional lability, somatic complaints and depression (Hachinski et al., 1975). Typically, MID patients are younger than AD patients with onset of dementia typically beginning in the 60s and the incidence among men is approximately double that in women (Morimatsu, Hirai, Muramatsu, and Yoshikawa, 1975; Tomlinson et al., 1970).

The first evidence of multi-infarct, or vascular, dementia is likely to be delirium or a small stroke followed by rapid deterioration (Sloane, 1980). Careful testing is needed at this stage to detect the intellectual disability. Following a bout of delirium, the patient may improve or fluctuate between orientation and confusion. Often, affected individuals cry and laugh inappropriately and easily, a condition known as emotional lability. Approximately 20 percent of vascular dementia patients experience seizures.

Three Major Subgroups of MID Patients

Making generalizations about patients with vascular dementia, without reference to the part of the vascular system involved, is impossible. For example, a patient with lacunes (small cavities of infarcted tissue) primarily in the basal ganglia is very different clinically from the individual with large vessel occlusion of the middle cerebral artery. The signs of MID patients reflect the location of the brain damage. Three major subgroups of MID have been distinguished (Rogers, Meyer, Mortel, Mahurin, and Judd, 1986). The first type is associated with a large cerebral infarction or chronic ischemia caused by large-vessel thrombotic strokes or multifocal adjacent embolic strokes. The second type is caused by many small, deep, subcortical lacunar infarctions, which occur most often in the middle cerebral arterial system. The third subgroup of MID patients have subcortical atherosclerotic encephalopathy (Binswanger's disease), which results from atherosclerosis of the penetrating cerebral arteries. Rogers and colleagues (1986) found the small pericapsular lacunar infarcts to be the most common form of MID.

Large Vessel Occlusion. An individual can suffer a large cortical infarct and not be demented. For dementia to be clinically discernible, multiple bilateral infarctions must have occurred. Infarctions

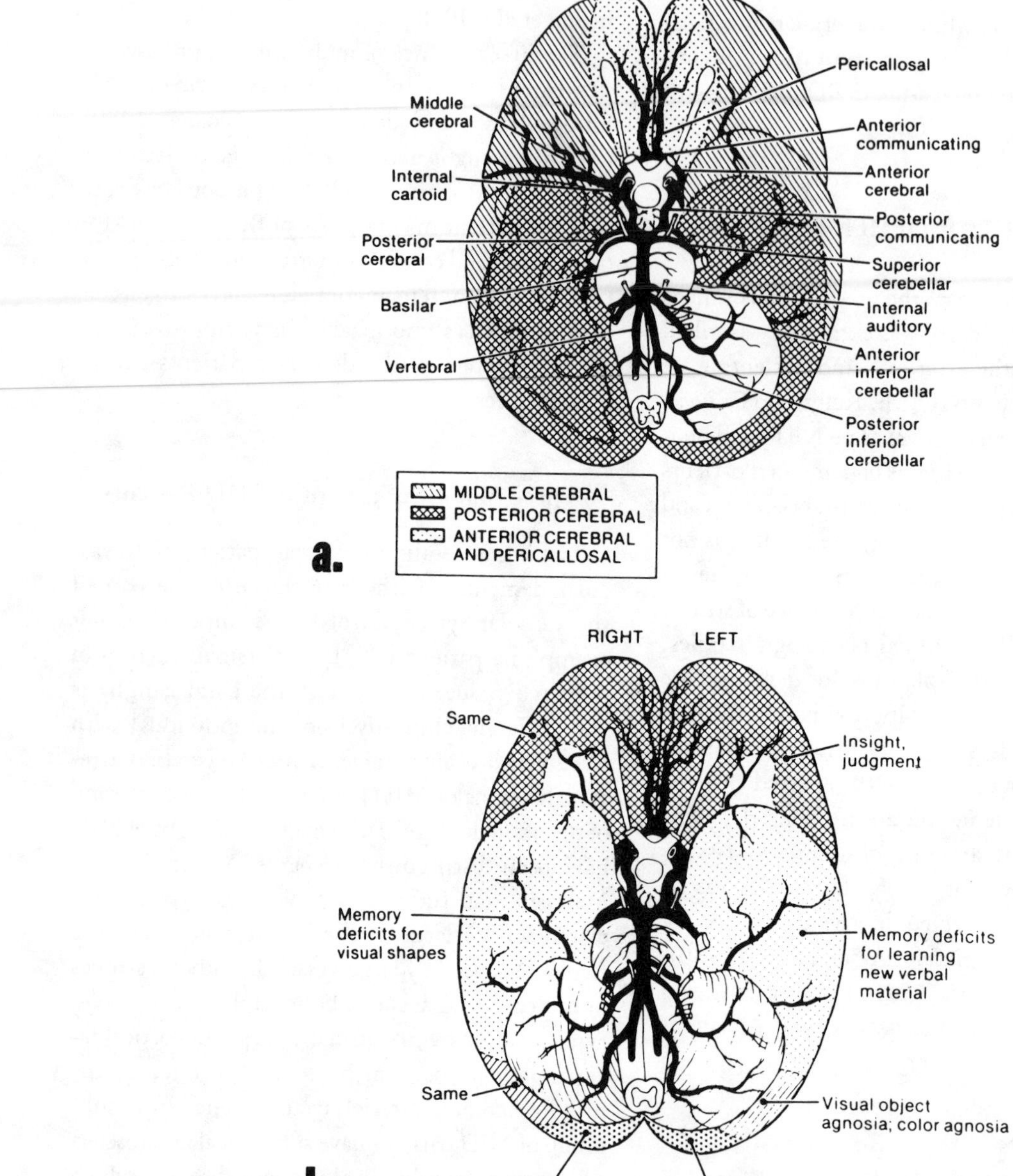

Figure 1-18. *A basal view of brain, cerebellum, and brain stem showing (a) the regions supplied by the major cerebral arteries and their branches, and (b) the psychophysiologic dysfunctions resulting from regional ischemias. (From Deshmukh, V.D., and Meyer, J.S. {1978}.* Noninvasive measurement of regional cerebral blood flow in man. *New York: SP Medical and Scientific Books, by permission. Copyright 1978 by Spectrum Publications, Inc.)*

are likely to predominate in brain regions supplied by the anterior, middle, or posterior cerebral arteries (Figures 1-18 and 1-19).

When the anterior arteries are affected, sensory and motor deficits in the contralateral legs may be present. Involvement of the left anterior artery is associated with transcortical motor aphasia (Alexander and Schmitt, 1980). Bilateral anterior cerebral artery occlusion may be associated with decreased initiative, loss of motivation, and psychomotor bradykinesia (Critchley, 1930).

Left middle cerebral artery (MCA) disease is likely to be manifested as aphasia and apraxia, in addition to dementia (Brust, Shafer, Richter, and Bruun 1976), whereas right MCA involvement is likely to result in visuospatial disorders, and deficits in the perception and production of emotionally intoned speech (Heilman, Scholes, and Watson, 1975; Tucker, Watson, and Heilman, 1977). Disease in either the right or the left middle cerebral artery can produce neglect syndrome, denial of weakness, and constructional disturbances (Benson and Barton, 1970; Cutting, 1978).

When the posterior portion of the middle cerebral artery is diseased, a condition that is hard to distinguish from AD can occur. Called angular gyrus syndrome, its features are fluent aphasia, alexia with agraphia, Gerstmann syndrome, and constructional deficits (Benson, 1979). The cluster of behaviors comprising Gerstmann syndrome traditionally includes acalculia, difficulty with left-right distinctions, and finger agnosia (Critchley, 1953).

Involvement of the posterior cerebral artery may result in contralateral hemianopsia. Lesions involving the right side are associated with visual hallucinations, palinopsia (abnormal recurring visual imagery), abnormalities in facial recognition and spatial disorientation (Cummings, Landis, and Benson, 1983; De Renzi, Scotti, and Spinnler, 1969). Left-sided lesions are typified by contralateral hemiparesis and hemisensory loss, anomia, and occasionally alexia without agraphia (Benson and Tomlinson, 1971). If occlusion occurs bilaterally, and there is destruction of the inferior medial temporal lobe, permanent severe amnesia may follow (DeJong, Itabashi, and Olson, 1969; Van Buren

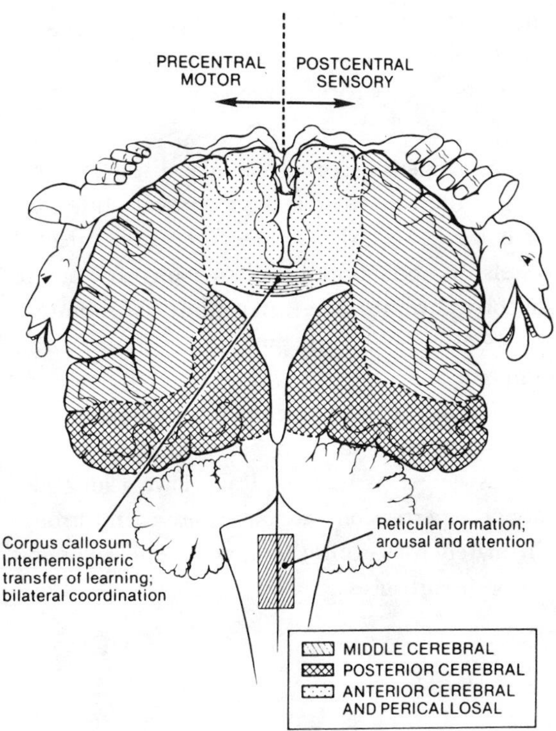

Figure 1-19. *A coronal section through brain, cerebellum, and brain stem, showing regions supplied by the major cortical arteries and the sensorimotor "homunculus." (From Deshmukh, V.D., and Meyer, J.S. (1978).* Noninvasive measurement of regional cerebral blood flow in man. *New York: SP Medical and Scientific Books, by permission. Copyright 1978 by Spectrum Publications, Inc.)*

and Borke, 1972). Other sequelae of bilateral occlusions in the posterior cerebral artery include cortical blindness, visual agnosia, and prosopagnosia, or difficulty in recognizing familiar faces (Albert, Soffer, Silverberg, and Reches, 1979; Benson, 1978; Damasio, Yamada, Damasio, Corbett, and McKee, 1980; Green and Lessell, 1977).

Lacunar State. Lacunes are small deep cavitary infarcts that occur in the small penetrating arteries of the basal ganglia, thalamus, brain stem, and deep cerebral white matter (Fisher, 1965; Mohr, 1982). They are almost always caused by hypertensive damage. The term, lacunar state, is applied to patients who have large numbers of lacunar infarctions. Associated with dementia in these patients are pseudobulbar palsy, dysarthria, dysphagia, weakness, bradykinesia, small-stepped gait, uncontrollable laughing and crying, hyperreflexia, and incontinence (Brust, 1983).

Binswanger's Disease. Vascular disease eventuating in multiple infarcts in subcortical white matter is the cause of Binswanger's disease. Affected vessels do not supply blood to the cortex but to subcortical white matter. According to Cummings and Benson (1983), in some cases, the posterior temporal and occipital white matter is more involved than the anterior white matter areas; in other patients, all white matter atrophies.

Binswanger patients typically have a long history of hypertension, vascular disease, and stroke. Ultimately they exhibit focal neurologic signs and motor disturbances.

Risk Factors for Vascular Dementia

The prominent risk factors for repeated strokes and dementia are hypertension, impaired cardiac functioning, diabetes, high-normal hemoglobin values, elevated serum cholesterol, and cigarette smoking (Cohen and Eisdorfer, 1984). Patients with hypertension develop cerebrovascular disease seven times more often than people with normal blood pressure. Librach, Schadel, Seltzer, Hert, and Yellin (1977) reported that hypertension, in persons without heart disease, increased the annual rate of stroke from 3.18 to 11.5 percent per 1000 persons. Cardiac disease is a potent predictor of stroke (Friedman, Loveland, and Ehrlich, 1968), and three out of four patients with cerebrovascular disease have one or more cardiac impairments.

Using data from the Framingham study of aging,

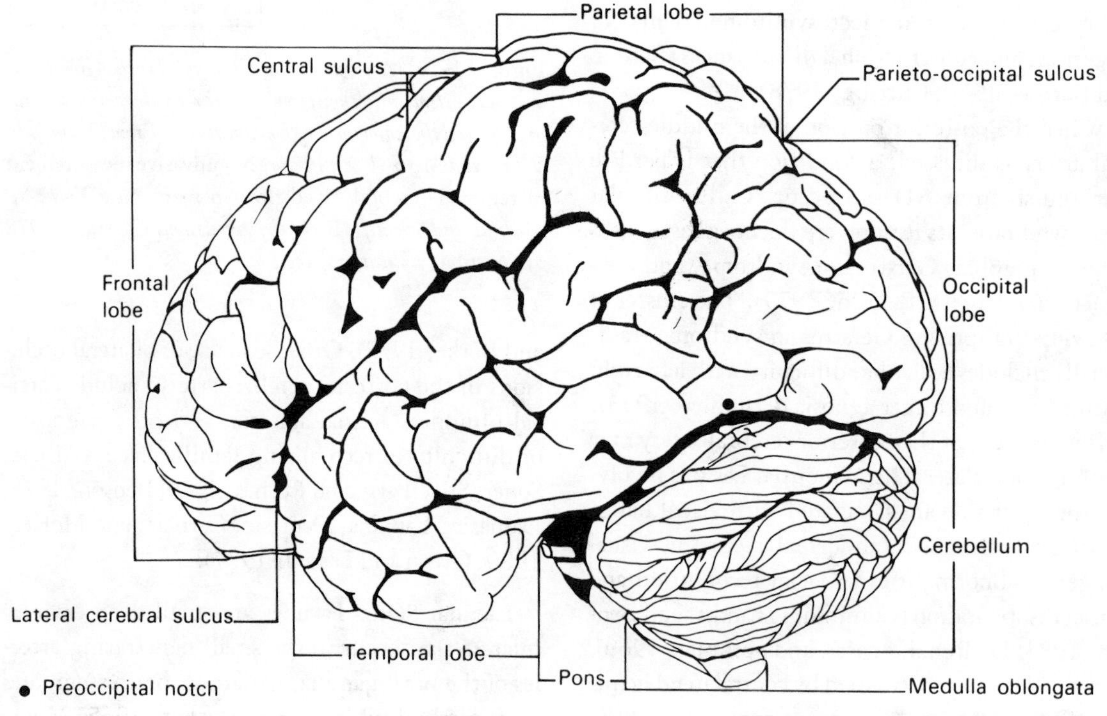

Figure 1-20. *Lobes of the cerebral hemisphere and other landmarks. (From Waddington, M.M. (1984).* Atlas of human intracranial anatomy. *Rutland, VT: Academy Books, by permission. Copyright 1984 by Margaret Miles Waddington.)*

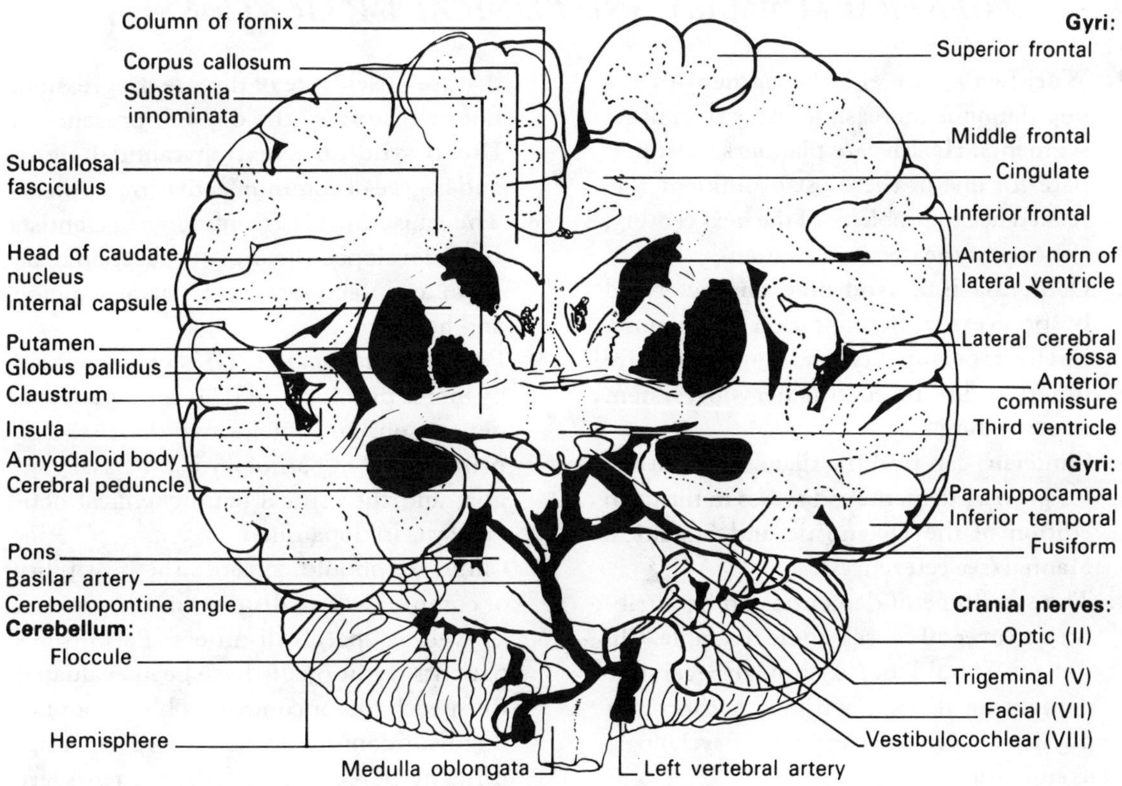

Figure 1-21. *A frontal view of the brain at the level of the anterior commissure. (From Waddington, M.M. (1984).* Atlas of human intracranial anatomy. *Rutland, VT: Academy Books, by permission. Copyright 1984 by Margaret Miles Waddington.)*

twice as much cerebrovascular disease was found in individuals with hemoglobin values higher than normal (Kannel, Gordon, Wolf, and McNamara, 1972). Also, whereas diabetic individuals had a two to three times greater risk for cerebrovascular disease (Wolf, Kannel, and Dawber, 1978), an only slightly higher risk was associated with obesity (Kannel, 1971).

CONCLUSION

Patients with dementia are the fastest growing neurobehaviorally disordered population. The prevalence of dementia is dramatically increasing worldwide, making care of demented patients one of the greatest health care challenges in the next century. The most prevalent dementing disease is AD, followed by vascular dementia. Another disease increasingly recognized as being associated with dementia is PD, though the rate of occurrence of dementia in PD patients is disputed. Three of the four major dementing diseases, AD, HD, and PD (vascular disease excepted) appear to have either common neuropathologic or neurochemical features that lead scientists to hope that a breakthrough in the understanding of one will lead to insights about the others.

GENERAL SUMMARY AND CLINICAL IMPLICATIONS

1. Worldwide, the elderly segment of the population is increasing faster than other segments. Health care planners must prepare for one of the most prominent age-related health problems of the next century, the care of the dementia patient.
2. Dementia is a syndrome characterized by progressive deterioration in memory, intellect, personality, and communicative function due to central nervous system degeneration.
3. Clinicians can find the diagnostic criteria for primary dementing diseases in the third edition of the Diagnostic and Statistical Manual (see references).
4. The syndrome of dementia can be attributed to over 50 causes, some treatable. Clinicians should not assume irreversible dementing disease without a thorough physical, neurologic, and neuropsychologic examination.
5. Clinicians are more likely to see patients with Alzheimer's dementia (AD) or vascular dementia than any other type.
6. Alzheimer's patients suffer deficiencies in critical neurochemicals and develop neuritic plaques, neurofibrillary tangles, and areas of granulovacuolar degeneration.
7. Alzheimer's patients may not represent a homogeneous population. Clinicians should be cognizant of potential variation in behavioral disorders as a function of age of disease onset, rate of disease progression, family history of the disease, presence of Down syndrome, extrapyramidal signs, and degree of communicative impairment.
8. The cause of AD is unknown. Scientists have developed theories of causation related to an infectious agent, metal toxicity, and heredity.
9. Parkinson's disease (PD) is characterized by motor problems, and for some patients, depression, and intellectual deficits. The primary site of pathology is the basal ganglia, and the critical neurochemical deficiency is in dopamine.
10. Clinicians should consider the possibility of communicative disorder in PD patients as well as speech disorders. Parkinson's patients traditionally have been evaluated for speech motor control problems but not linguistic communication disorders. A significant percentage of PD patients are known to develop intellectual deficits, and some, full dementia.
11. Patients with vascular dementia are a heterogeneous population. Clinicians should expect the behavioral problems and neurologic signs to vary with site of vascular pathology.
12. Vascular dementia patients typically have a history of hypertension, abrupt onset of mental status changes, and a fluctuating course.

BIBLIOGRAPHY

Cummings, J.L., and Benson, D.F. (1983). *Dementia: A clinical approach*. London: Butterworth.

Mayeux, R., and Rosen, W.G. (Eds.). (1983). *Advances in neurology: Vol. 38. The dementias*. New York: Raven.

Reisberg, B. (Ed.). (1983). *Alzheimer's disease: A standard reference*. New York: The Free Press.

REFERENCES

Adams, R.D., Fisher, C.M., Hakim, S., Ojemann, R.G., and Sweet, W.H. (1965). Symptomatic occult hydrocephalus with "normal" cerebrospinal fluid pressure. *New England Journal of Medicine, 273*, 117-126.

Adams, R.D., and Victor, M. (1977). *Principles of neurology*. New York: McGraw-Hill.

Adelstein, A.M., Downham, D.Y., Stein, Z., and Susser, M.W. (1968). The epidemiology of mental illness in an English city. Inceptions recognized by Salford Psychiatric Services. *Social Psychiatry, 3*, 47-49.

Adolfsson, R., Gottfries, C.G., Roos, B.E., and Winblad, B. (1979). Changes in brain catecholamines in patients with dementia of Alzheimer type. *British Journal of Psychiatry, 135*, 216-223.

Agnoli, A., Ruggieri, S., Meco, G., Casacchia, M., Denaro, A., Conti, L., Bedini, L., Stocchi, R., Fioravanti, M., Franzese, A., and Lazzari, R. (1984). An appraisal of the problem of dementia in Parkinson's disease. In R.G. Hassler and J.F. Christ (Eds.), *Advances in neurology: Vol 40. Parkinson-specific motor and mental disorders* (pp. 299-306). New York: Raven Press.

Åkesson, H.O. (1969). A population study of senile and arteriosclerotic psychoses. *Human Heredity, 19*, 546-566.

Alavi, A., Dann, R., Chawluk, J., Alavi, J., Kushner, M., and Reivich, M. (1986). Positron emission tomography imaging of regional cerebral glucose metabolism. *Seminars in Nuclear Medicine, 16*, 2-34.

Albert, E. (1968). On the nosology of senile dementia. In C. Muller and L. Ciompi (Eds.), *Senile dementia: Clinical and therapeutic aspects* (pp. 33-34). Bern, Switzerland: Hans Huber.

Albert, M.L., Soffer, D., Silverberg, R., and Reches, A. (1979). The anatomic basis of visual agnosia. *Neurology, 29*, 876-879.

Alexander, F.G., and Selesnick, S.T. (1966). *The history of psychiatry*. New York: Harper and Row.

Alexander, M.P., and Schmitt, M.A. (1980). The aphasia syndrome of stroke in the left anterior cerebral artery territory. *Archives of Neurology, 37*, 97-100.

American Psychiatric Association (1980). *Diagnostic and statistical manual of mental disorders* (3rd ed.). Washington, DC: Author.

Andrews, G.R., and Davidson, A.H. (1984). Aging and dementia in the developing world—a challenge for the future. In J. Wertheimer and M. Marois (Eds.), *Senile dementia: Outlook for the future* (pp. 479-490). New York: Alan R. Liss.

Arendt, T., Bigl, V., Arendt, A., and Tennstedt, A. (1983). Loss of neurons in the nucleus basalis of Meynert in Alzheimer's disease, paralysis agitans and Korsakoff's disease. *Acta Neuropathologica* (Berlin), *61*, 101-108.

Ayd, F.J. (1961). A survey of drug-induced extrapyramidal reactions. *Journal of the American Medical Association, 175*, 1054-1060.

Barchas, J.D., Akil, H., Elliott, G.R., Holman, R.B., and Watson, S.J. (1978). Behavioral neurochemistry: Neuroregulators and behavioral states. *Science, 200*, 964-973.

Behan, P.O., and Behan, W.M.H. (1979). Possible immunological factors in Alzheimer's disease. In A.I.M. Glen and L.J. Whalley (Eds.), *Alzheimer's disease: Early recognition of potential reversible deficits* (pp. 33-35). New York: Livingstone.

Benson, D.F. (1978). Amnesia. *Southern Medical Journal, 71*, 1221-1228.

Benson, D.F. (1979). *Aphasia, alexia, and agraphia* (pp. 169-170). London: Churchill Livingstone.

Benson, D.F., and Barton, M.I. (1970). Disturbances in constructional ability. *Cortex, 6*, 19-46.

Benson, D.F., Kuhl, D.E., Hawkins, R.A., Phelps, M.E., Cummings, J.L., Tsai, S.Y. (1983). The fluorodeoxyglucose 18F scan in Alzheimer's disease and multi-infarct dementia. *Archives of Neurology, 40*, 711-714.

Benson, D.F., and Tomlinson, E.B. (1971). Hemiplegic syndrome of the posterior cerebral artery. *Stroke, 2*, 559-564.

Berger, B., Tassin, J.P., Rancurel, G., and Blanc, G. (1980). Catecholaminergic innervation of the human cerebral cortex in presenile and senile dementia: Histochemical and biochemical studies. In E. Usdlin, T.L. Sourkes, and M.B.H. Youdin (Eds.), *Enzymes and neurotransmitters in mental disease* (pp. 317-322). New York: John Wiley.

Bergmann, K., Kay, D.W.K., Foster, E.M., McKechnie, A.A., and Roth, M. (1971). A follow-up study of randomly selected community residents to assess the effects of chronic brain syndrome and cerebrovascular disease. Excerpta Medica International Congress Series No. 274. *Psychiatry, 34*, 856-865.

Bernheimer, H., Birkmayer, W., Hornykiewicz, O.,

Jellinger, K., and Seitelberger, F. (1973). Brain dopamine and the syndromes of Parkinson and Huntington: Clinical, morphological and neurochemical correlations. *Journal of Neurological Sciences, 20*, 415-455.

Besdine, R.W. (1982). Dementia. In J.W. Rowe and R.W. Besdine (Eds.), *Health and disease in old age* (pp. 97-114). Boston: Little, Brown and Company.

Bird, E.D., and Iversen, L.L. (1974). Huntington's chorea. Post mortem measurement of glutamic acid, decarboxylase, choline acetyltransferase and dopamine in basal ganglia. *Brain, 97*, 457-472.

Blessed, G., Tomlinson, B.E., and Roth, M. (1968). The association between quantitative measures of dementia and of senile change in the cerebral grey matter of elderly subjects. *British Journal of Psychiatry, 114*, 797-811.

Boller, F., Mizutani, T., Roessmann, U., and Gambetti, P. (1980). Parkinson disease, dementia and Alzheimer's disease: Clinicopathological correlations. *Annals of Neurology, 7*, 329-335.

Bollerup, T.R. (1975). Prevalence of mental illness among 70-year-olds domiciled in nine Copenhagen suburbs: the Glostrup survey. *Acta Psychiatrica Scandinavica, 51*, 327-339.

Bolt, J.M.W. (1970). Huntington's chorea in the west of Scotland. *British Journal of Psychiatry, 116*, 259-270.

Bondareff, W., Baldy, R., and Levy, R. (1981). Quantitative computed tomography in senile dementia. *Archives of General Psychiatry, 38*, 1365-1368.

Bondareff, W., Mountjoy, C.Q., and Roth, M. (1981). Selective loss of neurones of origin of adrenergic projection to cerebral cortex (nucleus locus coeruleus) in senile dementia. *Lancet, 1*, 783-784.

Bowen, D.M., Smith, C.B., White, P., and Davison, A.N. (1976). Neurotransmitter-related enzymes and indices of hypoxia in senile dementia and other abiotrophies. *Brain, 99*, 459-496.

Brant-Zawadzki, M., Badami, J.P., Mills, C.M., Norman, D., and Newton, T.H. (1984). Primary intracranial tumor imaging: A comparison of magnetic resonance and CT. *Radiology, 150*, 435-440.

Brant-Zawadzki, M., Mills, C.M., and Davis, P.L. (1983). Applications of NMR to CNS disease. *Applied Radiology, 12*, 25-30.

Breitner, J.C.S., and Folstein, M.F. (1984). Familial Alzheimer dementia: A prevalent disorder with specific clinical features. *Psychological Medicine, 14*, 63-80.

Brody, H. (1955). Organization of the cerebral cortex. III. A study of aging in the human cerebral cortex. *Journal of Comparative Neurology, 102*, 511-556.

Brody, H. (1970). Structural changes in the aging nervous system. In H. T. Blumenthal (Ed.), *Interdisciplinary topics in gerontology: Vol. 7. The regulatory role of the nervous system in aging* (pp. 9-21). Basel: S. Karger.

Brody, J.A. (1984). An epidemiologist's view of the senile dementias—Pieces of the puzzle. In J. Wertheimer and M. Marois (Eds.), *Senile dementia: Outlook for the future* (pp. 383-393). New York: Alan R. Liss.

Broe, G.A., Akhtar, A.J., Andrews, G.R., Caird, F.I., Gilmore, A.J.J., and McLennan. W.J. (1976). Neurological disorders in the elderly at home. *Journal of Neurology, Neurosurgery, and Psychiatry, 39*, 362-366.

Brown, D.D. (1973). Involuntary movements. In L. Brain (Ed.), *Brain's clinical neurology* (4th ed. revised by R. Bannister) (p. 71). New York: Oxford University Press.

Brun, A., Gustafson, L., and Mittleman, F. (1978). Normal chromosome banding pattern in Alzheimer's disease. *Gerontology, 24*, 369-372.

Brust, J.C.M. (1983). Dementia and cerebrovascular disease. In R. Mayeux and W.G. Rosen (Eds), *The dementias* (pp. 131-147). New York: Raven.

Brust, J.C.M., Shafer, S.Q., Richter, R.W., and Bruun, B. (1976). Aphasia in acute stroke. *Stroke, 7*, 167-174.

Bruyn, G.W. (1968). Huntington's chorea: A historical, clinical, and laboratory synopsis. In P.J. Vinken and G.W. Bruyn (Eds.), *Handbook of clinical neurology: Vol. 6. Diseases of the basal ganglia* (pp. 298-378). Amsterdam: North-Holland.

Bryan, R.N. (1985). Imaging technique of the aging brain. In C.M. Gaitz and T. Samorajski (Eds.), *Aging 2000: Our health care destiny: Vol. 1. Biomedical issues* (pp. 197-201). New York: Springer-Verlag.

Bucci, L. (1963). A familial organic psychosis of Alzheimer type in six kinships of three generations. *American Journal of Psychiatry, 119*, 863-866.

Burger, P.C., and Vogel, F.S. (1973). The development of the pathologic changes of Alzheimer's disease and senile dementia in patients with Down's syndrome. *American Journal of Pathology, 73*, 457-476.

Carlsson, A., Adolfsson, R., and Aquilonius, S.M. (1980). Biogenic amines in brain in normal aging, senile dementia and chronic alcoholism. *Advances in Biochemical Psychopharmacology, 23*, 295-304.

Carter, C.O. (1969). Genetics of common disorders. *British Medical Bulletin, 25*, 52-57.

Charatan, F.B. (1984). Mental stimulation and deprivation as risk factors in senility. In H. Rothschild

(Ed.), *Risk factors for senility* (pp. 90-101). New York: Oxford University Press.

Chedru, F., and Geschwind, N. (1972). Disorders of higher cortical functions in acute confusional states. *Cortex, 8*, 395-411.

Chenoweth, B., and Spencer, B. (1986). Dementia: The experience of family caregivers. *The Gerontologist, 26*, 267-272.

Chou, S.M., and Martin, J.D. (1971). Kuru plaques in a case of Creutzfeldt-Jakob disease. *Acta Neuropathologica, 11*, 150-155.

Chui, H.C., Teng, E.L., Henderson, V.W., and Moy, A.C.L. (1985). Clinical subtypes of dementia of the Alzheimer type. *Neurology, 35*, 1544-1550.

Clough, C.G., Bergmann, K.J., and Yahr, M.D. (1984). Cholinergic and dopaminergic mechanisms in PD after long-term L-DOPA administration. In R.G. Hassler and J.F. Christ (Eds.), *Advances in neurology: Vol. 40. Parkinson-specific motor and mental disorders* (pp. 131-140). New York: Raven Press.

Cohen, D. , and Eisdorfer, C. (1984). Risk factors in late life dementias. In J. Wertheimer and M. Marois (Eds.), *Senile dementia: Outlook for the future* (pp. 221-237). New York: Alan R. Liss.

Cohen, D., Eisdorfer, C., and Leverenz, J. (1982). Alzheimer's disease and maternal age. *Journal of the American Geriatrics Society, 30*, 656-659.

Cook, R.H., Ward, B.E., and Austin, J.H. (1979). Studies in aging of the brain. IV. Familial Alzheimer's disease: Relation to transmissible dementia aneuploidy and microtubular defects. *Neurology (NY), 29*, 1402-1412.

Coyle, J.T., Price, D.L., and DeLong, M.R. (1983). Alzheimer's disease: A disorder of cortical cholinergic innervation. *Science, 219*, 1184-1190.

Crapper, D.R., Dalton, A.J., Skopitz, M., Scott, J.W., and Hachinski, V.C. (1975). Alzheimer degeneration in Down syndrome: Electrophysiologic alterations and histopathologic findings. *Archives of Neurology, 32*, 618-623.

Crapper, D.R., Krishnan, S.S., and Dalton, A.J. (1973). Brain aluminum distribution in Alzheimer's disease and experimental neurofibrillary degeneration. *Science, 180*, 511-513.

Crapper, D.R., Krishnan, S.S., and Quittkat, S. (1976). Aluminum neurofibrillary degeneration and Alzheimer's disease. *Brain, 99*, 67-79.

Creasy, M.R. (1974). Prenatal mortality of trisomy 21. *Lancet, 1*, 473.

Critchley, M. (1930). The anterior cerebral artery and its syndromes. *Brain, 53*, 120-165.

Critchley, M. (1953). *The parietal lobes*. London: Edward Arnold.

Cross, A.J., Crow, T.J., Perry, E.K., Perry, R.H., Blessed, G., and Tomlinson, B.E. (1981). Reduced dopamine-β-hydroxylase activity in Alzheimer's disease. *British Medical Journal, 282*, 93-94.

Cummings, J.L., and Benson, D.F. (1983). *Dementia: A clinical approach*. Boston, MA: Butterworth.

Cummings, J.L., Landis, T., and Benson, D.F. (1983, April). *Environmental disorientation: Clinical and radiologic findings*. Paper presented to the American Academy of Neurology, San Diego, CA.

Cutting, J. (1978). Study of anosognosia. *Journal of Neurology, Neurosurgery, and Psychiatry, 41*, 548-555.

Dalton, A.J., Crapper, D.R., Schlotterer, G.R. (1974). Alzheimer's disease in Down's syndrome: Visual retention deficits. *Cortex, 10*, 366-377.

Damasio, A.R., Yamada, T., Damasio, H., Corbett, J., and McKee, J. (1980). Central achromatopsia: Behavioral, anatomic, and physiologic aspects. *Neurology, 30*, 1064-1071.

Damasio, H., Eslinger, P., Damasio, A.R., Rizzo, M., Huang, H.K., and Demeter, S. (1983). Quantitative computed tomographic analysis in the diagnosis of dementia. *Archives of Neurology, 40*, 715-719.

Davies, P. (1979). Neurotransmitter-related enzymes in senile dementia of the Alzheimer type. *Brain Research, 171*, 319-327.

Davies, P. (1983). An update on the neurochemistry of Alzheimer disease. In R. Mayeux and W.G. Rosen (Eds.), *The dementias* (pp. 75-86). New York: Raven.

Davies, P., Katz, D.A., and Crystal, H.A. (1982). Choline acetyltransferase, somatostatin, and substance P in selected cases of Alzheimer's disease. In S. Corkin, K.L. Davis, J.H. Growdon, E. Usdin, and R.J. Wurtman (Eds.), *Aging: Vol. 19. Alzheimer's disease: A report of progress in research* (pp. 9-14). New York: Raven.

Davies, P., Katzman, R., and Terry, R.D. (1980). Reduced somatostatin-like immunoreactivity in cerebral cortex from cases of Alzheimer disease and Alzheimer senile dementia. *Nature, 288*, 279-280.

Davies, P., and Maloney, A.J.F. (1976). Selective loss of central cholinergic neurons in Alzheimer's disease. *Lancet, 2*, 1403.

Davies, P., and Terry, R.D. (1981). Cortical somatostatin-like immunoreactivity in cases of Alzheimer's disease and senile dementia of the Alzheimer type. *Neurobiology of Aging, 2*, 9-14.

Davies, P., and Verth, A.H. (1977). Regional distribution of muscarinic acetylcholine receptor in normal and Alzheimer type dementia brains. *Brain Research, 138*, 385-392.

Davis, K.L., and Mohs, R.C. (1982). Enhancement of memory processes in Alzheimer's disease with multiple-dose intravenous physostigmine. *American Journal of Psychiatry, 139,* 1421-1424.

DeJong, R.N., Itabashi, H.H., and Olson, J.R. (1969). Memory loss due to hippocampal lesions. *Archives of Neurology, 20*, 339-348.

DeRenzi, E., Scotti, G., and Spinnler, H. (1969). Perceptual and associative disorders of visual recognition. *Neurology, 19*, 634-642.

DeSmet, Y, Ruberg, M., Serdaru, M., DuBois, B., Lhermitte, F., and Agid, Y. (1982). Confusion, dementia and anticholinergics in Parkinson's disease. *Journal of Neurology, Neurosurgery, and Psychiatry, 45*, 1161-1164.

Dewhurst, K., Oliver, J., and McKnight, A. (1970). Socio-psychiatric consequences of Huntington's disease. *British Journal of Psychiatry, 116*, 255-258.

Direnfeld, L.K., Albert, M.L., Volicer, L., Langlais, P.J., Marquis, J., and Kaplan, E. (1984). Parkinson's disease. The possible relationship of laterality to dementia and neurochemical findings. *Archives of Neurology, 41*, 935-941.

Ditch, M., Kelly, F.J., and Fesnick, O. (1971). An ergot preparation (Hydergine) in the treatment of cerebrovascular disorders in the geriatric patient: Double-blind study. *Journal of the American Geriatrics Society, 19*, 208-217.

Divac, I. (1975). Magnocellular nuclei of the basal forebrain project to neocortex, brain stem and olfactory bulb. Review of some functional correlates. *Brain Research, 93*, 385-398.

Dongen, P.A.M. van (1981). The human locus coeruleus in neurology and psychiatry. *Progress in Neurobiology, 17*, 97-139.

Duffy, F.H., Albert, M.S., and McAnulty, G. (1984). Brain electrical activity in patients with presenile and senile dementia of the Alzheimer type. *Annals of Neurology, 16*, 439-448.

Duffy, P., Wolf, J., Collins, G., DeVoe, A.G., Streeten, B., and Cowen, D. (1974). Possible person-to-person transmission of Creutzfeldt-Jakob disease. *New England Journal of Medicine, 290*, 692-693.

Ehle, A.L., and Johnson, P.C. (1977). Rapidly evolving EEG changes in a case of Alzheimer disease. *Annals of Neurology, 1*, 593-595.

Engel, G.L., and Romano, J. (1959). Delirium: A syndrome of cerebral insufficiency. *Journal of Chronic Diseases, 9*, 260-277.

Erickson, J.D. (1978). Down's syndrome, paternal age, maternal age and birth order. *Annals of Human Genetics, 41*, 289.

Essen-Moller, E., Larsson, H., Uddenberg, C., and White, G. (1955). Individual traits and morbidity in a Swedish rural population. *Acta Psychiatrica et Neurologica Scandinavica Supplementum, 100*, 1-160.

Feldman, R.G., Chandler, K.A., Levy, L.L., and Glaser, G.H. (1963). Familial Alzheimer's disease. *Neurology, 13*, 811-824.

Finch, C.E. (1985). Alzheimer's disease: A biologist's perspective. *Science, 230*, 1109.

Fisher, C.M. (1965). Lacunes: Small, deep cerebral infarcts. *Neurology, 15*, 774-784.

Folstein, S.E., Abbott, M.H., Chase, G.A., Jensen, B.A., and Folstein, M.F. (1983). The association of affective disorder with Huntington's disease in a case series and in families. *Psychological Medicine, 13*, 537-542.

Folstein, M.F., and Breitner, J.C.S. (1981). Language disorder predicts familial Alzheimer's disease. *Johns Hopkins Medical Journal, 149*, 145-147.

Folstein, S.E., Franz, M.L., Jensen, B.A., Chase, A., and Folstein, M.F. (1983). Conduct disorder and affective disorder among offspring of patients with Huntington's disease. *Psychological Medicine, 13*, 45-52.

Foster, N.L., Chase, T.N., Fedio, P., Patronas, N.J., Brooks, R.A., and DiChiro, G. (1983). Alzheimer's disease: Focal cortical changes shown by positron emission tomography. *Neurology, 33*, 961-965.

Foster, N.L., Chase, T.N., Mansi, L., Brooks, R., Fedio, P., Patronas, N.J., and Dichiro, G. (1984). Cortical abnormalities in Alzheimer's disease. *Annals of Neurology, 16*, 649-654.

Fox, J.H., Topel, J.R., and Huckman, M.S. (1975). Use of computerized tomography in senile dementia. *Journal of Neurology, Neurosurgery and Psychiatry, 38*, 948-953.

Freemon, F.R. (1976). Evaluation of patients with progressive intellectual deterioration. *Archives of Neurology, 33*, 658-659.

Freyhan, F.A., Woodford, R.B., and Kety, S.S. (1951). Cerebral blood flow and metabolism in psychoses of senility. *Journal of Nervous and Mental Disorders, 113*, 449-459.

Friedland, R.P., Prusiner, S.B., Jagust, W.J., Budinger, T.F., and Davis, R.L. (1984). Bitemporal hypometabolism in Creutzfeldt-Jakob disease measured by positron emission tomography with 18 F-2-fluorodeoxyglucose. *Journal of Computer Assisted Tomography, 8*, 978-981.

Friedman, G.D., Loveland, D.B., and Ehrlich, S.P., Jr. (1968). Relationship of stroke to other cardiovascular disease. *Circulation, 38*, 533-541.

Gajdusek, D.C. (1977). Unconventional viruses and the origin and disappearance of kuru. *Science, 197*, 943-960.

Garron, D.C., Klawans, H.L., and Narin, F. (1972). Intellectual functioning of persons with idiopathic parkinsonism. *Journal of Nervous and Mental Disorders, 154*, 445-452.

Garruto, R.M., Yanagihara, R., and Gajdusek, D.C. (1985). Disappearance of high-incidence amyotrophic lateral sclerosis and parkinsonism dementia on Guam. *Neurology, 35*, 193-198.

Gibbs, C.J. Jr., and Gajdusek, D.C. (1978). Subacute spongiform virus encephalopathies: The transmissible virus dementias. In R. Katzman, R.D. Terry, and K.L. Bick (Eds.), *Alzheimer's disease: Senile dementia and related disorders* (pp. 559-575). New York: Raven.

Gibson, P.H. (1983). Form and distribution of senile plaques seen in silver impregnated sections in the brains of intellectually normal elderly people and people with Alzheimer-type dementia. *Neuropathology and Applied Neurobiology, 9*, 379-389.

Glenner, G.G., Ein, D., and Terry, R.D. (1972). The immunoglobulin origin of amyloid. *American Journal of Medicine, 52*, 141-147.

Glenner, G.G., and Wong, C.W. (1984) Alzheimer's disease and Down's syndrome: Sharing of a unique cerebrovascular amyloid fibril protein. *Biochemical and Biophysical Research Communications, 122*, 1131-1135.

Goodman, L. (1953). Alzheimer's disease. A clinicopathologic analysis of twenty-three cases with a theory on causation. *Journal of Nervous and Mental Diseases, 117*, 97-130.

Goudsmit, J., Marrow, C.H., Asher, D.M., Yanagihara, R.T., Masters, C.L., Gibbs, C.J. Jr., and Gajdusek, D.C. (1980). Evidence for and against the transmissibility of Alzheimer's disease. *Neurology, 30*, 945-950.

Green, G.J., and Lessell, S. (1977). Acquired central dyschromatopsia. *Archives of Opthalmology, 95*, 121-128.

Grubb, R.L., Raichle, M.E., Gado, M.H., Eichling, J.O., and Hughes, C.P. (1977). Cerebral blood flow, oxygen utilization, and blood volume in dementia. *Neurology, 27*, 905-910.

Gusella, J.F., Wexler, N.S., Conneally, P.M., Naylor, S.L., Anderson, M.A., Tanzi, R.E., Watkins, P.C., Ottina, K., Wallace, M.R., Sakaguchi, A.Y., Young, A.B., Shoulson, I., Bonilla, E., and Martin, J.B. (1983). A polymophic DNA marker genetically linked to Huntington's disease. *Nature, 306*, 234-238.

Gustafson, L., Brun, A., and Ingvar, D.H. (1977). Presenile dementia: Clinical symptoms, pathoanatomical findings and cerebral blood flow. In J.S. Meyer, H. Lechner, and M. Reivich (Eds.), *Cerebral vascular disease* (pp. 5-9). Amsterdam: Excerpta Medica.

Gustafson, L., and Risberg, J. (1974). Regional cerebral blood flow related to psychiatric symptoms in dementia with onset in the presenile period. *Acta Psychiatrica Scandinavica, 50*, 516-538.

Gustafson, L., and Risberg, J. (1979). Regional cerebral blood flow measurements by the 133 Xe-inhalation technique in differential diagnosis of dementia. *Acta Neurologica Scandinavica, 60* (Suppl. 72), 546-547.

Haase, G.R. (1977). Diseases presenting as dementia. In C.E. Wells (Ed.), *Dementia* (2nd ed.) (pp. 27-67), Philadelphia: F.A. Davis.

Hachinski, V.C., Iliff, L.D., Zilhka, E., duBoulay, G.H.D., McAllister, V.L., Marshall, J., Russell, R.W.R., and Symon, L. (1975). Cerebral blood flow in dementia. *Archives of Neurology, 32*, 632-637.

Hachinski, V.C., Lassen, N.A., and Marshall, J. (1974). Multi-infarct dementia. A cause of mental deterioration in the elderly. *Lancet, 2*, 207-210.

Hagberg, B., and Ingvar, D.H. (1976). Cognitive reduction in presenile dementia related to regional abnormalities in the cerebral blood flow. *British Journal of Psychiatry, 128*, 209-222.

Hagnell, O. (1970). Disease expectancy and incidence of mental illness among the aged. *Acta Psychiatrica Scandinavica Supplementum, 219*, 83-89.

Hakim, A.M., and Mathieson, G. (1979). Dementia in Parkinson's disease: A neuropathologic study. *Neurology, 29*, 1209-1214.

Halgin, R., Riklan, M., and Misiak, H. (1977). Levodopa, parkinsonism, and recent memory. *Journal of Nervous and Mental Disease, 164*, 268-272.

Harrison, M.J.G., and Marsden, C.D. (1977). Progressive intellectual deterioration. *Archives of Neurology, 34*, 199.

Hayden, M.R., MacGregor, J.M., Saffer, D.S., and Beighton, P.H. (1982). The high frequency of juvenile Huntington's chorea in South Africa. *Journal of Medical Genetics, 19*, 94-97.

Heilman, K.M., Scholes, R., and Watson, R.T. (1975). Auditory affective agnosia: Disturbed comprehension of affective speech. *Journal of Neurology, Neurosurgery and Psychiatry, 38*, 69-72.

Helgason, L. (1977). Psychiatric services and mental illness in Iceland. Incidence study (1966-1967) with 6-7 year follow-up. *Acta Psychiatrica Scandinavica Supplementum, 268*, 1-140.

Heston, L.L., Lowther, D.L.W., and Leventhal, C.M. (1966). Alzheimer's disease: A family study. *Archives of Neurology, 15*, 225-233.

Heston, L.L., and Mastri, A.R. (1977). The genetics of Alzheimer's disease: Association with hematologic malignancy and Down's syndrome. *Archives of General Psychiatry, 34*, 976-981.

Heston, L.L., Mastri, A.R., Anderson, E., and White, J. (1981). Dementia of the Alzheimer type: Clinical genetics, natural history, and associated conditions. *Archives of General Psychiatry, 38*, 1085-1090.

Heyman, A., Wilkinson, W.E., Hurwitz, B.J., Schmechel, D., Sigmon, A.H., Weinberg, T., Helms, M.J., and Swift, M. (1983). Alzheimer's disease: Genetic aspects and associated clinical disorders. *Annals of Neurology, 14*, 507-515.

Heyman, A., Wilkinson, W.E., Stafford, J.A., Helms, M.J., Sigmon, A.H., Weinberg, T. (1984). Alzheimer's disease: A study of epidemiologic aspects. *Annals of Neurology, 15*, 335-341.

Hirano, A., and Zimmerman, H.M. (1962). Alzheimer's neurofibrillary changes. *Archives of Neurology, 7*, 227-242.

Hoehn, M., and Yahr, M.D. (1967). Parkinsonism: Onset, progression and mortality. *Neurology, 17*, 427-442.

Hook, E.B., and Lindsjo, A. (1978). Down's syndrome in live births by single year maternal age in a Swedish study: Comparison with results from a New York State study. *American Journal of Human Genetics, 30*, 19-27.

Iqbal, K., Wisniewski, H.M., Grundke-Iqbal, I., Korthals, J.K., and Terry, R.D. (1975). Chemical pathology of neurofibrils: Neurofibrillary tangles of Alzheimer's presenile-senile dementia. *Journal of Histochemistry and Cytochemistry, 23*, 563-569.

Ishii, T. (1969). Enzyme histochemical studies of senile plaques and the plaque-like degeneration of arteries and capillaries. *Acta Neuropathologica, 14*, 250-260.

Jacoby, R.J., and Levy, R. (1980). Computed tomography in the elderly. 2. Senile dementia: Diagnosis and functional impairment. *British Journal of Psychiatry, 136*, 256-269.

Jankovic, J., and Fahn, S. (1980). Physiologic and pathologic tremors. *Annals of Internal Medicine, 93*, 460-465.

Jarvik, L.F., Altshuler, K.Z., Kato, T., and Blummer, B. (1971). Organic brain syndrome and chromosome loss in aged twins. *Diseases of the Nervous System, 32*, 159-169.

Jarvik, L.F., Ruth, V., and Matsuyama, S.S. (1980). Organic brain syndrome and aging: A six-year follow-up of surviving twins. *Archives of General Psychiatry, 37*, 280-286.

Jellinger, K. (1976). Neuropathological aspects of dementias resulting from abnormal blood and cerebrospinal fluid dynamics. *Acta Neurologica Belgica, 76*, 83-102.

Jervis, G.A. (1970). Premature senility in Down's syndrome. *Annals of the New York Academy of Sciences, 171*, 559-561.

Johannesson, G., Hagberg, B., Gustafson, L., and Ingvar, D.H. (1979). EEG and cognitive impairment in presenile dementia. *Acta Neurologica Scandinavica, 59*, 225-240.

Johansson, B., and Roos, B. (1967). 5-Hydroxyindolacetic and homovanillic acid levels in the cerebrospinal fluid of healthy volunteers and patients with Parkinson's syndrome. *Life Sciences, 6*, 1149-1154.

Kallmann, F.J. (1950). The genetics of psychoses: An analysis of 1232 twin index families. *Congres Internationale de Psychiatrie Rapports: Vol. 6* (pp. 1-27). Paris: Herman.

Kallmann, F.J. (1955). Genetic aspects of mental disorders in later life. In O.J. Kaplan (Ed.), *Mental disorders in later life* (2nd ed.) (pp. 26-46). Stanford, CA: Stanford University Press.

Kannel, W.B. (1971). Current status of the epidemiology of brain infarction associated with occlusive arterial disease. *Stroke, 2*, 295-318.

Kannel, W.B., Gordon, T., Wolf, P.A., and McNamara, P. (1972). Hemoglobin and the risk of cerebral infarction: The Framingham study. *Stroke, 3*, 409-420.

Kaszniak, A.W., Fox, J., Gandell, D.L., Garron, D.C., Huckman, M.S., and Ramsey, R.G. (1978). Predictors of mortality in presenile and senile dementia. *Annals of Neurology, 3*, 246-252.

Kaszniak, A.W., Garron, D.C., Fox, J.H., Bergen, D., and Huckman, M. (1979). Cerebral atrophy: EEG slowing, age, education, and cognitive functioning in suspected dementia. *Neurology, 29*, 1273-1279.

Katzman, R. (1978). Normal pressure hydrocephalus. In R. Katzman, R.D. Terry, and K.L. Bick (Eds.), *Aging: Vol. 7. Alzheimer's disease: Senile dementia and related disorders* (pp. 115-124). New York: Raven.

Kay, D.W.K., Beamish, P., and Roth, M. (1964). Old age mental disorders in Newcastle-upon-Tyne. Part I. A study of prevalence. *British Journal of Psychiatry, 110*, 146-158.

Kay, D.W.K., Bergmann, K., Foster, E.M., McKechnie, A.A., and Roth, M. (1970). Mental illness and hospital usage in the elderly: A random sample followed up. *Comprehensive Psychiatry, 11*, 26-35.

Kemper, T. (1984). Neuroanatomical and neuropathological changes in normal aging and in dementia. In M.L. Albert (Ed.), *Clinical neurology of aging* (pp. 9-52). New York: Oxford University Press.

Kidd, M. (1963). Paired helical filaments in electron microscopy of Alzheimer's disease. *Nature, 197*, 192-193.

Kievit, J., and Kuypers, H.G. (1975). Basal forebrain and hypothalamic connections to frontal and parietal cortex in the rhesus monkey. *Science, 187*, 660-662.

Klatzo, I., Wisniewski, H., and Streicher, E. (1965). Experimental production of neurofibrillary degeneration. I. Light microscopic observations. *Journal of Neuropathology and Experimental Neurology, 24*, 187-199.

Klawans, H.L. (1982). Behavioral alterations and the therapy of parkinsonism. *Clinical Neuropharmacology, 5*, 29-38.

Koller, W.C. (1984). Disturbance of recent memory in parkinsonian patients on anticholinergic therapy. *Cortex, 20*, 307-311.

Korczyn, A.D., and Goldberg, G.J. (1976). Extrapyramidal effects of neuroleptics. *Journal of Neurology, Neurosurgery, and Psychiatry, 39*, 866-869.

Koss, E., Friedland, R.P., Ober, B.A., and Jagust, W.J. (1985). Differences in lateral hemispheric asymmetries of glucose utilization between early- and late-onset Alzheimer's-type dementia. *American Journal of Psychiatry, 142*, 638-640.

Kuhar, M.H. (1976). The anatomy of cholinergic neurons. In A.M. Goldberg and I. Hanin (Eds.), *Biology of cholinergic function* (pp. 3-27). New York: Raven.

Kuhl, D.E., and Edwards, R.Q. (1963). Image separation radioisotope scanning. *Radiology, 80*, 653-662.

Kuhl, D.E., Edwards, R.Q., Ricci, A.R., and Reivich, M. (1973). Quantitative section scanning using orthogonal tangent correction. *Journal of Nuclear Medicine, 14*, 196-200.

Kuhl, D.E., Metter, E.J., and Riege, W.H. (1984). Patterns of local cerebral glucose utilization determined in Parkinson's disease by the [18F] fluorodeoxyglucose method. *Annals of Neurology, 15*, 419-424.

Kuhl, D.E., Phelps, M.E., Markham, C.H., Mettler, E.J., Riege, W.H., and Winter, J. (1982). Cerebral metabolism and atrophy in Huntington's disease determined by 18FDG and computed tomographic scan. *Annals of Neurology, 12,* 425-434.

Kurland, L.T. (1958). Epidemiology: Incidence, geographic distribution, and genetic considerations. In W. Field (Ed.), *Pathogenesis and treatment of parkinsonism* (pp. 5-43). Springfield, IL: Charles C Thomas.

Lange, H.W. (1981). Quantitative changes of telencephalon, diencephalon, and mesencephalon in Huntington's chorea, post-encephalitic, and idiopathic parkinsonism. *Verhandlungen Der Anatomischen Gesellschaft, 75*, 923-925.

Lange, H., Thorner, G., Hopf, A., and Schroder, K.F. (1976). Morphometric studies of the neuropathological changes in choreatic disease. *Journal of Neurological Sciences, 28*, 401-425.

Larsson, T., Sjögren, T., and Jacobson, G. (1963). Senile dementia: A clinical sociomedical and genetic study. *Acta Psychiatrica Scandinavica, 39*(Suppl. 167), 1-259.

Lassen, N.A., Munck, O., and Tottey, E.R. (1957). Mental function and cerebral oxygen consumption in organic dementia. *Archives of Neurology and Psychiatry, 6*, 245-256.

Lauter, H. (1985). What do we know about Alzheimer's disease today? *Danish Medical Bulletin, 31*(Suppl. 1), 1-21.

Lauter, H., and Meyer, J.E. (1968). Clinical and nosological concepts of senile dementia. In C. Muller and L. Ciompi (Eds.), *Senile dementia: Clinical and therapeutic aspects* (pp. 13-26). Bern, Switzerland: Hans Huber.

Leverenz, J., and Sumi, S.M. (1984). Prevalence of Parkinson's disease in patients with Alzheimer's disease. *Neurology, 34*(Suppl. 1), 101.

Libow, L.S. (1973). Pseudo-senility: Acute and reversible organic brain syndromes. *Journal of the American Geriatric Society, 21*, 112-120.

Librach, G., Schadel, M., Seltzer, M., Hert, A., and Yellin, N. (1977). Stroke: Incidence and risk factors. *Geriatrics, 32*, 85-91, 94-96.

Lieberman, A.N. (1974). Parkinson's disease: A clinical review. *American Journal of Medical Science, 267*, 66-80.

Lieberman, A., Dziatolowski, M., Kupersmith, M., Serby, M., Goodgold, A., Korein, J., and Goldstein, M. (1979). Dementia in Parkinson disease. *Annals of Neurology, 6*, 355-359.

Lipowski, Z.J. (1980). *Delirium. Acute brain failure in man*. Springfield, IL: Charles C. Thomas.

Lishman, W.A. (1978). *Organic psychiatry*. London: Blackwell Scientific Publications.

Loranger, A.W., Goodell, H., and McDowell, F.H., (1973). Parkinsonism, L-dopa, and intelligence. *American Journal of Psychiatry, 130*, 1386-1389.

Loranger, A.W., Goodell, H., McDowell, F.H., Lee, J.E., and Sweet, R.D. (1972). Intellectual impairment in Parkinson's syndrome. *Brain, 95*, 405-412.

Lott, I.T. (1982). Down's syndrome, ageing and Alzheimer's disease: A clinical review. *Annals of the New York Academy of Sciences, 396*, 15-27.

Lowenberg, K., and Waggoner, R.W. (1934). Familial organic psychosis (Alzheimer's type). *Archives of Neurology and Psychiatry, 31*, 737-767.

Malamud, N. (1972). Neuropathology of organic brain syndromes associated with ageing. In C.M. Gaitz (Ed.), *Ageing and the brain* (pp. 63-67). New York: Plenum.

Markesbery, W.R., Ehmann, W.D., Hossain, T.I.M., Alauddin, M., and Goodin, D.T. (1981). Instrumental neutron activation analysis of brain aluminum in Alzheimer's disease and aging. *Annals of Neurology, 10*, 511-516.

Marsden, C.D., and Harrison, M.J.G. (1972). Outcome of investigation of patients with presenile dementia. *British Medical Journal, 2*, 249-252.

Martilla, R.J., and Rinne, U.K. (1976). Dementia in Parkinson's disease. *Acta Neurologica Scandinavica, 54*, 431-441.

Martin, J.B. (1984). Huntington's disease: New approaches to an old problem. The Robert Wartenberg Lecture presented to the American Academy of Neurology. *Neurology, 34*, 1059-1072.

Masters, C.L., Gajdusek, D.C., and Gibbs, C.J., Jr. (1981). Creutzfeldt-Jakob disease virus isolations from the Gerstmann-Straussler syndrome with an analysis of the various forms of amyloid plaque deposition in the virus induced spongiform encephalopathies. *Brain, 104*, 559-587.

Mayeux, R., and Stern, Y. (1983). Intellectual dysfunction and dementia in Parkinson's disease. In R. Mayeux and W.G. Rosen (Eds.), *The dementias* (pp. 211-228). New York: Raven.

Mayeux, R., Stern, Y., and Spanton, S. (1985). Heterogeneity in dementia of the Alzheimer type: Evidence of subgroups. *Neurology, 35*, 453-461.

McDermott, J.R., Smith, A.I., Iqbal, K., and Wisniewski, H.M. (1977). Aluminum and Alzheimer's disease. *Lancet, 2*, 710-711.

McDermott, J.R., Smith, A.I., Iqbal, K., and Wisniewski, H.M. (1979). Brain aluminum in aging and Alzheimer disease. *Neurology, 29*, 809-814.

McDowell, F.H., Lee, J.E., and Sweet, R.D. (1978). Extrapyramidal disease. In A.B. Baker and L.H. Baker (Eds.), *Clinical neurology* (pp. 1-67). New York: Harper and Row.

McDowell, F.H., and Sweet, R.D. (1976). The ON-OFF phenomenon. In W. Birkmayer and O. Hornykiewicz (Eds.), *Advances in parkinsonism* (pp. 603-612). Basel: Editiones Roche.

McGeer, P.L. (1984). Aging, Alzheimer's disease, and the cholinergic system. *Canadian Journal of Physiology and Pharmacology, 62*, 741-754.

McGeer, P., and McGeer, E. (1975). Neurotransmitter synthetic enzymes. *Progress in Neurobiology, 2*, 69-117.

McKhann, G., Drachman, D., Folstein, M., Katzman, R., Price, D., and Stadlan, E.M. (1984). Clinical diagnosis of Alzheimer's disease: Report of the NINCDS-ADRDA work group under the auspices of the Department of Health and Human Services task force on Alzheimer's disease. *Neurology, 34*, 939-944.

Mesulam, M.M., and van Hoesen, G.W. (1976). Acetylcholinesterase-rich projections from the basal forebrain of the rhesus monkey to neocortex. *Brain Research, 109*, 152-157.

Mohr, J.P. (1982). Lacunes. *Stroke, 13*, 3-10.

Morimatsu, M, Hirai, S., Muramatsu, A., and Yoshikawa, M. (1975). Senile degenerative brain lesions and dementia. *Journal of the American Geriatric Society, 23*, 390-406.

Mortimer, J.A. (1983). Alzheimer's disease and senile dementia: Prevalence and incidence. In B. Reisberg (Ed.), *Alzheimer's disease* (pp. 141-148). New York: Free Press.

Mortimer, J.A., French, L.R., Hutton, J.T., and Schuman, L.M. (1985). Head injury as a risk factor for Alzheimer's disease. *Neurology, 35*, 264-267.

Mortimer, J.A., Pirozzolo, F.J., Hansch, E.C., and Webster, D.D. (1982). Relationship of motor symptoms to intellectual deficits in Parkinson's disease. *Neurology, 32*, 133-137.

Mortimer, J.A., Schuman, L.M., and French, L.R. (1981). The epidemiology of dementing illness. In J.A. Mortimer and L.M. Shuman (Eds.), *The epidemi-*

ology of dementia (pp. 3-23). New York: Oxford University Press.

Müller, H., and Schwartz, G. (1978). Electroencephalograms and autopsy findings in geropsychiatry. *Journal of Gerontology, 33*, 504-513.

Myers, G.C. (1982). The aging of populations. In R.H. Binstock, W.S. Chow, and J.H. Schulz (Eds.), *International perspectives on aging: Population and policy challenges*. New York: United Nations Fund for Population Activities.

Myers, R.H., Madden, J.J., Teague, J.L, and Falek, A. (1982). Factors related to onset age of Huntington's disease. *American Journal of Human Genetics, 34*, 481-488.

Myers, R.H., and Martin, J.B. (1982). Huntington's disease. *Seminars in Neurology, 2*, 65-72.

Naeser, M.A., Albert, M.S., and Kleefield, J. (1982). New methods in the CT scan diagnosis of Alzheimer's disease: Examination of white and gray matter mean CT density numbers. In S. Corkin, K.L. Davis, J.H. Growdon, E. Usdin, and R.J. Wurtman (Eds.), *Alzheimer's disease: A report of progress in research* (pp. 63-78). New York: Raven.

Nagai, T., McGeer, P.L., Peng, J.H., McGeer, E.G., and Dolman, C.E. (1983). Choline acetyltransferase immunohistochemistry in brains of Alzheimer's disease patients and controls. *Neuroscience Letters, 36*, 195-199.

Nagai, T., Pearson, T., Peng, J.H., McGeer, E.G., and McGeer, P.L. (1983). Immunohistochemical staining of the human forebrain with monoclonal antibody to human choline acetyltransferase. *Brain Research, 265*, 300-306.

Nakano, I., and Hirano, A. (1984). Parkinson's disease: Neuron loss in the nucleus basalis without concomitant Alzheimer's disease. *Annals of Neurology, 15*, 415-418.

Nee, L., Polinsky, R., Eldridge, R., Weingartner, H., Smallberg, S., and Ebert, M. (1983). A family with histopathologically confirmed Alzheimer's disease. *Archives of Neurology, 40*, 203-208.

Negrette, A. (1958). *Corea de Huntington*. Maracaibo, Venezuela: University of Zulia.

Newcombe, R.G., Walker, D.A., and Harper, P.S. (1981). Factors influencing age at onset and duration of survival in Huntington's chorea. *Annals of Human Genetics, 45*, 387-396.

Newman, R.P., and Calne, D.B. (1984). Diagnosis and management of Parkinson's disease. *Geriatrics, 39*, 87-96.

Nielsen, J. (1962). Geronto-psychiatric period—prevalence investigation in a geographically delimited population. *Acta Psychiatrica Scandinavica, 38*, 307.

Nobrega, F.T., Glattre, E., Kurland, L.T., and Okazaki, H. (1967). Genetics and epidemiology of Parkinson's disease. In A. Barbeau and J.R. Brunnette (Eds.), *Progress in neurogenetics* (pp. 474-485). Amsterdam: Excerpta Medica.

Obrist, W.D., Chivian, E. Cronquist, S., and Ingvar, D.H. (1970). Regional cerebral blood flow in senile and presenile dementia. *Neurology, 20*, 315-322.

Obrist, W.D., and Henry, C.E. (1958). Electroencephalograms and autopsy findings in geropsychiatry. *Journal of Gerontology, 33*, 504-513.

O'Connor, K.P., Shaw, J.C., and Ongley, C.O. (1979). The EEG and differential diagnosis in psychogeriatrics. *British Journal of Psychiatry, 135*, 156-162.

Olson, M.I., and Shaw, C.M. (1969). Presenile dementia and Alzheimer's disease in mongolism. *Brain, 92*, 147-156.

Owens, D., Dawson, J.C., and Lowsin, S. (1971). Alzheimer's disease in Down's syndrome. *American Journal of Mental Deficiency, 75*, 606-612.

Pearce, J.M.S. (1978). Aetiology and natural history of Parkinson's disease. *British Medical Journal, 2*, 1664-1666.

Penney, J.B., Young, A.B., Berent, S., Giordani, B.J., Jewett, D.M., Ehrenkaufer, R., and Hichwa, R. (1984). Positron emission tomography (PET) scanning in Huntington's disease: Studies of 18F-2-fluoro-2-deoxy-D-glucose [12FDG] uptake in 12 drug-free cases. *Society for Neuroscience Abstracts, 10*, 994.

Penrose, L.S. (1933). The relative effects of paternal and maternal age in mongolism. *Journal of Genetics, 27*, 219.

Perl, D.P., and Brody, A.R. (1980). Alzheimer's disease: X-ray spectrometric evidence of aluminum accumulation in neurofibrillary tangle-bearing neurons. *Science, 208*, 207-209.

Perry, E.K., Gibson, P.H., Blessed, G., and Tomlinson, B.E. (1977). Neurotransmitter enzyme abnormalities in senile dementia. *Journal of Neurological Sciences, 34*, 247-265.

Perry, E.K., and Perry, R.H. (1985). A review of neuropathological and neurochemical correlates of Alzheimer's disease. *Danish Medical Bulletin, 32*(Suppl. 1), 27-34.

Perry, E.K., Perry, R.H., Blessed, G., and Tomlinson, B.E. (1977). Necropsy evidence of central cholinergic deficits in senile dementia. *Lancet, 1*, 189.

Perry, E.K., Tomlinson, B.E., Blessed, G., Bergmann, K., Gibson, P.H., and Perry, R.H. (1978). Correlation of cholinergic abnormalities with senile plaques and mental test scores in senile dementia. *British Medical Journal, 2*, 1457-1459.

Perry, R.H., Candy, J.M., Perry, E.K., Irving, D., Blessed, G., Fairbairn, A.F., and Tomlinson, B.E. (1982). Extensive loss of choline acetyltransferase activity is not reflected by neuronal loss in the nucleus of Meynert in Alzheimer's disease. *Neuroscience Letters, 33*, 311-315.

Perry, T.L., Hansen, S., and Kloster, M. (1973). Huntington's chorea: Deficiency of gamma-aminobutyric acid in brain. *New England Journal of Medicine, 288*, 337-342.

Phelps, M.E. (1977). Emission computer tomography. *Seminars in Nuclear Medicine, 7*, 337-365.

Pollock, M., and Hornabrook, R.W. (1966). The prevalence, natural history and dementia of Parkinson's disease. *Brain, 89*, 429-448.

Pope, A., Hess, H.H., and Lewin, E. (1964). Microchemical pathology of the cerebral cortex in pre-senile dementia. *Transactions of the American Neurological Association, 89*, 15-16.

Portin, R., Raininko, R., and Rinne, U.K. (1984). Neuropsychological disturbances and cerebral atrophy determined by computerized tomography in parkinsonian patients with long-term levodopa treatment. In R.G. Hassler and J.F. Christ (Eds.). *Advances in neurology: Vol. 40. Parkinson-specific motor and mental disorders* (pp. 219-227). New York: Raven.

Powell, D., and Folstein, M.F. (1984). Pedigree study of familial Alzheimer's disease. *Journal of Neurogenetics, 1*, 189-197.

Pro, J.D., Smith, C.H., and Sumi, S.M. (1980). Presenile Alzheimer's disease: Amyloid plaques in the cerebellum. *Neurology, 30*, 820-825.

Price, D.L., Whitehouse, P.J., Struble, R.G., Clark, A.W., Coyle, J.T., DeLong, M.D., and Hedreen, J.C. (1982). Basal forebrain cholinergic systems in Alzheimer's disease and related dementias. *Neurosciences Communication, 1*, 84-92.

Prusiner, S.B. (1982). Novel proteinaceous infectious particles cause scrapie. *Science, 216*, 136-144.

Prusiner, S.B. (1984). Some speculations about prions, amyloid, and Alzheimer's disease. *New England Journal of Medicine, 310*, 661-663.

Rabins, P.V. (1981). The prevalence of reversible dementia in a psychiatric hospital. *Hospital and Community Psychiatry, 32*, 490-492.

Raichle, M.E., Hartman, B.K., Eichling, J.O., and Sharpe, L.G. (1975). Central noradrenergic regulation of cerebral blood flow and vascular permeability. *Proceedings of the National Academy of Sciences of the United States of America, 72*, 3726-3730.

Rajput, A.H., Offord, K.P., Beard, M., and Kurland, L.T. (1984). Epidemiology of parkinsonism: Incidence, classification and mortality. *Annals of Neurology, 16*, 278-282.

Rao, D.B., and Norris, J.R. (1972). A double-blind investigation of hydergine in the treatment of cerebrovascular insufficiency in the elderly. *Johns Hopkins Medical Journal, 130*, 317-324.

Rapoport, W.I. (1976). *Blood-brain barrier in physiology and medicine*. New York: Raven.

Reed, T., and Chandler, J. (1958). Huntington's chorea in Michigan. I. Demography and genetics. *American Journal of Human Genetics, 10*, 201-225.

Reisberg, B. (1981). *Brain failure*. New York: Free Press.

Reisine, T.D., Yamamura, H.I., Bird, E.D., Spokes, E., and Enna, S.J. (1978). Pre and postsynaptic neurochemical alterations in Alzheimer's disease. *Brain Research, 159*, 477-481.

Rinne, U.K. (1983). Problems associated with long-term levodopa treatment of Parkinson's disease. *Acta Neurologica Scandinavica Supplementum, 95*, 19-26.

Rinne, U.K., Sonninen, V., Siirtola, T., and Martilla, R. (1980). Long term responses of Parkinson's disease to levodopa therapy. *Journal of Neural Transmission, 16*, 149-156.

Risberg, J. (1985). Cerebral blood flow in dementias. *Danish Medical Bulletin, 1*(Suppl. 1), 48-50.

Risberg, J., and Gustafson, L. (1983). 133-Xe cerebral blood flow in dementia and neuropsychiatry research. In P.L. Magstrette (Ed.), *Functional radionuclide imaging of the brain*. New York: Raven.

Roberts, M.A., McGeorge, A.P., and Caird, F.I. (1978). Electroencephalography and computerized tomography in vascular and nonvascular dementia in old age. *Journal of Neurology, Neurosurgery, and Psychiatry, 41*, 903-906.

Rogers, J.D., Brogan, D., and Mirra, S. (1985). The nucleus basalis of Meynert in neurological disease: A quantitative morphological study. *Annals of Neurology, 17*, 163-170.

Rogers, R.L., Meyer, J.S., Mortel, K.F., Mahurin, R.K., and Judd, B.W. (1986). Decreased cerebral blood flow precedes multi-infarct dementia, but follows senile dementia of Alzheimer type. *Neurology, 36*, 1-6.

Ropper, A.H., and Williams, R.S. (1980). Relationship between plaques, tangles and dementia in Down syndrome. *Neurology, 30*, 639-644.

Rossor, M.N., Emson, P.C., Mountjoy, C.Q., Roth, M., and Iverson, L.L. (1980). Reduced amounts of immunoreactive somatostatin in the temporal cortex in senile dementia of Alzheimer's type. *Neuroscience Letters, 20*, 373-377.

Rossor, M.N., Iversen, L.L., Reynolds, G.P., Mountjoy, C.Q., and Roth, M. (1984). Neurochemical characteristics of early and late onset types of Alzheimer's disease. *British Medical Journal, 288*, 961-964.

Rossor, M.N., Svendsen, C., Hunt, S.P., Mountjoy, C.Q., Roth, M., and Iversen, L.L. (1982). The substantia innominata in Alzheimer's disease: A histochemical and biochemical study of cholinergic marker enzymes. *Neuroscience Letters, 28*, 217-222.

Roth, M. (1971). Classification and aetiology in mental disorders of "old age." Some recent developments. In D.W.K. Kay and A. Walk (Eds.), *Recent developments in psychogeriatrics* (pp. 1-18). Headley, London: British Journal of Psychiatry Special Publications (No. 6).

Ruberg, M., Ploska, A., and Javoy-Agid, F. (1982). Musarinic binding and choline acetyltransferase activity in Parkinsonian subjects with reference to dementia. *Brain Research, 232*, 129-139.

Rudelli, R., Strom, J.O., Welch, P.T., and Ambler, M.W. (1982). Posttraumatic premature Alzheimer's disease. *Archives of Neurology, 39*, 570-575.

Schade, B. (1982). Aging and old age in developing countries. In H. Thomae, and G.L. Maddox (Eds.), *New perspectives on old age. A message to decision makers* (pp. 98-112). New York: Springer.

Scheibel, A.B. (1978). Structural aspects of the aging brain. Spine systems and the dendritic arbor. In R. Katzman, R.D. Terry, and K.L. Bick (Eds.), *Alzheimer's disease: Senile dementia and related disorders* (pp. 353-373). New York: Raven.

Schoenberg, B.S., Anderson, D.W., and Haerer, A.F. (1985). Severe dementia: Prevalence and clinical features in a biracial U.S. population. *Archives of Neurology, 42*, 740-743.

Seltzer, B., and Sherwin, I. (1978). "Organic bain syndromes." An empirical study and critical review. *American Journal of Psychiatry, 135*, 13-21.

Seltzer, B., and Sherwin, I. (1983). A comparison of clinical features in early- and late-onset primary degenerative dementia. *Archives of Neurology, 40*, 143-146.

Shefer, V.F. (1972). Absolute number of neurons and thickness of the cerebral cortex during aging, senile and vascular dementia and Pick's and Alzheimer's disease. *Zhurnal Nevropatologii I Psikhiatrii Imeni S. Korsakova (Moskva), 72*, 1024-1029.

Sholl, D.A. (1956). *The organization of the cerebral cortex*. London: Methuen.

Shoulson, I. (1984). Huntington's disease: A decade of progress. *Neurologic Clinics, 2*, 515-526.

Shoulson, I., Plassche, W., and Odoroff, C. (1982). Huntington's disease: Caudate atrophy parallels functional impairment. *Neurology, 32*, A143.

Sjögren, T., Sjögren, H., and Lindgren, A.G.H. (1952). Morbus Alzheimer and Morbus Pick. A genetic, clinical and patho-anatomical study. *Acta Psychiatrica Scandinavica*, (Suppl. 82), 1-52.

Slater, E. and Cowie, V.A. (1971). *The genetics of mental disorders*. London: Oxford University Press.

Sloane, R.B. (1980). Organic brain syndrome. In J.E. Birren and R.B. Sloane (Eds.), *Handbook of mental health and aging* (pp. 554-590). Englewood Cliffs, NJ: Prentice-Hall.

Smith, C.M., Swash, M., and Hart, S. (1985). Cholinergic drugs and memory. In F.C. Rose (Ed.), *Interdisciplinary topics in gerontology: Vol. 20. Modern approaches to the dementias. Part II. Clinical and therapeutic aspects* (pp. 126-132). Basel: Karger.

Smith, G.F., and Berg, J.M. (1976). *Down's anomaly*. Edinburgh: Churchill Livingstone.

Smith, J.S., and Kiloh, L.G. (1981). The investigation of dementia: Results in 200 consecutive admissions. *Lancet, 1*, 824-827.

Solomon, P. (1961). *Sensory deprivation*. Cambridge, MA: Harvard University Press.

Sourander, P., and Sjögren, H. (1970). The concept of Alzheimer's disease and its clinical implications. In G.E.W. Wolstenholme and M. O'Connor (Eds.), *Alzheimer's disease and related conditions: A Ciba foundation symposium* (pp. 11-36). London: Churchill.

Stahl, W.L., and Swanson, P.D. (1974). Biochemical abnormalities in Huntington's chorea brains. *Neurology, 24*, 813-819.

Stefoski, D., Bergen, D., Fox, J., Morrell, F., Huckman, M., and Ramsey, R. (1976). Correlation between diffuse EEG abnormalities and cerebral atrophy in senile dementia. *Journal of Neurology, Neurosurgery, and Psychiatry, 39*, 751-755.

Stipe, J., White, D., and Van Arsdale, E. (1979). Huntington's disease. *American Journal of Nursing, 79*, 1428-1433.

Stober, T., Mussow, W., and Schimrigk, K. (1984). Bicaudate diameter: The most specific and simple CT parameter in the diagnosis of Huntington's disease. *Neuroradiology, 26*, 25-8.

Sulkava, R., and Amberla, K. (1982). Alzheimer's disease and senile dementia of Alzheimer type. *Acta Neurologica Scandinavica, 65*, 651-660.

Swanson, L.W., Connelly, M.A., and Hartman, B.K. (1976). Ultrastructural evidence for central monoaminergic innervation in paraventricular nucleus of hypothalamus. *Brain Research, 136*, 166-173.

Tagliavini, F., Pilleri, G., Bouras, C., and Constantinidis, J. (1984). The basal nucleus of Meynert in idiopathic Parkinson's disease. *Acta Neurologica Scandinavica, 69*, 20-28.

Terry, R. (1981). Clues to the cause of senile dementia. *Science, 211*, 1032.

Terry, R.D., and Davies, P. (1983). Some morphological and biochemical aspects of Alzheimer's disease. In D. Samuel, S. Algeri, S. Gershon, V.E. Grimm, and G. Toffano (Eds.), *Aging of the brain* (pp. 47-59). New York: Raven.

Terry, R.D., and Katzman, R. (1983). Senile dementia of the Alzheimer type. *Annals of Neurology, 14*, 497-506.

Terry, R.D., and Wisniewski, H.M. (1972). Ultrastructure of senile dementia and of experimental analogs. In C.M. Gaitz (Ed.), *Advances in behavioral biology: Vol. 3. Aging and the brain* (pp. 89-116). New York: Plenum Press.

Thase, M.E., Liss, L., Smeltzer, D., and Maloon, J. (1982). Clinical evaluation of dementia in Down's syndrome: A preliminary report. *Journal of Mental Deficiency Research, 26*, 239-244.

Tomlinson, B.E., Blessed, G., and Roth, M. (1968). Observations on the brains of non-demented old people. *Journal of Neurological Sciences, 7*, 331-356.

Tomlinson, B.E., Blessed, G., and Roth, M. (1970). Observations on the brains of demented old people. *Journal of Neurological Sciences, 11*, 205-242.

Tomlinson, B.E., and Henderson, G. (1976). Some quantitative cerebral findings in normal and demented old people. In R.D. Terry and S. Gershon (Eds.), *Neurobiology of aging*, (pp. 183-204). New York: Raven.

Tucker, D.M., Watson, R.T., and Heilman, K.M. (1977). Affective discrimination and evocation in patients with right parietal disease. *Neurology, 17*, 947-950.

Turnbull, C.J., and Aitken, J.A. (1983). Diagnosis and management of Parkinsonism in the elderly. *Age and Aging, 12*, 309-312.

Tyler, K.L., and Tyler, H.R. (1984). Differentiating organic dementia. *Geriatrics, 39*, 38-52.

United Nations. (1982). *Introductory document: Demographic considerations* (A/conf. 113/4). Prepared for the United Nations World Assembly on Aging, Vienna: Author.

United Nations Centre for Social Development and Humanitarian Affairs (1981). *Demographic aspects of the aging population in the Asian and Pacific region.* Hamburg: author.

U.S. Department of Health and Human Services Task Force on Alzheimer's Disease (1984). *Alzheimer's disease: A scientific guide for health professionals.* (NIH Publication No. 84-2251). Bethesda, MD: National Institute of Neurological and Communicative Disorders and Stroke.

U.S. Office of Technology Assessment (1985). *Technology and aging in America* OTA-BA-264. Washington, DC: U.S. Government Printing Office.

Van Buren, J.M., and Borke, R.C. (1972). The mesial temporal substratum of memory—anatomical studies in three individuals. *Brain, 95*, 599-632.

Wang, H.S., and Busse, E.W. (1969). EEG of healthy old persons: A longitudinal study: I. Dominant background activity and occipital rhythm. *Journal of Gerontology, 23*, 419-426.

Watson, C.P. (1979). Clinical similarity of Alzheimer and Creutzfeldt-Jakob disease. *Annals of Neurology, 6*, 368-369.

Weiner, W.J., Koller, W.C., Perlik, S., Nausieda, P.A., and Klawans H. (1980). Drug holiday and management of Parkinson's disease. *Neurology, 30*, 1257-1261.

Wheelan, L. (1959). Familial Alzheimer's disease. *Annals of Human Genetics, 23*, 300-310.

White, P., Goodhardt, M.J., Keet, J.P., Hiley, C.R., Caraso, L.H., Williams, I.E.I., and Bowen, D.M. (1977). Neocortical cholinergic neurons in elderly people. *Lancet, 1*, 668-671.

Whitehouse, P.J., Price, D.L., Clark, A.W., Coyle, J.T., and DeLong, M.R. (1981). Alzheimer disease: Evidence for selective loss of cholinergic neurons in the nucleus basalis. *Annals of Neurology, 10*, 122-126.

Wilcock, G.K., Esiri, M.M., Bowen, D.M., and Smith, C.C.T. (1983). The nucleus basalis in Alzheimer's disease: Cell counts and cortical biochemistry. *Neuropathology and Applied Neurobiology, 9*, 175-179.

Wing, J.K., and Hailey, A.M. (1972). *Evaluating a community psychiatric service. The Camberwell register 1964-1971.* London: Oxford University Press.

Wisniewski, H.M., and Merz, G.S. (1985). Neuropathology of the aging brain and dementia of the Alzheimer's type. In C.M. Gaitz and T. Samorajski (Eds.), *Aging 2000: Our health care destiny: Vol. 1. Bio-*

medical issues (pp. 231-243). New York: Springer-Verlag.

Wisniewski, H.M., Moretz, R.C., and Lossinsky, A.S. (1981). Evidence for induction of localized amyloid deposits and neuritic plaques by an infectious agent. *Annals of Neurology, 10*, 517-522.

Wisniewski, H.M., Narang, H.K., and Terry, R.D. (1976). Neurofibrillary tangles of paired helical filaments. *Journal of Neurological Sciences, 17*, 173-181.

Wisniewski, K., Howe, J., Williams, D.G., and Wisniewski, H.M. (1978). Precocious aging and dementia in patients with Down's syndrome. *Biological Psychiatry, 13*, 619-627.

Wolf, P.A., Kannel, W.B., and Dawber, T.R. (1978). Prospective investigations: The Framingham study and the epidemiology of stroke. In B.S. Schoenberg (Ed.), *Advances in neurology: Vol. 19. Neurological epidemiology: Principles and clinical applications* (pp. 107-120). New York: Raven.

Wolff, H.G., and Curran, D. (1935). Nature of delirium and allied states. *Archives of Neurological Psychiatry, 33*, 722-723.

Wright, A.F., and Whalley, L.J. (1984). Genetics, ageing, and dementia. *British Journal of Psychiatry, 145*, 20-38.

Yamaguchi, F., Meyer, J.S., Yamamoto, M, Sakai, S., and Shaw, T. (1980). Noninvasive regional cerebral blood flow measurements in dementia. *Archives of Neurology, 37*, 410-418.

Yates, C.M., Simpson, J., Maloney, A.F.J., Gordon, A., and Reid, A.H. (1980). Alzheimer-like cholinergic deficiency in Down's syndrome. *Lancet, 2*, 979.

Yerby, M.S., Sundsten, J.W., Larson, E.B., Wu, S.A., and Sumi, S.M. (1985). A new method of measuring brain atrophy: The effect of aging in its application for diagnosing dementia. *Neurology, 35*, 1316-1320.

Young, A.B., Shoulson, I., Penney, J.B., Starosta-Rubinstein, S., Gomez, F., Travers, H., Ramos-Arroyo, M.A., Snodgrass, S.R., Bonilla, E., Moreno, H., and Wexler, N.S. (1986). Huntington's disease in Venezuela: Neurologic features and functional decline. *Neurology, 36*, 244-249.

Zetusky, W.J., Jankovic, J., and Pirozzolo, F.J. (1985). The heterogeneity of Parkinson's disease: Clinical and prognostic implications. *Neurology, 35*, 522-526.

Chapter 2

Linguistic Communication, Cognition, and the Conceptual System

"Without concepts, mental life would be chaotic."
—(Smith and Medin, 1981)

Among the most fascinating of questions are how humans communicate, how the brain functions in linguistic communication, and the relationship of language and thought. These questions have been of historic interest to scientists and lay persons alike, because communicating is among the most complex of human behaviors and probably the most important.

As children, humans are intrigued with language and spend hours reciting riddles, rhyming words, and creating make-believe dialogues. As parents, they delight in their children's first words and youthful utterances, for it is through them that they glimpse the developing mind. For people of all ages, reading is a favorite pastime; they relish the experience of being carried by words to other worlds. As a society, Americans are captivated by the talk show and eagerly attend to what celebrities have to say, building an image of them from their words.

Most of us take for granted our ability to express our ideas linguistically until we are exposed to the tragedy of language loss. It is when someone we know has a stroke or a laryngectomy that we are awed by the importance of being able to communicate.

Persons with dementia gradually lose the ability to meaningfully communicate. To many clinicians these individuals are an unfamiliar clinical group, because it has been only recently that communicative impairment in dementia has been recognized. In fact, only in the last few years has there been widespread recognition of communicative disorder in dementia patients (de Ajuriaguerra and Tissot, 1975; Appell, Kertesz, and Fisman, 1982; Bayles, 1982, 1984, 1985; Bayles and Tomoeda, 1983; Cummings, Benson, Hill, and Read, 1985; Ferm, 1974; Irigaray, 1973; Obler, 1983; Obler and Albert, 1981; Wechsler, 1977), and the idea is still gaining acceptance. As yet, the feature of communicative impairment remains unspecified in the American Psychiatric Association Diagnostic and Statistical Manual (1980) as an always-present symptom of the dementia syndrome. Before explaining why persons with dementia always suffer communicative impairment, it is appropriate to define communication.

COMMUNICATION DEFINED

The first clarification that needs to be made is that when the term "communication" is used, the authors mean "intentional" communication. Persons with dementia, like other people, can unintentionally communicate by many means: their posture, facial expressions, and eye contact. It is intentional communication that is disordered, but to continue to use the term "intentional" would be burdensome; therefore, it will henceforth be assumed that the reader understands that it is implied.

Communication is the sharing of information by means of a symbol system; it is linguistic when words are used and nonlinguistic when other symbol systems, such as mathematical notation, are used. To communicate either linguistically or nonlinguistically, an individual must have an idea to share and a symbol system through which to purvey the idea. For example, the symphony conductor communicates ideas about tempo, loudness, and style by waving the baton in prescribed ways understood by the orchestra. The astronomer communicates the positions of celestial bodies by mathematical notation. These are examples of nonlinguistic forms of communication, and although nonlinguistic communication can be impaired as a consequence of dementing illness, the topic of this book is the nature of linguistic impairment and its relation to cognition. Nevertheless, an important point needing emphasis is that *the ability to (intentionally) communicate is impaired in dementing illness, be it linguistic or nonlinguistic.*

Meaningful communication requires the production and comprehension of ideas. The act of speaking, in and of itself, does not constitute communication, because that which is spoken may be structurally and semantically meaningless. Nor does knowing the grammar of a language insure the ability to communicate. One can know the rules for combining sounds into words, and words with each other, without being able to intentionally communicate. It is only when sounds and words have been structured in such a way that the idea of the speaker is derivable by the listener that communication occurs.

WHY IS COMMUNICATION IMPAIRED IN DEMENTIA?

In dementia, the capacity to form ideas deteriorates early, thereby affecting the ability to communicate. Simply stated, communication is impaired in persons with dementia because ideation is impaired.

The distinction between the terms "communication," "speech," and "language" are critical to the proper characterization of the effects of dementing illness. For our purposes, the word "speech" is used to refer to the motor production of sounds rather than an acoustic representation of language, and language is a symbol system by which sound is paired with meaning. Linguistic communication is the cognitive process of sharing ideas through language, rather than another symbol system. In dementing illnesses, the ability to communicate is affected more than speech and language.

Having distinguished communication, speech, and language, and having emphasized that communication is what is affected early in persons with dementia, the question of interest becomes, If communication is impaired because ideation is impaired, then why is ideation impaired? The authors would answer, because of the particular impairment of semantic and episodic memory.

Particular Impairment of Semantic and Episodic Memory

As this book develops, a case will be made for the claim that dementia patients suffer particular impairment of the mnemonic, conceptual, and inferential systems of the brain, the systems where ideas are born and where events and ideas are received and stored. To state the claim another way, in the parlance of psychologists, dementia patients suffer particular impairment of semantic memory (SM) and episodic memory (EM). Thus, it is necessary to be familiar with the contents and processes of semantic and episodic memory and how they relate to other forms of mental representation.

Mental Representation or Memory

Persons unfamiliar with psychologic theory and research in human memory typically assume that the term "memory" refers only to the recall of personally experienced events. However, scientific use of the term can refer to any mental representation. Thus, an individual's knowledge of word meaning, arithmetic operations, local geography, how to tie a shoe, and his or her personal history are types of memory. All involve stored mental representation. It is obvious that memory, thus defined, is not a single entity, nor does it serve a single psychologic function. Different types of memory have different rules of operation. Further, different memory systems have distinct neurologic substrates that can be differentially impaired by cerebral disease.

Information Processing Model of Memory. Until recently, a "linear" model of information processing has dominated memory research. In this model, illustrated in Figure 2-1, information is assumed to flow from input to output through a series of sequential stages. At the earliest stage of information registration is *sensory memory*, a preattentive and highly unstable system characterized by rapid decay of information. Perceptual and attentional processes serve to transfer information out of sensory memory and into the next stage, known as primary memory. *Primary memory* is also called short-term memory and is thought of as a labile, limited-capacity store, in which information is in conscious awareness. The next stage is *secondary memory*, or long-term memory, in which are stored an individual's enduring memories. The transfer of information from primary to secondary memory is hypothesized to occur if the information in primary memory is rehearsed (Murdock, 1974). If the information in primary memory is not rehearsed instantly, so that it can be stored in secondary memory, it will be lost.

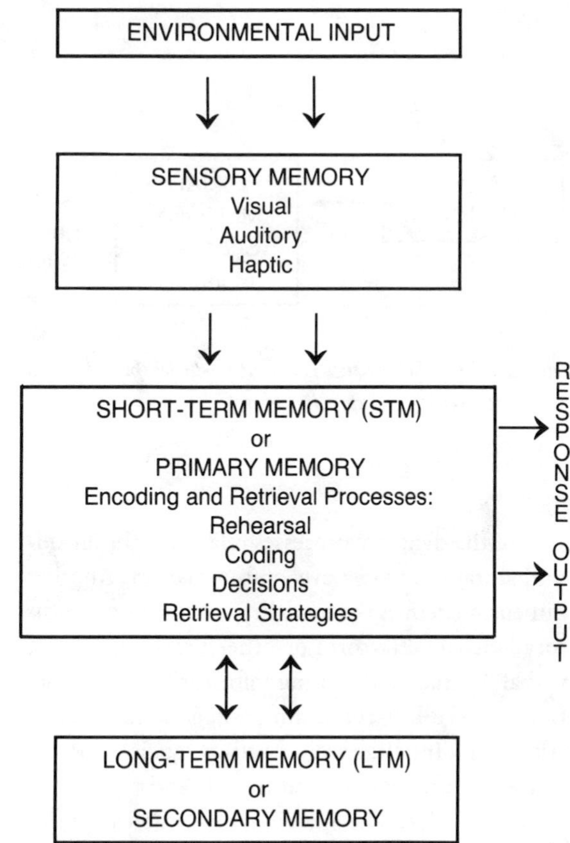

Figure 2-1. *Information processing through the memory system. (Modified from Atkinson, R.C., and Shiffrin, R.M., 1971).*

To understand the model, it may help to think of the example of looking up a telephone number. The seven digits of the number are approximately the size of the information capacity of the primary (short-term) store (Miller, 1956). If you rehearse the number, thus keeping it in consciousness, you will retain the mental representation, at least long enough to dial. With sufficient rehearsal, the number will be accessible for a longer period of time, because it will enter long-term, or secondary, memory. If rehearsal is interrupted because you are distracted, or engage in some other mental activity, the telephone number will be forgotten. Secondary, or long-term, memory is thus a repository of newly acquired and previously learned information. It is assumed to be more stable and of theoretically unlimited capacity. When information is retrieved from long-term memory, it is moved back into primary, or short-term, store, from which it can be used in some overt response (e.g., dialing the telephone).

In the linear information processing model, memory failures are attributed to factors such as reduced capacity of the hypothetical stores, particularly the short-term store, decay of information from one or more stores, a failure of the transfer processes (attention, rehearsal) by which information is moved between stores, or a combination of these factors.

In addition to the aforestated stages of memory in the information processing model, several other interacting dimensions are hypothesized. One con-

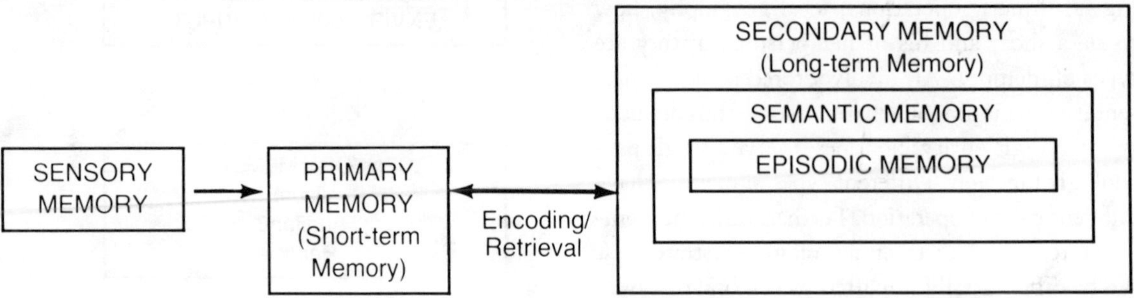

Figure 2-2. *Schematization of the relationship of the constructs of sensory memory, primary memory, secondary memory, semantic memory, and episodic memory.*

sists of the dynamic processes related to the encoding, storage, and retrieval of information. Another dimension defines the modality-specific (e.g., auditory, visual, olfactory) or other properties (e.g., verbal, spatial) of incoming information. The functioning of all of these dimensions of memory is affected by intelligence, education, socioeconomic status, and neurologic, hormonal, and physiologic states. Given the many factors that can influence memory, it is understandable that the level of functional memory is fluid and subject to both intra- and interpersonal variability.

Levels of Processing: An Alternative to the Memory Stores Model. Although the information processing model of memory has produced testable hypotheses, and investigators have been able to draw conclusions about the location of memory deficits in various types of patients, it has a basic limitation. That is, evidence has accumulated that the characteristics of the hypothesized stores vary considerably with changes in tasks, materials, and strategies, and it seems implausible that stores could vary with context. On the other hand, it is plausible that mental *processes* may vary according to changes in tasks, materials, and strategies (Craik, 1984). Consequently, the linear information processing model has been reconceptualized as a process-oriented, rather than a stores-oriented, system. What the linear information-processing model had seen as evidence of residence of information in primary memory is now seen as continued activation or "attention paid to" the information (Craik, 1984, p. 4). In this model, the distinctions between primary and secondary memory are now viewed in terms of encoding processes, retrieval processes, and their interaction. Therefore, rather than a series of discrete stages through which a mental representation is sequentially moved, memory is viewed as a continuous process.

Readers may be scratching their heads wondering how sensory, primary, and secondary memory relate to semantic and episodic. Didn't the text say that persons with dementia had particular impairment of semantic and episodic memory? A look at Figure 2-2 may clarify things. Semantic and episodic memory are terms for referring to the contents of secondary memory. The descriptor "semantic" means that the representation system is for concepts; "episodic" means that it is for personal events.

When information in primary memory is rehearsed and subsequently registered in secondary memory, it is stored with other similar memories. For example, new concepts are stored with those previously learned; a new procedure is stored with other procedures; a new word, with other words. When information in secondary memory is thought about, it is retrieved from secondary memory and brought into conscious awareness, or primary memory. The two-way arrows in the diagram signify that information is transferred, or encoded, from primary to secondary memory and retrieved from secondary memory when it is thought about. Encoding and retrieval processes involve highly similar mental operations.

Familiarity with the processes and types of memory are fundamental to understanding communication and normal aging, communication and dementia, and the relation of communicative to cognitive impairment in persons with dementia. However, because of their special significance, the terms "semantic" and "episodic" memory require further explication.

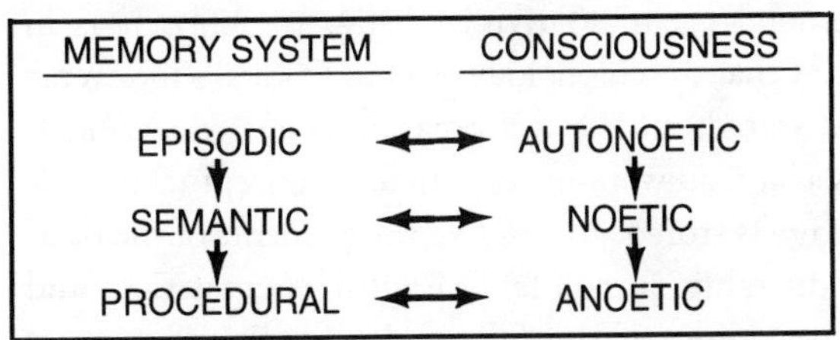

Figure 2-3. *Schematic arrangement of three memory systems and three kinds of consciousness.* Note. *An arrow means "implies." (From Tulving, E. (1985). How many memory systems are there?* American Psychologist, 40, *385–398, by permission. Copyright 1985 by the American Psychological Association, Inc.)*

Semantic Memory Further Defined

Semantic memory is that domain in the nervous system in which concepts are represented and inferential processing takes place. The term SM was introduced by Quillian (1966), who proposed a theory about human semantic processing, and was adopted by other psychologists to refer to a long-term memory store in which conceptual knowledge is represented. (Cohen, 1983; Tulving, 1972; Wickelgren, 1979). Tulving (1985) elaborated the concept of SM as being one of two parts of a tripartite memory system (Figure 2-3), in which conscious processing occurs. Tulving described SM as a subcomponent of the unconsciously operating procedural memory system.

According to Tulving (1985), procedural memory (PM) enables organisms to retain "learned connections between stimuli and responses, including those involving complex stimulus patterns and response chains" (p. 389). It is the most elemental of the memory systems and the only system capable of independent operation. Within PM is stored an individual's knowledge of how to do things, plans, and skills, whereas within SM is stored factual knowledge of the world, sometimes referred to as declarative knowledge. Anderson (1976) describes the distinction between procedural and declarative knowledge as analogous to the computer scientist's distinction between program and data. Procedural knowledge is the program; declarative, the data.

Contents are Recoded Representations of the World. The contents of SM are different from the external sensory information received from the world (Yates, 1985). Sensory information received from the world is analyzed, transduced, and coded in a form readable by SM processors. The transmission of sensory information is carried out by a central system that is separate from SM. Yates (1985) emphasized the importance of this fact when he wrote that "the central claim of cognitive psychology is that information about the world is coded in the form of mental representations that are distinct from external information and sensory information" (p. 249).

According to Wickelgren (1979), SM is the "highest-level, most abstract, cognitive modality which integrates the verbal and non-verbal strands" (p. 19). Input from the perceptual modalities is accessed, actively cross-referenced, indexed, and sorted in SM. Although its exact structure is debated by scholars, consensus exists that it is a cognitive store in which knowledge is coded in an abstract way independently of the input modality. It is the functional system in which ideation and inferential processing consciously occur. A synonym for SM is the "central system," a term introduced by Fodor (1983).

Episodic Memory Defined

Episodic memory (EM) is a "system that receives and stores information about temporally dated episodes or events, and temporal–spatial relations among them" (Tulving, 1984, p. 223). It is in EM that the chronology of an individual's life events is stored, such as information about educational, social, and work history. In SM, conceptual knowledge is stored, things like the elements of the periodic table, principles of English composition, and the causes of the fall of the Ferdinand Marcos regime. Episodic and semantic memory are highly interdependent systems, because information is transferred between them, and both types of knowledge are used in thinking. Knowing your responsibilities as best man at a wedding involves SM; remembering what you did and who you met at the wedding involves EM. As will be discussed in later chapters, dementia patients show marked impairment in EM. In part, this impairment is due to the abnormally rapid forgetting of events stored in EM, similar to that seen in amnesic patients with medial temporal lobe damage. However, much of the impairment in EM seems attributable to problems in the access to, and structure of, SM.

Is SM a Modular System?

A much discussed issue among cognitive scientists is whether SM, or the central system, is modular. It is not necessary to also inquire whether EM is a modular system, because EM is a subset of SM.

Modularity is a construct that attributes to a cognitive faculty a set of unique characteristics (Fodor, 1983), those listed in Table 2-1. Familiarity with the modularity concept is crucial to an understanding of the prominent theories about the structure of the mind, theories to which the data from dementia patients ultimately will be related (See Chapter 3). Remember, the central claim of this book is that in dementia, SM, or the central system, is particularly impaired—a claim that makes reference to the attributes of modularity.

TABLE 2-1. Definitional Criteria for Modularity

1. Domain specificity
2. Mandatory operation
3. Limited access by the central system to the mental representations that input systems compute
4. Fast processing rate
5. Informational encapsulation
6. Shallow outputs
7. Association with fixed neural architecture
8. Characteristic and specific breakdown patterns
9. Characteristic pace and sequencing of ontogeny

Adapted from Fodor (1983).

The most widely discussed theory about the modularity of mind is that of Fodor's (1983), which is of interest to us on two counts. First, it is a general theory about the structure of human cognition; second, it is a particular theory about how language is processed. Fodor's theory, very simply stated, is that humans have two types of cognitive systems: modular perceptual systems, of which there are at least six, and one nonmodular central system. In the modular perceptual input systems of hearing, sight, touch, taste, smell, and language, sensory information is encoded into mental representations understood by the central system. The function of the nonmodular central system is to "fix beliefs" and "plan intelligent action." Fodor's central system construct is roughly equivalent to the construct of SM described earlier in this chapter. The central system is an inferential faculty with access to the output of all the perceptual systems, output that is used in problem-solving and the building of beliefs. What is crucial for the reader to understand is that the data from dementia patients may demonstrate the particular impairment of the central system, or, to use the more familiar term, semantic memory. That SM undergoes particular impairment is a major theme in this book. Such an allegation contradicts Fodor's claim that the nonmodular central system lacks a characteristic and specific breakdown pattern. Indeed, if it can be shown that SM (or the central system in Fodorean theory) is particularly impaired, the view that the central system is entirely nonmodular may need modification, or the criterion that only a modular system can have a characteristic and specific breakdown pattern must be reconsidered. However, before the reader can evaluate the credibility of the claim that SM is particularly impaired in dementing diseases, it is necessary to understand the criteria that define modularity, gain a deeper appreciation of the nature of SM, and become familiar with the performance patterns of dementia patients.

Fodor's Definitional Criteria for Modularity

Domain Specificity. Domain specificity means that the system is specially designed to process a certain kind of information. In the case of hearing, the input "module" is designed to receive and process sound waves; in the case of the visual "module," information about light energy is processed. In the language "module," language is processed.

Operation is Mandatory. "Mandatory" refers to the obligatory processing by the input module of the stimuli it is uniquely prepared to receive. As Fodor (1983) says, "You can't help hearing an utterance of a sentence (in a language you know) as an utterance of a sentence, and you can't help seeing a visual array as consisting of objects distributed in three-dimensional space" (pp. 52-53).

Only Limited Access by the Central System to the Mental Representations That Input Systems Compute. As information is moved from the bottom of an input module to the top, its representation changes. The points in the module where this occurs are called "interlevels" by Fodor. He theorizes that the central system does not have conscious access to information at these interlevels. For example, during language comprehension, the central system is ignorant of the module's analysis of the acoustic features of sounds and the syntactic form of the word strings.

Input Systems are Fast. Because Fodor does not know precisely where the activities of the input system modules leave off and those of the central system begin, specification of the amount of time required by each system to perform its unique analysis has been impossible. However, input modules are described as "fast," faster than central systems because they, unlike central systems, are not concerned with belief.

Input Systems are Informationally Encapsulated. More than any other, this attribute is the essence of modularity. To be informationally encapsulated is to be limited in the kind of information available during processing. The input modules do not draw upon the full range of the organism's knowledge, beliefs, and desires to perform their function. They have access only to information from within the domain to which they are dedicated. In the case of the language input module, syntactic and phonologic information is processed, but semantic and pragmatic information are unavailable.

Input Systems Have Shallow Outputs. To have shallow output is to have output that is mandatory, fast, and relevant to the perceptual encoding of stimuli. In terms of language, shallow output is the production by the language module of only a linguistic and logical form analysis (subject-verb-object) of the linguistic stimuli it receives. For example, the language module does not recover the social function of utterances. Recovery of the social function of an utterance requires pragmatic knowledge, to which the language module is not privy.

Input Systems are Associated with Fixed Neural Architecture. Each input system is associated with a characteristic neural architecture. Hard-wired neuronal connections attend only to certain kinds of information and are limited to the further transport of that information through the module. Fodor (1983) says, "Neural architecture, I'm suggesting, is the natural concomitant of informational encapsulation" (p. 99). This is an oft-quoted phrase of Fodor's because it has special significance. Fodor is emphasizing that the way a system is built has a lot to do with the type of information it can process. Cells and systems of cells are biologically limited in the kinds of information they can process. The neural architecture of cells and systems of cells in input modules limits the information to which they have access.

Input Systems Exhibit Characteristic and Specific Breakdown Patterns. Deficits associated with brain injury or disease represent "patterned failures of functioning—i.e., they cannot be explained by mere quantitative decrements in global, horizontal capacities like memory, attention, or problem solving" (p. 99). An example is aphasia, which according to Fodor's model represents a breakdown in the language module.

Ontogeny Exhibits a Characteristic Pace and Sequencing. Though environment has some influence on the development of the processing characteristics of the input modules, by and large the developmental course of the system is biologically determined.

Modularity does not appear to be an all-or-none state, and as Marshall (1984) notes, the principle of modularity as defined by Fodor does not particularize which aspects of human cognition are likely to be modular. Whereas the authors agree with Fodor that the perceptual input systems are computationally and informationally constrained in ways that the central system, or SM, is not, they do not agree that the central system cannot be particularly, or in Fodor's terms "selectively," impaired.

The issue of modularity of mental structure is a complex provocative topic on which one could write an entire book, as Fodor (1983) did. However, for our purposes, it is necessary not to delineate the full scope of the modularity debate but rather to familiarize the reader with the criteria Fodor uses to define modularity so they can be meaningfully evaluated. What is necessary is to provide the reader with a fuller account of the nature of semantic memory and its associated processes.

MORE ABOUT THE STRUCTURE OF SEMANTIC MEMORY

Semantic memory is a hierarchically organized representational system (Figure 2-4) that can be activated by input from perceptual input systems. It is the highest faculty in the cognitive system and the point in the information processing chain where information from the perceptual systems is interrelated. Information from the verbal, spatial, and other perceptual input systems ultimately will be interrelated within semantic memory, for it is in SM that intermodality representation of knowledge occurs. Verbal and nonverbal information is synthesized, and thought occurs.

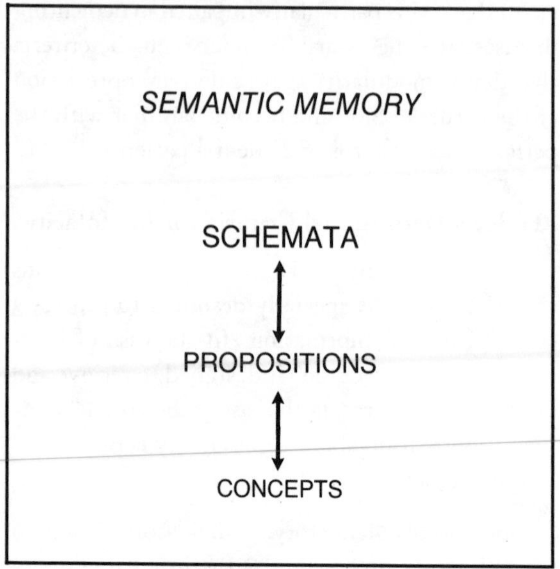

Figure 2-4. *Semantic memory: a hierarchically organized representational system.*

Concept is the Elemental Unit of SM

The word "semantic" in the phrase "semantic memory" has probably made some readers think that the contents of semantic memory are words. However, the elemental unit is not a word but a concept. A concept has been acquired, according to Schlesinger (1977), "only to the extent that one knows what belongs to it and what does not" (p. 156). "For someone to have a concept entails that all instances of the concept elicit a common response" (Schlesinger, 1977, p. 157). For example, "hammer," "axe," "saw," "screwdriver," and "pliers" all elicit the concept "tool." Halford (1982) defines concepts as representations of general classes or categories of objects and events. Concepts are constructs we form about the world. As Smith and Medin (1981) wrote in their book about categories and concepts, "Without concepts, mental life would be chaotic. If we perceived each entity as unique, we would be overwhelmed by the sheer diversity of what we experience and unable to remember more than a minute fraction of what we encounter" (p. 1).

If the suggestion is unconvincing that concepts, as opposed to words, form the elemental structural unit of SM, consider that humans can conceptualize things for which they have no words. For example, you can conceptualize the following, for which no word exists: an amorphous mass of gelatinous material about the size of a basketball seeming to have a self-contained propulsion system that enables it to continually change shape. Words help us conceptualize and indeed are so helpful that much, if not most, of our thinking is done in words. When linguistically obtained knowledge is stored, however, the words through which the knowledge was conveyed are rarely remembered; instead, we remember the concepts expressed by the words.

Other evidence that the units of semantic memory are not in a one-to-one correspondence with words is that many concepts can be referred to by a single word. Consider the word "net." "Net" is associated with the concept of a tennis court barrier, a fisherman's tool, what is left after expenses, and a material used to make prom formals, just to name a few of its associations. Conversely, one concept can be associated with many words. For example, the concept "religion" is represented by Protestantism, Catholicism, Judaism, Buddhism, and so forth.

Concepts can be activated by words, but conceptual activation can occur nonlinguistically as well. For example, a picture of a parallelogram may activate the spatial concepts of parallel lines and lines of equal length. These concepts could be recreated using language, but a drawing could also be made. Every day, individuals obtain new information by nonlinguistic means, and unless the need arises, much of this knowledge is never given linguistic representation.

Conceptual learning occurs throughout life as the individual makes inferences and forms abstractions about the world. Through concepts we can represent the ways in which objects, events, and states are alike. These representations enable us to think beyond the information given, for "once we have assigned an entity to a class on the basis of its perceptible attributes, we can infer some of its nonperceptible attributes" (Smith and Medin, 1981, p. 1). Sometimes the meaning of a concept is derived through its association with another known concept, sometimes concepts are defined for us, and sometimes their meaning is inferred from the propositions in which they occur.

Concepts are Stored in a Categorical Hierarchy. As our knowledge of concepts is elaborated, it is thought to be stored systematically in a categorical hierarchy. Miller (1971) observed that when individuals sort words into categories, hierarchical structures emerge. Tulving and Pearlstone (1966) used cueing techniques to demonstrate categorical organization of memory. Subjects learned, on a single trial, lists of words belonging to explicitly stated conceptual categories. Immediate recall of words was tested in two conditions. In the cued condition, subjects were provided with a response form on which the conceptual categories were printed in the order they were originally presented. In the noncued condition, category names were not given on the response form as retrieval cues. Recall of the list of words was significantly better in the cued recall condition.

Wickens (1970) demonstrated that less interference occurs in learning lists of words when new lists contain words from a different category. Deese (1962) reported word clustering in free-association experiments. Meyer and Schvaneveldt (1971) found that when subjects were presented with two related words, such as "rain" and "umbrella," and asked to state whether the two strings of letters were real words, their responses were faster than when the two stimulus words were unrelated in meaning. The results of such experiments demonstrate that concepts are not represented haphazardly in SM but are associated in such a way that thinking of one causes us to think of another, or makes it more likely that we will think of another. Words activate concepts, and words that are associated with related concepts come themselves to be associated. Take, for example, the words "swimming," "rowing," "diving," "sailing," and "canoeing"; all are associated with each other because they are conceptually related as water sports.

Other Units, the Proposition and Schema

Although the concept is the elemental structural unit in semantic memory, it is not the only unit. Propositions and schemata are also thought to be represented. A proposition can be defined as a relational expression that is grammatically analogous to a clause and comprises a relational term, such as a verb, and one or more nouns or noun phrases that function as subjects and objects of the relation. For example, the following are propositions:

The Titanic sank.
The arms race escalated.
Christa McAuliffe is an American hero.

These propositions have been given linguistic representation, though not all propositions are translated into words.

Evidence for the Psychologic Reality of Propositions. Considerable evidence for the psychologic reality of propositions comes from the literature on information processing. For example, regardless of the grammatical form of a sentence, it is reducible to the same constituent propositions; that is, it makes no difference whether the propositions are couched in a complex syntactic frame, a compound construction, or a simple construction (Bransford and Franks, 1971; Wang, 1977). People can recognize when two sentences or clauses are equivalent paraphrases because they perceive the relational expression, or proposition, contained in them. The following two sentences, which are equivalent paraphrases, illustrate this fact.

1. A strong desire of Barry's is to purchase an acre of land with a panoramic view of Tucson.
2. Barry really wants to buy an acre-sized lot with a valley-wide view of the "Old Pueblo."

It is the relational expression, or proposition, that is important and stored in SM, not the form (Anderson, 1974; Garrod and Trabasso, 1973). Bransford, Barclay, and Franks (1972) demonstrated the importance of meaning in an experiment in which they showed that if a previously heard sentence is changed so it no longer describes the original proposition, listeners detect the change. If, instead, the alteration does not affect the events expressed in the sentence, the same physical change will go unnoticed.

Sachs (1967) demonstrated that people remember meaning and ultimately forget the grammatical form in which it was expressed. Thus, concepts and propositions are retained, not syntax. Sachs had subjects listen to 24 taped passages of prose, after which they were asked to decide whether a particular sentence was identical to one in the passage or changed in some way. Some of the test sentences were identical, others were identical only in meaning, and others expressed altered meaning. Subjects had to make these judgments after intervals of 0, 80, and 160 syllables of connected discourse. When the test sentence followed the passage immediately, recognition of both structure and meaning was excellent. When the retention interval was increased, meaning recognition was still excellent, but recognition of syntactic changes had dropped to near-chance levels.

Anderson and Bower (1973) studied recall of sentences composed of two propositions and reported that subjects recall a proposition better when they are provided with a cue word from that same proposition than when they are provided with a cue word from the other. The findings of this study suggest that propositions are units of storage within SM. If one word from a stored proposition is provided, it stimulates recall of the rest of the concepts and words in the proposition because they are stored together.

Kintsch and Glass (1974) demonstrated that it is the number of propositions, rather than the number of words, that affects the memorability of the meaning of a sentence. Related to this finding is one by Kintsch and Keenan (1973), who demonstrated that the study time needed for learning textual meaning is dependent on the number of propositions, not words. The greater the number of propositions, the longer the time required to learn the meaning.

In summary, propositions are relational expressions that if translated into a linguistic form are like a clause. The relation expressed is what is important and remembered; the grammatical form of the relation is forgotten.

Schemata. When we attend to the different tasks that constitute our days, concepts and propositions related to the task at hand are activated. In other words, a schema is formed. A schema is an attentional set formed by the simultaneous activation of a group of related concepts (Figure 2-5).

Schemata are thought to be another structural unit of semantic memory. People have a schema for a variety of activities, for example, playing cards, being part of a wedding party, or making an appointment with the doctor. Certain concepts and propositions are associated with each of these activities and are activated when we participate in them. The process of building new schemata involves learning the associations between a particular set of concepts and propositions. For example, in bridge we learn that the rules of partnerships affect seating arrangements, that the number and distribution of cards is related to particular bids, and that certain types of food are considered appropriate for serving. Schemata activate concepts and propositions, and concepts and propositions activate schemata.

THUNDER . . . .
LIGHTNING . . . . . .
BLACK CLOUDS . STORM SCHEMA ACTIVATED
RAIN DROPS . . . .
WIND . . . .

Figure 2-5. *How a schema is activated.*

The interactivation that occurs between the elements of SM make us more efficient processors of information. We learn to expect and anticipate certain events and kinds of information in particular contexts. This is a very important point. An understanding of the process of interactivation will enable us to better understand the way in which thought occurs and the ultimate dissolution of communicative functioning in dementia.

Activation of the Structural Units of Semantic Memory

A concept helpful for understanding the ways in which concepts, propositions, and schemata can be activated is to remember that each can be excited by a source external to the organism or from within SM. The sights and sounds of the world can trigger the activation process, as can the individual's needs and desires. Consider first the activation of concepts.

Activation of Concepts and Propositions

The concepts and propositions in SM can be activated by verbal and nonverbal stimuli originating at both higher and lower levels of the nervous system. When concepts and propositions are activated from sensory stimuli processed in a perceptual system and transmitted to SM, the activation is said to have occurred from the bottom up. When propositions or schemata activate concepts, the activation is said to be from the top down. Finally, concepts can activate other concepts just as propo-

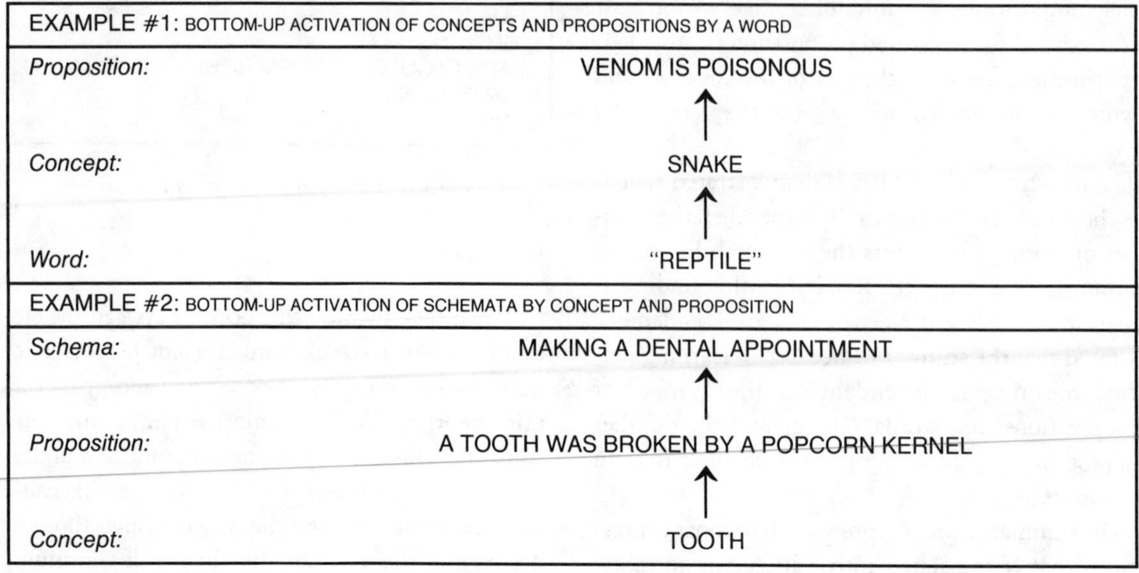

Figure 2-6. *Bottom-up activation.*

sitions and schemata can activate other propositions and schemata. This type of activation is horizontal. Examples of the different types of activation may make the process easier to remember.

Bottom-up Activation. An example of bottom-up activation (Figure 2-6) is the activation of the concept of "snake" and the proposition "venom can be poisonous" from the stimulus word "reptile."

Words are not the only stimuli that activate concepts and propositions, but they are among the most common. Things you see, feel, hear, and smell activate concepts. Seeing a brand new Ferrari sports car may activate the concept of wealth, and snow may trigger thoughts of skiing. The smell of roasting chestnuts may activate the concept of Christmas.

Often new concepts are learned by virtue of their inclusion in propositions. In childhood, many concepts are learned this way. The authors recently learned the concept "rad," a term that means desirable, good, and fun because of its inclusion in the following propositions uttered by a teenager:

1. "The ski trip was totally rad, I got a great tan and five days of powder skiing."
2. "Mr. Nelson is a rad teacher, he never gives homework."

Top-down Activation. Not only can concepts be activated from the bottom up, they are activated from the top down, by propositions and schemata (Figure 2-7). Consider that communicative acts can have a larger frame of reference, that is, a schema. For example, you might say, "How about Chinese" when discussing where to eat. The frame of reference, or schema, is choosing a place to eat, and the uttering of "How about Chinese" is one part of a larger communicative event. Linguists, psychologists, computer simulation scholars, and speech–language pathologists recognize that a framework larger than the word or proposition exists and have used various terms to describe this larger unit, such as *plan* (Abelson, 1975; deBeaugrande, 1979, 1980; Cohen, 1978; Schank and Abelson, 1977), *frame* (Charniak, 1975; Minsky, 1975; Winograd, 1975), *schema* (Adams and Collins, 1979; Bartlett, 1932; Freedle and Hale, 1979; Kintsch, 1977; Rumelhart, 1975), *script* (Minsky, 1975; Selz, 1922), and *macrostructure* (van Dijk, 1980). Regardless of the term used, theorists recognize that subcomponents of communication are affected by a larger set of associations. For our purposes, this larger set of associations will be referred to as a schema.

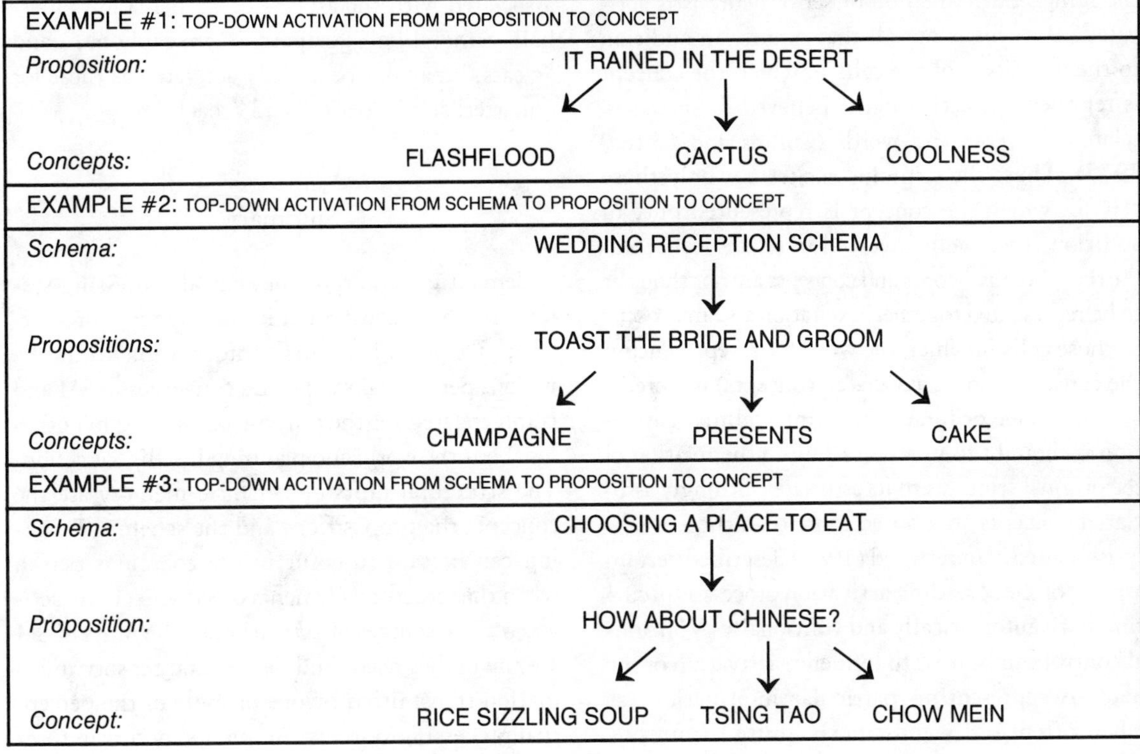

Figure 2-7. *Top-down activation.*

When the associations constituting a schema are activated in SM, they guide our comprehension. Consider the associations constituting the "dining-out schema"; the mind becomes focused on considerations like what would taste good, types of restaurants and their location, price, and popularity. Schemata are important for the recognition of individual utterances as part of a text and influence the way in which information is comprehended.

Horizontal Activation. Another way concepts are activated is horizontally, by each other. The concept "cactus" might activate other concepts, such as "sharp," "saguaro," and "jelly." Each of us has unique associations for the words we know and some associations that are shared by many other people in our culture. Most Americans associate the concept of "bacon" with "eggs" because of their similar cultural experiences, but only poetry fanciers are likely to have an association between an egg and the poet Günter Grass, or musicians between the violin and Itzhak Perlman.

How Does Activation of the Structural Elements of SM Occur?

Consider that the human cortex is a vastly interconnected neuronal network in which one nerve cell may communicate with thousands of others (Eccles, 1977). Then, conceptualize the nerve cell as an entity specialized for information processing (Kent, 1981) with a means of receiving, transmitting, and processing information. Kent describes a nerve cell as "performing the same function as a logical gate in a digital machine or an operational amplifier in an analog machine" (p. 6). In fact, it is a very versatile device capable of doing either of these jobs.

Although scientists lack sufficient data concerning the relation between cognition and cellular neurophysiology, it seems that when a concept is being thought about, a neuron or set of neurons is activated. But this is not all that occurs. In addition to the activation of the cells in which the concept is represented, activation is believed to spread to related concepts and words (Collins and Loftus, 1975). Thus, the stimulus excites not only those cells in which the concept is represented but, in addition, those cells involved in related concepts. Further, because words and concepts are not thought to be represented together, excitation also may occur in those cells in which the word form representing the concept (and its associated concepts) is stored.

The degree or frequency of intercellular activation is thought to vary according to the relation of the original stimulus to its associates. Strongly associated concepts are excited more than those weakly associated. Underwood (1982) described certain aspects of the spreading activation process as occurring both automatically and volitionally. Volitional control can be used to influence activation of the neurons representing particular information, as when attention is consciously shifted from one object or event to another.

To apply the theory of spreading activation to information processing, it can be predicted that spreading activation should facilitate the processing of the second word of a pair if the concepts expressed by the two words are associated. Further, it should facilitate processing even when the first word is unattended and is presented very shortly before the second word. Both predictions have been verified experimentally. Neely (1977) found that words presented 250 ms or 2 s prior to a related word facilitated the making of a lexical decision about the second word if the words were associated. Fowler, Wolford, Slade, and Tassinary (1981) reported facilitation by words that were not available to awareness and that were presented immediately prior to a second word.

The levels of activation for all the neurons activated in response to a particular stimulus are not the same. The degree of neuronal activation varies for many reasons, among them the strength of the association between the stimulus and its associates, the recency with which the neurons have been previously activated, and the context. The neurons associated with the aspects of a schema for a football game, like "goalpost," "megaphone," and "cleats," may not be as fully activated as those for "quarterback," "team," and "coach."

Summary

Semantic memory is the central processing system in which conceptual knowledge is represented and thinking occurs. Information from the various perceptual modalities converges in SM and is interrelated for the purpose of forming hypotheses about the world and planning intelligent action. The structural units of semantic memory are the concept, the proposition, and the schema. Thinking can be said to occur in the conscious person when the structural elements of SM are serially activated. The sources of activation to the units of SM are the body's needs and desires and sensory information transmitted by one or more of the perceptual processing systems. Activation occurs in three ways: from the bottom up, from the top down, and horizontally (Figure 2-8).

When a concept is activated, associated concepts, propositions, and schemata are also activated, or primed. This priming effect is an efficient way for the nervous system to increase the speed of response during an activity. It seems to operate on the assumption that if a particular concept is needed by the central processor, then other related concepts might also be needed; therefore, they are alerted to be ready for recall.

Verbal communication is the linguistic representation of thought and occurs when the relations between concepts, propositions, and schemata are translated into a linguistic symbol system. Communication in the strict sense requires thought by both the speaker/writer and listener/reader and can be subdivided into the processes of information comprehension and information expression. As a prelude to discussing the types of deficits dementia patients have in comprehending and producing linguistic information, it is necessary to consider what it means to comprehend and produce linguistic information.

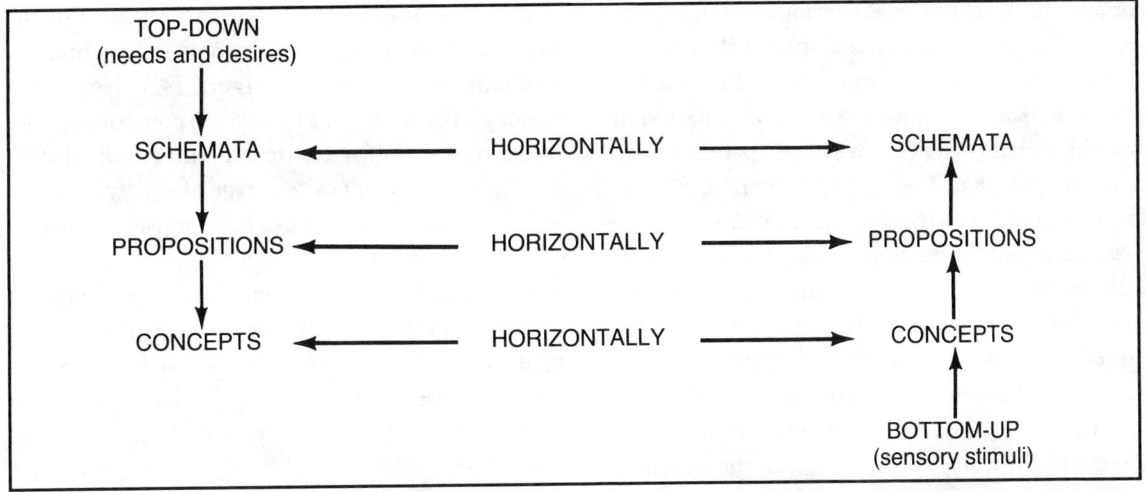

Figure 2-8. *Ways in which elements of semantic memory can be activated.*

COMPREHENSION OF LINGUISTIC INFORMATION

Linguistic comprehension ultimately involves deriving the right concepts and propositions, and the interconceptual and interpropositional relations. Linguistic comprehension is the product of sequential and parallel processes that involve many parts of the nervous system. For example, the perception of a spoken concept or proposition can be traced from its detection by the auditory system in which feature, segmental, and word analyses occur to the level of semantic memory. During its journey through the nervous system, linguistic stimuli undergo lexical, structural, and logical analyses, the output of which is a conceptual set, a propositional set, or both.

These analyses involve sounds, syntax, meaning, and use, and certain of them are less vulnerable to the effects of dementing illness, most notably those that are predominantly phonologic (involving sounds) and syntactic (involving sentence structure). Whitaker (1976) was the first to emphasize the dissociation in dementia of phonologic and syntactic analyses from semantic analysis. Whitaker's severely demented patient could echo sentences correctly and even spontaneously correct errors of syntax and phonology without processing meaning. A possible explanation for why certain analytic processes are better preserved is that they occur in different parts of the nervous system and vary in the degree to which conscious processing is needed. Phonologic and syntactic information may be processed unconsciously by nervous system processors that are active without the individual's conscious awareness (the "language module" in Fodor's theory), because these rules are finite and predictable by adulthood. Such an explanation seems credible when it is remembered that there is evidence that the amount of cortex involved in certain linguistic functions appears to vary in relation to the function's complexity.

Ojemann (1983) has argued, on the basis of cortical stimulation data, that after the nervous system has developed competence with a language, certain processes such as naming utilize smaller areas of the primary cortex (that is not to say that they are not assigned to deeper structures). Ojemann uses a procedure in which electric stimulation is applied to areas of exposed cortex while the patient is engaged in an activity such as speaking. If the application of current to an area disrupts the ongoing language task, the area is thought to be important for the activity in which the patient was engaged. The electric stimulation acts like a temporary lesion.

Through such techniques, Ojemann and others have been able to create a functional map of the cortex.

Ojemann and Whitaker (1978) studied the disruption of naming through cortical stimulation in three bilingual patients. Two of the patients were more competent in English; the other, in Dutch. They observed that the area where naming in the least competent language was altered was "substantially larger than the area in which naming of the same objects in the more competent language was altered" (p. 194). Ojemann and Whitaker theorized that "the area of cortex utilized for a particular language process may be greater for functions of greater difficulty. Over time, as one develops competence with a language, simple processes such as naming, utilize smaller primary cortical areas" (p. 194). It may be the case that syntactic and phonologic rules mastered in early childhood are finite and predictable and therefore do not require conscious mediation in the adult for their correct application. Then too, the authors speculate that if it were possible to map the amount of cortical area subserving syntactic and phonologic analysis, the area would be very small.

Unlike phonologic and syntactic analyses, no algorithm exists for predicting the semantic content of utterances, a fact that makes conscious mediation essential for linguistic comprehension. And, though it is true that much of what is said can be anticipated from the content of that previously uttered, the topic can change abruptly at any time. Certainly it is a fact that the length of any sentence is potentially infinite, because of the recursive properties of language; nevertheless, the potentially endless structure is predictable. Recursiveness is a property that allows language users to continue to add elements, such as noun phrases, to a sentence indefinitely (Figure 2-9). However, although the length of a sentence is potentially limitless, the types of syntactic structures available for use are not. The opposite is true of content; nothing limits the ideas that can be expressed. Context and expectation help us predict linguistic content, and sensitivity to context and expectancy require conscious processing. In fact, both sensitivity to context and the ability to develop expectancies are vital processes in linguistic comprehension, ones that should be discussed in greater detail.

The clown laughed.

The clown, with the big red nose, laughed.

The clown, in the tiny car, with the big red nose, laughed.

The clown, with the big red nose, in the tiny car, laughed at the dog.

Figure 2-9. *Recursive properties of human natural language.*

Sensitivity to Context

The context of a communicative event biases the interpretation of information exchanged. Context can be defined as the physical setting, the emotional climate, the social organization between participants, and the purpose underlying the communicative event. Enumeration of the influences of context on communication would be an endless task; however, an example may make it clear why comprehension requires contextual sensitivity. For example, the phrase "I know him" means quite different things in the context of a police lineup, the identification of a lost person, vouching for a check, or admitting someone to an illegal gambling party. From just this one example, it can be seen that the physical setting, the purpose underlying the communicative event, the emotional climate, and the social organization among participants can alter the way in which the linguistic input is analyzed.

Tracking these variables is a complex constructive process, and the participants need to be attentive to phonetic and paraverbal features such as pitch, intonation, gestures, facial expressions, and emotional loading of words. It is our ability to analyze context that enables us to develop appropriate expectations about the linguistic information that is forthcoming.

Expectations Facilitate Comprehension

The process of forming expectations results from the intellectual process of relating past experience to immediate experience. It involves being able to identify commonalities between a particular context and a past event in such a way that a reasonable prediction can be made about what propositions will follow. Not only in listening and reading are expectations formed about what will follow, but also when nonlinguistic information is being processed. Expectancies are based on stored knowledge of the world. The more new stimuli match existing conceptual knowledge, the easier they are to process. Weisstein and Harris (1974) found that a line in a context of other lines was more accurately remembered later when the lines in which it was originally nested resembled a single three-dimensional object rather than a flat-appearing, disconnected figure. Organization of the pattern into a three-dimensional object seemed to be a more important variable than the structural form or position of the target line. The spatial representation of the world contained in SM is considered to be three-dimensional; thus, the three-dimensional pattern was more meaningful and produced a facilitating effect (Lanze, Weisstein, and Harris, 1982). Similarly, objects are identified faster when embedded in a coherent scene than when the scene is jumbled (Biederman, 1972; Biederman, Glass, and Stacey, 1973; Biederman, Rabinowitz, Glass, and Stacey, 1974). A scene is coherent when it is a reasonable match to a stored representation about the world.

Our stored representations about the world guide us in interpreting new information and influence the way in which new information is processed. Jenkins (1977) reported that the same story with three different titles was interpreted in three different ways. A finding such as this is credible because language users assign different interpretations to sentences depending upon the context in which they are produced. The following sentences taken individually have a quite different meaning than when they are analyzed together in relation to context.

A. I'm here to collect the money.
B. Give me what you owe.
C. I promise you, you'll wish you had.

Neither sentences A nor B are threats, but together with sentence C, the speaker's intention to threaten the hearer becomes clear. A statement, a command, and a promise add up to a threat in this instance. If you were to witness this communicative interchange and it took place between two men one of whom was glowering over the other, you would be quite sure of your conclusion.

When miscommunication occurs, people find themselves systematically reviewing the context of the communicative event in terms of their expectations to discover where the breakdown occurred. All of the activities involved in contextual analysis and the building of expectancies require conscious processing by numerous cognitive systems. But, there is even more to comprehension. Assuming that contextual analysis and the building of expectancies has occurred, a final conclusion must still be reached, which is to say that a set of propositions must be derived. The propositions we derive from a communicative interchange, be it a conversation, a lecture, a story, or a chapter, require inference.

The Ability to Infer is Fundamental to Comprehension

An inference is a conclusion derived from an analysis of facts and premises. During listening and reading, a selection process is occurring; that is, not everything that is heard or read is stored. Most likely to be stored is the moral or point of the discourse. The point of the discourse is a higher-level semantic structure, which we shall call the macrostructure (after van Dijk, 1980). A macrostructure is the overall idea expressed in a discourse, the most memorable element derivable (van Dijk and Kintsch, 1975; 1977; Kintsch and van Dijk, 1978). Less memorable are the exact words and syntax. Macrostructures are necessary to provide a full account of a discourse or text. These aspects of a text can not be accounted for at the sentence level but represent a synthesis of the content of many sentences. Although macrostructures have propositional form, they cannot be expressed by a single clause or sentence but rather require a sequence of sentences. To comprehend the macrostructure of a discourse, inferential maneuvers are necessary.

Seven basic types of inferential maneuvers (Wickelgren, 1979) are employed in thinking and are basic to the comprehension of language. The types of inference are as follows:

Equivalence and reference: Inferring when two concepts are synonymous. Example: If *Amadeus* won the Oscar for best movie in 1985, and the best movie of 1985 was filmed in Czechoslovakia, then *Amadeus* was filmed in Czechoslovakia.

Implication: Inferring that propositions true of a superordinate concept are true of all examples of that concept. Example: "Two gray hills" rugs are objects of Indian art; Indian art is valuable; "two gray hills" rugs are valuable.

Coimplication: Knowing whether *p* implies *q* and *q* implies *p*. Example: A mature ovary of a flowering plant is a fruit; the peach is a mature ovary of a flowering plant; therefore, a peach is a fruit.

Negation and contradiction: Inferences of the following form: If Nebraska is flat, Nebraska is not mountainous. If Nebraska is not Arizona, and North Platte is in Nebraska, North Platte is not in Arizona.

Disjunction: Inferring the relation between two or more alternatives of a compound proposition. Example: Tyler will go skiing or to the beach over spring break; Tyler will not go skiing; therefore, Tyler will go to the beach.

Quantification: Inferences of the following form: Maserati is a sports car; Maseratis go fast; therefore, some sports cars go fast. A cat is a mammal; a cat can't fly; therefore, not all mammals can fly.

Linear Orderings: Inferring transitive relations: x is $>y$; y is $>z$; thus x is $>z$. Dave is thinner than Ed; Ed is thinner than Steve; therefore, Dave is thinner than Steve.

The exercise of thinking through these examples of the types of inferences people make produces a sense of appreciation for the capacity of the central system to relate new to old information.

Summary

Comprehension necessarily involves inference, a process whereby old information is related to new information. Comprehension depends on the ability of an individual to infer and cannot be accomplished without the existence of an associative neuronal network in which knowledge of the world is represented and interrelated, a network that can be accessed.

Comprehension is facilitated to the degree that the information to be processed can be predicted from the context and the past experience of the individual: an inferential process. Hearers/readers form expectancies that guide the interpretation of sensory stimuli. In linguistic communication, misunderstanding occurs when what is said or read does not match the expectancy of the listener/reader.

During the dynamic reconstructive process of comprehension, the nervous system selects certain aspects of information for encoding. Not everything heard or read is stored; rather, selected elements are encoded. As was emphasized earlier in the chapter, dementia patients ultimately suffer impairment in all cognitive processes, but the degree of impairment at different stages varies, making the explication of impaired comprehension quite challenging.

PRODUCTION OF LINGUISTIC INFORMATION: IDEATION, TRANSLATION, IMPLEMENTATION

Ideation

Ideation begins the process of producing meaningful linguistic output. Of greatest importance in the formation of an idea are physical needs and emotional states. A critical difference between computer programs and human programs is that human thinking, as Neisser (1963) says, "begins in an intimate association with emotion and feelings which is never entirely lost" (p. 195). Indeed, Vygotsky (1934/1962) appreciated this relation and wrote the oft-quoted passage, "To understand another's speech, it is not sufficient to understand his words—

we must understand his thought. But even that is not enough—we must also know its motivation. No psychological analysis of an utterance is complete until that plane is reached" (Vygotsky, 1934/1962, p. 151). Ideas result from the ability of the mind to activate concepts, propositions, schemata and link them in interesting ways to each other and to new perceptual experience. It is because SM is an associative network that ideas can be developed. The sequential development of ideas can be said to define thought, of which there are many kinds: associating, imagining, reviewing, planning, problem-solving, and considering, to name a few.

Translation

Once an idea or idea sequence has been generated, it must be translated into a linguistic symbol system for communication to occur. The point to be underscored is that a translation process occurs; that is, ideation and thinking are done in a different language than what is seen on the written page or heard in a lecture. The brain appears to have a language of its own, a machine language, as Fodor (1975) says, a language of thought, the output of which is translatable into human natural language. In dementia, the numerous morphologic and neurochemical changes in the brain eventuate in disruption of the machine language, the language of thought.

When an idea or intention is formed, it is translated into a linguistic representation through a process of word selection and phrase composition. Further, when information to be shared is complex, a plan may be needed in which decisions are made about the appropriate sequence of speech acts. For example, if the speaker's purpose is to convince the loan officer at the bank to lend the speaker a large sum of money, neither the first nor any other speech act should be a threat.

Implementation

Implementation refers to the process whereby the linguistic representation of an idea is realized in speech or writing. Although the activation and coordination of the respiratory, phonatory, and articulatory systems is complicated, it is generally accomplished without conscious planning. Like many other automatically executed processes, the implementation process is not difficult for the Alzheimer's dementia patient. Patients with a subcortical pathologic condition and dementia may experience implementation problems. The Parkinson's patient frequently experiences difficulty initiating the motor movements needed in speech and writing because of a pathologic condition in the basal ganglia, an area of the brain that helps control movement.

Summary

The production of meaningful linguistic information requires ideation, the integrity of the language of thought, and the ability to translate machine language into natural language. Humans possess the incredible ability to combine the conceptual, propositional, and schematic knowledge in semantic memory to generate new ideas. Indeed, the most important task undertaken by the theorist in the development of a model of the mind and how it works is accounting for the ability of the human organism to produce and comprehend that which is new.

The specification of the structure and processing capabilities of SM provides a framework for discussion of the decline in linguistic communication abilities of the dementia patient. Chapter 3 contains performance data from the literature, which demonstrate that dementia patients have trouble comprehending linguistic information because they have difficulty deriving the correct proposition(s). They experience gradual deterioration of their inferential capabilities and disruption in the contents of semantic memory.

Persons with dementia have trouble producing linguistic information because they have trouble thinking, generating, and ordering ideas, in part because information-processing capabilities of SM are disturbed. Consider that this is a quite different explanation of linguistic incompetency from that generally given for patients with focal lesions and aphasia. Understanding the likely causes of linguistic incompetency in dementia patients is absolutely essential for developing appropriate testing strategies, forming realistic expectations of the patients, planning a support system for caregivers, and inspiring techniques that will enable patients with mild dementia to maximize their ability to function outside of an institution.

GENERAL SUMMARY AND CLINICAL IMPLICATIONS

1. Dementia is a syndrome, that is, a cluster of symptoms. The dementia syndrome is characterized by a progressive decline in intellectual and communicative functioning and accompanied by personality change. Alzheimer's disease (AD) is the most common cause of irreversible dementia.
2. Clinicians need a set of organizing principles to guide them in the interpretation of the behavioral changes typical of dementia, evaluation of dementia patients, and counseling of dementia patient caregivers.
3. When considering the dementia patient, clinicians need to differentiate between disorders of speech, language, and communication. Speech is one of many modalities used to express thoughts and ideas. Language is a symbol system used in the transmission of ideas. Communication is the sharing of ideas with or without words.
4. In patients with mild and moderate AD, clinicians should expect greater impairment in the ability to communicate than in speech or language.
5. Communication is impaired early in victims of AD because of the particular impairment of semantic memory (SM).
6. Semantic memory (SM), or the central system, contains an individual's conceptual knowledge, as well as propositional and schematic knowledge, and is the domain in the nervous system where thought occurs.
7. The contents of SM can be activated in a variety of ways, and as individual concepts are activated, so also are their associates.
8. External information perceived by the sensory systems is transduced and carried to SM, where it will be indexed and used in the formulation of ideas. In dementia, the particular impairment of SM diminishes the patient's ability to formulate and remember ideas, the basis of meaningful communication.
9. Episodic memory is the repository for information about temporally dated events and is the system by which an individual's chronologic history is stored. It is prominently impaired early in dementia. An interesting relation between the episodic and semantic memory deficits of dementia patients is that deficits in semantic memory may prevent the registration of information in episodic memory.
10. Linguistic comprehension is a complex multistage process that involves deriving the right concepts and propositions and interconceptual and interpropositional relations.
11. Comprehension often requires sensitivity to context. Contextual cues help us interpret utterances and form expectations about upcoming information.
12. When we make inferences, we relate old, previously stored information to information we recognize as new, and take into account contextual cues, all of which facilitate comprehension.
13. Linguistic comprehension deteriorates in dementing illness because of a decrease in the individual's sensitivity to context and ability to form expectations, make infer-

ences, and distinguish given and new information.

14. **The production of linguistic information begins with an idea that is translated into a linguistic symbol system.**
15. **Ideation and thinking are done in a different language from what is seen on the page or heard in a lecture.**
16. **Dementia patients have trouble producing meaningful communication because of deficits in ideation and the ability to translate ideas into linguistic symbols.**

REFERENCES

Abelson, R. (1975). Concepts for representing mundane reality in plans. In D. G. Bobrow and A. Collins (Eds.), *Representation and understanding. Studies in cognitive science* (pp. 273-309). New York: Academic Press.

Adams, M.J., and Collins, A. (1979). A schema-theoretical view of reading. In R.O. Freedle (Ed.), *New directions in discourse processing* (pp. 1-22). Norwood, NJ: Ablex Publishing Company.

Ajuriaguerra, J. de, and Tissot, R. (1975). Some aspects of language in various forms of senile dementia: Some comparisons with language in childhood. In E.H. Lenneberg and E. Lenneberg (Eds.), *Foundations of language development: A multidisciplinary approach: Vol. 1* (pp. 323-339). New York: Academic Press.

American Psychiatric Association (1980). *Diagnostic and statistical manual of mental disorders* (3rd ed.). Washington, DC: Author.

Anderson, J.R. (1974). Retrieval of propositional information from long-term memory. *Cognitive Psychology*, 6, 451-474.

Anderson, J.R. (1976). *Language, memory and thought*. Hillsdale, NJ: Lawrence Erlbaum Associates.

Anderson, J.R., and Bower, G.H. (1973). *Human associative memory*. Washington, DC: Winston.

Appell, J., Kertesz, A., and Fisman, M. (1982). A study of language functioning in Alzheimer patients. *Brain and Language, 17*, 73-91.

Atkinson, R.C., and Shiffrin, R.M. (1971). The control of short-term memory. *Scientific American, 225*, 82-90.

Bartlett, F. (1932). *Remembering*. Cambridge, England: Cambridge University Press.

Bayles, K.A. (1982). Language function in senile dementia. *Brain and Language, 16*, 265-280.

Bayles, K.A. (1984). Language and dementia. In A. Holland (Ed.), Recent advances: Speech, hearing, and language pathology (pp. 209-244). San Diego, CA: College-Hill Press.

Bayles, K.A. (1985). Communication in dementia. In H. Ulatowska (Ed.), *The aging brain* (pp. 157–173). Austin, TX: PRO-ED.

Bayles, K.A., and Tomoeda, C.K. (1983). Confrontation naming impairment in dementia. *Brain and Language, 19*, 98-114.

Beaugrande, R. de (1979). Text and sentence in discourse planning. In J.S. Petofi (Ed.), *Text vs. sentence* (pp. 467-494). Hamburg: Buske.

Beaugrande, R. de (1980). The pragmatics of discourse planning. *Journal of Pragmatics, 4*, 15-42.

Biederman, I. (1972). Perceiving real-world scenes. *Science, 177*, 77-80.

Biederman, I., Glass, A.L., and Stacey, E.W. Jr. (1973). Searching for objects in real word scenes. *Journal of Experimental Psychology, 97*, 22-27.

Biederman, I., Rabinowitz, J., Glass, A., and Stacey, E.W. Jr. (1974). On the information extracted from a glance at a scene. *Journal of Experimental Psychology, 103*, 597-600.

Bransford, J., Barclay, J., and Franks, J. (1972). Sentence memory: A constructive versus interpretive approach. *Cognitive Psychology, 3*, 193-209.

Bransford, J.D., and Franks, J.J. (1971). The abstraction of linguistic ideas. *Cognitive Psychology, 2*, 331-350.

Charniak, E. (1975). *Organization and inference in a framelike system of common sense knowledge*. Castagnola, Switzerland: Institute for Semantic and Cognitive Studies.

Cohen, G. (1983). *The psychology of cognition* (2nd ed.). New York: Academic Press.

Cohen, P.R. (1978). *On knowing what to say: Planning speech acts*. Unpublished doctoral dissertation (CS-TR 118), University of Toronto, Toronto.

Collins, A.M., and Loftus, E.F. (1975). A spreading-activation theory of semantic processing. *Psychological Review, 82*, 407-428.

Craik, F.I.M. (1984). Age differences in remembering. In L.R. Squire and N. Butters (Eds.), *Neuropsychology of memory* (pp. 3-12), New York: Guilford Press.

Cummings, J.L., Benson, D.F., Hill, M. A., and Read,

S. (1985). Aphasia in dementia of the Alzheimer type. *Neurology, 35*, 394-397.

Deese, J. (1962). On the structure of associative meaning. *Psychological Review, 69*, 161-175.

Dijk, T.A. van. (1980). *Macrostructures*. Hillsdale, NJ: Lawrence Erlbaum Associates.

Dijk, T.A. van, and Kintsch, W. (1975). Comment on se rappelle et on resume des histoires. *Langages, 40*, 98-116.

Dijk, T.A. van, and Kintsch, W. (1977). Cognitive psychology and discourse: Recalling and summarizing stories. In W.U. Dressler (Ed.), *Current trends in textlinguistics* (pp. 61-80). Berlin and New York: deGruyter.

Eccles, J.C. (1977). *The understanding of the brain*. New York: McGraw-Hill.

Ferm, L. (1974). Behavioral activities in demented geriatric patients. *Gerontologica Clinica, 16*, 185-194.

Fodor, J. (1975). *The language of thought*. New York, NY: Thomas Y. Crowell.

Fodor, J.A. (1983). *The modularity of the mind*. Cambridge, MA: The MIT Press.

Fowler, C.A., Wolford, G. Slade, R., and Tassinary, L. (1981). Lexical access with and without awareness. *Journal of Experimental Psychology: General, 110*, 341-362.

Freedle, R.O., and Hale, G. (1979). Acquisition of new comprehension schemata for expository prose by transfer of a narrative schema. In R.O. Freedle (Ed.), *New directions in discourse processing* (pp. 121-136). Norwood, NJ: Ablex Publishing Company.

Garrod, S., and Trabasso, T. (1973). A dual-memory information processing interpretation of sentence comprehension. *Journal of Verbal Learning and Verbal Behavior, 12*, 155-167.

Halford, G.S. (1982). *The development of thought*. Hillsdale, NJ: Lawrence Erlbaum Associates.

Irigaray, L. (1973). *Le langage des dements*. The Hague: Mouton.

Jenkins, J. (1977, May). *Context conditions meaning*. Paper presented at a meeting of the Midwestern Psychological Association, Chicago, IL.

Kent, E.W. (1981). *The brains of men and machines*. New York: McGraw-Hill.

Kintsch, W. (1977). On comprehending stories. In M.A. Just and P.A. Carpenter (Eds.), *Cognitive processes in comprehension*. Hillsdale, NJ: Lawrence Erlbaum Associates.

Kintsch, W., and Glass, G. (1974). Effects of propositional structure upon sentence recall. In W. Kintsch (Ed.), *The representation of meaning in memory* (pp. 140-151). Hillsdale, NJ: Lawrence Erlbaum Associates.

Kintsch, W., and Keenan, J.M. (1973). Reading rate and retention as a function of the number of propositions in the base structure of sentences. *Cognitive Psychology, 5*, 257-274.

Kintsch, W., and van Dijk, T.A. (1978). Towards a model of discourse comprehension and production. *Psychological Review, 85*, 363-394.

Lanze, M., Weisstein, N., and Harris, J. (1982). Perceived depth vs. structural relevance in the object superiority effect. *Perception and Psychophysics, 31*, 376-382.

Marshall, J.C. (1984). Multiple perspectives on modularity. *Cognition, 17*, 209-242.

Maynard, D.W. (1980). Placement of topic changes in conversation. *Semiotica, 30*, 263-290.

Meyer, D.E., and Schvaneveldt, R.W. (1971). Facilitation in recognizing pairs of words: Evidence of a dependence between retrieval operations. *Journal of Experimental Psychology, 90*, 227-234.

Miller, G.A. (1956). The magical number seven, plus or minus two: Some limits on our capacity for processing information. *Psychological Review, 63*, 81-97.

Miller, G.A. (1971). Empirical methods in the study of semantics. In D.D. Steinberg and L.A. Jakobovits (Eds.), *Semantics: An interdisciplinary reader* (pp. 569-585). Cambridge, MA: Cambridge University Press.

Minsky, M. (1975). A framework for representing knowledge. In P.H. Winston (Ed.), *The psychology of computer vision* (pp. 211-217). New York: McGraw-Hill.

Murdock, B.B., Jr. (1974). *Human memory: Theory and data*. Hillsdale, NJ: Lawrence Erlbaum Associates.

Neely, J.H. (1977). Semantic priming and retrieval from lexical memory: Roles of inhibitionless spreading activation and limited attention. *Journal of Experimental Psychology: General, 106*, 226-254.

Neisser, U. (1963). The imitation of man by machine. *Science, 139*, 193-197.

Obler, L.K. (1983). Language and brain dysfunction in dementia. In S. J. Segalowitz (Eds.), *Language functions and brain organization* (pp. 267-282). New York: Academic Press.

Obler, L.K., and Albert, M.L. (1981). Language and aging: A neurobehavioral analysis. In D.S. Beasley and G.A. Davis (Eds.), *Aging: Communication processes and disorders* (pp. 107-121). New York: Grune and Stratton.

Ojemann, G.A. (1983). Brain organization for language from the perspective of electrical stimulation mapping. *The Behavioral and Brain Sciences, 2*, 189-230.

Ojemann, G.A., and Whitaker, H. (1978). The bilingual brain. *Archives of Neurology, 35*, 409-412.

Quillian, M.R. (1966). *Semantic memory*. Unpublished doctoral dissertation. Carnegie Institute of Technology. (Reprinted in part in M. Minsky (Ed.), (1968). *Semantic information processing*. Cambridge, MA: MIT Press.

Rumelhart, D. (1975). Notes on a schema for stories. In D. Bobrow and A. Collins (Eds.), *Representation and understanding* (pp. 211-236). New York: Academic Press.

Sachs, J.S. (1967). Recognition memory for syntactic and semantic aspects of connected discourse. *Perception and Psychophysics, 2*, 437-444.

Schank, R.C. (1977). Rules and topics in conversation. *Cognitive Science, 1*, 421-442.

Schank, R., and Abelson, R. (1977). *Scripts, plans, goals, and understanding*. Hillsdale, NJ: Lawrence Erlbaum Associates.

Schlesinger, I. (1977). The role of cognitive development and linguistic input in language acquisition. *Journal of Child Language, 4*, 153-169.

Selz, O. (1922). *Zur Psychologie des produktiven Denkens und Irrtums*. Bonn: Cohen.

Smith, E.E., and Medin, D.L. (1981). *Categories and concepts*. Cambridge, MA: Harvard University Press.

Tulving, E. (1972). Episodic and semantic memory. In E. Tulving and W. Donaldson (Eds.), *Organization of memory* (pp. 381-403). New York: Academic Press.

Tulving, E. (1984). Elements of episodic memory (precis). *The Behavioral and Brain Sciences, 7*, 223-268.

Tulving, E. (1985). How many memory systems are there? *American Psychologist, 40*, 385-398.

Tulving, E., and Pearlstone, Z. (1966). Availability versus accessibility of information in memory for words. *Journal of Verbal Learning and Verbal Behaviour, 5*, 381-391.

Underwood, G. (1982). Attention and awareness in cognitive and motor skills. In G. Underwood (Ed.), *Aspects of consciousness: Vol. 3. Awareness and self-awareness* (pp. 111-145). New York: Academic Press.

Vygotsky, L.S. (1962). *Thought and language*. Cambridge, MA: MIT Press (First published in 1934).

Wang, M.D. (1977). Frequency of effects in the abstraction of linguistic ideas. *Bulletin of the Psychonomic Society, 9*, 303-306.

Wechsler, A.F. (1977). Presenile dementia presenting as aphasia. *Journal of Neurology, Neurosurgery, and Psychiatry, 40*, 303-305.

Weisstein, N., and Harris, C.S. (1974). Visual detection of line segments: An object-superiority effect. *Science, 186*, 752-755.

Whitaker, H.A. (1976). A case of isolation of the language function. In H. Whitaker and H.A. Whitaker (Eds.), *Perspectives in neurolinguistics and psycholinguistics: Vol. 2, Studies in neurolinguistics*. (pp. 1-58). New York: Academic Press.

Wickelgren, W.A. (1979). *Cognitive psychology*. Englewood Cliffs, NJ: Prentice-Hall.

Wickens, D.D. (1970). Encoding categories of words: An empirical approach to meaning. *Psychological Review, 77*, 1-15.

Winograd, T. (1975). Frame representations and the declarative-procedural controversy. In D. Bobrow and A. Collins (Eds.), *Representation and understanding*. (pp. 185-210). New York: Academic Press.

Yates, J. (1985). The content of awareness is a model of the world. *Psychological Review, 92*, 249-284.

Chapter 3

The Effects of Dementing Illness on Communication

As the title says, this chapter contains specific information about how communication is affected in dementing illnesses. Such information could be presented in a recipe-like fashion with few interpretative comments, and although a recipe-like recitation of dementing illness effects would be easy, it would shortchange the clinician responsible for educating professional and personal caregivers. It turns out to be the case that the performance data of dementia patients have import for the most fundamental and interesting issue in psychology, the structure of the human mind. The data from the study of communicative function in the dementia patient may lead scientists to modify currently popular models of memory and language. Clinicians who appreciate the theoretic issues to which the data of dementia patients relate will be better prepared to interpret patient behavior, predict behavioral sequelae, and conceptualize and conduct research with dementia patients. Thus, the authors have elected to organize the performance data around two theoretic premises: first, that the contents and processes of SM deteriorate in dementing illness, and second, that the data from communication studies of dementia substantiate a conceptualization of SM as a cognitive faculty in which concepts, but not their linguistic representations, are stored.

To activate within the reader the critical concepts required to follow the discussion of the first premise, that the contents and processes of SM deteriorate in the development of dementia, the reader is invited to consider two questions:

1. What would constitute evidence for deterioration in the contents of SM?
2. What would constitute evidence for deterioration in the processes of SM?

When a patient fails to comprehend or produce conceptual, propositional, or schematic information, either the contents of SM or the ability to use the information in SM is gone; perhaps both. A moment's reflection is likely to convince readers of the difficulty, if not impossibility, of thinking of a task in which the integrity of SM and conceptual knowledge is evaluated without simultaneous evaluation of SM processing, especially if the task is intentional. Nonetheless, just because it is hard to envision a paradigm in which the contents and processes of SM can be separately evaluated, it does not mean they are the same thing.

Because of the heuristic value of the notion that

the contents and processes of SM have deteriorated, an admittedly arbitrary criterion has been adopted by the authors to decide whether the performance data from a myriad of language/communication studies offer evidence about the integrity of conceptual knowledge or processing capabilities.

CRITERION FOR INTERPRETING PERFORMANCE DATA

Evidence Related to SM Contents

As evidence about the patency of SM contents, only those paradigms in which subjects were required to recognize or recall a single concept will be considered. Such paradigms include confrontation naming, vocabulary, pantomime, and word association.

The rationale for this criterion is that dementia patients correctly answer some of the items in the aforementioned types of tests, thereby demonstrating that processing skills are functional, at least occasionally. When subjects fail some items and complete others on these tests, they do not necessarily have a SM processing problem. The more probable explanation would seem to be that their errors represent deterioration in conceptual knowledge.

Convincing evidence that these intermittent errors represent conceptual, rather than processing, deficits, would be repeated errors on the same concepts in different types of tests or in repetitions of the same test. If it were the case that the errors were the result of processing deficits, then one would expect the errors to be random. Huff, Corkin, and Growdon (in press) addressed just this question. They asked whether the errors on confrontation naming tests were random, or the same items consistently missed in different types of tests. They compared patterns of error in a confrontation naming test and a name recognition test using the same objects in 23 patients with mild to moderate dementia. Items on which a patient made a semantic error in a name recognition test were less likely to be named in a confrontation naming test. Huff and colleagues concluded that because errors were consistently made on the same items in the two tests, semantic information is lost in patients with AD.

Evidence Related to SM Processing

In tasks like reading comprehension, discourse production, and linguistic reasoning, where multiple concepts, propositions, and schemata are simultaneously activated, the presence of bizarrely juxtaposed, nonrelated ideas implicates impaired processing, notably the inability to generate and order meaningful ideas. Consider the following letter received by our colleague Tom Slauson, a few days after testing an AD patient.

> August 19, 1985
>
> Dear Mr. Slauson,
>
> Your recent Note is much appreciated and I am most interested in the coming of more data such as I have had for about a year. Having read Alzheimer's from end to end it would be a treat to brighten some stillness of mine own!
>
> Indeed Miss Caffrey was a great help to me for I think I enlarged a few names somewhat with pleasure that she sent out. I shall hope to find her again soon.
>
> Perhaps I should tell you that I have no desire to leave Tucson at any time, nor has my wife. We have our own home, have owned Rancho del Norte from '56 to '70. I have been a victim since about two and one half years with the dying out, but it works slowly and I feel fine.
>
> Forgive me for going ahead of you—I thought I would get just a bite and let go.
>
> With every good wish,

For this individual, the capacity to meaningfully relate concepts, propositions, and schemata is clearly impaired. While it is true that conceptual deterioration, as well as processing deficiencies, contribute to the production of the disordered discourse in this letter, no method exists for quantifying the degree to which each is responsible. In the next section, studies indicative of diminishment in the contents of SM will be reviewed, followed by studies indicative of impaired processing.

EVIDENCE FOR DETERIORATION IN THE CONTENTS OF SM

Confrontation Naming Deficits

In a confrontation naming task, the subject is given an object, a picture, or a drawing of an object and asked to provide the name. In addition to recording the frequency with which the correct name is provided, the time needed to respond correctly can also be recorded.

Numerous authors report a significantly impaired naming ability in dementia patients (Bayles and Tomoeda, 1983a; Kirshner, Webb, and Kelly, 1984; Lawson and Barker, 1968; Overman, 1979; Rochford, 1971; Schmitt and Mitchell, 1984). The only point of controversy seems to be in the degree to which confrontation naming is impaired early in the dementia syndrome. Though some authors argue that it is the most prominent early clinical feature (Kirshner et al., 1984), others consider it to be less characteristic of early communicative impairment than other deficits (Appell, Kertesz, and Fisman, 1982; Bayles, 1982; Benson, 1979; Obler, 1983). Both conceptualizations may be correct, that is, a subpopulation of dementia patients may have prominent early confrontation dysnomia because of greater damage to the neural substrates for naming in the language dominant hemisphere. In Chapter 1, mention was made of the considerable variation among dementia patients in the degree of hypometabolism between the two cerebral hemispheres as demonstrated by glucose uptake during positron emission tomography (Haxby, Duara, Grady, Cutler, and Rapoport, 1985; Koss, Friedland, Ober, and Jagust, 1985). Patients with left perisylvian damage and hypometabolism may have greater confrontation naming problems early in dementia.

Influence of Misperception on Misnaming. A controversial issue related to the interpretation of the misnamings of dementia patients is the degree to which misnaming is caused by misperception. Lawson and Barker (1968) formally studied the naming ability of 100 dementia patients and 40 normal volunteers and found that both groups had longer latencies for object naming, particularly for less common objects. Further, when the function of the stimulus items was demonstrated, naming was facilitated, an observation that lead to the hypothesis that perceptual impairment caused the misnaming. Like Lawson and Barker, Rochford (1971) concluded that dementia patients are "perceptually off-course." He presented 23 dementia patients with an eight-item naming test and classified their responses as correct, misrecognized, unclassifiable, or no response. The most frequent response of Rochford's subjects was misrecognition, occurring 55 percent of the time. Thirty-five percent of the errors made were attributed to the naming of an object similar in appearance to the stimulus item, a finding that Rochford interpreted as evidence of perceptual impairment.

More recently, Kirshner et al. (1984) argued that although most naming errors of dementia patients are perceptual, linguistic factors also contribute. In a study of 12 Alzheimer's patients, four types of stimuli, each more abstract than its predecessor, were presented for naming: the actual object, a black-and-white photograph, a line drawing, and a masked line drawing. Half of the 40 stimulus items were associated with high-frequency words and half with low-frequency words; half were short and half long. Thus, the authors were interested in the following issues: first, the effect of the perceptual strength of the stimulus items on naming accuracy; second, the relation of naming accuracy to word frequency and length; and third, the relation of naming dysfunction to degree of language and cognitive deficit in dementia.

Overall, dementia patients made significantly more errors than normal subjects, and the level of perceptual difficulty significantly influenced the rate of misnaming. Further, word frequency, but not length, significantly influenced naming accuracy. The authors concluded that perceptual problems figured more prominently in misnaming than linguistic problems because more errors were made on the perceptually degraded stimuli. This conclusion is surprising because of the finding that in fact, normal subjects made more perceptual errors than the dementia patients (56.9 percent vs 35.7 percent). Had the reverse been true, the conclusion would have more impact and credibility. Then too, it is not surprising that perceptual errors became more common as the stimuli became more imperceptible. It is well known that stimuli vary in their strength and ability to arouse concepts (Goodglass, 1980). Weaker stimuli make concept arousal harder in a naming task. Therefore, the findings of the study are not unexpected. Greater difficulty should be expected, and was observed, for naming degraded stimuli.

Finally, the published report of the findings of the study did not make it clear whether mild dementia patients had a significantly higher misnaming rate than normals. The authors reported that overall, dementia patients had a significantly higher misnaming rate, but all patients were grouped together regardless of severity. The authors did not specify whether mild dementia patients had a significantly higher misnaming rate than normal subjects. It may have been the case that high error rates, in more severely demented patients, obscured the *lack* of a significant difference between mildly demented patients and normal subjects in misnaming rate. Additionally, because all dementia patients were combined regardless of severity, the effect of the perceptual characteristics of the stimuli on naming, as a function of dementia severity, was obscured.

Misperception May Not Be the Primary Cause of Misnaming. In a study by Bayles and Tomoeda (1983a) of the misnamings of dementia patients, the performances of 61 patients were analyzed. Only 8.6 percent of all errors were found to be visually similar and otherwise unrelated to the target word. This suggests that misperception may have some relation to misnaming, though not a prominent one. Bayles and Tomoeda used a classification system in which the following types of responses were noted:

Stimulus: PEACH

I. No response
II. Unrelated response .... shoes
    (not linguistically or visually related)
III. Related response
    A. Visually related .... ball
    B. Linguistically related
        1. Phonemically similar .... pear
        2. Semantically associated
            a. Same category .... plum
            b. Function .... food
            c. Part .... pit
            d. Attribute .... fuzzy
            e. Superordinate .... fruit
            f. Context .... orchard

Semantically Associated Misnaming Was Most Common. The most common type of response was one that was semantically associated, occurring 65 percent of the time among AD patients. Typically, the name of another item from the same category was substituted for the correct response. Schmitt and Mitchell (1984) also used a system of classification similar to the one used by Bayles and Tomoeda (1983a) and observed more semantically than visually related errors. Finally, 66 percent of the naming errors made by AD subjects in Kempler's study (1984) were semantically related to the target, while only 15 percent were visual errors.

The controversy about the influence of misperception on naming raises an interesting point in relation to the claim that data obtained in confrontation naming studies can be interpreted as providing information about the integrity of conceptual knowledge in SM. If misnaming occurs because of misperception (and although we do not think it routinely does, it seems reasonable that that might account for some instances), then it would be inappropriate to conclude that the misnamed concept was *not* in SM. Indeed, the concept might exist, but not be aroused because of perceptual deficits.

Adding more fuel to the fire, the authors wish to suggest yet another reason why an instance of misnaming may not mean that the concept no longer exists in SM, namely, that object naming may not require activation of the concept associated with a name. If conceptual activation can be bypassed in the naming process, then naming may not be a test of conceptual knowledge. And indeed, evidence has accumulated from studies of reading and semantic priming, in normal subjects and persons with dementia, that the name of a thing may be retrievable from the mental dictionary without activating its associated concept.

Naming Without Conceptual Processing

Evidence From Reading Studies. Numerous researchers have observed the phenomenon of dementia patients reading words they no longer understand (Irigaray, 1973; Schwartz, Marin, and Saffran, 1979; Whitaker, 1976). Halpern, Darley, and Brown (1973) reported a marked impairment in reading comprehension as the most distinguishing characteristic of dementia patients in their comparative study of patients with dementia, aphasia, apraxia, and the "language of confusion." Also, Whitaker's (1976) famous patient, HCEM, could read aloud when semantic knowledge was severely compromised, as could WLP, the well-known patient of Schwartz, Saffran and Marin (1980). Schwartz and colleagues noted that WLP read effortlessly but "appended comments that emphasized the discrepancy between her ability to pronounce the target and to comprehend it (e.g., 'hyena . . . hyena . . . what in the heck is that?')" (p. 261). These data suggest the existence of a brain circuit between graphemes, word forms, and phonologic codes that bypasses the meaning processing system.

Some may argue that bypassing conceptual analysis during confrontation naming is not analogous to bypassing conceptual analysis during reading because in confrontation naming, a visual form, rather than the sounds associated with a string of letters, elicits the word. More specifically, in reading, phonetic rules are used to derive words from a series of letters. However, deriving words by sounding out letters is not the only way people read. People read by recognizing the visual configuration of words. This is called reading by sight (Bower, 1970). Most of us have a subset of words that we recognize by sight, particularly foreign words for which we lack knowledge of the phonetic rules of the language. Rehabilitation specialists teach the sight method of reading to individuals with hearing problems or phonologic encoding deficits. The critical point is that because reading can be done by sight, the process of retrieving a word based on the memory of a visual configuration, rather than sound or meaning, is analogous to naming an object by matching its visual configuration to a word.

Dementia patients read without processing meanings by using both the phonetic and sight methods. WLP, the dementia patient of Schwartz and colleagues (1980), was able to read words spelled phonetically, as well as those whose spelling was not phonetic, and pairs of similarly spelled words that are pronounced differently (e.g., cost and post). Thus, because dementia patients can read by sight, it seems reasonable to suggest that they might also match the visual features of an object with its associated word form without activating the associated concept.

Evidence from Semantic Priming Studies. Data from the semantic priming literature provide evidence of the existence of two channels for word access, one in which the stimuli evoke a concept that is subsequently associated with a word form, and a second in which the word form is accessed before the concept. For example, Bowles and Poon (1985) presented the following five types of primes in a word retrieval task in which subjects had to produce a target word: semantically related words, unrelated words, orthographically similar words, words with the same first two letters as the target word, and neutral primes consisting of a series of x's. Primes that were orthographically and phonemically related to the target words were found to facilitate word retrieval, whereas semantically related and unrelated primes inhibited retrieval. These findings are consistent with those of several other researchers (Brown, 1979; Roediger, Neely, and Blaxton, 1983). Bowles and Poon explained these findings by reasoning that information in the mental dictionary is organized orthographically and phonemically and is therefore different from information in SM, which is organized conceptually. The inhibition in naming after the presentation of semantically related words reflects subject preference for using orthographic and phonemic information. When given a choice, subjects preferred orthographic and phonemic information to semantic. Bowles and Poon point out that in priming paradigms, in which orthographically and phonemically related primes are not included with semantically related primes, the semantically related primes are facilitating (Fischler and Goodman, 1978; Meyer and Schvaneveldt, 1971; Meyer, Schvaneveldt, and Ruddy, 1975). Again, the critical point is the existence of two access routes to words, one of which could explain the production of a word in the absence of access to its conceptual representation.

Summary

The primary issue discussed in this section is whether confrontation naming can be accomplished without conceptual analysis, not whether dementia patients perform inferiorly on confrontation naming tasks; they do. Although the degree of dysnomia early in the dementia syndrome, and the contribution of misperception to dysnomia, remain points of debate, consensus exists that naming is impaired and worsens as the dementia syndrome progresses. Whether the performance of dementia patients on confrontation naming tasks can be used to demonstrate a deterioration in the conceptual structure of SM is equivocal.

The use of confrontation naming data for this purpose has been called into question by the fact that dementia patients can produce words without regard for meaning; they do so in reading and appear to do so in spontaneous discourse. The preserved oral reading ability of severely intellectually impaired dementia patients is evidence of the ability of the nervous system to access the lexicon without conceptual processing. The fact that such access is available in reading suggests that it may be available in naming as well.

Evidence from the semantic priming studies of Bowles and Poon (1985) suggests mechanisms by which the matching of a word form to a visual configuration might be accomplished without necessarily accessing the concept. If the data substantiate that word forms and their access are separable from conceptual representation, they have implications for the theory of the structure of SM. That is, either SM does not contain the word forms, or they are separately represented from conceptual information within SM.

OTHER EVIDENCE OF DETERIORATION OF THE CONTENTS OF SM

Progressively Diminishing Vocabulary

Expressive and receptive vocabulary progressively decline during the course of dementia (de Ajuriaguerra and Tissot, 1975; Ernst, Dalby, and Dalby, 1970). In expressive vocabulary tests, subjects define words presented by the examiner. Unlike confrontation naming, a correct response cannot be given without concept activation, because in this task the examiner is asking for the conceptual representation of the word.

Probably the most frequently given and best known expressive vocabulary test is the vocabulary subtest of the Wechsler Adult Intelligence Scale. The test was given to a subset of the AD patients (7 mild, 7 moderate AD patients, and 19 normal elderly) who participated in the Tucson study of dementia and communication. Performance scores are presented in Table 3-1. Moderate AD patients were significantly impaired, compared with normal subjects.

A receptive vocabulary test commonly used in the study of dementia patients is the Peabody Picture Vocabulary Test (PPVT) (Dunn, 1959). In this measure, subjects must select, from among four black and white line drawings, the one depicting the word spoken by the examiner. The PPVT was used in both the Chicago (Kaszniak and Wilson, 1985) and the Tucson (Bayles, 1985) studies of dementia patients, and in both, significant differences were obtained between patients with mild dementia and normal subjects (Tables 3-2 and 3-3).

Table 3-1. Performance of Dementia Patients and Elderly Controls on the WAIS Vocabulary Subtest—Tucson Study

Groups	N	$\bar{X}$	SD
Normals	19	60.26	8.87
Mild AD	7	42.29	17.05
Moderate AD	7	24.27*	25.18

*Moderate AD subjects performed significantly differently from controls at p = .05 level.

Table 3-2. Performance of Dementia Patients and Elderly Controls on the Peabody Picture Vocabulary Test—Chicago Study

Groups	N	Year 1	Year 2	Year 3
Normals	32			
$\bar{X}$		138.56	137.28	137.51
SD		14.34	12.68	16.04
Dements	20			
$\bar{X}$		116.10	113.70	101.10
SD		21.87	22.09	27.47

Group $F(1,57) = 35.17$ ($p < .01$).
Year $F(2,56) = 5.15$ ($p < .01$).
Interaction $F(2,56) = 7.74$ ($p < .01$)

However, because the selection of the correct drawing in the PPVT, depends upon visual perceptual ability, as well as word knowledge, knowledge of vocabulary is said to be confounded with visual perceptual ability. To determine if visual perceptual disorders were responsible for the diminished performances of dementia patients, 35 Alzheimer's subjects in another study (Bayles, Boone, Tomoeda, and Slauson, 1986) were asked to orally define the words missed during the test. Beginning with the easiest item, the examiner told the subject the word and asked for an oral definition. Only three subjects were able to provide a correct definition of a word missed during the standard administration of the test, leading Bayles and colleagues to conclude that lack of knowledge of the word definition, rather than visual perceptual problems, accounts for the majority of PPVT errors.

Table 3-3. Performance of Dementia Patients and Elderly Controls on the Peabody Picture Vocabulary Test—Tucson Study

Groups	N	$\bar{X}$	SD
Normals	33	136.03	14.00
Mild AD	16	121.50*	16.93
Moderate AD	14	103.29*+	21.20

*Mild AD and moderate AD subjects performed significantly differently from controls at $p < .01$.
+Moderate AD subjects performed significantly differently from mild AD subjects at $p < .01$.

Diminished Ability to Comprehend and Produce Pantomime

Another type of conceptual knowledge, though frequently overlooked, is how to use common objects. By demonstrating the functional use of objects through pantomime, dementia patients can reveal their understanding of concepts. In a pantomimic comprehension test, the subject must identify the object, or picture of the object, from among several choices that the examiner is demonstrating. In pantomimic expression, the subject is shown an object and asked to demonstrate its use without words.

In an elaborate study, Langhans (1985) attempted to determine whether persons with AD demonstrate a disturbance of pantomime recognition, expression, or both compared with healthy aged control subjects and to determine the relation of performance on measures of pantomime to performance on measures of cognition and language. Thirty AD subjects participated, 5 with mild, 17 with moderate, and 8 with severe dementia according to performance on the Mental Status Questionnaire (Goldfarb, 1975).

Subjects with mild AD did not differ significantly from control subjects in performing tasks of pantomime recognition or pantomime expression, though patients with moderate and severe AD did. According to Langhans, the poorer performance by patients with moderate and severe AD was not due to ideomotor apraxia, or a central symbolic disorder, but rather to cognitive decline. Ideomotor apraxia was defined as difficulty executing an act in the absence of difficulty formulating the ideas of the act to be performed. Patients with ideomotor apraxia have difficulty when asked to imitate an act or perform it on command, but not in spontaneous execution. The AD patients in the Langhans study did not have difficulty imitating acts or performing them on command.

Langhans reasoned that if the impaired performance of AD patients on the expressive pantomime test results from a central symbolic disorder, both nonverbal and verbal symbolic abilities should associate more closely with each other than with other cognitive/intelligence or praxis variables. Such was not the case; performance on pantomime tasks was most closely associated with performance on cognitive tasks.

Naming and verbal (word) recognition tasks were also administered to study participants because Langhans reasoned that if the same items were in error for both the verbal and pantomime recognition, as well as the naming and pantomime expression measures, it would serve as evidence of a central symbolic disorder. Therefore, 23 common items on each of these measures were compared.

Error comparisons made on the verbal and pantomime recognition measures revealed that in only 3 of the 690 instances were the same items in error. Of the two tasks, pantomime recognition proved harder. When performances on the naming and pantomime expression measures were compared, 81 of the 690 instances were in error, or 11.7 percent. Langhans concluded that being able to name a pictured object does not predict ability to pantomime the object's use. However, if a subject cannot name an item, the probability is great that the subject also cannot pantomime its use. Of the 138 errors made on the naming task, 95 percent were also in error by the same subject on the pantomime expression measure. AD subjects performed extremely well on the verbal recognition measure; only 9 errors were made out of 690 responses, and one severe AD subject accounted for 5 of the 9 errors. In contrast, 172 of 690 responses, or 24.9 percent, were incorrect on the pantomime recognition measures, indicating that the pantomime recognition task was more difficult than the verbal recognition task.

Changes in the Patterns of Word Associations

Other evidence for deteriorated conceptual structure comes from studies of the word associations given by dementia patients. In word association paradigms the common hypothesis is that if conceptual knowledge is intact, strongly associated words, as defined by word association norms, will be elicited.

Gewirth, Shindler, and Hier (1984) gave 38 patients with dementia of various causes, a word association test in which the stimuli were equal numbers of nouns, verbs, adjectives, and adverbs. Each of the subject's responses to a stimulus word was classified as to whether the response was one of the three most frequent in the word association norms of Palermo and Jenkins (1964) and whether it was a paradigmatic, syntagmatic, idiosyncratic, or unrelated response.

Paradigmatic responses are words of the same word class that are semantically related to the stimulus and typically include antonyms, synonyms, and coordinates. Syntagmatic responses are words from different grammatical classes that typically occur sequentially in sentence structure (Clark and Clark, 1977), such as ". . . kittens meow," "the fog horn . . .," "laughing loudly . . .," and ". . . lapped the warm milk."

Because the particular cause of dementia appeared to have no effect on type of associative response in this study, etiologically different dementia cases were grouped together and stratified according to severity. The effect of severity on the type of word association responses given was prominent. The greater the severity of dementia, the lower the frequency with which one of the three most common associates of the stimulus words was given, a finding interpreted as indicative of disruption in the conceptual network. Further, a marked increase was observed in the number of idiosyncratic responses. Interestingly, the number of syntagmatically related responses did not significantly diminish, suggesting that syntactic knowledge was less affected than conceptual or paradigmatic knowledge.

Other Viewpoints About the Integrity of SM

Though the dominant view is that conceptual knowledge deteriorates in dementia, not everyone agrees. Grober, Buschke, Kawas, and Fuld (1985) suggest that the contents of semantic memory are intact in demented patients but that the organization of conceptual knowledge is disrupted. In their study, 20 AD patients were given a group of concepts and a list of possible attributes and non-attributes. Subjects had to identify which attributes were associated with a particular concept and order them according to saliency. Because AD patients could identify the attributes but not order them, Grober and colleagues concluded that the SM concepts were intact.

Nebes, Martin, and Horn (1984) also concluded that the contents of SM are intact, but for a different reason. They used a semantic priming paradigm in which the dependent variable was the time it took subjects to name tachistoscopically presented words. They hypothesized that if the structure of SM is intact in dementia patients, then the effect of semantic priming should be equivalent to that seen in normal subjects. That is, words following a semantically related prime would be named faster because of their having been activated by the prime. Nebes and associates observed that although the dementia patients performed more slowly than normal subjects, the difference between the speed of their responses, when the primes were related and unrelated, was of the same magnitude as observed in normal subjects, thereby indicating an equivalent priming effect. Nebes and colleagues interpreted this to be evidence for the integrity of the contents of SM in dementia.

Before the finer points of this study are discussed, it is important to recognize that the naming paradigm may not test the integrity of semantic memory (Lupker, 1984). Lupker has demonstrated that naming is primarily accomplished by accessing the lexical (word associative memory) system rather than the conceptual system (for a more in-depth discussion of Lupker's research, see "Evidence from Semantic Priming," this chapter). However, if the assumption is made that the naming paradigm does activate semantic memory—that is, conceptual memory—there are still other questions about the conclusions of Nebes and colleagues. First, the erosion of conceptual knowledge in dementia does not occur abruptly. It is a gradual process spanning months and years. In the early stages, patients can be expected to recognize attributes or experience a semantic priming effect because most concepts are still intact. Then, as the dementing process continues, the priming effect weakens. However, even in patients with very severe dementia, the effect might occasionally be present for particular concepts; not all concepts are lost at the same rate. What is not clear from the published report of the study by Nebes and colleagues is whether the dementia patients always correctly named the target word. This information is important because if some of the target words were not named by dementia patients, that could constitute evidence of deterioration of SM. On the other hand, if all the target words were named, the study results may still not constitute evidence that *all* concepts are intact, but rather only those concepts that were tested.

Subsequent to the aforementioned study, Nebes, Boller, and Holland (1986) conducted an investigation of the use of semantic context by AD patients from which was obtained more convincing evidence of the structural integrity of SM. Among the tasks used was a category decision task in which young normal subjects, older normal subjects, and AD patients were given the name of a semantic category in the form of a question: "Bird, is this a bird?" Afterwards a single noun was presented tachistoscopically. The word remained visible until the subject responded, "yes," it was an example of the category, or "no," it was not. The time required to make a judgment was the dependent variable. The stimulus words varied as to whether they were highly associated examples of the category, minimally associated, or unrelated. The results showed no evidence of a disproportionate loss in dementia patients of weaker semantic associations. The effect of exemplar associative strength on decision time was the same in dementia patients as in normal subjects. Nebes and colleagues concluded that in both normally aging persons and AD patients, knowledge about category membership is preserved, even for more atypical members of the category. In this study the error rates for dementia patients were presented, and they were only slightly higher than those for the young and older normal subjects.

Another priming study in which the findings

were interpreted as demonstrating the sparing of SM, a study partially motivated by the data of Nebes and colleagues, is that of Brandt, Spencer, McSorley, and Folstein (1986). In a clever two-part paradigm, 34 AD patients were asked to remember a set of target words and subsequently were given an ostensibly unrelated word-association task composed of 20 words. Ten of the words on the word-association test were selected so that their third most common associates were items on the previously given free recall test. These words were considered to be "biased," since one of their common associates had previously been activated by the free recall test. The frequency with which subjects gave a common associate of the words on the word association task was recorded. The extent to which subjects gave the third most common associate was taken as an indication of implicit memory.

In comparison with normal subjects, the dementia patients freely recalled significantly fewer words. Whereas the normal subjects averaged 5.33 items, AD patients recalled only 1.97. Of interest, however, was the large and statistically significant difference in the frequency with which the third most frequent associate was given by both the AD patients and the normal subjects in the word association task. Both groups gave the third most frequent associate significantly more often than other associates. The authors concluded that the mental representation of lexical items, and their common semantic associations, may be weakened in AD, but not disorganized. The fact that dementia patients named associates of concepts they did not remember demonstrates strikingly that activation can occur unconsciously even in the brain with a pathologic condition. Perhaps the persistence of the activation of concepts that are unconsciously stimulated causes the perseveration so common among brain-injured individuals.

It should be mentioned that not all investigators have obtained a positive effect for semantically related primes. Margolin and Friedrich (1985) used picture primes in a lexical decision task, a task in which subjects must decide if a string of letters constitute a real word. Subjects viewed 35 mm slide pairs presented via a microcomputer-controlled tachistoscope. The first slide was a simple line drawing of an object. The second was a letter string, which formed either a real word or a pronounceable nonword. In one condition, the picture and word were identical; in another, they were exemplars of the same class (cat/dog); in the third, they were unassociated, and in the fourth (neutral) condition, the prime was a nonsense design. An absence of semantic priming was observed in the AD patients, who were similar in degree of anomia to a group of stroke patients, in whom a priming effect was observed. A priming effect was observed in normal subjects as well.

A provocative finding from the priming literature comes from a study by Ober and Shenaut (1986) who reported "negative" priming in dementia patients. Nine patients with AD varying in severity from mild to moderate (mean score on the Mattis Dementia Rating Scale of 110.44, SD = 15.19) were asked to indicate whether a string of letters presented on a CRT screen formed a real word. The dependent variable was the amount of time required to make the lexical decision. For the semantic priming manipulation, each target word was used as its own control, enabling Ober and Shenaut to determine whether differences in reaction time existed between a target primed by a semantically related item and the same word primed by an unrelated item.

Normal control subjects were 25 ms faster in making an affirmative decision about a word that was preceded by a semantically related word than one preceded by an unrelated word. AD subjects were 59 ms slower responding to words that had been semantically primed. Ober concluded that AD patients experienced an interference effect from semantically related primes, probably from lateral inhibition, and believed the finding to be indicative of the preservation of associative relations within semantic memory.

Although provocative, the conclusion of Ober and Shenaut must be accepted cautiously, first, because of the small number of AD subjects; second, because of the wide variance in severity of dementia as evident by the large standard deviation on the Mattis Dementia Rating Scale; and third, because associative relations between concepts may exist, but not in the same manner as in healthy brains. Clearly, the AD patients were disordered, or they would have performed like the normal subjects. The fact that they performed significantly differently—that is, it took them significantly longer to name target words—is evidence that some aspect of SM, contents, or processes is disordered. In patients with mild dementia, SM is not empty (it may never be empty even in patients with very severe dementia), and the prime may have elicited some associated activation but only enough to generate confusion; therefore the response times increased.

Summary. The priming literature, though complex, is fascinating because it may be the best paradigm for answering the question whether the structure, as well as the processes, of SM deteriorate in dementia. At present, the results are mixed, and any firm conclusions would be premature. It is apparent, however, that information known premorbidly is treated differently from new information by the dementing nervous system. It may be that in mild dementia the priming effect will be detectable because the deterioration of conceptual knowledge is slight. In moderate and advanced dementia the effect may be diminished or negative because the primes are in some way familiar to the nervous system, but because of processing difficulties, conceptual deterioration, or both, the information is not processed in a normal way.

Before the evidence of the deterioration of the processes of SM is reviewed, the information presented in support of the claim that the contents of SM deteriorate will be summarized. Taken together, the reports of deterioration in the ability of dementia patients to name on confrontation, define, recognize, and associate words, and recognize and produce pantomime, suggest the possibility that the conceptual network, as well as the processes associated with using that network, is disrupted in dementing illness. The disruption occurs gradually, and in patients with mild dementia may be difficult to detect. By the time dementia is advanced, however, the inability of affected individuals to meaningfully use objects, or even imitate their use, leads us to suspect that conceptual knowledge deteriorates.

DETERIORATION IN THE PROCESSES OF SM

An elemental process of SM is the ability to infer. Inferences are conclusions based on the analysis of the relation(s) between two or more concepts, propositions, or schemata, and are fundamental to logical thought. Without an inferential mechanism, memory would be useless. Evidence of deterioration in the inferential capacity of dementia patients comes from many sources, among them studies of response latency, reading comprehension, and linguistic reasoning.

Evidence of Impaired Inferential Processing: Diminished Reading Comprehension Ability

The marked deterioration of reading comprehension in dementia patients was mentioned earlier, though not formally reviewed. Reading ability was explored in two of the well-known case studies of dementia patients, that of WLP, the patient of Schwartz et al. (1980), and Warrington's (1975) three agnosic patients. In WLP, a progressive deterioration in reading was observed during the 30 months when she was observed. Early in that period, when she could pronounce words like "liquor," "watch," "police," and "shoe," she was, nevertheless, unable to match the words to objects, nor could she sort printed object names with others from the same superordinate category. The disparity between her ability to read and comprehend became more evident later when she could fluently read the names of uncommon animals that she no longer recognized.

Like WLP, Warrington's agnosic patients with progressive dementia read words for which they were profoundly agnosic. As an aside, Warrington (1975) noted that the mechanical aspects of reading were intact and that the phonetic rules of English appeared to be a factor in whether the stimulus

Table 3-4. Performance of Dementia Patients and Elderly Controls on the BDAE Word-Picture Matching Subtest—Chicago Study

Groups	N	Year 1	Year 2	Year 3
Normals	39			
$\bar{X}$		9.97	9.92	9.92
SD		0.16	0.27	0.27
Dements	20			
$\bar{X}$		9.00	8.45	6.70
SD		1.34	1.73	2.79

Group $F(1,57) = 54.78$ ($p < .01$).
Year $F(2,56) = 7.70$ ($p = .01$).
Interaction $F(2,56) = 13.75$ ($p < .01$).

Table 3-6. Performance of Dementia Patients and Elderly Controls on the BDAE Oral Sentence-Reading Subtest—Chicago Study

Group	N	Year 1	Year 2	Year 3
Normals	39			
$\bar{X}$		9.72	9.59	9.67
SD		(0.72)	(0.68)	(0.53)
Dements	23			
$\bar{X}$		9.39	8.43	7.04
SD		(0.89)	(1.47)	(2.82)

Group $F(1,60) = 35.89$ ($p < .01$).
Year $F(2,59) = 8.39$ ($p < .01$).
Interaction $F(2,59) = 11.16$ ($p < .01$)

words were readable. Words whose pronunciation conformed to the general rules of English pronunciation were readable. However, when the agnosic patients were given the Nelson Reading Test (Nelson, 1962), a test containing words that are not spelled phonetically, their reading skills deteriorated, suggesting they were using a phonetic route only for access to the mental lexicon. The question might arise why the patient WLP could read words that were not spelled phonetically whereas Warrington's agnosic patients could not. The answer is that unlike Warrington's patients, WLP did not have a visual agnosia and could therefore read using the sight method. For Warrington's patients, the only intact input channel was the phonetic channel.

Table 3-5. Performance of Dementia Patients and Elderly Controls on the BDAE Word-Reading Subtest—Chicago Study

Groups	N	Year 1	Year 2	Year 3
Normals	39			
$\bar{X}$		29.97	30.00	29.69
SD		(0.16)	(0.00)	(1.15)
Dements	25			
$\bar{X}$		29.08	28.20	24.68
SD		(3.45)	(5.75)	(8.30)

Group $F(1,62) = 9.60$ ($p < .01$).
Year $F(2,61) = 6.20$ ($p < .01$).
Interaction $F(2,61) = 7.25$ ($p < .01$).

In the Chicago longitudinal study, reading ability was investigated using the BDAE word reading, word to picture matching, and oral sentence reading subtests. Mild dementia patients were significantly different from normal subjects at the time of initial testing in their performance on all three measures (Tables 3-4, 3-5, and 3-6). Further, a significant performance decline was observed on each reading test.

Reading comprehension of words, sentences, and paragraphs was investigated in 13 mild and 22 moderate dementia patients by Bayles et al. (1986) who devised a reading task in which stimuli in the word reading section were used in the composition of sentences and a paragraph. At each level (word, sentence, paragraph), mild AD patients performed significantly more poorly than normal elderly subjects (Table 3-7).

Linguistic Reasoning: Impaired in Dementia

The ability to reason linguistically has typically been investigated in three types of paradigms: verbal associative reasoning, linguistic disambiguation, and sentence judgment and correction.

Verbal Associative Reasoning Tasks. Linguistic reasoning tasks are inferential enterprises; thus, it is not surprising that the performance of dementia patients progressively deteriorates. One of the first

Table 3-7. Performance of Dementia Patients and Elderly Controls on the Reading Comprehension Task—Andrus Study

Group	N	Task			
		Word	Sentence	Paragraph	Total
Normals	26				
$\bar{X}$		7.35	6.38	2.85	17.27
SD		1.67	1.50	0.61	1.28
Mild AD	13				
$\bar{X}$		5.69*	3.92*	1.15*	10.92*
SD		1.49	2.06	1.14	3.35
Moderate AD	22				
$\bar{X}$		2.68*+	1.05*+	0.23*+	3.95*+
SD		2.51	1.68	0.43	4.19

*Mild AD and moderate AD subjects performed significantly differently from controls at $p < .01$ level.
+Moderate AD subjects performed significantly differently from mild AD subjects at $p < .01$ level.

reasoning tests to be used in dementia research was the Similarities subtest of the WAIS (Wechsler, 1955, 1981), in which individuals must explain how two things are alike. As the test progresses, the two objects for which a commonality must be identified become increasingly unrelated. For example, the first object pair is orange and banana; the last is fly and tree.

Similarities was the most discriminating of the WAIS subtests, after Block Design, discriminating AD patients from those with MID (Perez, Gay, and Taylor, 1975). The finding of the discriminant value of Block Design and Similarities subtests accords with the results of Crookes (1974).

Table 3-8. Performance of Dementia Patients and Elderly Controls on the WAIS Similarities Subtest—Tucson Study

Group	N	$\bar{X}$	SD
Normals	33	17.06	3.76
Mild AD	16	11.50*	5.70
Moderate AD	14	5.07*+	3.71

*Mild AD and moderate AD subjects performed significantly differently from controls at $p = .05$ level.
+Moderate AD subjects performed significantly differently from mild AD subjects at $p = .05$ level.

In the Tucson study of AD patients, the Similarities subtest was included as part of the assessment battery. The results of subject performance, according to dementia severity, are presented in Table 3-8. Patients with mild AD were significantly inferior to normal subjects in their ability to perform this verbal associative reasoning task.

Linguistic Disambiguation Tasks. In the seminal study of communication and dementia by the University of Arizona team, a linguistic disambiguation test was included, and it has been retained in some form as a test of reasoning in all subsequent studies (the most recent form is discussed in Chapter 7). The disambiguation of linguistically ambiguous sentences requires a variety of inferential maneuvers: lexical, structural and logical.

Lexical Ambiguity. In lexically ambiguous sentences, one of the words in the sentence can be meaningfully interpreted in more than one way, as in "The boy found a *bat*" or "The *solution* seemed clear in chemistry class." To perceive the ambiguity, the subject must identify the ambiguous word and verify both interpretations within the context of the sentence.

Structural Ambiguity. In sentences with structural ambiguity, the way in which the words are chunked can be meaningfully varied, as in "He told me to go without hesitation" and "She asked how old George was." In the first sentence, the phrase "without hesitation" can modify "told" or "go," in the second sentence, the word "old" can be grouped with "how" or "George."

Logical Ambiguity. Logically ambiguous sentences permit different interpretations in who or what was the actor and who or what was the recipient of the action, as in "The duck is ready to eat" and "Kurt wants the presidency more than Sara." It is our knowledge of the world that enables us to see the two interpretations. We know that ducks can eat and be eaten, and Kurt could want the presidency or Sara, and Sara could want the presidency, and Kurt could want the presidency more than Sara wants Kurt to have the presidency.

Because sentences can be designed to have a lexical, structural, or logical ambiguity, our rationale has been that the types of sentences missed by dementia patients would provide evidence about the relative vulnerability, in dementia, of certain linguistic operations. Up to a point, this has been true. The performance of dementia patients has demonstrated that lexical analysis is better preserved than structural and logical analysis. This finding accords with the general finding of many researchers that those language analysis tasks which are easiest for normal subjects are less likely to be impaired in dementing illness. Normals have less difficulty performing lexical disambiguation than structural or logical.

An Aside. An interesting piece of information obtained from the use of the linguistic disambiguation task is that contrary to what generative grammar theory would predict, logical ambiguities are not the hardest to disambiguate (MacKay, 1966; McKay and Bever, 1967). In our studies, normal subjects, as well as dementia patients, do not find them harder than structural ambiguities. Indeed, most subjects disambiguate logical and structural ambiguities with about the same degree of accuracy (a slight trend has been observed for structural ambiguity to be harder).

Back to the Point. The important point is that the capacity of mild dementia patients to perform a disambiguation task, when compared with normal elderly individuals matched for age and education, declines (Table 3-9). Thus, the task has proved useful for early differential diagnosis.

Table 3-9. Performance of Dementia Patients and Elderly Controls on the 30-item Sentence Disambiguation Task—Tucson Study

Group	N	Mean % Correct	SD
Normals	33	75.09	19.34
Mild AD	16	46.69*	26.87
Moderate AD	14	9.36*+	16.27

*Mild AD and moderate AD subjects performed significantly differently from controls at $p < .01$.

+Moderate AD subjects performed significantly differently from mild AD subjects at $p < .01$.

In its most recent revision, the disambiguation test was shortened from 30 to 10 items, and paraphrases for the ambiguous sentences were professionally illustrated to create a nonoral form in which subjects can choose the two sentence meanings from among two sets of four choices. Not surprisingly, the visual form of the test is easier than the oral nonvisual form. The performance of mild AD patients compared with normal subjects on both the oral and the visual portions was significantly poorer (Table 3-10). However, the fact remains that dementia patients are less able to use their linguistic reasoning, or inferential skills, to complete the task.

The reduction in the difficulty of this task appears to have improved its diagnostic value. When the shortened illustrated version of the test was compared with the longer oral form in an Australian study (Portsmouth, 1985), the ten item task was found to correctly classify a larger percentage of the subjects, 82 as opposed to 73 percent.

Table 3-10. Performance of Dementia Patients and Elderly Controls on the 10-Item Sentence Disambiguation Task—Andrus Study

Groups	N	$\bar{X}$	SD
Normals	27	7.46	2.12
Mild AD	13	2.69*	2.53
Moderate AD	23	1.17*	1.90

*Mild AD and moderate AD subjects performed significantly differently from controls at $p < .01$.

Sentence Judgment and Correction Tasks. The use of sentence judgment and correction tasks has given scientists insights about the dissociation between syntactic and conceptual analyses. The ability to make phonologic and syntactic judgments is more durable than semantic judgment, perhaps because it is less inferential.

In 1975, de Ajuriaguerra and Tissot reported performance results of dementia patients on a sentence judgment and correction task. Stimulus sentences contained one of two types of errors: morphosyntactic mistakes such as "Peter and John has left"; and logical errors, demonstrated by the use of conjunctions such as "why" and "too" and autonomous monemes such as "yesterday," e.g., "It is raining for I cannot go out." Sentences with morphosyntactic mistakes generally were corrected, whereas those with illogicalities were "either overlooked or inadequately corrected" (p. 333).

Whitaker's (1976) use of a sentence correction paradigm vividly revealed the isolability of grammatical (phonologic and syntactic) analysis from semantic. Whereas her patient, HCEM, automatically echoed corrections to syntactically and phonologically anomalous sentences, with no apparent appreciation of having made a correction, semantic errors were undetected.

In 1982, Bayles and Boone studied the selective correction phenomenon in a larger group of 35 dementia patients. Patients were given a sentence judgment and correction task comprising three sets of ten ill-formed sentences: phonologically, syntactically, and semantically. Within each group of ten incorrect sentences were three correct sentences. In the case of phonologically anomalous sentences, the subject was asked to state whether the sentence was spoken correctly and if not, to correct it. When subjects had difficulty correcting a sentence, because of poor task comprehension, they were asked to repeat it, though not in a word by word fashion. It was expected that the mildly demented individuals would be able to correct sentences with phonologic and syntactic errors but make significantly more errors than normal subjects on those with semantic errors. In Table 3-11 are the mean scores of dementia patients and normal subjects on the judgment and correction portions of the test.

Table 3-11. Performance of Dementia Patients and Elderly Controls on the Sentence Judgment and Correction Test

	Controls (N = 28)		AD (N = 35)	
Task	$\bar{X}$	SD	$\bar{X}$	SD
Phonology judgment	8.5	(1.7)	5.6*	(3.5)
Phonology correction	5.6	(1.6)	3.6*	(2.4)
Syntax judgment	12.2	(1.2)	9.4*	(4.4)
Syntax correction	8.7	(1.1)	6.4*	(2.9)
Semantics judgment	9.8	(0.5)	7.0*	(3.8)
Semantics correction	6.9	(0.6)	4.1*	(2.5)

*p = .001.

Patients with more severe dementia, who were unable to judge the well-formedness of the sentences, were expected, nonetheless, to spontaneously correct syntactic and phonologic errors when they repeated the sentences after the examiner. Most did. The seven severely demented study participants, who did not comprehend the nature of the task, were asked to repeat each sentence to ascertain whether they would make a spontaneous correction. Six made spontaneous corrections of syntax and phonology; in no case was a semantic error spontaneously corrected.

The performance of AD patients was significantly poorer than that of normal subjects on all aspects of the task. Error rates associated with the judgment and correction of phonologically anomalous sentences were greater than expected because of an inability to control for ambient noise. Patients were tested in a variety of settings (home, hospital, speech clinic), and the noise level was beyond the examiner's control.

Schwartz and colleagues (1979) used a sentence

correction test with WLP, their well-known patient with progressive dementia. WLP was unable to use semantic context in the written disambiguation of spoken homophones (i.e., nun–none, nose–knows, blue–blew) but could use modest syntactic cues to guide lexical selection. Schwartz and colleagues interpreted these results as being consistent with the relative preservation of syntactic operations coincident with marked semantic deterioration.

Ideation: Another Fundamental Process of SM

Ideation is the mind's ability to link concepts and propositions with each other and new information. Impoverished ideational capacity is a hallmark of dementia (Bayles, 1984; 1986; Bayles and Tomoeda, 1983b, Obler, 1983). Tasks in which ideational impairment is prominent include generative naming and the production of oral and written discourse.

Deterioration in Generative Naming Ability. In a test of generative naming, the subject is asked to generate instances of a particular category, for example, animals, items in a supermarket, or words that begin with a certain letter. Early in dementia, patients are able to conceptualize the task but typically name fewer exemplars than do normal subjects (Bayles and Tomoeda, 1983b; Cummings, Benson, Hill, and Read, 1985; Langhans, 1985; Martin and Fedio, 1983; Miller and Hague, 1975; Rosen, 1980; Weingartner et al., 1981). As dementia worsens, the number of unrelated examples increases and the number of acceptable examples falls. Ultimately patients seem unable to conceive of strategies for thinking of examples. Performance on generative naming tasks is strongly correlated with performance on memory tests (Weingartner et al., 1981).

Generative Naming: A Better Predictor of Early Dementia. Compared with confrontation naming, generative naming is more sensitive to the effects of early dementia (Bayles and Tomoeda, 1983b; Benson, 1979). In the study by Appell and colleagues (1982) the AD patients were "much better at naming objects than at word fluency, i.e., ability to produce a list of words belonging to a particular category" (p. 82). Similar results were obtained in the Tucson study, in which generative naming was found superior to confrontation naming for discriminating patients with mild dementia from normal subjects.

Martin, Brouwers, Cox, and Fedio (1985) gave a generative naming test to 14 AD patients. Patients were instructed to name as many items as possible that could be bought in a supermarket (Mattis Dementia Rating Scale; Mattis, 1976). Whereas both normal subjects and AD subjects tended to produce items from one category, for example vegetables, before switching to another category such as fruit, the AD patients generated significantly fewer category items.

Cummings and colleagues (1985) presented 30 Alzheimer's type dementia patients and 70 normal subjects with a word list generation task as part of an extensive language evaluation. AD subjects produced significantly fewer animal names (3.37) than did control subjects (23.20). Langhans (1985) found that the FAS Verbal Fluency Test was the only task, from among 13 cognitive, praxis, and language measures, to differentiate mild AD patients from normal subjects.

Generative naming tasks were included in both the Chicago and the Tucson studies of language and dementia. In the Chicago study the animal naming subtest from the BDAE (Goodglass and Kaplan, 1976) was used; in the Tucson study the FAS Verbal Fluency Test (Borkowski, Benton, and Spreen, 1967) was used. The typical performance of mild and moderately impaired dementia patients in these studies has been summarized in Tables 3-12 and 3-13. Notice the steep decline in response rate with dementia severity.

A related finding comes from a study of the "generation effect" by Mitchell, Hunt, and Schmitt (1986). The generation effect refers to the fact that internally generated information is more memorable than information received from external sources (Slameck and Graf, 1978). Mitchell and colleagues hypothesized that if the generation effect is due to SM processing, then AD patients should fail to exhibit it because of a putative deterioration in SM generative capacity. Subjects were asked to read sentences aloud and either generate an object to com-

Table 3-12. Performance of Dementia Patients and Elderly Controls on the BDAE Animal-Naming Subtest—Chicago Study

Group	N	Year 1	Year 2	Year 3
Controls	39			
X̄		18.59	19.10	18.36
SD		4.85	4.27	5.21
Dementia	23			
X̄		10.61	8.26	5.52
SD		4.31	4.32	3.65

Group $F(1,60) = 117.43$ ($p < .0001$).
Year $F(2,59) = 5.91$ ($p < .005$).
Interaction $F(2,59) = 6.74$ ($p < .002$).

plete the sentence or read the one furnished by the examiner. After an intervening task, a recall test was given and subjects had to indicate whether the subject–object pair presented by the examiner came from a sentence they had generated or one provided by the examiner that they read. As predicted, dementia patients did not exhibit a generation effect. Although dementia patients were similar to normal subjects in their ability to identify subject-object pairs provided by the examiner, recall for internally generated objects was significantly less than for normal controls.

Disordered Oral and Written Discourse. The production of meaningful oral or written discourse requires conceptual activation and processing. Concepts must be linked and propositions formed and ordered in the proper sequence. Because written discourse is harder to generate than oral for normal individuals and persons with dementia, direct comparison of the two types is inappropriate.

Oral Discourse. Both the content and form of oral discourse are influenced by the type of elicitation procedure employed. For example, when subjects are asked to describe common objects, discourse syntax is likely to be simple and repetitive, as in, "It is sharp, and shiny, and useful. It's a nail." When the task is to orally describe a procedure, much of the syntax will be designed to mark the sequence of steps defining the procedure. Often discourse is elicited through picture description, an approach that may elicit more elaborate syntax and logical forms, especially if the picture has a moral or gist.

The aspect of discourse that has proved most descriptive of dementing illness effects is the number of ideas produced (Bartol, 1979; Bayles, 1982; Horner, Heyman, Kanter, Royall, and Aker, 1983; Ripich, Spinelli, and Terrell, 1983; Santo Pietro and Berman, 1984). Whereas the number of words generated may not diminish, the number of ideas expressed does. Other discourse characteristics typical of dementia include reduced phrase length and an increase in the number of repetitions, irrelevancies, and intrusions (Horner et al., 1983), diminished vocabulary diversity (Bayles, 1986) more frequent use of indefinite reference (Kempler and Curtiss, 1983; Obler, 1983), and "omission of all the terms implicit in the extralinguistic situation" (de Ajuriaguerra and Tissot, 1975, p. 329).

Bartol (1979) describes the discourse of dementia patients as empty and replete with stereotypies. Stereotypies are highly predictable, overused phrases. Kirshner, Webb, Kelly, and Wells (1984) wrote that the "spontaneous speech typically remains fluent and composed of normal grammatical structure, although the content of speech becomes devoid of abstract content" (p. 496). Irigaray (1973) and Obler (1983) mention the overuse of indefinite reference, as does Kempler (1984), whose discourse analysis revealed pronouns with no antecedents and deictic (referential) terms with no clear or recoverable points of reference. Circumlocution is another oft-noted feature of the language of dementia (Obler, 1983; Critchley; 1964). Critchley observed that dementia patients seem to form appropriate

Table 3-13. Performance of Dementia Patients and Elderly Controls on FAS-Word Fluency Measure—Tucson Study

Groups	N	X̄	SD
Controls	21	36.48	12.19
Mild AD	9	23.33*	11.20
Moderate AD	8	12.88*	15.00

*Mild AD and moderate AD subjects performed significantly differently from controls at $p < .05$.

semantic intentions, but as their memory for recent events deteriorates, their intentions are forgotten and they stop in the midst of an utterance.

As dementia severity worsens, utterance content becomes more disordered (Bayles, 1984; Bayles and Tomoeda, 1983a; Santo Pietro and Berman, 1984). Notice, in the following samples, the dramatic difference between the discourse content of patients with mild dementia and those with more severe dementia.

Discourse Sample 1: Mild AD

Button: This is a button, it's round. It has an indented round circle in the middle. And then it has a triangle around the little eye holes. And it's gray. I don't know the size, perhaps three quarters of an inch. I don't see, know anything else. Did I say gray, yeah.

Nail: Well, some people call it a, a straight pin but I've never used that expression. I call it a stick pin, but this is an unusually stout one. They're usually finer, and it's gray, grayish metal. Is that alright? I never say straight pin or straight hair, but I did even say, well, did you ever see a crooked one?

Discourse Sample 2: Moderate AD

Button: Well, this is very good to keep your clothes together. Yes, I guess your clothes together would be buttons. It's a button and it's, uh, very important to, uh, in fact just yesterday, no last night, I sewed one on the inside and one on the outside because it was, uh, it was outside of my, it was a dress.

Envelope: It is a piece of paper and attached to it is another paper of some kind and, uh, the surfaces are a-all seem to be shiny n-not necessarily shiny but, uh, uh, they aren't hacked up in any way. They are, they're, uh, for the purposes of showing what is being done by this paper.

Table 3-14. Performance of Dementia Patients and Elderly Controls on the Verbal Description Task—Tucson Study

Group	N	$\bar{X}$	SD
Controls	33	37.00	9.22
Mild AD	16	21.75*	9.05
Moderate AD	14	13.57*	4.62

*Mild AD and Moderate AD subjects performed significantly differently from controls at $p < .05$.

Discourse Sample 3: Severe AD

Nail: It's a nail that got caught in a purse. Apparently somebody stepped on it real good. It makes animals mad when you touch it in them. That's what stops the beating up of little koala bears. It has a nice movement to be had. And I can't feel any breaks in it.

Pin: Well, it's, uh, w-crewnut, you know. Uh hun, ye. What you call a crew-neck, because it's almost howl-neck. I trust you can't find it so good otherwise.

These discourse samples were elicited in a verbal description task. Subjects were asked to describe, as completely as possible, a nail, a button, a marble, and an envelope. Subject responses were audiorecorded and later transcribed for analysis. A count was made of the number of relevant information units produced. As can be seen in Table 3-14, the number of units distinguished the normal subjects from those with mild AD and subjects with mild from those with moderate dementia.

Written Discourse. Because of the value of the aforementioned verbal description task, other discourse production tasks have been added to the Ari-

Table 3-15. Performance of Dementia Patients and Elderly Controls on the Written Description Task—Andrus study

		Information Units		Gist	
Groups	N	$\bar{X}$	SD	$\bar{X}$	SD
Control	25	32.44	9.98	16.40	6.25
Mild AD	9	9.56*	6.71	4.89*	6.17
Moderate AD	19	1.79*+	4.30	1.05*	3.22

*Mild AD and moderate AD subjects performed significantly differently from controls at $p < .05$.
+Moderate AD subjects performed significantly differently from mild AD subjects at $p < .05$.

zona test battery, notably, written explanations of Norman Rockwell paintings. In the written description task, dementia patients not only produced fewer ideas but failed to derive the gist of the pictures (Table 3-15). The samples of the written discourse of dementia patients (Figure 3-1) reveal an increase in sentence fragments, perseverations, and a decrease in vocabulary diversity.

Summary

An aforestated purpose of this chapter was the documentation of the claim that the contents and processes of SM progressively deteriorate in dementing illness. Toward that end, a substantial literature was reviewed that depicts the progressive impairment in linguistic communication of dementia patients. Documentation was provided of problems in confrontation naming, vocabulary, pantomime, word associations, reading comprehension, verbal associative reasoning, linguistic disambiguation, sentence judgment and correction, generative naming, and oral and written discourse. Findings from each of these paradigms were interpreted as evidence of conceptual deterioration or processing deficits. The authors are fully cognizant of the arbitrariness of interpreting the performance data as evidence of either deterioration in conceptual knowledge, or the ability to use that knowledge, but believe in the heuristic value of this conceptualization for greater understanding of the behavioral changes seen in dementia patients. Consideration of the published literature in this way forces the reader to think about the nature of SM, or the mind; the assumptions of popular research paradigms; and the variables likely to confound data interpretation. Though the designation of a particular research finding as being supportive of one or the other claims is debatable, the existence of the deterioration is not.

THE DETERIORATION OF SM: IMPLICATIONS FOR MODULARITY THEORY

If the central system, or SM, is particularly impaired, that fact has significance for how modularity is defined. Recall that Fodor, (1983) in his book *Modularity of the Mind,* makes the claim that the mind consists of at least six modular perceptual input systems and a nonmodular central system. The perceptual input systems receive and transduce sensory information into a form readable by the central system. The nonmodular central system is responsible for fixing belief and planning intelligent action. Three important definitional criteria of modularity are, according to Fodor, that they have fixed neural architecture (are hard wired, that is, have "privileged paths of informational access" [Fodor, 1983, p. 98]), can be selectively impaired, and have a characteristic pattern of breakdown. Central systems, on the other hand, do not have fixed neural architecture, cannot be selectively impaired, and do not have a characteristic pattern of breakdown. It is in relation to these three features that the evidence from dementia patients is noteworthy, for the authors contend that the performance of dementia patients demonstrates the particular impairment of the central system, a characteristic pattern of breakdown, and therefore a fixed neural architecture.

Dementia: Particular Impairment of SM. The literature reviewed in this chapter is offered as evidence of the particular impairment of the central system. Indeed, analysis of the performance data from dementia patients shows that they gradually lose the ability to decide what is true or false about the world and to plan intelligently, though they retain the ability to receive and transduce sensory information. It is the dissociability between grammatical processing abilities and communication that makes the particular impairment of the central system, or SM, apparent. Dementia patients suffer impairment in the ability to communicate while retaining considerable knowledge of language. This point has been emphasized throughout the book. Dementia patients process word forms, syntax, and phonology, but not meaning and use. Thus, in patients with mild and moderate dementia, the language module, as Fodor presents it, appears preserved.

Remember that in Fodor's model language is identified as one of the perceptual modules. The

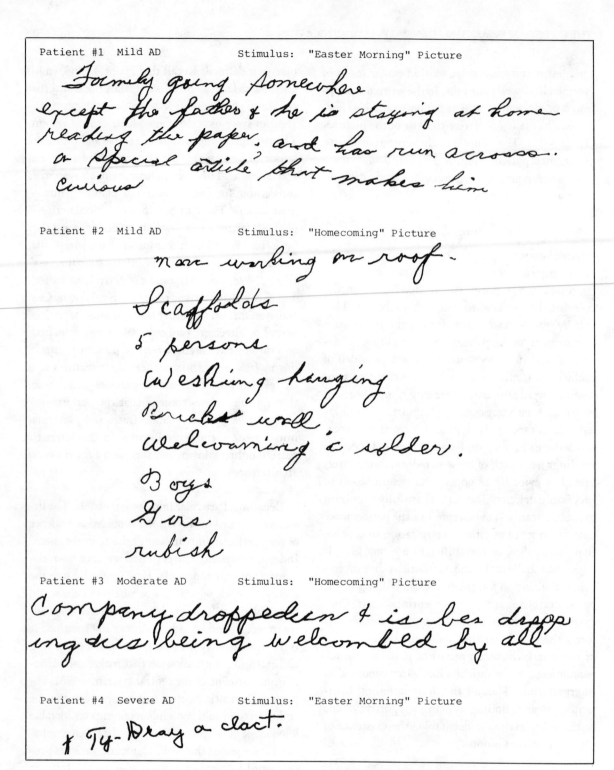

Patient #1 Mild AD Stimulus: "Easter Morning" Picture

Family going somewhere
except the father & he is staying at home
reading the paper, and has run across
a special article that makes him
curious

Patient #2 Mild AD Stimulus: "Homecoming" Picture

man working on roof.
Scaffolds
5 persons
Washing hanging
Bricks wall
Welcoming a solder.
Boys
Girs
rubish

Patient #3 Moderate AD Stimulus: "Homecoming" Picture

Company droppedein & is bes dropp
ing dus being welcombed by all

Patient #4 Severe AD Stimulus: "Easter Morning" Picture

& Ty-Dray a clact.

Figure 3-1. *Written discourse samples of dementia patients.*

language module specifies, for any utterance in its domain, "its linguistic and maybe its logical form. It is implicit . . . that it does no more than that—e.g., that it does not recover speech-act potential (except, perhaps, insofar as speech-act potential may be correlated with properties of form, as in English interrogative word order)" (Fodor, 1983, p. 90).

The neuropathologic and neurochemical changes associated with Alzheimer's dementia appear to result from particular impairment in the cellular circuits dependent upon certain neurochemicals. One such circuit originates in the basal forebrain and involves widespread areas of cortex and subcortex, a circuit that depends upon the neurotransmitter acetylcholine for operation. The authors recognize that the data currently available about the neurochemistry of dementia are insufficient to completely define the central system, but the progress made in the last decade from the study of dementia patients is encouraging.

FURTHER CONCEPTUALIZATION OF SM

During the introduction to the chapter, the reader was advised of its organization around the defense of two major theoretical claims: first, that the contents and processes of SM deteriorate in dementing illness, and second, that the data from communication studies of dementia substantiate a conceptualization of SM as a conscious and nonconscious cognitive faculty in which concepts, but not their linguistic representations are stored. This second claim will now be discussed.

The discussion will have two parts. In the first, the evidence for characterizing SM as both a conscious and nonconscious cognitive faculty will be considered, and in the second, the evidence for the dissociability of conceptual knowledge and its linguistic representation will be further discussed.

SM: A Conscious and Nonconscious Conceptual Store

The logic of the argument that SM processes conceptual information at both a conscious and nonconscious level will take the following form:

1. Conceptual knowledge is represented in SM.
2. Analysis of meaning requires activation of conceptual knowledge.
3. Certain aspects of meaning analysis occur at a nonconscious level.
4. Therefore, conscious and nonconscious analyses of meaning are carried out in SM.

In Chapter 2, the concept was defined as the elemental structural unit of SM, and though the psychological reality of conceptual knowledge is not in dispute, the functional characteristics of the conceptual processing system are. One debatable characteristic is whether SM is only a conscious system, as Tulving (1985) argues. It will be argued that the data from the study of semantic priming, and the resolution of lexical ambiguity, suggest it is not.

Evidence from Semantic Priming

Semantic priming is the phenomenon in which a stimulus (e.g., a word, string of letters, category name) facilitates a target response (e.g., naming a word, deciding if a string of letters is a word, providing an example of a category), because the target is semantically related to the stimulus. For example, the word "rain" is processed faster after the stimulus "umbrella" than after the stimulus "apple."

Facilitation, which results in a faster response after a semantically related prime, is thought to occur because the concept activated by the original stimulus activates related concepts as well. This process, described as spreading activation (Quillian, 1962, 1967), occurs without the subject's awareness (Hasher and Zacks, 1979; Posner and Snyder, 1975). Although individuals can initiate a systematic, consciously directed search of semantic memory, the priming effect occurs subconsciously.

The idea of activation spreading throughout the conceptual network was used by Quillian (1962, 1967) as a model for how to build a computer program that would simulate human semantic processing. Since Quillian proposed his theory, numerous investigators have studied priming effects, and most often they have used one of four paradigms: word naming, lexical decision, category instance generation, and multiple categories.

Word Naming. In the word naming paradigm, subjects are asked to name a word, called a target, that is preceded by a stimulus (the stimulus can be a related word, unrelated word, letter, nonsense word, etc.) as fast as possible. When the target words are preceded by a semantically related word stimulus, subjects are able to name them faster (Warren, 1977; Katz and Feldman, 1983) than when the stimulus is unrelated.

Lexical Decision. In the lexical decision paradigm, subjects are asked to judge whether strings of letters following a prime are real words. The prime may be related or unrelated to the target, which may or may not be a word. When the prime is semantically related, subjects make faster judgments (Fischler and Goodman, 1978; Meyer and Schvaneveldt, 1971; Meyer, Schvaneveldt, and Ruddy, 1975; Morton, 1969).

Category Instance Generation. In the category instance generation paradigm (Freedman and Loftus, 1971), subjects must provide an instance of a category that begins with a given letter or is characterized by a given adjective. In this paradigm, the presentation order of the category name is varied. In one condition, subjects are given the category name first, for example, "transportation," then a letter such as "R," after which they are asked to provide an instance of the category, one of which might be "rickshaw." In another condition, subjects are given the letter (or an adjective) first, such as "A," and then the name of the category, for example, "transportation," and then asked to provide an exemplar. In yet another condition, the adjective is given first. Freedman and Loftus (1971) observed that subjects are faster when the category is presented first; they reasoned that the specification of the category caused the activation of the concept embodied in the category and certain related concepts, as well. When, however, a letter or adjective was given first, the activation spread to a much larger set of concepts making the retrieval of an exemplar more time-consuming. For example, consider the multiplicity of concepts the letter "A," or an adjective like "green," would activate.

Multiple Categories. Juola and Atkinson (1971) reported an increase in reaction time with multiple categories. They used a task in which subjects had to decide whether a stimulus word belonged to one of a variable number of categories, as compared with judging whether a stimulus word was the same as one of a variable number of target words. Juola and Atkinson argued that each additional target category adds more instances that must be searched, whereas each additional target word adds only one: the word itself.

Additional evidence that human semantic processing might be something like the conceptualizations of Quillian, and later Collins and Loftus (1975), comes from the reports of interference effects in semantic priming when multiple semantically related primes are given. It appears that when the relations between concepts are primed, inhibition of activation of competing relations also occurs (Roediger and Neely, 1982; Blaxton and Neely, 1983; Brown, 1981). Therefore, when multiple semantically related primes are presented, the priming effect is diminished because of interference with the inhibition process.

A question that has probably arisen in the reader's mind is whether the data from these different research paradigms are interpretable in the same way, namely as evidence of semantic (conceptual) priming. Is it possible that semantic memory is not what is activated? Could activation be occurring in lexical memory instead? According to some scholars (Fodor, 1983; Forster, 1981; Lupker, 1984), the answer to these questions is yes, and the data that are thought to be misinterpreted come from the naming paradigm.

Naming Priming May Only Access Lexical Memory. Forster (1981) and Lupker (1984) reason that when the target words named in the naming paradigm are semantically (that is, conceptually) related to the prime, they are also related as word associates. Lupker writes, "what might appear to be semantic priming in naming tasks would be really nothing more than the effect of uncontrolled associative relationships. At present there appears to be no clear resolution of this issue since in most studies using the naming task the word pairs were specifically selected for their high associative strength (e.g., Becker and Killion, 1977; Meyer et al., 1975)" (p. 710).

To critically test whether conceptual, as opposed to lexical, memory is primed, the researcher would have to demonstrate a priming effect with stimulus pairs that are related semantically but *not* associatively, for example, "spatula and spoon," "goat and cat." Although spatula and spoon are both kitchen utensils, and goat and cat are both animals, spatula is not a typical associate of spoon or vice versa; neither is an individual likely to say goat if the stimulus is cat. Lupker's purpose (1984) was to test whether a priming effect is obtained for stimulus pairs that are conceptually but not associatively related. Lupker used the "name the prime-name the target task" of Irwin and Lupker (1983), which was designed to eliminate, as far as possible, any associative strength between the word pairs while preserving semantic relations. Reaction times were measured for naming nonrelated (neither semantically or associatively) word pairs (primes and targets) and compared with reaction times for naming semantically (only) related pairs.

Sixteen college students were told they would see a series of word pairs and to say each word as rapidly as possible when it appeared. When the results of the study were analyzed, little, if any, facilitation was obtained when targets were preceded by semantically similar primes. Lupker concluded that simple semantic similarity provides little facilitation in a naming task, a finding that supports Fodor's (1983) suggestion that priming in naming tasks is essentially an associative phenomenon.

Lupker (1984) subsequently conducted a lexical decision task in an attempt to demonstrate semantic priming for nonassociated word pairs. He theorized that if a priming effect could be produced in a lexical decision task, it would be strong evidence that the effects of a semantic relationship depend on the task and that many pervious accounts of priming are too simple. Using 18 college students, he obtained a significant semantic priming effect and concluded that the amount of priming provided by pairs related semantically, but not associatively, is task dependent. Lupker suggests that there are two primeable processes, a "preaccess process" and a "postaccess process." The preaccess process that can "be facilitated by activation spreading along the links of a network of direct associations" (p. 727). Semantic relations between infrequently associated concepts would have no influence in this network, which is what occurs in naming. The "postaccess process" is more susceptible to the influences of semantic relations. In a lexical decision task, not only do subjects have to pronounce the letter string (preaccess process), but they must make a decision about whether it is a real word (postaccess process).

The fact that the interpretation of data from the naming paradigm studies is debatable does not negate, however, the fact that priming can occur in both semantic and lexical memory, independently or concurrently. The consistent reports of priming effects in a variety of paradigms are compelling evidence that the process of linguistic comprehension originates with, and is facilitated by, a process of activation within lexical and semantic memory of related words and concepts. Although scholars debate about the inferences that can be drawn from the different models, consensual agreement exists that the activation or priming occurs subconsciously. Therefore, the characterization of SM as only a conscious system seems inaccurate.

Resolution of Linguistic Ambiguity: Evidence for Nonconscious Lexical Processing?

Consider that the nervous system may be capable of processing all possible meanings of ambiguous words and sentences without the language user's awareness. This is the major debatable issue related to the processing of linguistic ambiguity. Are all readings of an ambiguous word or sentence processed when an instance of lexical ambiguity is encountered, or do natural language contexts constrain the lexical retrieval process in such a way that only contextually appropriate meaning is accessed? Reaction time studies have been a popular paradigm for studying this issue, the theory being that if all meanings are accessed before one is selected, then processing time is longer. Foss (1970) and Foss and Jenkins (1973) reported that subjects took more time to respond to the presence of a particular phoneme at the beginning of a word if it was preceded by an ambiguous word. Using the same technique, Cairns and Kamerman (1975) obtained similar results. Further, they demonstrated that reaction time differences disappeared when words containing target phonemes did not immediately follow the ambiguous words.

Mehler, Segui, and Carey (1978) questioned the results of these studies, suggesting that word length was a possible artifact, one that could account for the increase in response time that Foss and Jenkins attributed to the activation of all possible meanings. Mehler and colleagues argued that the ambiguous words used by Foss and Jenkins and by Cairns and Kamerman were generally shorter than the unambiguous words, an important fact because longer words are thought to be more redundant. In long words it is primarily the initial syllable(s) that influence perception. After the processing of the initial syllable(s), the word is likely to be identified, making the amount of information provided in the final syllables redundant. Thus, the processing of a long word can be completed before the final syllable. Mehler and colleagues reasoned that if the ambiguous prime is a long word, then, at the moment when the target word is processed, the processing load is light (because the system is processing the redundant portion of the long word) and the mechanism can respond more quickly. On the other hand, with short words, the processor is likely to be highly loaded when the target word appears because short words have less redundancy. Therefore reaction time is increased. Thus, Mehler and colleagues controlled the length and frequency of words preceding the target phoneme of a word and found that ambiguity of a word preceding the target did not cause an increase in the time required for phoneme detection. These results contradicted the hypothesis of Foss and Jenkins that an ambiguous word necessarily increases reaction time processing. Subsequently, similar findings were reported by Newman and Dell (1978).

Another type of study, in which multiple activation was reported, was conducted by Holmes, Arwas, and Garrett (1977). They used a "rapid serial visual presentation" technique in which subjects were presented with a sentence at a rate of 16 words per second. Subjects were to report as many words as possible, and the number reported was considered to represent the subjects' ability to organize the input sentence. Holmes and associates found that fewer words were recalled from sentences containing ambiguous words, even when these were biased towards one meaning.

Semantic Priming Paradigms and the Study of Ambiguity. More recently, semantic priming paradigms have been used to determine which readings of an ambiguous word are accessed. If a particular reading is accessed, then priming of targets related to that meaning should exist. Most recent studies employ one of two priming techniques. The first method compares the recognition of target words that are primed by ambiguous and unambiguous words; the second method uses ambiguous primes only, followed by targets that are related to one or the other meaning of the ambiguous prime.

In the first method, equal facilitation of the target responses by ambiguous or unambiguous words suggests that both meanings have been retrieved in the ambiguous case. This results from the fact that if only one meaning were activated, one would expect facilitation equal to half that seen in the unambiguous condition, because the meaning consistent with the target would be activated by chance on half the trials (Simpson and Burgess, 1985). Equal facilitation has been reported for ambiguous and unambiguous primes (Holley-Wilcox and Blank, 1980; Seidenberg, Tananhaus, Leiman, and Bienkowski, 1982).

Simpson (1981) used the second method, in which ambiguous primes are followed by targets related to one or the other meaning, and reported greater priming effects for words related to the dominant meaning of the homograph (saw, lead) than for those related to the subordinate meaning (Simpson, 1981). Simpson's result led to the conclusion that in the absence of context, only the most frequent meaning of an ambiguous word is retrieved. However, Simpson and Burgess (1985) suggest that the interpretation of the results in Simpson's study may be confounded by its design. Subjects were required to make lexical decisions to both the prime and target, the consequence of which was that the amount of elapsed time between the prime and target varied across trials and was often long. During the interval between the presentation of the prime and target, all the meanings of the prime could have been retrieved and reviewed and all but the most frequent suppressed. Many investigators favor a model in which an exhaustive meaning analysis is said to occur before one meaning is selected (Onifer and Swinney, 1981; Seidenberg et al., 1982; Swinney, 1979; Tanenhaus, Leiman, and Seidenberg, 1979). These investigators have reported that after ambiguous primes, words related to either meaning are responded to more quickly than unrelated targets. But, when the prime–target interval is lengthened, only the meaning that is consistent with the context shows facilitation, compared with unrelated targets.

Most Favor the Multiple Activation Theory. As yet, most language scientists favor the exhaustive search explanation of the processing of ambiguous words in sentential contexts (Simpson and Burgess, 1985). Initially all meanings are retrieved, but subsequently context is used to select the appropriate meaning (Onifer and Swinney, 1981; Seidenberg et al., 1982; Swinney, 1979; Tanenhaus et al., 1979; Yates, 1978). Simpson and Burgess (1985), by manipulating the interval between the onset of the prime and the target, concluded that while all meanings are retrieved, when homographs are presented alone, the meanings become available in the order of their frequency.

The Point in Relation to SM. What is salient to our argument is that all the meanings of lexically ambiguous words appear to be processed before one is favored (and the others suppressed), and this operation occurs subconsciously. To state the argument another way, semantic memory contents are activated and processes employed without the language user's awareness. These facts about nonconscious processing of linguistic ambiguity, together with the evidence of a nonconscious semantic priming effect, result in a paradoxical situation in relation to the definition of SM. Remember that SM is conceptualized as both a conscious system (Tulving, 1985) and the system in which conceptual information is processed. But, given the evidence from semantic priming and linguistic disambiguation, it would seem that either SM has a nonconscious component or another system processes conceptual information. In the opinion of these authors, the most parsimonious explanation is that SM is both a conscious and nonconscious system.

SM: A Conceptual, But Not a Lexical Store

The defense of SM as a store that contains concepts, but not their lexical representation, will consist of the following argumentation:

1. If concepts and their linguistic representations (words) have a shared representation in neuronal circuitry, they would not be dissociable.
2. Evidence from a variety of sources demonstrates the dissociability of concepts and words.
3. Therefore, concepts and words do not have a shared representation in neuronal circuitry.

The concept of dissociability is the key to understanding this argument. In terms of this issue, dissociability means the degree to which aspects of cognition can be separately impaired. Vania and Hintikka (1984) write that "central to . . . cognitive science today is the assumption that the organization of cognitive processes is revealed through the dissociation of their function" (p. *x*). The pervasive finding, indeed the common thread in the literature on dementia and communication, is that words are dissociable from the concepts they represent. Indeed, this is the most interesting aspect of the data obtained in the study of dementia patients. Dementia patients read words they no longer comprehend, utter words meaninglessly, and unknowingly correct grammatical errors. The meaning and use systems of linguistic communication are particularly impaired and dissociated from grammatical aspects of language. Yet, the repository for word forms remains, ultimately to be accessed by an intentionless mind. The study of the dementia patient has left us with a tantalizing unanswered question: where are the words? If they are not represented with the concepts, where are they?

GENERAL SUMMARY AND CLINICAL IMPLICATIONS

1. **A theoretic model characterizing the cognitive and communicative dysfunctions of dementia patients is proposed. It is argued that dementia patients suffer particular impairment in the processes and likely the contents, of semantic memory (SM).**
2. **Clinicians who appreciate the theoretic issues to which the data from dementia patients relate will be better prepared to interpret patient behavior and predict the course of behavioral change.**
3. **The difficulty dementia patients have defining words, naming objects and items in a category, pantomiming, and associating words may be evidence of deterioration in the contents of SM.**
4. **Deterioration of SM processes becomes obvious in tasks requiring dementia patients to create, relate, and order ideas. Examples of such tasks are reading comprehension, verbal associative reasoning, linguistic disambiguation, generative naming, and oral and written discourse.**
5. **The mechanical aspects of reading, writing, and speaking are largely spared in early and moderate dementia. Sometimes dementia patients are thought to have greater communicative competency than they actually do because of their ability to talk and read aloud.**
6. **The fact that dementia patients can read words without processing meaning, and produce grammatical but nonsensical verbal utterances, suggests that concepts and their lexical representations are stored separately. Clinicians must be careful about concluding that conceptual knowledge is intact from performance on a confrontation naming (or priming naming task) only. Naming may access only lexical and not semantic memory.**
7. **Within SM, some processing of meaning appears to occur without the language user's conscious awareness, notably the disambiguation of linguistic ambiguity and semantic (conceptual) priming.**
8. **Nonconscious meaning processing suggests that SM should be conceptualized as both a nonconscious and a conscious system.**

REFERENCES

deAjuriaguerra, J., and Tissot, R. (1975). Some aspects of language in various forms of senile dementia (comparisons with language in childhood). In E.H. Lenneberg and E. Lenneberg (Eds.), *Foundations of Language Development: Vol. 1* (pp. 323-339). New York: Academic Press.

Appell, J., Kertesz, A., and Fisman, M. (1982). A study of language functioning in Alzheimer's patients. *Brain and Language, 17*, 73-91.

Bartol, M.A. (1979). Nonverbal communication in patients with Alzheimer's disease. *Journal of Gerontological Nursing, 5*, 21-31.

Bayles, K.A. (1982). Language function in senile dementia. *Brain and Language, 16*, 265-280.

Bayles, K.A. (1984). Language and dementia. In A. Holland (Ed.), *Recent advances: Speech, hearing and language pathology* (pp. 209-244). San Diego, CA: College-Hill Press.

Bayles, K.A. (1985, February). *Effects of dementing illness on communicative function*. Paper presented as part of symposium to the International Neuropsychological Society, San Diego, CA.

Bayles, K.A. (1986). Management of neurogenic communication disorders associated with dementia. In R. Chapey (Ed.), *Language intervention strategies in adult aphasia* (pp. 462-473). Baltimore, MD: Williams and Wilkins.

Bayles, K.A., and Boone, D.R. (1982). The potential of language tasks for identifying senile dementia. *Journal of Speech and Hearing Disorders, 47*, 210-217.

Bayles, K.A., Boone, D.R., Tomoeda, C.K., and Slauson, T.J. (1986). [Neurogenic communication disorders in adults: Andrus study]. Unpublished raw data.

Bayles, K.A., and Tomoeda, C.K. (1983a). Confrontation naming impairment and dementia. *Brain and Language, 19*, 98-114.

Bayles, K.A., and Tomoeda, C.K. (1983b). Confrontation and generative naming abilities of dementia patients. In R.H. Brookshire (Ed.), *Proceedings of the clinical aphasiology conference* (pp. 304-315). Minneapolis, MN: BRK Publishers.

Becker, C.A., and Killion, T.H. (1977). Interaction of visual and cognitive effects in word recognition. *Journal of Experimental Psychology: Human Perception and Performance, 3*, 389-401.

Benson, D.F. (1979). Neurologic correlates of anomia. In H. Whitaker and H.A. Whitaker (Eds.), *Studies in Neurolinguistics, Vol. 4* (pp. 293-328). New York: Academic Press.

Blaxton, T.A., and Neely, J.H. (1983). Inhibition from semantically related primes: Evidence of category-specific inhibition. *Memory and Cognition, 11*, 500-510.

Borkowski, J.G., Benton, A.L., and Spreen, O. (1967). Word fluency and brain damage. *Neuropsychologia, 5*, 135-140.

Bower, T.G.R. (1970). Reading by eye. In H. Levin and J.P. Williams (Eds.), *Basic studies in reading* (pp. 134-146). New York: Basic Books.

Bowles, N.L., and Poon, L.W. (1985). Effects of priming in word retrieval. *Journal of Experimental Psychology, 11*, 272-283.

Brandt, J., Spencer, M., McSorley, P., and Folstein, M.F. (1986, February). *Memory activation and implicit remembering in Alzheimer's disease*. Paper presented at the meeting of the International Neuropsychological Society, Denver, CO.

Brown, A.S. (1979). Priming effects in semantic memory retrieval processes. *Journal of Experimental Psychology: Human Learning and Memory, 5*, 65-77.

Brown, A.S. (1981). Inhibition in cued retrieval. *Journal of Experimental Psychology: Human Learning and Memory, 7*, 204-215.

Cairns, H.S., and Kamerman, J. (1975). Lexical information processing during sentence comprehension. *Journal of Verbal Learning and Verbal Behavior, 14*, 170-179.

Clark, H.H., and Clark, E.V. (1977). *Psychology and language*. New York: Harcourt Brace Jovanovich.

Collins, A.M., and Loftus, E.F. (1975). A spreading activation theory of semantic processing. *Psychological Review, 82*, 407-428.

Critchley, M. (1964). The neurology of psychotic speech. *British Journal of Psychiatry, 110*, 353-364.

Crookes, T.G. (1974). Indices of early dementia on WAIS. *Psychological Reports, 34*, 734.

Cummings, J.L., Benson, D.F., Hill, M., and Read, S. (1985). Aphasia in dementia of the Alzheimer type. *Neurology, 34*, 394-397.

Dunn, L.M. (1959). *The Peabody Picture Vocabulary Test* (original edition). Circle Pines, MN: American Guidance Service.

Ernst, B., Dalby, M.A., and Dalby, A. (1970). Aphasic disturbances in presenile dementia. *Acta Neurologica Scandinavica, 46*(Suppl. 43), 99-100.

Fischler, I., and Goodman, G.O. (1978). Latency of associative activation in memory. *Journal of Experimental Psychology: Human Perception and Performance, 4*, 455-470.

Fodor, J.A. (1983). *The modularity of the mind*. Cambridge, MA: The MIT Press.

Forster, K.I. (1981). Priming and the effects of sentence and lexical contexts on naming time: Evidence for autonomous lexical processing. *Quarterly Journal of Experimental Psychology, 33A*, 465-495.

Foss, D.J. (1970). Some effects of ambiguity upon sentence comprehension. *Journal of Verbal Learning and Verbal Behavior, 9*, 699-7006.

Foss, D.J., and Jenkins, C.M. (1973). Some effects of context on the comprehension of ambiguous sentences. *Journal of Verbal Learning and Verbal Behavior, 12*, 577-589.

Freedman, J.L., and Loftus, E.F. (1971). Retrieval of

words from long-term memory. *Journal of Verbal Learning and Verbal Behavior, 10*, 107-115.

Gewirth, L.R., Shindler, A.G., and Hier, D.B. (1984). Altered patterns of word association in dementia and aphasia. *Brain and Language, 21*, 307-317.

Goldfarb, A. I. (1975). Memory and aging. In R. Goldman and M. Rockstein (Eds.), *The physiology and pathology of human aging*. New York: Academic Press.

Goodglass, H. (1980). Disorders of naming following brain injury. *American Scientist, 68*, 647-655.

Goodglass, H., and Kaplan, E. (1976). *The assessment of aphasia and related disorders*. Philadelphia: Lea and Febiger.

Grober, E., Buschke, H., Kawas, C., and Fuld, P. (11985). Impaired ranking of semantic attributes in dementia. *Brain and Language, 26*, 276-286.

Halpern, H., Darley, F.L., and Brown, J.R. (1973). Differential language and neurological characteristics in cerebral involvement. *Journal of Speech and Hearing Disorders, 38*, 162-173.

Hasher, L., and Zacks, R.T. (1979). Automatic and effortful processes in memory. *Journal of Experimental Psychology: General, 108*, 356-388.

Haxby, J.V., Duara, R., Grady, C.L., Cutler, N.R., and Rapoport, S.I. (1985). Relations between neuropsychological and cerebral metabolic asymmetries in early Alzheimer's disease. *Journal of Cerebral Blood Flow and Metabolism, 5*, 193-200.

Holley-Wilcox, P., and Blank, M.A. (1980). Evidence for multiple access in the processing of isolated words. *Journal of Experimental Psychology: Human Perception and Performance, 6*, 75-84.

Holmes, V.M., Arwas, R., and Garrett, M.F. (1977). Prior context and the perception of lexically ambiguous sentences. *Memory and Cognition, 5*, 103-110.

Horner, J., Heyman, A., Kanter, J., Royall, J.B., and Aker, C.R. (1983, February). *Longitudinal changes in spoken discourse in Alzheimer's dementia*. Paper presented at the annual meeting of the International Neuropsychological Society, Mexico City, Mexico.

Huff, F.J., Corkin, S., and Growdon, J.H. (in press). Semantic priming and anomia in Alzheimer's disease. *Brain and Language*.

Irigaray, L. (1973). *Le language des dements*. The Hague: Mouton.

Irwin, D.I., and Lupker, S.J. (1983). Semantic priming of pictures and words: A levels of processing approach. *Journal of Verbal Learning and Verbal Behavior, 22*, 45-60.

Juola, J.F., and Atkinson, R.C. (1971). Memory scanning for words versus categories. *Journal of Verbal Learning and Verbal Behavior, 14*, 215-239.

Kaszniak, A.W., and Wilson, R.S. (1985, February). *Longitudinal deterioration of language and cognition in dementia of the Alzheimer's type*. Paper presented as part of a symposium at the International Neuropsychological Society meeting, San Diego, CA.

Katz, L., and Feldman, L.B. (1983). Relation between pronunciation and recognition of printed words in deep and shallow orthographies. *Journal of Experimental Psychology: Learning, Memory and Cognition, 9*, 157-166, 1983.

Kempler, D. (1984). *Syntactic and symbolic abilities in Alzheimer's disease*. Unpublished doctoral dissertation, University of California, Los Angeles, CA.

Kempler, D., and Curtiss, S. (1983, October). *Selective preservation of syntax in Alzheimer's patients*. Paper presented at the 8th annual Boston University Conference on Language Development, Boston, MA.

Kirshner, H.S., Webb, W.G., and Kelly, M.P. (1984). The naming disorder of dementia. *Neuropsychologia, 22*, 23-30.

Kirshner, H.S., Webb, W.G., Kelly, M.P., and Wells, C.E. (1984). Language disturbance: An initial symptom of cortical degenerations and dementia. *Archives of Neurology, 41*, 491-496.

Koss, E., Friedland, R.P., Ober, B.A., and Jagust, W.J. (1985). Differences in lateral hemispheric asymmetries of glucose utilization between early- and late-onset Alzheimer's-type dementia. *American Journal of Psychiatry, 142*, 638-640.

Langhans, J.J. (1985). *Pantomime recognition and expression in persons with Alzheimer's disease*. Unpublished doctoral dissertation, University of Arizona, AZ.

Lawson, J.S., and Barker, M.G. (1968). The assessment of nominal dysphasia in dementia: The use of reaction-time measures. *British Journal of Medical Psychology, 41*, 411-414.

Lupker, S.J. (1984). Semantic priming without association: A second look. *Journal of Verbal Learning and Verbal Behavior, 23*, 709-733.

MacKay, D.G. (1966). To end ambiguous sentences. *Perception and Psychophysics, 1*, 426-436.

MacKay, D.G., and Bever, T.G. (1967). In search of ambiguity. *Perception and Psychophysics, 2*, 193-200.

Margolin, D.I., and Friedrich, F.J. (1985, October). *Picture priming in anomia*. Poster presented at the 23rd meeting of the Academy of Aphasia, Pittsburgh, PA.

Martin, A., Brouwers, P., Cox, C., and Fedio, P. (1985). On the nature of the verbal memory deficit in Alzheimer's disease. *Brain and Language, 25*, 323-341.

Martin, A., and Fedio, P. (1983). Word production and comprehension in Alzheimer's disease: The breakdown of semantic knowledge. *Brain and Language, 19*, 124-141.

Mattis, S. (1976). Mental status examination for organic mental syndrome in the elderly patient. In L. Bellak, and T.B. Karasu (Eds.), *Geriatric psychiatry* (pp. 77-121). New York: Grune and Stratton.

Mehler, J., Segui, J., and Carey, P. (1978). Tails of words: Monitoring ambiguity. *Journal of Verbal Learning and Verbal Behavior, 17*, 29-37.

Meyer, D.E., and Schvaneveldt, R.W. (1971). Facilitation in recognizing pairs of words: Evidence of a dependence between retrieval operations. *Journal of Experimental Psychology, 90*, 227-234.

Meyer, D.E., Schvaneveldt, R.W., and Ruddy, M.G. (1975). Loci of contextual effects on word recognition. In P.M.A. Rabbitt and S. Dornic (Eds.), *Attention and performance: Vol. 5*. (pp. 98-118). London: Academic Press.

Miller, E., and Hague, F. (1975). Some characteristics of verbal behaviour in presenile dementia. *Psychological Medicine, 5*, 255-259.

Mitchell, D.B., Hunt, R.R., and Schmitt, F.A. (1986). Generation effects and reality monitoring: Evidence from dementia and normal aging. *Journal of Gerontology, 41*, 79-84.

Morton, J. (1969). Interaction of information in word recognition. *Psychological Review, 76*, 165-178.

Nebes, R.D., Boller, F., and Holland, A. (1986). Use of semantic context by patients with Alzheimer's disease. *Psychology and Aging, 1*, 261–269.

Nebes, R.D., Martin, D.C., and Horn, L.C. (1984). Sparing of semantic memory in Alzheimer's disease. *Journal of Abnormal Psychology, 93*, 321-330.

Nelson, M.J. (1962). *The Nelson Reading Test*. New York: Houghton Mifflin.

Newman, J.E., and Dell, G.S. (1978). The phonological nature of phoneme monitoring: A critique of some ambiguity studies. *Journal of Verbal Learning and Verbal Behavior, 6*, 364-371.

Ober, B.A., and Shenaut, G.K. (1986). *Semantic prime inhibition of lexical decision in Alzheimer's-type dementia*. Manuscript submitted for publication.

Obler, L.K. (1983). Language and brain dysfunction in dementia. In S. Segalowitz (Ed.), *Language functions and brain organization* (pp. 267-282). New York: Academic Press.

Onifer, W., and Swinney, D.A. (1981). Accessing lexical ambiguities during sentence comprehension: Effects of frequency of meaning and contextual bias. *Memory and Cognition, 9*, 225-236.

Overman, C. (1979, November). *Naming performance in geriatric patients with chronic brain syndrome*. Paper presented to the annual meeting of the American Speech and Hearing Association, Washington, DC.

Palermo, D.S., and Jenkins, J.J. (1964). *Word association norms: Grade school through college*. Minneapolis: University of Minnesota Press.

Perez, F.I., Gay, J.R., and Taylor, R.L. (1975). WAIS performance of neurologically impaired aged. *Psychological Reports, 37*, 1043-1047.

Portsmouth, L. (1985). *The application of sentence disambiguation tasks to the identification of senile dementia*. Unpublished bachelor of science thesis. Western Australian Institute of Technology.

Posner, M.I., and Snyder, C.R.R. (1975). Attention and cognitive control. In R.L. Solso (Ed.), *Information processing and cognition: The Loyola symposium*. Hillsdale: Lawrence Erlbaum Associates.

Quillian, M.R. (1962). A revised design for an understanding machine. *Mechanical Translation, 7*, 17-29.

Quillian, M.R. (1967). Word concepts: A theory and simulation of some basic semantic capabilities. *Behavioral Science, 12*, 410-430.

Ripich, D.N., Spinelli, F.M., and Terrell, B.Y. (1983, November). *Patterns of discourse cohesion in Alzheimer's disease*. Paper presented at the annual meeting of the American Speech-Language Hearing Association, Cincinnati, OH.

Rochford, G. (1971). A study of naming errors in dysphasic and demented patients. *Neuropsychologia, 9*, 437-445.

Roediger, H.L., and Neely, J.H. (1982). Retrieval blocks in episodic and semantic memory. *Canadian Journal of Psychology, 36*, 213-242.

Roediger, H.L., Neely, J.H., and Blaxton, T.A. (1983). Inhibition from related primes in semantic memory retrieval: A reappraisal of Brown's (1979) paradigm. *Journal of Experimental Psychology: Learning, Memory, and Cognition, 9*, 478-485.

Rosen, W.G. (1980). Verbal fluency in aging and dementia. *Journal of Clinical Neuropsychology, 2*, 135-146.

Santo Pietro, M.J., and Berman, R. (1984, November). *Analysis of connected speech in institutionalized elderly with and without senile dementia*. Paper presented at the annual meeting of the American Speech-Language Hearing Association, San Francisco, CA.

Schmitt, F.A., and Mitchell, D.B. (1984 February). *Naming speed, retrieval efficiency, and facilitation in dementia of the Alzheimer's type*. Paper presented at the annual meeting of the International Neuropsychological Society, Houston, TX.

Schwartz, M.F., Marin, O.S.M., and Saffran, E.M. (1979). Dissociations of language function in dementia: A case study. *Brain and Language, 7*, 277-306.

Schwartz, M.F., Saffran, E.M., and Marin, O.S.M. (1980). Fractionating the reading process in dementia: Evidence for word specific print-to-sound associations. In M. Coltheart, K. Patterson, and J.C. Marshall (Eds.), *Deep dyslexia* (pp. 259-269). London: Routledge and Kegan Paul.

Seidenberg, M.A., Tanenhaus, M.K., Leiman, J.M., and Bienkowski, M. (1982). Automatic access of the meanings of ambiguous words in context: Some limitations of knowledge-based processing. *Cognitive Psychology, 14*, 489-537.

Simpson, G.B. (1981). Meaning dominance and semantic context in the processing of lexical ambiguity. *Journal of Verbal Learning and Verbal Behavior, 20*, 120-136.

Simpson, G.B., and Burgess, C. (1985). Activation and selection processes in the recognition of ambiguous words. *Journal of Experimental Psychology: Human Perception and Performance, 11*, 28-39.

Slameck, N.J., and Graf, P. (1978). The generation effect: Delineation of a phenomenon. *Journal of Experimental Psychology: Human Learning and Memory, 4*, 592-604.

Swinney, D.A. (1979). Lexical access during sentence comprehension: (Re)consideration of context effects. *Journal of Verbal Learning and Verbal Behavior, 18*, 645-659.

Tanenhaus, M.K., Leiman, J.M., and Seidenberg, M.S. (1979). Evidence for multiple stages in the processing of ambiguous words in syntactic contexts. *Journal of Verbal Learning and Verbal Behavior, 18*, 427-440.

Tulving, E. (1985). How many memory systems are there? *American Psychologist, 40*, 385-398.

Vania, L., and Hintikka, J. (1984). *Cognitive constraints on communication: Representations and processes*. Boston: D. Reidel.

Warren, R.E. (1977). Time and the spread of activation in memory. *Journal of Experimental Psychology: Human Learning and Memory, 3*, 458-466.

Warrington, E.K. (1975). The selective impairment of semantic memory. *Quarterly Journal of Experimental Psychology, 27*, 635-657.

Wechsler, D. (1955). *Manual for the Wechsler Adult Intelligence Scale*. New York: The Psychological Corporation.

Wechsler, D. (1981). *Manual for the Wechsler Adult Intelligence Scale-Revised*. New York: The Psychological Corporation.

Weingartner, H., Kaye, W., Smallberg, S.A., Ebert, M.H., Gillin, J.C., and Sitaram, N. (1981). Memory failures in progressive idiopathic dementia. *Journal of Abnormal Psychology, 90*, 187-196.

Whitaker, H.A. (1976). A case of isolation of the language function. In H. Whitaker and H.A. Whitaker, (Eds.), *Studies in neurolinguistics: Vol. 2* (pp. 1-58). New York: Academic Press.

Yates, J. (1978). Priming dominant and unusual senses of ambiguous words. *Memory and Cognition, 6*, 636-643.

Chapter 4

Linguistic Communication: Interetiologic and Longitudinal Considerations

Few comparative studies of communicative function in patients with etiologically different dementias have been conducted; therefore, specification of differences in the effects of the disease on communicative functioning must be tentative. A methodologic problem associated with interetiologic comparison is equating the severity of dementia in subjects with different diseases. Are mild AD and PD patients comparable? Are moderate PD patients comparable with moderate HD patients? Does mild dementia in multi-infarct dementia and AD patients mean the same thing? When interetiologic comparisons are being made, it is not obvious how severity of dementia should be defined. In intraetiologic studies, it is most often specified in terms of functional or mental status. However, if functional status (the ability to carry out activities of daily living) is used in making interetiologic comparisons, the question arises how patients with motor problems, such as PD and HD patients, can reasonably be compared with Alzheimer's patients in whom motor function is preserved until late in the disease course. If severity is defined in terms of mental status and the dependent measure in the research study is a mental function, then the researcher must select one or more psychologic states or functions that have credibility as being equally vulnerable in the dementing diseases being compared. Presently, consensus is lacking as to what these psychologic states and functions are.

Methods for establishing the severity of dementia have varied among investigators, and in many studies, severity has been ignored or poorly specified. Unfortunately, no objective physiologic measure exists by which it can be determined. One nonphysiologic measure often considered is duration of illness. As a criterion for equating severity of dementia, however, duration of illness is problematic, not only because the progression rate of different dementing diseases varies, but because the rate of progression varies in individuals with the same disease. Then too, many individuals are uncertain of when the dementing disease actually began. Families in a study by Chenoweth and Spencer (1986) were asked when they first recognized the symptoms of dementia. They reported having difficulty pinpointing the first symptoms. Many families reported the year prior to the first certain symptom as upsetting because of frequent misunderstandings between the patient and other family members. Finally, when a group of individuals can be identified who appear to have had the same time of onset, the assumption cannot be made that they have deteriorated equally. The importance and difficulty of specifying severity of dementia in interetiologic comparisons must be borne in mind when evaluating research results.

INTERETIOLOGIC COMPARISON OF AD, PD, AND HD

The Tucson Study

At the University of Arizona a comparative study of communicative function in Alzheimer's, Parkinson's, and Huntington's disease patients was conducted. Because the study purpose was to provide a description of communicative function in dementia patients, it was imperative that the measure used to establish severity of dementia not judge severity by assessing communicative skill. To do so would have made the study tautologic. The study began in 1979 before the availability of dementia rating scales in which communicative function was not a criterion for severity determination. Therefore, severity of dementia was determined in three other ways: first, rating on a behavioral inventory; second, performance on nonlinguistic psychologic tests; and third, the rating of the examining neurologist. The psychologic tests employed were Block Design, a visuospatial constructive subtest of the WAIS, and Goldfarb's Mental Status Questionnaire (1975), a ten-item test of orientation to time, place, and person. The behavioral inventory was devised by the investigators and considered the ability of subjects to assume responsibility for their personal affairs and execute the activities of daily living. The examining neurologist was instructed to exclude language and communicative functioning from consideration when specifying severity on a five-point scale that ranged from mild to severe. Only individuals who were capable of taking psychometric tests were accepted as study participants. None of the sample were institutionalized, and all were ambulatory.

Patients who were designated as having mild dementia were like patients who receive a rating of three or four on the Global Deterioration Scale for Dementia (Reisberg, Ferris, and Crook, 1982). Subjects with moderate dementia were like patients who receive a five or six on this scale. Patients with mild dementia had some disorientation, memory defects, difficulty in concentrating, and a decreased ability to handle finances and independent travel. Patients with moderate dementia could no longer manage without assistance because of marked disorientation and memory failure.

One hundred subjects participated in the study, 31 with AD, 15 with PD, 21 with HD, and 33 normal elderly individuals. Analysis of the demographic characteristics of the sample (Table 4-1), showed them to be comparable in education, intelligence, and age (with the exception of HD for age).

Subjects were given a variety of linguistic communication measures to test the comprehension, expression, and processing of linguistic information (Table 4-2). It was hypothesized that of the measures administered in the study, those which were active (not a pointing or fill-in-the-blank task), nonautomatic, generative, and dependent upon reasoning would best discriminate dementia patients from normal subjects. The obtained results supported this hypothesis. For example, regardless of etiology, all mild groups were more impaired on the FAS Verbal Fluency Measure, a test of generative naming ability developed by Borkowski, Ben-

Table 4-1. Demographic Characteristics of Subjects in the Tucson Study

Groups	N	Age*	Male	Female	Years of Education*	Estimated+ IQ*
Elderly controls	33	70	12	21	13	115
Alzheimer's disease	31	71	19	12	12	113
Parkinson's disease	15	69	13	2	14	117
Huntington's disease	21	43	11	10	13	115

*Groups not significantly different on these variables (with the exception of Huntington's disease on age).

+Based on regression equation developed by Wilson, Rosenbaum, and Brown (1979).

Table 4-2. Measures Constituting the Communication Test Battery in the Tucson Study

NONLINGUISTIC

Mental Status Questionnaire (MSQ): ten-question test of orientation to time, place, and person

Block Design: WAIS subtest designed to evaluate visuospatial construction ability by having subject manipulate blocks to match increasingly difficult pictured patterns

Forward Digit Span (DS): WAIS subtest of memory for gradually increasing strings of numbers

Nonsense Syllable Learning Test (NSLT): test of ability to learn the correct serial order of six nonsense syllables in six trials

LINGUISTIC

Confrontation Naming Task (CN): 20-item test of ability of subjects to name common objects from colored pictures

FAS Word Fluency Measure (FAS): test of ability to name as many words as possible beginning with each of three letters (F, A, S) in 1 minute, respectively

Peabody Picture Vocabulary Test (PPVT): receptive vocabulary test in which subjects select, from among four line drawings, the correct visual representation of increasingly difficult words spoken by the examiner

Vocabulary: WAIS subtest of ability to orally define a list of increasingly difficult words

Similarities: WAIS subtest of verbal associative reasoning in which subjects explain a common feature of increasingly dissimilar objects

Sentence Correction Task: test of ability to judge and correct sentences with syntactic and semantic errors;
Abbreviations for components of the test:
Sentence Correction—Syntactic Judgment (SCSJ)
Sentence Correction—Syntactic Correction (SCSC)
Sentence Correction—Semantic Judgment (SCSeJ)
Sentence Correction—Semantic Correction (SCSeC)

Sentence Disambiguation Task (SDT): 30-item test of ability of subjects to explain five types of ambiguous sentences

Verbal Description Task (VDES): test of ability to produce oral descriptive discourse

Story-Retelling Task (SR-1, SR-2): test of ability of subjects to recount information contained in a short story composed of 16 information units immediately after hearing it (SR-1) and in a delayed condition (SR-2)

Pragmatics Task (Prag): four part test of ability to use context in utterance interpretation

ton, and Spreen (1967), than on Sentence Judgment and Correction. In generative naming, individuals had to generate examples of items within a category, whereas in the sentence judgment and correction task, subjects identified and corrected anomalous sentences in a group of sentences read by the examiner.

Other tasks that differentiated each of the three groups of mild dementia patients (AD, PD, HD) from normal subjects were the Similarities subtest of the WAIS (Wechsler, 1958), the Sentence Disambiguation Test, Verbal Description, and Story-Retelling. When the performance of moderately demented individuals, irrespective of etiology, was compared with that of normal subjects, significant differences were found on all measures.

Best Test for Discriminating Each Group of Dementia Patients from Normals. Discriminant function analyses (stepwise, maximum significance of F to enter $p = .05$; minimum significance of F to remove $p = .10$) were calculated to answer the question of what test, or test combination, best differentiated each etiologically unique dementia patient group from normal subjects (Table 4-3). When the comparison was between all AD patients and normal subjects, the Verbal Description Task

Table 4-3. Best Tests for Discriminating Dementia Patients from Normals Using Discriminant Function Analysis in the Tucson Study

Group	Variable	% Variance Explained
AD vs. normals	VDES	54
	SR-1	12
	Prag	3
PD vs. normals	FAS	53
	SDT	7
HD vs. normals	FAS	67
	SCSeC	7
	SDT	4

Maximum significance of F to enter = 0.05.
Minimum significance of F to remove = 0.10.

was best, accounting for 54 percent of the explained variance. It was followed by Story-Retelling, which accounted for 12 percent, and the Pragmatics Task, 3 percent. When the discriminant function analysis was calculated using PD patients and normal subjects, the FAS Verbal Fluency Measure was most discriminating, explaining 53 percent of the variance, and was followed by Sentence Disambiguation, at 7 percent. Similarly, the FAS Verbal Fluency Measure best discriminated HD patients from normal subjects, explaining in this case 67 percent of the variance. When discriminant function analyses were used to classify each group of dementia patients and normal subjects, classification was done with at least 93 percent accuracy.

Results of Interetiologic Comparisons: More Similarities Than Differences. When patients with mild etiologically different dementia were compared with each other, the singular significant difference obtained was between the AD and HD patients on the Sentence Disambiguation Test. Mild HD patients performed more poorly.

When moderately demented groups were compared, no significant differences were obtained between moderate AD and PD patients, and moderate PD and HD patients. As was the case with the comparison of mildly demented patients, the only significant differences were between AD and HD patients, in this case, on the Verbal Description and Confrontation Naming tests. On both tasks the AD patients performed more poorly.

The number of significant intergroup differences obtained in this study was surprisingly small. Clearly, the performances of patients with etiologically different dementia were more similar than different, and severity of dementia better predicted performance than etiology. The lack of prominent differences between the performance of patients with etiologically different dementia, controlled for severity, is similar to the finding of Mayeux, Stern, Rosen, and Benson (1983). In their comparative study, 123 patients with either AD, HD, or PD were given a brief quantitative neuropsychologic assessment. Although patients with HD and PD were less intellectually deteriorated than those with AD, when intergroup comparisons were made between groups of patients similar in overall intellectual function, no distinct performance patterns were observed.

Similarities of HD to AD Patients Surprising

Whereas reports of interetiologic differences among AD, HD, and PD patients are not uncommon, they have resulted primarily from studies concerned with functions other than communication. Then too, in some of the studies in which conclusions about interetiologic differences have been drawn, interetiologic comparisons were not actually done. Rather, the results of one study were compared with those previously reported in the literature. Butters, Sax, Montgomery, and Tarlow (1978), who compared recently diagnosed with advanced HD patients on intelligence, memory, and naming, reported that only confrontation naming remained intact. On a verbal fluency test, both groups of HD patients generated fewer words than normal subjects, but neither group performed significantly differently from normal subjects on the confrontation naming task. Butters and colleagues (1978) concluded that the intact naming ability of the HD patients "suggests that their intellectual deterioration is not as widespread as in other 'dementing' disorders" (p. 588). It must be mentioned, however, that the advanced HD patients in this study showed severe decreases on verbal IQ scores as well as on full-scale and performance IQ.

Josiassen, Curry, and Mancall (1983) reported less deterioration in verbal ability in HD patients as compared with other cognitive functions. These investigators administered 36 measures to seven recently diagnosed HD patients, nine moderately advanced HD patients, and 48 individuals at risk but asymptomatic. Verbal performance scores on the WAIS did not discriminate between the groups. The authors concluded that verbal disorders were not as prominent in HD as in patients with other dementing disorders. However, they also noted that subtle verbal changes might be observed if a comprehensive language examination were given.

Recent Reports of Lexical Access and Semantic Memory Deficits. Although many investigators have concluded that language is largely spared in HD patients, several have reported impaired performance on tasks reputed to involve lexical access or semantic knowledge (Josiassen, Curry, Roemer, DeBease and Mancall, 1982; Josiassen et al., 1983; Butters, Wolfe, Granholm and Martone, 1986). Although these investigators reported diminished performance by HD patients on verbal fluency and verbal associative reasoning tests, they argued that the processes by which acquired knowledge is manipulated are more impaired than language knowledge and account for the diminished performance.

Recently, Smith, White, Lyon, Granholm, and Butters (in press) attempted to minimize performance factors to explore the semantic networks in patients with mild and moderately advanced HD. They employed a free association paradigm in which target responses to particular stimulus items were either primed or not primed. Both free association and priming activities are considered largely automatic and do not require active manipulation of knowledge (Posner and Snyder, 1975; Hasher and Zacks, 1979). The strength and type of relation between the stimulus and target words were systematically varied in such a way that half of the targets were strongly associated with their corresponding stimuli, and half were only moderately related. Subjects were first asked to rate the degree of relatedness of 12 word pairs and then provide a verbal association to words that had and had not been stimulus items in the priming task. This design permitted the investigators to establish primed and nonprimed hit rates for each type of word pair (strongly or moderately related, and unrelated).

A positive priming effect was found for all three groups (mild HD, moderate HD, normal subjects) regardless of the strength of association or type of relation. No overall group differences were found in the degree to which enhanced activation was maintained from the priming task to the free association task. This finding alone seems to suggest that the system of spreading activation in semantic networks remains intact throughout the mild–moderate stages of HD. However, Smith and colleagues found an important qualitative difference between groups, namely, that the strength of association influenced subjects' hit rates. While HD patients showed no impairment in the ability to prime, there was a progressive decline in the degree to which association strengths of word pairs affected priming of semantic relations.

Smith and colleagues concluded that HD patients suffer breakdown in the organization of the "lexicosemantic representational system." They buttressed their conclusion with additional evidence from a series of language tests, given to these same subjects, which evaluate lexical access and knowledge of specific semantic properties of words. The language tests included the FAS test of letter fluency and category fluency (animals) developed by Benton (1968), the Boston Naming Test (Kaplan, Goodglass, and Weintraub, 1983), and the WAIS-R Vocabulary subtest (Wechsler, 1981). Significantly poorer performances were observed in mild HD patients compared with normal subjects on all of these measures; the results were similar to those from the aforementioned Tucson study. The findings from these two studies suggest that communicative impairment is likely to be a prominent feature of HD.

INTERETIOLOGIC COMPARISONS OF HD, AD, AND KORSAKOFF'S DISEASE PATIENTS

Butters and colleagues (1983) investigated the degree to which patients with alcoholic Korsakoff syndrome (KS), HD, AD, or right-hemisphere damage were able to use explicit verbal cues to associate specific human and animal figures with particular scenic backgrounds. Their results suggest that patients with HD and right-hemisphere damage can be distinguished from patients with KS and AD by their ability to employ verbal mediators to facilitate contextual memory. Patients with HD and right-hemisphere damage were better able to use verbal information. Butters and colleagues write,

> the results with the present picture-context memory task suggest that the dementias (like the amnesias) should not be treated as a single disorder. The HD patients can utilize language as a mnemonic for circumventing their pictorial memory problems, whereas patients with Alzheimer's Disease have lost the opportunity to use language in this constructive manner due to the aphasic symptoms (e.g. anomia) usually apparent early in the disease process. (p. 319)

Moss, Albert, Butters and Payne (1986) compared HD, alcoholic KS, and AD patients with normal subjects on a task designed to assess recognition memory for different classes of stimuli, among them verbal. No significant differences were observed among the three patient groups in ability to recognize new spatial, colored, patterned, or facial stimuli. However, HD patients performed significantly better (near normal) than the other two groups when verbal stimuli were used. In a subsequent recall test for verbal stimuli, AD, HD, and KS patients were equally impaired at the shorter delay (15 s), but when the delay lasted for 2 minutes, HD and KS patients performed significantly better than AD patients. This pattern of recall performance suggests that patients with AD, unlike patients with HD or KD, experience an abnormally rapid rate of forgetting. There was no significant difference among the HD or KS patients or normal subjects in the degree of loss between retention trials. Huntington's patients were, however, more likely to remember additional, previously unrecalled words from the verbal recognition trial than either KS or AD patients or normal subjects.

AD AND PICK'S DISEASE

Like AD patients, Pick's disease patients develop communication disorders, though the pattern of linguistic deterioration is different. Patients with AD have been described as developing fluent aphasias (Albert, 1981; Cummings, 1982; Goodman, 1953), and ultimately palilalia (repetition of a phrase or word with increasing rapidity) and logoclonia (repetition of the final syllable of a word), whereas the linguistic changes typical of Pick's patients include auditory agnosia, excessive use of verbal stereotypies, echolalia (Cummings, 1982; Cummings and Duchen, 1981; Ferraro and Jervis, 1936; Kahn and Thompson, 1933-34; Wechsler, Verity, Rosenschein, Fried, and Scheibel, 1982), and late-stage mutism.

Holland, McBurney, Moossy, and Reinmuth (1985) have provided the most comprehensive account to date of the deterioration of language in a Pick's disease patient, a man known as Mr. E. They conducted a retrospective study of his language ability from the time of his first speaking difficulty in 1967 to his death 12½ years later. A postmortem examination was performed, and Mr. E. was found to have neuropathologic features typical of Pick's disease and neurofibrillary tangles but no neuritic plaques.

In the early stages of the disease, his speech became slower, more deliberate, and interspersed with inordinately long pauses. Then, Mr. E. began to substitute lower-frequency words for words of higher frequency, a tendency that continued throughout the language dissolution process. In a speech/language evaluation in 1971, he was found to have language formulation and word finding problems though his responses were clear and concise. Particularly troublesome was what appeared to be a progressive auditory agnosia. After 1971, Mr. E. became more and more reluctant to talk, preferring to communicate in writing. From the letters written in his last years of life, it is apparent that Mr. E. retained memory for names of people and environments. In the final 24 months, marked personality changes occurred; he became increasingly passive, impulsive, and exhibited poor judgment.

Holland and colleagues point out that the pattern of impairment in Mr. E. is dissimilar from the neuropsychologic deterioration observed in Alzheimer's dementia. Unlike AD patients, Mr. E. first lost the formal syntactic elements of language, but throughout the course of the disease he appeared to retain access to the semantic store, a fact clearly revealed in the letters he wrote.

Hereditary Dysphasic Dementia

A condition similar to both Pick's and AD is referred to by Morris, Cole, Banker, and Wright (1984) as "hereditary dysphasic dementia." This condition affects the elder members of successive generations within a family and is characterized by progressive deterioration of language and cognitive abilities. In addition, paralysis agitans (tremor, slowing of movement, weakness, and resting tremor associated with parkinsonism) coexists secondary to neuronal depigmentation and depletion in the substantia nigra.

Morris and colleagues (1984) described hereditary dysphasic dementia as a condition that lies between Alzheimer's and Pick's diseases on the spectrum of dementing illnesses. They investigated its features in a German immigrant family. Ten affected individuals in three generations were studied. Signs and symptoms were similar in all affected family members and consisted of "insidious appearance of memory defects, intellectual decline, and behavioral and personality changes. Various abnormalities of speech and language were generally recognized soon after, but occasionally the dysphasic disturbances were the initial indication of disease" (Morris et al., 1984, p. 457).

The dysphasia was characterized by hesitancy of speech, decrease in spontaneous output, and dysnomia. The most prominent dysphasic characteristic was diminished verbal fluency. Morris and associates observed overt paraphasic errors, deficits in auditory and visual comprehension, dysgraphia, alexia, and defects in repetition. Within 5 years

Table 4-4. The Pick-Alzheimer Spectrum of Primary Cortical Dementia

Pick's Disease	Hereditary Dysphasic Dementia	Alzheimer's Disease
	Pathologic Findings	
Lobar atrophy	Focal atrophy	Generalized atrophy
Spongiform degeneration	Spongiform degeneration	Granulovacuolar degeneration
Tangles	Plaques	Plaques and tangles
Argyrophillic (Pick) inclusions		
Pick cells		Hirano bodies
	Communication Profile	
Slow, deliberate speech	Nonfluent speech	Fluent speech
Dysnomia	Dysnomia	Dysnomia
Defect in auditory comprehension	Defect in auditory comprehension	Defect in auditory comprehension
Decrease in spontaneous output and mutism	Decrease in spontaneous output and mutism	Quantity of output generally preserved; mutism in very late stage
Breakdown of syntactic aspect of language		Syntactic processes generally preserved
Reading comprehension generally preserved	Reading comprehension problems	Reading comprehension problems
Communicative deficits more pronounced than memory	Memory and cognitive deficits proportional to communicative	Memory and cognitive deficits proportional to communicative

of dysphasic signs, some affected individuals were globally aphasic, others mute.

A complete neuropathologic study of four patients with hereditary dysphasic dementia was possible and revealed asymmetric focal cerebral atrophy that was most prominent in frontal and anterior temporal lobes. As might be expected from the marked dysphasia, the left perisylvian region was more damaged than the right. Cortical gray matter appeared "soft and mottled," and white matter was firm and rubbery. The substantia nigra "demonstrated symmetrical pallor, gliosis, and faint yellowish-brown discoloration" (Morris et al., 1984, p. 458). Additionally, conspicuous spongiform degeneration of the superficial external layers of cerebral cortex was noted. Finally, Pick cells were absent, but neuritic plaques were discovered in significant numbers throughout the cortex.

Other scientists have reported similar dementia patients whose signs do not in a strict sense meet the criteria of either Pick's or AD. Kim, Collins, Parisi, Wright, and Chu (1981) described an Italian family in which 4 of 10 individuals in the same generation developed dysphasia, dementia, and parkinsonian signs, as well as bulimia (excessive eating). Neuropathologic examination was conducted on three of the four affected individuals, and changes similar to those described by Morris and colleagues (1984) were observed, although neurofibrillary tangles, neuritic plaques, Pick cells, and Pick bodies were absent.

Thus, Morris and colleagues suggested that primary cortical dementias "be considered in the context of a spectrum of cerebral disorders in which the unifying abnormality is degenerative nerve cell death" (p. 464). A continuum can be observed in terms of both pathologic findings and communication behaviors (Table 4-4).

AD AND MID

A large scale study of neuropathologically well-defined MID patients has not been done, nor has a large-scale comparative study of MID and AD patients. As noted in Chapter 1, MID patients have variable signs depending upon the locus of pathologic changes within the vascular system. Yet, in most comparative studies of MID and AD patients, MID patients are not grouped according to locus and extent of vascular pathologic changes.

Perez, Gay, and Taylor (1975) did differentiate between patients with vertebrobasilar arterial insufficiency and MID in a comparative study of AD and vascular dementia. However, patients with etiologically different dementias were not matched for severity. AD patients were significantly better educated and tended to be younger. Performance on the short form of the WAIS was the dependent variable. Perez and colleagues reported significant quantitative but not qualitative differences in cognitive performance among the groups. In their discussion of results, they noted that further study using memory and language measures would "probably increase the understanding of the dementias" (p. 1047). Brinkman (1983) attempted to replicate the findings of Perez and colleagues but was unsuccessful. He analyzed the WAIS IQ and subtest scores of 20 MID and 16 DAT patients matched for age, education, and dementia severity and found no significant differences.

Fuld, Katzman, Davies, and Terry (1982) compared MID, AD, and other dementia patients for frequency of intrusive errors produced during performance on five neuropsychological measures. An intrusion was defined as "an inappropriate recurrence of a response (or type of response) from a preceding test item, test, or procedure" (p. 156). The major finding reported by these investigators was the association of frequency of intrusions with large numbers of senile plaques, low choline acetyltransferase levels, and the clinical diagnosis of AD. Interestingly, intrusive errors were not made exclusively by AD patients. Whereas 90 percent of the AD patients made intrusive errors, 57 percent of the MID patients did as well.

Hier, Hagenlocker, and Shindler (1985) investigated possible differences in the language characteristics of AD and MID patients. Twenty-six individuals with AD, 13 with MID, and 20 with aphasia due to focal brain damage were given the Vocabulary Subtest of the WAIS, the Ammons Test of Receptive Vocabulary (Ammons and Ammons, 1977), the Logicogrammatical Sentence Comprehension Test (Wiig and Semel, 1974), a 20-item confrontation naming task, and a generative naming test. Finally, a speech sample was elicited. After data analysis, Hier and associates described the MID patients as "laconic" because they used fewer words and fewer unique words than AD patients and were more likely to have syntactic deficits. These investigators concluded that

> the relatively random but diffuse loss of neurons that characterizes AD may take a particularly heavy toll on the complex semantic networks that make up the mental lexicon. On the other hand, the focal loss of neurons that occurs in stroke-related dementia appears to have a greater adverse effect on the complexity of syntax than on accessing substantive words in the lexicon (p. 125).

CORTICAL AND SUBCORTICAL DEMENTIAS

The studies mentioned thus far in the chapter are not the only interetiologic comparisons of dementia patients. Other important studies will be mentioned in this section. The studies yet to be mentioned are related to the explication of the cortical–subcortical distinction as a way of classifying dementing diseases. Many scholars prefer to classify dementing diseases according to the distribution of pathologic changes. Patients with HD, those with supranuclear palsy, and some PD patients with subcortical pathologic changes are said to have subcortical dementia, whereas patients with AD or Pick's disease are said to have cortical dementia. Whitehouse (1986) reports that the term "subcortical dementia" was used first in 1974 by Albert, Feldman, and Willis, and again in 1975 by McHugh and Folstein to describe

> a clinical syndrome believed to be characteristic of progressive supranuclear palsy, normal pressure hydrocephalus, and Huntington's disease. In these conditions, impairment in memory and learning were associated with slowness of intellectual function, inertia, and apathy but not with difficulties in language, perception, and praxis, symptoms which were more characteristic of cortical dementias such as Alzheimer's disease and Creutzfeldt-Jakob disease (Whitehouse, 1986, p. 1).

Since its introduction, the term has been applied to demented patients with PD (Albert, 1978), Wilson's disease (Cummings and Benson, 1983), MID (Cummings and Benson, 1983), and the dementia associated with depression (Caine, 1981; McHugh and Folstein, 1979).

Obler and Albert (1981) describe differences in the speech and language behaviors between patients with subcortical and cortical dementia, the most important of which is the common occurrence of speech problems in the population with subcortical dementia. In cortically demented individuals, at least in the mild stages, speech is not adversely affected because the motor strip is spared. Another difference described by Obler and Albert is the appropriate use of language. Whereas patients with subcortical dementia tend to use language appropriately, those with cortical dementing disease do not. Then too, subcortical dementia patients have better language comprehension. Among cortical dementia patients, anomic errors are more common and include verbal and sometimes literal paraphasias.

Mildworf (1978) conducted a study of the linguistic ability of 38 Parkinson's patients, 10 patients with HD, and 42 normal elders, age-matched with the PD patients. Although her study is unpublished, it is reported and described by Obler and Albert (1981). PD patients performed inferiorly, though not significantly worse in a statistical sense, to normal subjects on the Boston Naming Test and the Body-Part Naming subtest off the BDAE. On both measures, Huntington's disease patients performed significantly more poorly than normal subjects and PD patients. Further, HD patients performed significantly more poorly on a test of generative naming. Whereas both PD and HD subjects could perform a serial speech task, subjects in both groups had difficulty stopping after a complete recitation of months of the year. Additionally, they were unable to name the months in reverse order. When asked to write a description

Table 4-5. Features That Distinguish Cortical and Subcortical Dementias

Characteristic	Subcortical	Cortical
	MENTAL STATUS	
Language	No aphasia	Aphasia
Memory	Forgetful (difficulty retrieving learned material)	Amnesia (difficulty learning new material)
Cognition	Impaired (poor problem-solving produced by slowness, forgetfulness, and impaired strategy and planning)	Severely disturbed (based on agnosia, aphasia, acalculia, and amnesia)
	Slow processing time	Response time relatively normal
Personality	Apathetic	Unconcerned or euphoric
Mood	Affective disorder common (depression or mania)	Normal
	MOTOR SYSTEM	
Speech	Dysarthric	Normal*
Posture	Abnormal	Normal, upright*
Gait	Abnormal	Normal*
Motor speed	Slow	Normal*
Movement disorder	Common (chorea, tremor, rigidity, ataxia)	Absent
	ANATOMY	
Cortex	Largely spared	Involved
Basal ganglia, thalamus, mesencephalon	Involved	Largely spared
	METABOLISM	
Fluorodeoxyglucose scan	Subcortical hypometabolism (cortex largely normal)	Cortical hypometabolism (subcortical metabolism less involved)
	NEUROTRANSMITTERS	
Preferentially involved	Hungington's disease: -amino-butyric acid Parkinson's disease: dopamine	Alzheimer's disease: acetylcholine

*Motor system involvement occurs late in the course of Alzheimer's disease and Pick's disease.
(From Cummings, J.L., and Benson, D.F. (1984). Subcortical dementia. Review of an emerging concept. *Archives of Neurology, 41,* 874–879, by permission.

of the BDAE Cookie-Theft picture, responses of PD patients were similar to those of normal subjects. Huntington's patients able to complete the task wrote telegrammatic sentences.

The results of this study are hard to interpret for two reasons. First, the dementia patients were not controlled for severity; second, it is unclear whether the PD patients had dementia. Not all PD patients develop dementia, and indeed the prevalence of dementia in PD is in dispute. In the description of this study by Obler and Albert (1981), it is not specified whether the PD patients had dementia, some intellectual impairment, or no intellectual impairment, or if they were a mixed group.

An excellent description of the features of cortical and subcortical dementia can be found in the highly recommended book *Dementia: A Clinical Approach*, by Cummings and Benson (1983). When comparing cortical and subcortical dementia patients, Cummings and Benson describe speech output (number of words) in AD as normal, in dramatic contrast to the altered output of subcortical dementia patients. According to Benson (1983), the clinical differences between patients with subcortical and cortical dementia are so striking that the conditions should be accepted as two distinct dementia types. Table 4-5 is reprinted from Cummings and Benson (1984), who summarize the major features that differentiate cortical and subcortical disorders.

Cummings and Benson (1983) go on to differentiate patients with acute confusional states from those with cortical and subcortical dementias. In acute confusional states, speech tends to be slurred, while language is generally normal; the opposite is true in cortical dementia. When speech and language deficits are associated with acute confusional state, they are usually apparent in naming and writing. Acute confusional state shares with subcortical dementia the features of motor abnormalities, speech impairment, and attentional disorder.

Cortical-Subcortical Dichotomy: A Controversial Distinction

The subcortical-cortical distinction, although popular, is not universally accepted. Some scientists question whether anatomic terms like "subcortical" are appropriate descriptors for clinical syndromes. Cummings and Benson (1984), however, emphasize that subcortical dementia is a clinical, rather than anatomic concept. Freedman (1984) writes that although the term "subcortical dementia" may be unsatisfactory from the standpoint of anatomy, it is not necessarily invalid as a clinical entity. Whitehouse (1986) asserts that the type of study necessary to determine the validity of the distinction between subcortical and cortical has yet to be done. Whitehouse makes the point that whereas researchers have reported neuropsychologic differences between the dementias of AD, PD, and HD, no one has yet demonstrated the validity of the concept of subcortical dementia. The authors of this book would add that as yet, no one has demonstrated the validity of the concept of subcortical dementia in a controlled study in relation to speech, language, and communication disorders.

Another criticism of the dichotomy is that the defining characteristics of each dementia type are not exclusive to that type. For example, the major difference between cortical and subcortical dementia is said to be the lack of aphasia, agnosia, and apraxia in the subcortical type. Yet, language and visuospatial problems are known to occur in both PD and HD patients (Boller et al., 1984; Matison, Mayeux, Rosen, and Fahn, 1982; Pirozzolo, Hansch, Mortimer, Webster, and Kuskowski, 1982; Scott, Caird, and Williams, 1984; Stern, Mayeux, and Rosen, 1984; Villardita, Smirni, LePira, Zappala, and Nicoletti, 1982). Conversely, damage to subcortical structures has been associated with aphasia (Albert, 1984; Damasio, Damasio, Rizzo, Varney, and Gersh, 1982; Riklan and Levita, 1970).

Yet another criticism with the cortical–subcortical distinction is made by Whitehouse (1986). Whitehouse argues that the terms "subcortical" and "cortical" emphasize the independence of these anatomic, regions while neurochemical and neuropathologic studies are showing a relation between them. AD patients, or cortical dementia patients, have been found to have subcortical pathologic changes in the nucleus basalis of Meynert (Arendt, Bigl, Arendt, Tennstedt, 1983; Rogers, Brogan, and Mirra, 1985; Tagliavini and Pilleri, 1983; Whitehouse, Price, Clark, Coyle, and DeLong, 1981) the nucleus locus coeruleus (Forno, Barbour, and Norville, 1978; Hirano and Zimmerman, 1962; Perry et al., 1981), the raphe nucleus (Curcio and Kemper, 1984), the amygdala (Corsellis, 1970; Herzog and Kemper, 1980; Hooper and Vogel, 1976), and the thalamus, hypothalamus, and mamillary body (McDuff and Sumi, 1985). Similarly, PD patients, or subcortical dementia patients, have degeneration of neurons in the cortex (Alvord, 1968; Boller, Mizutani, Roessmann, and Gambetti, 1980; Gaspar and Gray, 1984; Hakim and Mathieson, 1979; Jellinger and Grisold, 1982), as do HD patients (Bruyn, Bots, and Dom, 1979; Forno and Jose, 1973; McCaughey, 1961).

Cummings and Benson (1984), proponents of the dichotomy, recognize as important the criticism that most dementing diseases are associated with pathologic changes in both cortical and subcortical brain areas. Their rejoinder is that no acceptable alternative nomenclature has been devised, and the "terminologic shortcomings do not abrogate the basic tenet that diseases involving primarily subcortical structures produce intellectual deficits distinguishable from those associated with the diseases involving predominantly cortical structures" (p. 875).

A Different Approach to Classifying Dementia Patients. Rather than trying to define the behavioral characteristics associated with different dementia-producing diseases, Mesulam (1985) looked for the existence of behavioral patterns that transcend etiologic boundaries. He discerned several different profiles of mental state alterations. The first clinically identifiable group is patients in whom amnesia is a major feature; the diagnosis is generally AD. The second group of patients have salient aphasia, agnosia, and apraxia and may be Pick's or AD patients. The third behavioral profile defines those patients whose preponderant problems are in motivation and comportment, and the diagnosis is obscure; AD patients are least common in this group.

SUMMARY

Although many interetiologic studies have been conducted, few have been done for the purpose of investigating linguistic communication ability in patients with etiologically different dementias. Thus, little can be definitively stated about critical interetiologic differences. One exception is the much greater probability of a motor speech problem in patients with HD or PD because of pathologic changes in the basal ganglia. In terms of language and communicative function, the picture is less certain. Bayles (1985) found many more likenesses than differences between PD, HD, and AD in performance on a variety of communication tasks.

Not only are the similarities between etiologically different patients in communication test performance important (Bayles, 1985) so also is the fact that each of the three types of dementia patients were extensively impaired in communicative functioning. Each group of mildly demented patients exhibited impairment in verbal associative reasoning, generative naming, linguistic disambiguation, verbal description, and story-retelling. Additionally, each group of moderately impaired individuals exhibited impairment in confrontation naming, vocabulary, sentence judgment and correction, and language use.

The similarities and differences between AD and Pick's disease patients were discussed in this section. At present, a formal study of both types of patients has not been reported, to our knowledge, and differences must be inferred from the descriptions of published case histories. The most prominent difference, mentioned by Holland and co-workers (1985), is the greater loss of formal syntactic knowledge early in Pick's disease. In AD, syntactic knowledge generally holds, and the most prominent early defect is semantic.

A disorder similar to both Alzheimer's and Pick's diseases is one that Morris and associates (1984) call "hereditary dysphasic dementia." The condition is characterized by loss of verbal fluency, dysnomia, paraphasia, late stage mutism, and global aphasia.

From the comparative investigations of AD and MID patients, it appears that MID patients are more likely to experience a loss of specific linguistic rules. Far more typical of AD is the gradual deterioration of semantic memory and ideation. MID patients with focal damage have focal neurologic signs and the classic aphasia syndromes.

A popular dichotomy is the cortical-subcortical distinction, in which AD patients, with predominantly cortical pathologic changes, are distinguished from patients with dementia and subcortical pathologic changes secondary to HD, PD, supranuclear palsy, and normal pressure hydrocephalus. Though the terms "cortical" and "subcortical dementia" are widely used, they are controversial. The controversy arises from the fact that the pathologic changes of cortical dementing diseases extends to subcortical structures, and the pathologic changes of subcortical dementias extends to the cortex. Proponents of the use of these terms recognize them as somewhat misleading, but argue that their imperfection is dwarfed by their heuristic value.

After this review of differences in the nature of linguistic impairment in patients with etiologically different dementias, it is now appropriate to consider what intraetiologic differences might exist.

INTRAETIOLOGIC DIFFERENCES IN LINGUISTIC COMMUNICATION DEFICITS AMONG DEMENTIA PATIENTS

Alzheimer's Disease

Gillian Cohen (1983) has argued persuasively that the time has come to give more attention to specifying the variability, rather than the similarity, in information processing skills among individuals—a view we support, particularly in relation to the study of dementia patients. In their clinical experience, Albert and Moss (1984) report having examined three types of AD patients: (1) patients with striking memory impairment, defective processing of abstractions, set shifting, and naming deficits, (2) patients with dramatic and progressive language impairment and associated, though less striking, memory and abstraction problems, and (3) patients with dramatic visuospatial deficits early in the disease course, and some other cognitive problems, which again are less striking. Numerous variables have been identified as affecting the nature of linguistic communicative impairment in AD patients, among them distribution of morphologic change, age at disease onset, familial history, and rate of disease progression.

Distribution of Morphologic Changes. A variable that logically may affect the nature of linguistic communicative impairment in AD patients is distribution of pathologic changes within the brain. Although it is true that the neuropathologic change in dementing illness is diffuse, it is not necessarily symmetric. Using positron emission tomography, several investigators (Chase et al., 1984; Friedland et al., 1983; Haxby, Duara, Grady, Cutler, and Rapoport, 1985) demonstrated that individuals with Alzheimer's disease vary in the degree of hypometabolism in homologous regions of the cerebral hemispheres. Whereas the temporoparietal areas in both cerebral hemispheres generally have the greatest hypometabolism, they are not symmetrically impaired. Chase and colleagues (1984) found a close association between WAIS verbal IQ scores and cortical metabolism in the left cerebral hemisphere, especially in the left temporal lobe. WAIS performance IQ scores correlated best with metabolism in the right hemisphere, particularly with that of the right parietal lobe. Similarly, Haxby and associates 1985) have observed visuospatial deficits with greater right temporoparietal hypometabolism, and language deficits with greater left hypometabolism.

Age at Disease Onset. Another potential contributor to differences in AD patients is age at disease onset. Seltzer and Sherwin (1983) suggested a "possible heightened selective vulnerability of left hemisphere" in early-onset AD. They reported language disturbance with early onset of AD and described these patients as significantly more likely to show abnormalities in spontaneous speech and verbal comprehension, object naming, and writing. On the other hand, Sulkava and Amberla (1982) reported no significant differences in impressive and expressive speech between early and late onset. Constantinidis (1978) observed language loss in both senile and presenile AD patients, although language dissolution in individuals with the presenile form was described as quicker in onset, more serious, and less regular in chronologic evolution. Like Seltzer and Sherwin (1983), Sourander and Sjögren (1970) and Lauter and Meyer (1968) associated language problems with the early form.

Albert and Moss (1984) found that presenile and senile AD patients (equated on the Mattis Dementia Rating Scale for severity) differed on the Boston Naming Test. The senile AD patients performed significantly worse in relation to age-matched controls.

Familial History. A familial history of AD is yet another variable suspected of being linked with special clinical characteristics. An aggregation of AD patients within the same family suggests genetic influences in disease development. Some authors have associated the familial form with specific linguistic characteristics. Breitner and Folstein (1984) reported language disturbance and apraxia in 78 percent of their familial cases and a sevenfold increase in lifetime dementia risk for relatives of language-disordered DAT probands versus controls. The Breitner and Folstein finding is very provocative, but Heyman and colleagues (1984) were unable to replicate it.

Rate of Disease Progression. Language has been related to progression rate by Kaszniak and associates (1978), who reported overall accuracy of simple sentence production to differentiate AD patients who died within a 1-year follow-up from those still surviving (both groups had equivalent length of dementia history). To date, systematic and comprehensive evaluation of communicative function in relation to these distinguishing variables has not been done.

To summarize, patterns of morphologic change, age of disease onset, familial history, and rate of disease progression appear to have the potential to affect the nature and rate of dissolution of communicative functioning. With the potential effects of these variables in mind, the question of how language changes over time as dementia worsens will now be addressed.

RESULTS OF LONGITUDINAL STUDIES OF LANGUAGE CHANGE

Even fewer longitudinal studies have been completed than interetiologic investigations, and of those completed, only two were expressly for the purpose of documenting change in communicative function: the Chicago study (Kaszniak and Wilson, 1985) and the Tucson study (Bayles, 1985). The Chicago study, conducted by Drs. Kaszniak and Wilson at Rush-Presbyterian-St. Luke's Medical Center, is also the largest completed longitudinal investigation. A description of the methodology and results of the Chicago and Tucson studies will dominate this section. However, data from the study by Berg and colleagues (1984) will be reviewed, as well as data from a smaller longitudinal study by Horner, Heyman, Kanter, Royall, and Aker (1983) of change in spoken discourse among AD patients.

The Chicago Longitudinal Study

A major purpose of the Chicago longitudinal study was to document changes in communicative and other cognitive functions in Alzheimer's dementia patients. Recruited for participation were 122 subjects: 62 AD patients and 60 normal controls. All subjects received physical and neurologic examinations, computed tomographic (CT) scan, electroencephalogram (EEG), psychiatric interview, and extensive neuropsychologic evaluation. The 62 AD participants met the criteria established in the DSM-III for primary degenerative dementia. Only patients with a history of cognitive decline and an absence of focal pathologic changes, major systemic illness, delirium, and psychotic symptoms and signs were accepted for participation. To deselect patients suspected of having vascular disease and dementia, the Hachinski ischemic scale (Hachinski, Lassen and Marshall, 1974) was used. None of the AD subjects were institutionalized when the study began. Study participants were examined annually for the 5-year duration of the study. During the first 4 years, new subjects were added. Eight AD patients and 14 controls entered in year 4 and therefore received only two examinations. The longest period over which subjects were followed up was 3 years, with 31 AD patients and 39 normal control subjects remaining in the 3-year follow-through sample. Demographic data for longitudinal participants and those lost to followup are presented in Table 4-6. No significant differences were found in age, sex, education, physical and neurologic examination, initial memory performance, or mental status scores between the two groups.

Generally, Alzheimer's subjects were mildly impaired at the time of their inclusion in the study (although a few would probably be classified within the mild to moderate range by current standards). All were living in the community, none required assistance with the basic self-care activities, and all were capable of participating in 2 days of testing.

Four measures were used to evaluate communicative function: the Boston Diagnostic Aphasia Examination (BDAE) (Goodglass and Kaplan, 1972), the Northwestern Word Latency Naming Test (Rutherford, 1972), the Peabody Picture Vocabulary Test (PPVT) (Dunn, 1965), and the Auditory Comprehension Test for Sentences (ACTS) (Shewan, 1979). As discussed elsewhere in this volume, the BDAE is a comprehensive language examination battery, which surveys fluency, auditory comprehension, naming, oral reading, repetition, automatic speech, reading comprehension, writing, and music. The Northwestern Word Latency Naming Test is a visual confrontation naming task that involves the sequential presentation of 63 pictures of common objects with three temporally separated, reordered repetitions, the subject being required to name each object. The PPVT is a receptive vocabulary test, and the ACTS is a 42-item auditory comprehension test in which sentence length, word frequency, and syntactic complexity are systematically varied. In addition, the Wechsler Memory Scale (Wechsler, 1945) and a 24-item mental status examination were administered.

To identify initial group performance differences on cognitive and communicative measures, as well as possible differences between longitudinal and nonlongitudinal (i.e., those who could not be followed up for a full 3 years) subjects, a series of two-way (group by dropout) analyses of variance (ANOVA) were computed for each cognitive and language measure. Significant group main effects ($p < .05$) were obtained for all dependent measures, confirming pervasive impairment of memory and language functions in AD patients compared with normal elderly subjects. On only 2 of the 45 variables, PPVT and BDAE written spelling to dicta-

Table 4-6. Demographic Description of Subjects Followed Up for Three Annual Examinations Versus Subjects Lost to Follow-Up in the Chicago Study

	Sample Followed Up		Sample Lost to Follow-Up	
	Controls	AD	Controls	AD
Age	69.28	68.81	68.86	66.70
Education	10.82	11.81	13.10	10.80
Sex*				
Female	17.6%	18.5%	9.2%	11.8%
Male	15.1%	7.6%	9.2%	10.9%
Race*				
White	32.0%	23.5%	18.5%	22.7%
Black	0.8%	2.5%	0.0%	0.0%
Illness length (months)	—	33.14	—	44.18

*Expressed as percentage of total sample.

tion, were nonlongitudinal AD patients (patients lost to follow-up) different in initial performance from longitudinal subjects. Nonlongitudinal subjects showed slightly better performance. No significant main effects of followed-up versus not followed-up (collapsing across AD and control subjects) were obtained; thus, it can be concluded that the sample available for reexamination at each of the three annual evaluations is representative of the entire sample originally enrolled in the study.

Significant group main effects were obtained for all dependent memory and linguistic communication variables at the initial examination, and the magnitude of their corresponding *F* ratios ranged from relatively small (5.49 on the Boston Repetition of Word subtest) to very large (243.84 for the Wechsler Memory Scale Raw Score total). Though the magnitude of *F* ratios is a function of the magnitude of group differences *and* variability in task performance, the wide range of F ratios does suggest differential impairment of the various memory and communicative functions assessed by the dependent measures. To help the reader appreciate the level of AD patient functioning at the time of initial evaluation, and the degree to which performance on the various measures of language and communication changed over time, the performance of subjects on several language measures has been graphed. The performance graphs have been combined into two figures (Figures 4-1 and 4-3). The slope of each graph represents change in the group average over time.

Characteristics of Conversational Speech. The flow of speech of AD patients was not found to be abnormal at any time during the course of the study. In relation to Speech Melody, Phrase Length, Articulatory Agility, Grammatical Form, Word Finding, and Frequency of Paraphasic Errors in Running Speech, AD patients demonstrated only mild to moderate impairment (Figure 4-2). Multivariate analyses of variance were computed to test for differential deterioration over time in the AD versus control group. Among the characteristics of conversational speech, only Grammatical Form and Frequency of Paraphasia in Running Speech showed significant interaction effects.

Auditory Comprehension. At the initial testing, moderate to severe impairment was observed on the BDAE subtests examining auditory comprehension. Moderate deficit was apparent in AD patients when they were asked to point to pictured objects or body parts in response to a spoken word, and for two- and three-step verbal commands. Severe deficit was apparent when AD patients attempted to answer logical questions (e.g., Will a board sink in water?) and demonstrate comprehension of brief stories read to them.

A similar pattern of AD patient impairment was apparent on the PPVT and ACTS. Auditory comprehension of single words was moderately impaired at the time of initial evaluation and deteriorated significantly over time. Comprehension of sentence-length spoken phrases was, however, more severely impaired at the first examination, as determined by performance on the ACTS, and continued to significantly deteriorate over time.

Naming: Generative and Confrontation. Severe impairment was observed, at the time of initial evaluation, in the ability to generate examples of a semantic category (in this case, animals). The amount of deterioration over 3 years can be seen in Figure 4-3.

Mild to moderate impairment was observed on the Boston Visual Confrontation Naming, Boston Responsive Naming, and Northwestern Word Naming tests at the initial evaluation (Figure 4-3), and performance on all four tests deteriorated during the course of the study. Most confrontation naming errors were perseverations of previously correct naming responses or names semantically related to the target name (e.g., "lock" for "key"). Phonemic substitutions and neologisms were rare.

Repetition. Difficulty with repetition appeared to be a function of task difficulty. Patients had mild difficulty repeating words, slightly more difficulty repeating simple common phrases, and marked problems with unusual phrases (e.g., "The Chinese fan had a rare emerald"). Failures on the latter task are not necessarily attributable to short-term

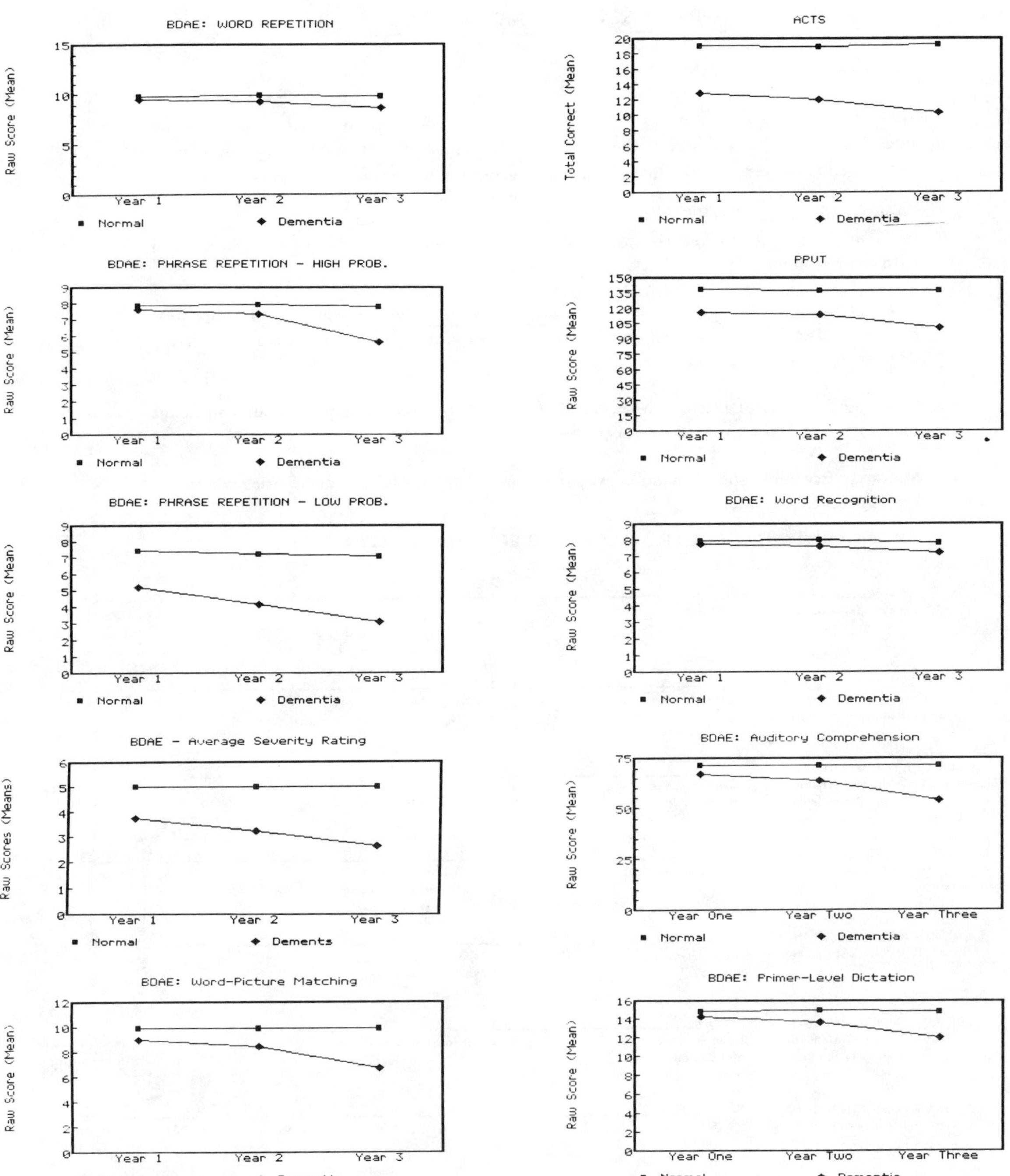

Figure 4-1. *Performance of Chicago study subjects on various language/communication measures.*

APHASIA SEVERITY RATING SCALE

0. No usable speech or auditory comprehension.

1. All communication is through fragmentary expression; great need for inference, questioning and guessing by the listener. The range of information which can be exchanged is limited, and the listener carries the burden of communication.

2. Conversation about familiar subjects is possible with help from the listener. There are frequent failures to convey the idea, but patient shares the burden of communication with the examiner.

3. The patient can discuss almost all everyday problems with little or no assistance. However, reduction of speech and/or comprehension make conversation about certain material difficult or impossible.

4. Some obvious loss of fluency in speech or facility of comprehension, without significant limitation on ideas expressed or form of expression.

5. Minimal discernible speech handicaps; patient may have subjective difficulties which are not apparent to listener.

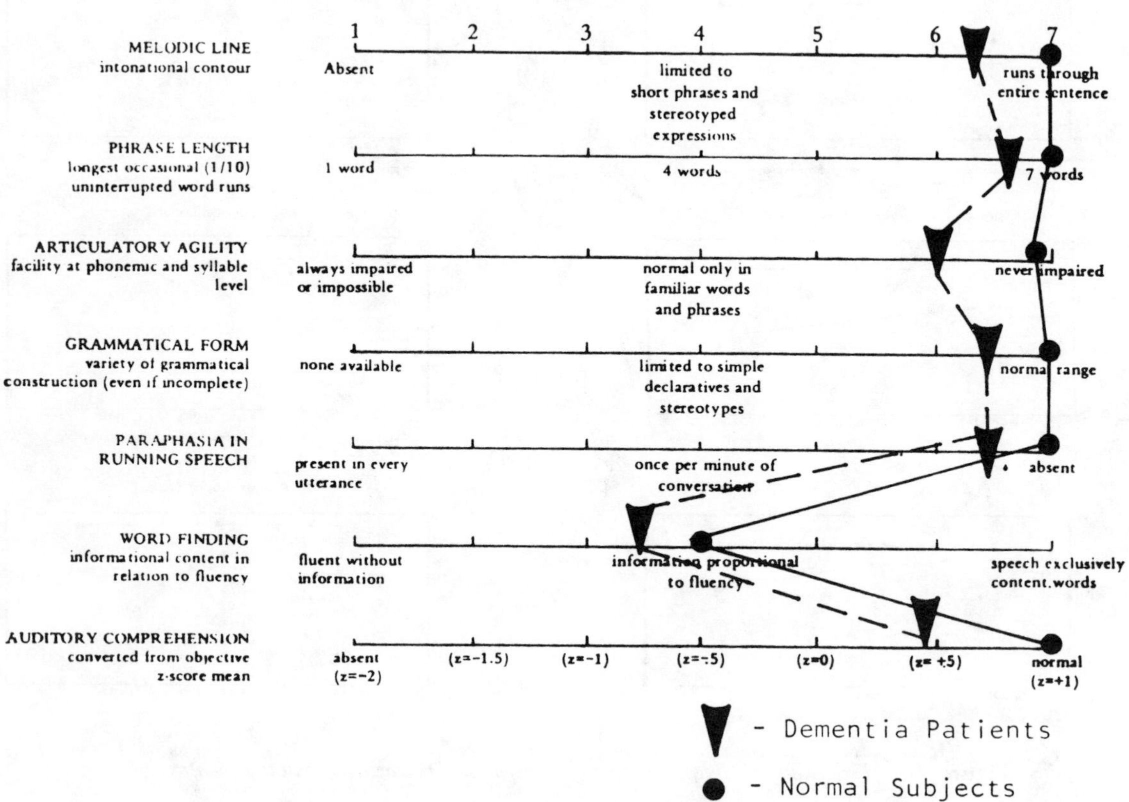

Figure 4-2. *Performance of Chicago study subjects on BDAE conversational speech measures at year 1 examination.*

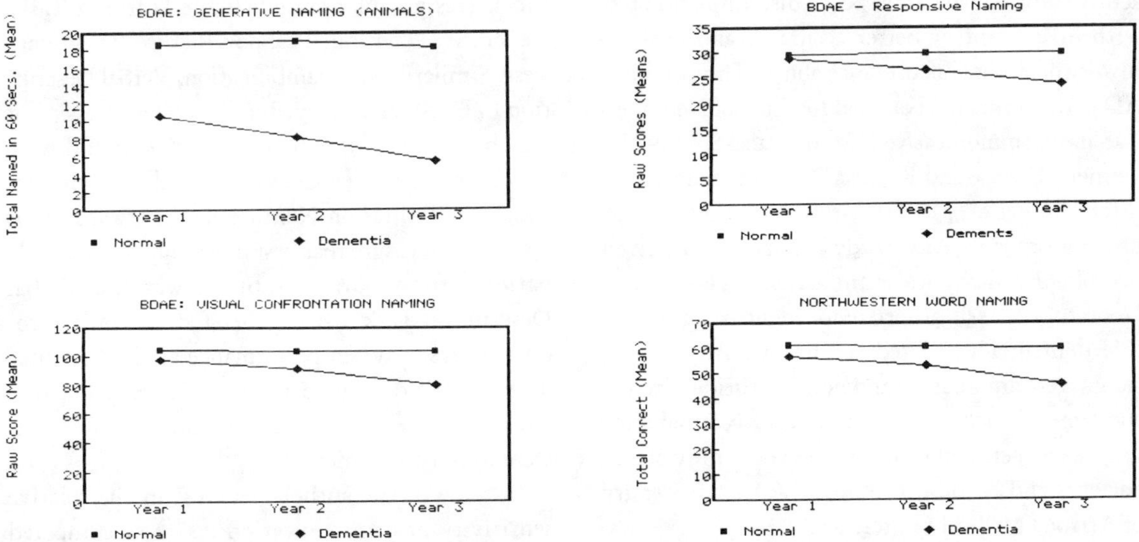

Figure 4-3. *Performance of Chicago study subjects on naming tasks.*

memory defects, because the AD patients were relatively successful repeating high probability phrases of equivalent length.

Reading and Writing. Patients could perceive written material and read aloud, but comprehension of written material was poor. Orthography of writing was initially only mildly defective, but writing to dictation and narrative writing were moderately impaired. All aspects of reading and writing deteriorated significantly during the study.

Summary. In AD subjects in the Chicago study, deficits were apparent across a broad range of communicative functions: naming, repetition, comprehension, reading, and writing. At initial examination of patients, early in the course of the disorder, the form (articulatory agility, phrase length, grammar, and so on) of conversational speech was relatively normal, but it became more impaired as the disease worsened. Content defects, however, were noticeable early and markedly increased with the evolution of dementia. Naming problems, particularly generative, were prominent early and worsened over the 3 years. Repetition was good in the early stages when words or simple phrases were being repeated, but impaired when unusual phrases were given. With the exception of the orthographic aspects, writing was moderately impaired early and deteriorated steadily over the 3 years.

Tucson Longitudinal Study of Communicative Change in Dementia

One of the purposes of the 3-year Tucson study was to document the nature of linguistic dissolution in AD patients over time. Thirty-one AD subjects and 33 normal elderly control subjects were selected for participation. New subjects were added until the end of the 2nd year. Subjects were tested every 6 months, and the longest unit of time over which longitudinal analysis was feasible turned out to be 18 months. Of the original sample, 13 AD patients and 20 normal subjects were evaluated over the course of 18 months. Potential differences between the subjects who participated in the longitudinal portion and those who did not were considered, but no significant differences in age, years of education, or estimated premorbid intelligence were found. The most common reasons for subject attrition were death, development of another serious illness, and intellectual deterioration sufficient to make them untestable.

All study participants had to be native speakers of English, be of normal estimated premorbid intelligence, be able to read newsprint, have auditory acuity sufficient to pass a speech discrimination test with 80 percent or better accuracy, and have no history of alcohol or substance abuse. The sample of AD patients met the National Institute of Neurological and Communicative Disorders and Stroke-Alzheimer's Disease and Related Disorders Association (McKhann et al., 1984) criteria for clinical diagnosis of probable AD. Study participants received neurologic and physical examinations, CT scan, and laboratory tests appropriate for identifying reversible dementia-associated conditions. All AD patients were ambulatory and noninstitutionalized at the time of inclusion in the study. Normal subjects were recruited from spouses and family of AD patients and hospital volunteers at the University of Arizona Medical Center.

Severity of dementia was determined using results of neurologic examination, nonlinguistic neuropsychologic testing, and scores on a behavioral inventory of the capacity to perform activities of daily living and accept responsibility for management of personal affairs. Seven of the AD patients were mildly impaired (GDS = 3 or 4) and six were moderately impaired (GDS = 5 or 6). The average score of mild AD patients on the 10-question Mental Status Questionnaire (Goldfarb, 1975) was 7.4 (of a possible 10), and for moderates, 6.0.

The test battery, which was designed in 1979, included psychologic measures reputed to be sensitive to dementia, notably Block Design and Forward Digit Span subtests of the WAIS, the Nonsense Syllable Learning Task (Alexander, 1973), and a variety of communication tasks (Table 4-2). The rationale for test selection was based on a desire to evaluate receptive and expressive functions in each linguistic domain (phonologic, syntactic, semantic, and pragmatic), in addition to linguistic reasoning, naming, vocabulary, and propositional language. According to the literature available at the commencement of the study, dementia patients were described as having difficulty with propositional language, though knowledge of specific linguistic rules was well preserved.

Using analysis of variance, a significant performance difference was observed between *mild* dementia patients and normal subjects on the following: Block Design, Nonsense Syllable Learning Task, Generative Naming, Peabody Picture Vocabulary Test, Similarities, Disambiguation, Verbal Description (VDES), and Story-Retelling. Those tasks for which a significant difference was *not* found were as follows: Sentence Correction Task, Pragmatics Task, Confrontation Naming, and Forward Digit Span. The measure that best discriminated mild AD patients from normal subjects was the Verbal Description Task, a self-generated, discourse production task. When performance at time of entry of *moderately* demented individuals was compared with that of normal subjects, significant differences were found on all measures.

Because of the authors' interest in the relative sensitivity of communication tasks, as compared with a select group of neuropsychologic tasks, for discriminating dementia, a composite variable, "LING," representing linguistic performance, was created for each subject. All of the communication measures were used, except Verbal Description, because it is an open-ended test with no ceiling score.

The discriminant power of this variable was compared with that of the four cognitive measures. Would the composite score, LING, better discriminate dementia patients than one of its subcomponents or the psychologic measures used in the study? LING was found to be best for differentiating dementia patients from normal subjects (Table 4-7). Alone, it classified normal subjects and AD patients with 85 percent accuracy. When combined with performance on the Verbal Description Task, the accuracy of classification increased to 93 percent. When the discrimination was between PD and normal subjects, and HD and normal subjects, LING alone or LING and VDES were better than LING and a nonlinguistic psychologic measure. Thus, language measures were found to be effective for discriminating mild dementia and more effective than the small set of psychologic measures (i.e., Block Design, Forward Digit Span, Nonsense Syllable Learning Task, and Mental Status Questionnaire).

When the first and last LING scores of AD patients were compared, five patients had slightly, but not significantly, higher scores after 18

Table 4-7. Results of Discriminant Function Analysis in the Tucson Study

Group	Analysis	Selected Variable	Classification Accuracy Rate (Percent)
AD and controls	LING alone		85
	LING and VDES		93
	LING and NL	None	93
PD and controls	LING alone		83
	LING and VDES		83
	LING and NL	None	81
HD and controls	LING alone		81
	LING and VDES		81
	LING and NL	None	80

NL, Nonlinguistic psychologic measures: Block Design, Forward Digit Span, Nonsense Syllable Learning Task, and Mental Status Questionnaire.

months. The scores of one individual did not change, and the scores of seven were significantly lower. The measures on which the greatest deterioration occurred were, in order; Confrontation Naming, Sentence Disambiguation, Block Design, Verbal Description, and the Peabody Picture Vocabulary Test.

Summary. The data from the Tucson longitudinal study revealed that language content is affected before form, generative naming before confrontation naming, and propositional use of language before automatic use. Further, phonologic and syntactic judgments are more easily made than semantic and pragmatic. Knowledge of vocabulary is significantly impaired early and gradually diminishes as dementia worsens. Finally, the data suggest that measures of communicative function are as efficacious as Block Design, a visuospatial constructive task, and the Nonsense Syllable Learning Task, a learning task for discriminating mildly and moderately demented persons.

Other Longitudinal Reports

Horner and associates (1983) investigated changes in spoken discourse over a 1-year period in 12 AD patients who were "moderately-advanced" at the time of first testing. Subjects were asked to give a verbal description of the well-known "Cookie-Theft" picture from the BDAE (Goodglass and Kaplan, 1972). Samples were evaluated for fluency, frequency of nouns and adjectives, instances of repetition, perseveration, irrelevancy, number of words, concept productivity, grammatical completeness, speech sound integrity, and semantic completeness.

At the end of a year, 7 of the 12 patients remained stable in overall severity of language impairment, as measured by analysis of performance in relation to the aforementioned variables. Of the five individuals who worsened, the most significant changes occurred in fluency, the frequency of nouns and adjectives, and repetitions and perseverations. Verbal fluency and frequency of use of nouns and adjectives decreased, and the number of repetitions and perseverations increased.

Berg and colleagues (1984) studied 43 community-dwelling patients with mild AD to examine the usefulness of clinical, psychometric, CT, EEG, and visual evoked potentials in predicting the clinical course of dementia over a year. In addition to the physiologic and radiographic measures, subjects were given numerous clinical scales, specifically the Short Portable Mental Status Questionnaire of Pfeiffer (1975), the Dementia Scale of Blessed, Tomlinson, and Roth (1968), the Initial Subject Protocol based upon the Clinical Dementia Rating devised at Washington University (Hughes, Berg, Danziger, Coben, and Martin, 1982), and the Face-Hand Test (Fink, Green, and Bender, 1952). Additionally, communicative function was assessed with six verbal tasks derived from the BDAE, including the Rating Scale Profile of Speech Characteristics from the subject's description of the Cookie-Theft picture, Oral Naming, Word Discrimination, and Written Expression from pictured items, Reading Comprehension, Reception (yes-or-no responses to five oral questions), and Body-Part Identification.

Of the 43 mild AD patients studied, 21 remained unchanged at the end of the year, 16 had advanced to the moderate stage of dementia, 5 were rated severely demented, and 1 was lost to follow-up.

Table 4-8. Summary of Clinical Impressions and Research Reports on Communicative Impairment in Early Mild Dementia Patients

Rating Scale	Score	Rating Scale	Score
Global Deterioration Scale (range 1–7, normal = 1)	3–4	Mattis Dementia Rating Scale (range 0–142, normal = 142)	120–130
Mini-Mental Status Examination (range 0–30, normal = 30)	16–24	Blessed's Dementia Scale (range 0–28, normal = 0)	9–19
Goldfarb's Mental Status Questionnaire (range 0–10, normal = 0)	3–6	Clinical Dementia Rating (range 0–3, normal = 0)	1

	Degree of Deficit				
	Little or None	Minimal	Moderate	Prominent	Severe
Contents of SM					
Conceptual knowledge		*----------	----------*		
Propositional knowledge		*----------	----------*		
Schematic knowledge		*----------*			
Processes of SM					
Ideation		*----------	----------*		
Inferencing		*----------	----------*		
Reasoning		*----------	----------*		
Association		*----------	----------*		
Contents of EM					
Verbal			*----------	----------*	
Nonverbal			*----------	----------*	
Processes of EM					
Encoding			*----------	----------*	
Retention			*----------	----------*	
Retrieval			*----------	----------*	
Lexical knowledge					
Form	*----------*				
Orthographic	*----------*				
Phonologic	*----------*				
Class	*----------*				
Definition		*----------	----------*		
Linguistic knowledge					
Phonologic	*----------*				
Syntactic	*----------*				
Semantic		*----------	----------*		
Pragmatic		*----------	----------*		
Automatic language use	*----------*				
Propositional language use		*----------	----------*		

Table 4-8. *(continued)*

Communicative Skills/Functions					
	Little, If Any, Deterioration	Deterioration		Little, If Any, Deterioration	Deterioration
Confrontation naming		X	Articulation (AD only)	X	
Misperception	X		Phrase length	X	
Generative naming		X	Grammar	X	
Reading comprehension			Linguistic disambiguation		X
Word		X	Verbal associative reasoning		X
Sentence		X	Sentence judgment		
Paragraph		X	Phonologic error	X	
Vocabulary		X	Syntactic error	X	
Pantomime recognition	X		Semantic error		X
Pantomime expression		X	Sentence correction		
Repetition			Phonologic	X	
Word	X		Syntactic	X	
Low-probability phrases		X	Semantic		X
High-probability phrases	X		Oral and written discourse		
Word association			Number of ideas		X
Paradigmatic		X	Number of words	X	
Syntagmatic	X		Vocabulary diversity		X
			Use of reference		X
			Cohesion		X
			Auditory discrimination of word pairs	X	

Longer estimated duration of illness was associated with moderate or severe dementia. One of the most accurate predictors of dementia severity at the end of the year was performance on the communication measures, or aphasia tests.

DISSOLUTION OF COMMUNICATIVE FUNCTION IN DEMENTIA: A SUMMARY

The results of studies reviewed in this chapter have been summarized and related to the various stages of dementia as defined by several dementia severity rating scales (Tables 4-8, 4-9, and 4-10). In the top section of Tables 4-8 and 4-9 are specified the range of values associated with early mild and moderate dementia, respectively. In the middle section is specified the degree of deficit in the contents and processes of semantic memory, episodic memory, lexical knowledge, linguistic knowledge, and automatic and propositional language systems. In the continuation of Tables 4-8 and 4-9 (top of pp. 123 and 125, respectively) is a summary of the specific types of communicative tasks on which deficits have been reported, and a gross estimate of the degree of impairment based upon the authors' clinical impressions and integration of available research reports. In Table 4-10, a brief description of the nature of the impairment in common communicative functions is provided.

Early Mild Stage

In the mild stage, the duration of which is variable, typically lasting 1 to 3 years, communication deficits are frequently overlooked. Errors made

Table 4-9. Summary of Clinical Impressions and Research Reports on Communicative Impairment in Moderate Dementia Patients

Rating Scale	Score	Rating Scale	Score
Global Deterioration Scale (range 1–7, normal = 1)	5–6	Mattis Dementia Rating Scale (range 0–142, normal = 142)	90–120
Mini-Mental Status Examination (range 0–30, normal = 30)	8–15	Blessed's Dementia Scale (range 0–28, normal = 0)	20–28
Goldfarb's Mental Status Questionnaire (range 0–10, normal = 0)	7–8	Clinical Dementia Rating (range 0–3, normal = 0)	2

	Degree of Deficit				
	Little or None	Minimal	Moderate	Prominent	Severe
Contents of SM					
Conceptual knowledge			*--------	--------*	
Propositional knowledge			*--------	--------*	
Schematic knowledge			*---------------*		
Processes of SM					
Ideation			*--------	--------*	
Inferencing			*--------	--------*	
Reasoning			*--------	--------*	
Association			*--------	--------*	
Contents of EM					
Verbal					*---------------*
Nonverbal					*---------------*
Processes of EM					
Encoding					*---------------*
Retention					*---------------*
Retrieval					*---------------*
Lexical knowledge					
Form	*--------	--------*			
Orthographic	*--------	--------*			
Phonologic	*--------	--------*			
Class	*--------	--------*			
Definition			*--------	--------*	
Linguistic knowledge					
Phonologic	*---------------*				
Syntactic		*---------------*			
Semantic			*---------------*		
Pragmatic			*--------	--------*	
Automatic language use		*---------------*			
Propositional language use			*--------	--------*	

Table 4-9. *(continued)*

Communicative Skills/Functions					
	Little, If Any, Deterioration	Deterioration		Little, If Any, Deterioration	Deterioration
Confrontation naming		X	Articulation (AD only)	X	
Misperception		X	Phrase length	X	
Generative naming		X	Grammar		X
Reading comprehension			Linguistic disambiguation		X
Word		X	Verbal associative reasoning		X
Sentence		X	Sentence judgment		
Paragraph		X	Phonologic error	X	
Vocabulary		X	Syntactic error	X	
Pantomime recognition		X	Semantic error		X
Pantomime expression		X	Sentence correction		
Repetition			Phonologic	X	
Word	X		Syntactic		X
Low-probability phrases		X	Semantic		X
High-probability phrases		X	Oral and written discourse		
Word association			Number of ideas		X
Paradigmatic		X	Number of words	X	
Syntagmatic		X	Vocabulary diversity		X
			Use of reference		X
			Cohesion		X
			Auditory discrimination of word pairs	X	

by patients in the comprehension and production of linguistic information are presumed by most listeners to be the everyday performance errors that people make when they are tired, distracted, or nervous. Listeners automatically correct such errors and think nothing of them. (If the reader doubts the existence of these errors, make a tape recording and transcription of an ordinary conversation, preferably your own!)

Most linguistic communication errors made by dementia patients in the early stage are conceptual and can be detected by discourse analysis. A review of the discourse content will reveal ideational impoverishment, shrinking vocabulary, frequent irrelevancies, perseverations, and intrusions. Syntax, or the structure of language, is essentially unaffected. The most sensitive measures for detecting the disordered communication are verbal description, generative naming, vocabulary, reading comprehension, verbal associative reasoning, and linguistic disambiguation.

Moderate Stage

Patients in the moderate stages of dementia, whose duration can range from 2 to 10 years, have prominent communication problems that are no longer mistaken for performance errors. The marked deterioration in the contents and processes of semantic and episodic memory are readily apparent in a variety of tasks, among them poor generative naming and worsening confrontation naming, inability to comprehend what has been read, diminished receptive and expressive vocabularies, difficulty pro-

Table 4-10. Summary of Clinical Impressions and Research Reports on Communicative Impairment in Severe Dementia Patients

Communicative Skill	Degree of Deficit	Comments
Naming	Severe dysnomia; anomia	
Reading: words	Severely impaired comprehension; mechanics of oral reading may be spared	
Pantomime recognition	Severely impaired	
Pantomime expression	Severely impaired	
Written discourse	Severe impairment of both ideation and orthography	
Vocabulary	Severely limited	Continued access to a diverse lexicon is evident in some late-stage patients
Repetition	Variable impairment	Ranges from echolalia to mutism; some patients may correctly repeat common words and short, familiar phrases; occasional spontaneous correction of grammatical errors
Sentence judgment	Severely impaired	Phonologic, syntactic, and semantic errors are not typically corrected by advanced patients
Oral discourse	Variety of impairments	Characterized by palilalia, echolalia, perseveration, sentence fragments, jargon, neologisms; discourse is empty and vague, lacking cohesion, with few definite references; prosody, cadence, and social language stereotypies may be spared disproportionately to other verbal abilites; number of expressed ideas is severely depressed in all advanced patients, yet the total number of words produced varies greatly; some patients lose all oral–verbal abilities and appear mute
Auditory discrimination of word pairs	Little or no impairment	Repetition indicates accurate perception of speech sounds, although the same–different discrimination is invariably lost

ducing pantomime, errors in the repetition of high as well as low probability phrases, verbal associative reasoning deficits, and confusion with sentence disambiguation. Yet, moderately affected patients (with AD) talk fluently, read aloud effortlessly, produce generally grammatical utterances, and respond to many of the social conventions governing communicative interchanges. As was the case with mildly demented patients, analysis of linguistic content, rather than form, is best for quantifying the communicative impairment of this stage.

Severe Stage

Late-stage dementia patients are disoriented for time, place, and person and typically are unable to take formal psychometric tests. Nevertheless, considerable variation exists in the communicative characteristics of patients with late-stage dementia, variation that is undoubtedly due to differences in the distribution and type of pathologic changes. To date, however, a large systematic study of late-stage dementia patients, with postmortem follow-up, has not been reported as far as we know.

In an ongoing longitudinal study at the University of Arizona, supported by the National Institute of Mental Health, severe AD patients are being examined. The examination consists of a series of semistructured interviews in which the abilities of the patient to name, discriminate, repeat, imitate, read, write, pantomime, and participate in a conversation are rated. Although in some patients the mechanics of speaking, reading, and writing are intact, the linguistic output is typically incoherent. Occasionally a well known phrase will be interspersed amidst the nonsensical babble, and it will seem as though the individual is momentarily lucid. Many severely demented patients retain access to the mental lexicon after the conceptual system has become essentially nonfunctional. Other patients appear to lose access to both lexical and semantic memory. Perseveration, echolalia, and palilalia are chronic in this severity group.

GENERAL SUMMARY AND CLINICAL IMPLICATIONS

1. Interetiologic comparisons of dementia patients are complicated by the methodologic problems involved in controlling dementia severity. When evaluating the dementia research literature, clinicians should consider how effectively dementia severity was specified and controlled.
2. The use of the terms "mild," "moderate," and "severe" varies across investigators.
3. Clinicians and researchers should use the validated dementia rating scales to determine severity.
4. Regardless of the cause of dementia, patients have difficulty with tasks requiring abstract thinking, reasoning, and understanding of logical relationships.
5. Dementia patients with diseases affecting motor control, such as Parkinson's and Huntington's patients, are likely to have speech motor control problems and dysarthria.
6. Intraetiologic variation among AD patients is likely to occur as a result of the age of disease onset, family history of AD, rate of disease progression, and presence of extrapyramidal signs.
7. Three groups of AD patients have been distinguished clinically: those in whom memory problems are most prominent, those in whom aphasia is most prominent, and those in whom visuospatial impairment is most prominent.
8. Parkinson's patients are highly variable. Some have little, if any, intellectual deterioration; others have circumscribed deficits; others, a full dementia.
9. Although Huntington's disease (HD) patients always develop a frank dementia, qualitative differences may exist between the dementias of HD and AD.
10. Few interetiologic studies of communicative functions have been conducted. In one such study of AD, PD, and HD patients, many similarities were observed in linguistic communication profiles. Regardless of etiology, deficits were apparent in verbal associative reasoning, linguistic disambiguation, verbal description, story-retelling, and generative naming.
11. Alzheimer's patients, hereditary dysphasic dementia patients, and Pick's patients may represent a spectrum of disorders. Alzheimer's patients have greater difficulty with language content than form; and Pick's patients appear to have greater form than content problems. Hereditary dysphasic dementia patients may exhibit motor impairment and a reduction in the amount of spontaneous speech.
12. The dementias are sometimes subcate-

gorized as cortical and subcortical. Alzheimer's patients are said to have cortical dementia, HD and PD patients are said to have subcortical. The site of the most prominent pathologic changes dictates the classification. The distinction is controversial because it is anatomically based. AD patients are known to have subcortical pathologic changes, and HD and PD patients are known to have cortical changes.

13. Results of longitudinal studies of dementia patients reveal that language content is affected before form, semantic and pragmatic knowledge before phonologic and syntactic, generative before confrontation naming, sentence correction before judgment, low-probability phrase repetition before high-probability, and defining before naming.
14. In dementia, certain aspects of either communicative or cognitive functions may be more impaired than others. However, clinicians generally can expect the degree of communicative impairment to be proportional to overall cognitive impairment.

REFERENCES

Albert, M.L., (1978). Subcortical dementia. In R. Katzman, R.D. Terry, and K.L. Bick (Eds.), *Aging: Vol. 7. Alzheimer's disease: Senile dementia and related disorders* (pp. 173-180). New York: Raven Press.

Albert, M.L. (1981). Changes in language with aging. *Seminars in Neurology, 1*, 43-46.

Albert, M.L. (1984). The controversy of subcortical dementia. *Neurosurgery Update Series, 5*, 2-8.

Albert, M.L., Feldman, R.G., and Willis, A.L. (1974). The "subcortical dementia" of progressive supranuclear palsy. *Journal of Neurology, Neurosurgery, and Psychiatry, 37*, 121-130.

Albert, M.S., and Moss, M. (1984). The assessment of memory disorders in patients with Alzheimer's disease. In L.R. Squire and N. Butters (Eds.), *Neuropsychology of memory* (pp. 236-246). New York: Guilford Press.

Alexander, D.A. (1973). Some tests of intelligence and learning for elderly psychiatric patients: A validation study. *British Journal of Social and Clinical Psychology, 12*, 188-193.

Alvord, E.C. Jr. (1968). The pathology of parkinsonism. In J. Minckler (Ed.), *Pathology of the nervous system: Vol. 1.* (pp. 1152-1161). New York: McGraw-Hill.

Ammons, R.B., and Ammons, C.H. (1977). The Quick Test (QT) provisional manual. *Psychological Reports, 11*, 111-161.

Arendt, T., Bigl, V., Arendt, A., and Tennstedt, A. (1983). Loss of neurons in the nucleus basalis of Meynert in Alzheimer's disease, paralysis agitans, and Korsakoff's disease. *Acta Neuropathologica* (Berlin), *61*, 101-108.

Bayles, K.A. (1985, February). *Effects of dementing illnesses on communicative function.* Paper presented as part of a symposium at the International Neuropsychological Society Meeting, San Diego, CA.

Benson, D.F. (1983). Subcortical dementia: A clinical approach. In R. Mayeux, and W.G. Rosen (Eds.), *The dementias* (pp. 185-194). New York: Raven Press.

Benton, A.L. (1968). Differential behavioral effects in frontal lobe disease. *Neuropsychologia, 6*, 53-60.

Berg, L., Danziger, W.L., Storandt, M., Coben, L.A., Gado, M., Hughes, C.P., Knesevich, J.W., and Botwinick, J. (1984). Predictive features of mild senile dementia of the Alzheimer's type. *Neurology, 34*, 563-569.

Blessed, G., Tomlinson, B.E., and Roth, M. (1968). The association between quantitative measures of dementia and of senile change in the cerebral grey matter of elderly subjects. *British Journal of Psychiatry, 114*, 797-811.

Boller, F., Mizutani, T., Roessman, U., and Gambetti, P. (1980). Parkinson disease, dementia, and Alzheimer disease: Clinicopathological correlations. *Annals of Neurology, 7*, 329-335.

Boller, F., Passafiume, D., Keefe, N.C., Rogers, K., Morrow, L., and Kim, Y. (1984). Visuospatial impairment in Parkinson's disease: Role of perceptual and motor factors. *Archives of Neurology, 41*, 485-490.

Borkowski, J.G., Benton, A.L., and Spreen, O. (1967). Word fluency and brain damage. *Neuropsychologia, 5*, 135-140.

Breitner, J.C.S., and Folstein, M.F. (1984). Familial Alzheimer dementia: A prevalent disorder with specific clinical features. *Psychological Medicine, 14*, 63-80.

Brinkman, S. (1983, October). *Neuropsychological differences between Alzheimer's disease and multi-infarct dementia.* Paper presented at the Talland Memorial Conferencve on Clinical Memory Assessment of Older Adults, Wakefield, MA.

Bruyn, G.W., Bots, G.T.A.M., and Dom, R. (1979). Huntington's chorea: Current neuropathological status. In T.N. Chase, N.S. Wexler, Barbeau, A. (Eds.), *Advances in Neurology: Vol. 23. Huntington's disease* (pp. 83-93). New York: Raven Press.

Butters, N., Albert, M.S., Sax, D.S., Miliotis, P., Nagode, J., and Sterste, A. (1983). The effect of verbal elaborators on the pictorial memory of brain-damaged patients. *Neuropsychologia, 21*, 307-323.

Butters, N., Sax, D., Montgomery, K., and Tarlow, S. (1978). Comparison of the neuropsychological deficits associated with early and advanced Huntington's disease. *Archives of Neurology, 35*, 585-589.

Butters, N., Wolfe, J., Granholm, E., and Martone, M. (1986). An assessment of verbal recall, recognition, and fluency abilities in patients with Huntington's disease. *Cortex, 86*, 11-32.

Caine, E.D., (1981). Pseudodementia. *Archives of General Psychiatry, 38*, 1359-1364.

Chase, T.N., Fedio, P., Foster, N.L., Brooks, R., DiChiro, G., and Mansi, L. (1984). Wechsler Adult Intelligence Scale performance. Cortical localization by fluorodeoxyglucose F18-positron emission tomography. *Archives of Neurology, 41*, 1244-1247.

Chenoweth, B., and Spencer, B. (1986). Dementia: The experience of family caregivers. *The Gerontologist, 26*, 267-272.

Cohen, G. (1983). *The psychology of cognition* (2nd ed.). New York: Academic Press.

Constantinidis, J. (1978). Is Alzheimer's disease a major form of senile dementia? Clinical, anatomical, and genetic data. In R. Katzman, R.D. Terry, and K.L. Bick (Eds.), *Alzheimer's disease: Senile dementia and related disorders* (pp. 15-25). New York: Raven Press.

Corsellis, J.A.N. (1970). The limbic areas in Alzheimer's disease and in other conditions associated with dementia. In G.E.W. Wolstenholme and M. O'Connor (Eds.), *Alzheimer's disease and related conditions* (pp. 37-50). London: Churchill.

Cummings, J.L. (1982). Cortical dementias. In D.F. Benson and D. Blumer (Eds.), *Psychiatric aspects of neurologic disease. Vol. 2.* (pp. 93-120). New York: Grune and Stratton.

Cummings, J.L., and Benson, D.F. (1983). *Dementia: A clinical approach.* Boston: Butterworth.

Cummings, J.L., and Benson, D.F. (1984). Subcortical dementia: Review of an emerging concept. *Archives of Neurology, 41*, 874-879.

Cummings, J., and Duchen, L. (1981). Klüver-Bucy syndrome in Pick disease: Clinical and pathologic correlations. *Neurology, 31*, 1415-1422.

Curcio, C.A., and Kemper, T. (1984). Nucleus raphe dorsalis in dementia of the Alzheimer type: Neurofibrillary changes and neuronal packing density. *Journal of Neuropathology and Experimental Neurology, 43*, 359-368.

Damasio, A.R., Damasio, H., Rizzo, M., Varney, N., and Gersh, F. (1982). Aphasia with nonhemorrhagic lesions in the basal ganglia and internal capsule. *Archives of Neurology, 39*, 15-20.

Dunn, L.M. (1965). *The expanded manual for the Peabody Picture Vocabulary Test.* Circle Pines, MN: American Guidance Service.

Ferraro, A., and Jervis, G.A. (1936). Pick's disease. Clinico-pathologic study and report of two cases. *Archives of Neurology and Psychiatry, 36*, 739-767.

Fink, M., Green, M.A., and Bender, M.B. (1952). The face-hand test as a diagnostic sign of organic mental syndrome. *Neurology, 2*, 46-58.

Forno, L.S., Barbour, P.J., and Norville, R.L. (1978). Presenile dementia with Lewy bodies and neurofibrillary tangles. *Archives of Neurology, 35*, 818-822.

Forno, L.S., and Jose, C. (1973). Huntington's chorea: A pathological study. In A. Barbeau, T.N. Chase, and G.W. Paulson (Eds.), *Advances in Neurology: Vol. 1. Huntington's chorea 1872-1972* (pp. 453-370). New York: Raven Press.

Freedman, M. (1984). Cortical and subcortical dementia. *Annals of Neurology, 15*, 506-507.

Friedland, R.P., Budinger, T.F., Ganz, E., Yano, Y., Mathis, C.A., Koss, E., Ober, B.A., Huesman, R.H., and Derenzo, S.E. (1983). Regional cerebral metabolic alterations in dementia of the Alzheimer's type: Positron emission tomography with [18F]fluorodeoxyglucose. *Journal of Computer Assisted Tomography, 7*, 590-598.

Fuld, P.A., Katzman, R., Davies, P., and Terry, R.D.

(1982). Intrusions as a sign of Alzheimer dementia. Chemical and pathological verification. *Annals of Neurology, 11*, 155-159.

Gaspar, P., and Gray, F. (1984). Dementia in idiopathic Parkinson's disease: A neuropathological study of 32 cases. *Acta Neuropathologica* (Berlin) *64*, 43-52.

Goldfarb, A.I. (1975). Memory and aging. In R. Goldman and M. Rockstein (Eds.), *The physiology and pathology of human aging*. New York: Academic Press.

Goodglass, H., and Kaplan, E. (1972). *The assessment of aphasia and related disorders*. Philadelphia: Lea and Febiger.

Goodman, L. (1953). Alzheimer's disease. A clinicopathologic analysis of twenty-three cases with a theory on causation. *Journal of Nervous and Mental Disease, 117*, 97-1330.

Hachinski, V.C., Lassen, N.A., and Marshall, J. (1974). Multi-infarct dementia: A cause of mental deterioration in the elderly. *Lancet, 2*, 207-210.

Hakim, A.M., and Mathieson, G. (1979). Dementia in Parkinson disease: A neuropathologic study. *Neurology, 29*, 1209-1214.

Hasher, L., and Zacks, R.T. (1979). Automatic and effortful processes in memory. *Journal of Experimental Psychology: General, 108*, 356-388.

Haxby, J.V., Duara, R., Grady, C.L., Cutler, N.R., and Rapoport, S.I. (1985). Relations between neuropsychological and cerebral metabolic asymmetries in early Alzheimer's disease. *Journal of Cerebral Blood Flow and Metabolism, 5*, 193-200.

Herzog, A.G., and Kemper, T.L. (1980). Amygdaloid changes in aging and dementia. *Archives of Neurology, 37*, 625-629.

Heyman, A., Wilkinson, W.E., Stafford, J.A., Helms, M.J., Sigmon, A.H., and Weinberg, T. (1984). Alzheimer's disease: A study of epidemiologic aspects. *Annals of Neurology, 15*, 335-341.

Hier, D.B., Hagenlocker, K., and Shindler, A.G. (1985). Language disintegration in dementia: Effects of etiology and severity. *Brain and Language, 25*, 117-133.

Hirano, A., and Zimmerman, H.M. (1962). Alzheimer's neurofibrillary changes: A topographic study. *Archives of Neurology, 37*, 625-629.

Holland, A.L., McBurney, D.H., Moossy, J., and Reinmuth, O.M. (1985). The dissolution of language in Pick's disease with neurofibrillary tangles: A case study. *Brain and Language, 24*, 36-58.

Hooper, M.W., and Vogel, F.S. (1976). The limbic system in Alzheimer's disease: A neuropathologic investigation. *American Journal of Pathology, 85*, 1-20.

Horner, J., Heyman, A., Kanter, J., Royall, J.B., and Aker, C.R. (1983, February). *Longitudinal changes in spoken discourse in Alzheimer's dementia*. Paper presented at the International Neuropsychological Society Meeting, Mexico City, Mexico.

Hughes, C.P., Berg, L., Danziger, W.L., Coben, L.A., and Martin, R.L. (1982). A new clinical scale for the staging of dementia. *British Journal of Psychiatry, 140*, 566-572.

Jellinger, K., and Grisold, W. (1982). Cerebral atrophy in Parkinson syndrome. *Experimental Brain Research Supplement, 5*, 26-35.

Josiassen, R.C., Curry, L.M., and Mancall, E.L. (1983). Development of neuropsychological deficits in Huntington's disease. *Archives of Neurology, 40*, 791-796.

Josiassen, R., Curry, L., Roemer, R., DeBease, C., and Mancall, M.L. (1982). Patterns of intellectual deficit in Huntington's disease. *Journal of Clinical Neuropsychology, 4*, 173-183.

Kahn, E., and Thompson, L.J. (1933-1934). Concerning Pick's disease. *American Journal of Psychiatry, 90*, 937-946.

Kaplan, E., Goodglass, H., and Weintraub, S. (1983). *Boston Naming Test*. Philadelphia: Lea and Febiger.

Kaszniak, A.W., Fox, J., Gandell, D.L., Garron, D.C., Huckman, M.A., and Ramsey, R.G. (1978). Predictors of mortality in presenile and senile dementia. *Annals of Neurology, 3*, 246-252.

Kaszniak, A.W., and Wilson, R.S. (1985, February). *Longitudinal deterioration of language and cognition in dementia of the Alzheimer's type*. Paper presented as part of a symposium at the International Neuropsychological Society Meeting, San Diego, CA.

Kim, R.C., Collins, G.H., Parisi, J.E., Wright, A.W., and Chu, Y.B. (1981). Familial dementia of adult onset with pathologic findings of a "nonspecific" nature. *Brain, 104*, 61-78.

Lauter, H., and Meyer, J.E. (1968). Clinical and nosological concepts of senile dementia. In C. Muller, and L. Ciompi (Eds.), *Senile dementia: Clinical and therapeutic aspects* (pp. 13-26). Bern, Switzerland: Hans Huber.

Matison, R., Mayeux, R., Rosen, J., and Fahn, S. (1982). "Tip-of-the-tongue" phenomenon in Parkinson disease. *Neurology, 32*, 567-570.

Mayeux, R., Stern, Y., Rosen, J., and Benson, D.F. (1983). Is "subcortical dementia" a recognizable clinical entity? *Annals of Neurology, 14*, 278-283.

McCaughey, W.T.E. (1961). The pathologic spectrum of Huntington's chorea. *Journal of Nervous and Mental Disease, 133*, 91-103.

McDuff, T., and Sumi, S.M. (1985). Subcortical degeneration in Alzheimer's disease. *Neurology, 35*, 123-126.

McHugh, P.R., and Folstein, M.F. (1975). Psychiatric syndromes of Huntington's chorea: A clinical and phenomenologic study. In D.F. Benson and D. Blumer (Eds.), *Psychiatric aspects of neurologic disease* (pp. 267-286). New York: Grune and Stratton.

McHugh, P.R., and Folstein, M.F. (1979). Psychopathology of dementia: Implications for neuropathology. In R. Katzman (Ed.), *Congenital and acquired cognitive disorders* (pp. 17-30). New York: Raven Press.

McKhann, G., Drachman, D., Folstein, M., Katzman, R., Price, D., and Stadlan, E.M. (1984). Clinical diagnosis of Alzheimer's disease: Report of the NINCDS-ADRDA work group under the auspices of the Department of Health and Human Services task force on Alzheimer's disease. *Neurology, 34*, 934-944.

Mesulam, M-M. (1985). Dementia: Its definition, differential diagnosis, and subtypes. *Journal of the American Medical Association, 253*, 2559-2561.

Mildworf, B. (1978). *Cognitive function in elderly patients*. Unpublished Masters Thesis, Hebrew University, Jerusalem, Israel.

Morris, J.C., Cole, M., Banker, B.Q., and Wright, D. (1984). Hereditary dysphasic dementia and the Pick-Alzheimer spectrum. *Annals of Neurology, 16*, 455-466.

Moss, M.B., Albert, M.S., Butters, N., and Payne, M. (1986). Differential patterns of memory loss among patients with Alzheimer's disease, Huntington's disease, and alcoholic Korsakoff's syndrome. *Archives of Neurology, 43*, 239-246.

Obler, L.K., and Albert, M.L. (1981). Language and aging: A neurobehavioral analysis. In D.S. Beasley and G.A. Davis (Eds.), *Aging: Communication processes and disorders* (pp. 107-121). New York: Grune and Stratton.

Perez, F.I., Gay, J.R.A., and Taylor, R.L. (1975). WAIS performance of neurologically impaired aged. *Psychological Reports, 37*, 1043-1047.

Perry, E.K., Tomlinson, B.E., Blessed, G., Perry, R.H., Cross, A.J., and Crow, T.J. (1981). Neuropathological and biochemical observations on the noradrenergic system in Alzheimer's disease. *Journal of Neurological Sciences, 51*, 279-287.

Pfeiffer, E. (1975). A short portable mental status questionnaire for the assessment of organic brain deficit in elderly patients. *Journal of the American Geriatrics Society, 23*, 433-441.

Pirozzolo, F.J., Hansch, E.C., Mortimer, J.A., Webster, D.D., and Kuskowski, M.A. (1982). Dementia in Parkinson disease: A neuropsychological analysis. *Brain and Cognition, 1*, 71-83.

Posner, M.I., and Snyder, C.R.R. (1975). Attention and cognitive control. In R.L. Solso (Ed.), *Information processing and cognition* (pp. 55-85). Hillsdale, NJ: Lawrence Erlbaum Associates.

Reisberg, B., Ferris, S.H., and Crook, T. (1982). Signs, symptoms, and course of age-associated cognitive decline. In S. Corkin, K.L. Davis, J.H. Growdon, E. Usdin, and R.L. Wurtman (Eds.), *Aging: Vol. 19. Alzheimer's disease: A report of progress* (pp. 177-181). New York: Raven Press.

Riklan, M., and Levita, E. (1970). Psychological studies of thalamic lesions in humans. *Journal of Nervous and Mental Disorders, 150*, 251-265.

Rogers, J.D., Brogan, D., and Mirra, S.S. (1985). The nucleus basalis of Meynert in neurological disease: A quantitative morphological study. *Annals of Neurology, 17*, 163-170.

Rutherford, D. (1972). *The Northwestern Word Latency Test*. Evanston, IL: Northwestern University Press.

Scott, S., Caird, F.I., and Williams, B.O. (1984). Evidence for an apparent sensory speech disorder in Parkinson's disease. *Journal of Neurology, Neurosurgery, and Psychiatry, 47*, 840-843.

Seltzer, B., and Sherwin, I. (1983). A comparison of clinical features in early- and late-onset primary degenerative dementia. One entity or two? *Archives of Neurology, 40*, 143-146.

Shewan, C.M. (1979). *Auditory Comprehension Test for Sentences*. Chicago: Biolinguistics Clinical Institutes.

Smith, S., White, R., Lyon, L., Granholm, E., and Butters, N. (in press). Priming semantic relations in patients with Huntington's disease. *Brain and Language*.

Sourander, P., and Sjögren, H. (1970). The concept of Alzheimer's disease and its clinical implications. In G.E.W. Wolstenholme and M. O'Connor (Eds.), *Alzheimer's disease and related conditions* (pp. 11-36). London: Churchill.

Stern, Y., Mayeux, R., and Rosen, J. (1984). Contribution of perceptual motor dysfunction to construction and tracing disturbances in Parkinson's disease. *Journal of Neurology, Neurosurgery, and Psychiatry, 47*, 983-989.

Sulkava, R., and Amberla, K. (1982). Alzheimer's disease and senile dementia of Alzheimer type. A neuropsychological study. *Acta Neurologica Scandinavica, 65*, 651-660.

Tagliavini, F., and Pilleri, G. (1983). Neuronal counts in basal nucleus of Meynert in Alzheimer disease and in simple senile dementia. *Lancet, 1*, 469-470.

Villardita, C., Smirni, P., LePira F., Zappala, G., and Nicoletti, F. (1982). Mental deterioration, visuoperceptive disabilities and constructional apraxia in Parkinson's disease. *Acta Neurologica Scandinavica, 66*, 112-120.

Wechsler, D. (1945). A standardized memory scale for clinical use. *Journal of Psychology, 19*, 87-95.

Wechsler, D. (1958). *The Wechsler Adult Intelligence Scale* (4th ed.). Baltimore: Williams and Wilkins.

Wechsler, D. (1981). *Wechsler Adult Intelligence Scale-Revised Manual.* New York: Harcourt, Brace, Jovanovich.

Wechsler, A.F., Verity, M.A., Rosenschein, S., Fried, I., and Scheibel, A.B. (1982). Pick's disease. A clinical, computed tomographic, and histopathologic study with Golgi impregnation observations. *Archives of Neurology, 39*, 287-290.

Whitehouse, P.J. (1986). The concept of subcortical and cortical dementia: Another look. *Annals of Neurology, 19*, 1-6.

Whitehouse, P.J., Price, D.L., Clark, A.W., Coyle, J.T., and DeLong, M.R. (1981). Alzheimer disease: Evidence for selective loss of cholinergic neurons in the nucleus basalis. *Annals of Neurology, 10*, 122-126.

Wiig, E.H., and Semel, E.M. (1974). Development of comprehension of logico-grammatical sentences by grade school children. *Perceptual and Motor Skills, 38*, 171-176.

Wilson, R.S., Rosenbaum, G., and Brown, G. (1979). The problem of premorbid intelligence in neuropsychological assessment. *Journal of Clinical Neuropsychology, 1*, 49-53.

Chapter 5

Linguistic Communication and Normal Aging

"Old age is not a disease, it is strength and survivorship, triumph over all kinds of vicissitudes and disappointments, trials and illnesses."

Maggie Kuhn, 1979

The elderly endure many stereotypes, among them being decrepit, feeble, and sick. Although only a small percentage of elderly are affected by mental status changes, many people consider pathologic senility synonymous with old age. One ability that is not part of the "declines with age" stereotype is communicative functioning. We do not expect to be unable to communicate when we are aged, and generally that expectation is valid. In the course of this chapter, data will be reviewed that demonstrate that certain of the processes important in communication do diminish with age, but the diminishment is small and more common in the old old or the sick old.

The general question whether aging affects the ability to linguistically communicate can best be answered by addressing three specific issues:

Issue 1: Aging and the contents and processes of SM.

Issue 2: Aging and linguistic knowledge.

Issue 3: Aging and the mechanics of communication.

Discussion of these three issues will constitute the remainder of this chapter. The reader is advised that the literature related to the first issue contains contradictory results and complicated studies, particularly in relation to processing ability and age. The conclusion emphasized at the end of this complex section is that a modest amount of data suggests that the contents of SM deteriorate with age, and considerable data suggest some deterioration in the processes of SM. However, in the opinion of these authors, age effects on processing capacities do not handicap individuals in normal everyday communication.

ISSUE 1: AGE EFFECTS ON THE CONTENTS AND PROCESSES OF SEMANTIC MEMORY

Preservation of Conceptual Knowledge

The elemental unit of SM is the concept (see Chapter 2 for a discussion of the contents of SM). Concepts are the building blocks used to form propositions and schemata, the other components of SM. These units, which can be given linguistic representation, constitute an individual's knowledge of the world. To date, the bulk of scientific evidence suggests that conceptual knowledge is maintained across the span of adulthood, and indeed, it seems intuitively reasonable that an individual's knowledge of concepts is enriched by experience. Some empirical evidence supports this intuition, evidence from studies of the performance of adults on vocabulary tests.

Vocabulary

The study of vocabulary is the most researched aspect of communicative competency. Not only is vocabulary reputed to be maintained with age (Lewinsky, 1948; Shakow and Goldman, 1938; Thorndike and Gallup, 1944); some researchers report vocabulary growth (Owens, 1953; Fox, 1947). One of these researchers was Fox, who compared the performance of persons in their 40s and 70s on the Vocabulary subtest of the WAIS, an expressive vocabulary test. In this test, individuals are given a word and asked to provide a definition. Points are awarded in relation to the appropriateness of the synonym or quality of description. An age effect was not found in the ability of subjects to define words or choose the correct definition in a multiple-choice task.

Bayles, Tomoeda, and Boone (1985) investigated the possibility of an age effect on receptive vocabulary using the *Peabody Picture Vocabulary Test–Revised* (PPVT-R) (Dunn and Dunn 1981). In this test subjects are required to select the correct visual representation, from among four choices, of a word presented orally by the examiner. Ten subjects in each decade of life from the third to the eighth, who were group matched for intelligence and years of education, participated in the study. As can be seen in Figure 5-1, mean scores for each group were very similar. Subjects in their 50s performed best, but not significantly better in a statistical sense than subjects in any other decade.

Some investigators suspect that the failure to find age-related differences in vocabulary might be due to the way in which data from vocabulary studies are analyzed. Botwinick and Storandt (1974) considered that a qualitative analysis of the definitions given by the elderly might reveal differences in the extent of semantic knowledge. Thus, they under-

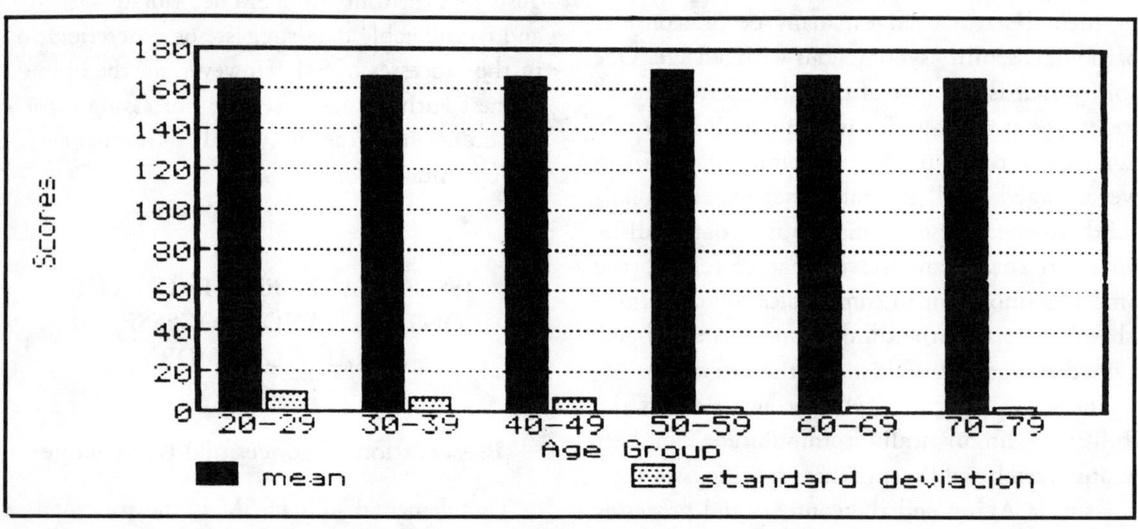

Figure 5-1. *Mean scores and standard deviations on the Peabody Picture Vocabulary Test—Revised in Decades Study. (Based on data from Bayles, Tomoeda, and Boone, 1985.)*

took an analysis of the types of responses given by 24 young and 24 older subjects matched for quantitative WAIS Vocabulary scores. In the older group, subjects ranged in age from 62 to 83 years and had a mean age of 70.58; young subjects ranged in age from 17 to 20 with a mean of 18.42 years. Test responses were analyzed using a six-point scale with 6 awarded for a superior synonym, 5 for a good explanation, 4 for an inferior synonym, 3 for a poor explanation, 2 for a description or specification of use, and 1 for an illustration. Using multivariate analysis, a significant age difference was found in the frequency of responses given in various descriptive categories. Botwinick and Storandt observed that young adults more frequently gave superior synonyms, and individuals in the seventh and eighth decades were more likely to produce multiword responses, that is, explanations, descriptions, and illustrations.

The earlier research of two other individuals, Feifel (1949) and Ricks (1958), supports the conclusion of Botwinick and Storandt that aging affects vocabulary. Both investigators qualitatively analyzed responses on the Stanford-Binet (Terman and Merrill, 1937) vocabulary test, and both observed deterioration in the quality of responses.

Lexical decision tasks also have been used to study age effects on conceptual and lexical knowledge and their access. Unlike vocabulary tests in which the examinee is given a word and asked to provide a definition, in a lexical decision task a string of letters must first be recognized as a word form, after which the meaning is accessed. In a lexical decision task, the individual is given a string of letters and must judge whether it constitutes a real word. To perform the task, individuals must match an orthographic representation to the mental store of orthographic representations. When the input string is a word known to the individual, verifying it as a word is simple. Responses on vocabulary tasks take longer because additional time is required to retrieve the conceptual information after the lexical form is recognized (Kramer and Jarvik, 1979).

Though age does not appear to affect lexical decision making, it does affect lexical access when the input is not orthographic but conceptual. In a lexical decision task, in which subjects had to decide whether a string of letters was a word, Howard (1983) reported that word retrieval from the orthographically organized lexical network did not differ for old and young subjects. In this task the stimulus, a letter string, provides the complete orthographic information concerning the target word; therefore, word retrieval is easy if the word is known by the subject.

However, when the definition rather than the word name is given first, and the subject has to provide the name of the word, an age effect obtains. In the first part of a two-part study by Bowles and Poon (1985), 24 young and 24 old subjects were given a string of letters and asked to decide if it was a real word. The authors interpreted the information processing route in this task to go from lexical to conceptual, and no age effect was found for either accuracy or response latency. In the second part of the study, 18 young and 18 elderly persons were given the definition of a target word and asked to name it. For this processing route, conceptual to lexical, an age effect was observed. Younger subjects were superior in word retrieval, as measured by the number of words correctly named, and response latency. Bowles and Poon interpreted the findings as evidence that older adults "have a specific deficit in accessing word-name information in an orthographically organized lexical network given stimulus information that is conceptual rather than orthographic" (p. 71). "The difficulty . . . must reflect a specifically directional breakdown in the connection from the semantic network to the lexical network" (p. 76). This deficit is more commonly known as the "tip-of-the-tongue" phenomenon and is one occasionally experienced by everyone. Graduate students frequently experience the phenomenon in tests: "Let's see, what's the term for the phenomenon of not being able to think of the words to express what you want to say, but the words are right there?"

Summary

In summary, then, conceptual knowledge as assessed by vocabulary tests appears to be well maintained throughout adulthood. However, in advanced age, individuals may be more inclined to define a word by giving a multiword explanation of its meaning rather than a superior synonym. In light of results from vocabulary and lexical decision studies, what may deteriorate is access to lexical knowledge if the route of activation is from conceptual to orthographic rather than orthographic to conceptual.

Preservation of Propositional Knowledge

What evidence exists that propositional knowledge is maintained with age? Remember, a typical proposition is comprised of two concepts and a relational term. "The Papago Indian Reservation is the size of the state of Connecticut" and "Pralines are made in New Orleans" are propositions. A method for ascertaining whether propositional knowledge is impervious to age effects is the study of sentence comprehension. A simple sentence with subject-verb-object construction is a linguistically represented proposition. If elderly adults comprehend sentences in the same way that young and middle-aged adults do, then propositional knowledge and its access can be considered intact.

Sentence Comprehension

Sentence comprehension ability as a function of age has been studied by several investigators, but the outcomes have differed (Table 5-1). Among those who reported no significant age effect was Shewan (1979), author of the Auditory Comprehension Test for Sentences (ACTS). As part of the standardization of the ACTS, Shewan analyzed age effects on sentence comprehension and observed no significant variability in sentence comprehension ability in adults whose ages ranged from 21 to 76 years.

Borod, Goodglass, and Kaplan (1980) studied comprehension using the auditory comprehension subtests of the Boston Diagnostic Aphasia Examination (BDAE), (Goodglass and Kaplan, 1972). Among the auditory comprehension subtests is a task in which a series of one-sentence commands is given, a task on which an age effect was not found. An age effect was reported on the sentence and paragraph reading tasks and in the repetition of low-probability phrases. Deterioration in propositional knowledge cannot be assumed to be the sole explanation of a diminished performance on the two latter tasks, however; memory deficits also may have contributed.

Table 5-1. Summary of Research on Sentence Comprehension and Aging

Ways Measured	Presence of Age Effect
ACTS auditory sentence comprehension (Shewan, 1979)	No
BDAE auditory sentence comprehension	No
BDAE sentence and paragraph reading comprehension	Yes
BDAE repetition of low-probability sentences (Borod et al., 1980)	Yes
Phrase to picture matching (Nebes, 1976)	No
Sentence completion of improbable sentences (Obler, Nicholas et al., 1985)	Yes
Auditory sentence comprehension of syntactically difficult and low predictability sentences (Obler, Fein et al., 1985)	Yes
Sentence disambiguation (Bayles et al., 1985)	No
Demonstration of sentence comprehension by figure manipulation (Feier and Gerstman, 1980)	Yes for subjects > 60 years old

Nebes (1976) investigated the capacity of the elderly to translate verbal propositions into a pictorial code. Elderly adults (mean age = 69) took longer than young adults (mean age = 19) to match phrases to pictures and pictures to pictures, but of the two tasks, the phrase-to-picture verification took longer. However, the phrase-to-picture verification proved longer for the younger subjects as well. In fact, the time difference between the two conditions was the same for both the young and old subject groups, a finding that led Nebes to argue that aging affects processing time rather than comprehension.

Among those reporting an age effect on sentence comprehension were Obler, Nicholas, Albert, and Woodward (1985), who analyzed the performance of 16 men and 16 women in their 30s, 50s, 60s, and 70s on the Speech Perception in Noise test developed by Kalikow, Stevens, and Elliott (1977). In this test, subjects have to write the final word of a sentence. Stimulus sentences are presented over speech babble noise. In half the sentences, the identity of the final word is cued by other words in the sentence (e.g., "A rose bush has prickly *thorns*"), while in the remaining sentences, no semantic cue is given. A linear decline in scores with age was observed. Further, final words with low predictability were more difficult than high-predictability words. The investigators obtained a significant age-by-predictability interaction; elderly subjects performed more poorly on the low-predictability words.

In a follow-up study conducted by Obler, Fein, Nicholas, and Albert (1985), two general questions about aging effects on language comprehension were addressed. The first question was whether certain syntactic sentence types were more difficult to comprehend with age, and the second was whether semantically unlikely sentences were more difficult. Data related to the accuracy and latency of subject performance were analyzed for subjects from four age groups: 30s (N = 24), 50s (N = 27), 60s (N = 25), and 70s (N = 18). The results were consistent with those from previous studies in which comprehension was found to diminish with age. Further, a preferential decline was observed for comprehending syntactically difficult and semantically improbable sentences. Of the syntactic forms evaluated, the easiest to most difficult were as follows: single negative, active comparative, embedded, passive, double negative. A significant main effect was reported for reaction time, with older subjects requiring more time to judge the harder syntactic types and unlikely sentences. However, no age–by–syntactic-type interaction was obtained, which Obler and colleagues interpreted to mean that older adults have a motor or cognitive slowing that affects all material equally.

Studying the ability to disambiguate different types of ambiguous sentences is another approach to assessing the patency of propositional knowledge. However, in a disambiguation paradigm, sentence comprehension is confounded with linguistic reasoning ability. Nevertheless, because an age effect was not found, the disambiguation study will be described. Bayles and colleagues (1985) administered 21 linguistically ambiguous sentences and nine unambiguous sentences to ten normal individuals in each decade of life from the third through the eighth. Study participants were group matched for intelligence and education. Subjects were told that many of the sentences had more than one meaning and to explain both meanings in their own words. Three practice sentences were given. Sentences were presented both visually and auditorially. The results of subject performance are presented in Figure 5-2. No significant decrements were found as a function of aging.

Feier and Gerstman (1980) studied sentence comprehension by having subjects enact a series of sentences by manipulating small animal and human figures. Stimulus sentences were structurally complex, and each contained a relative clause. Four subject groups, balanced for sex and education, participated: young adults (18–25 years), and three groups of older adults (52–58; 63–69; and 74–80). No significant intergroup differences were apparent until the 60s. Significant performance differences were noted between subjects in their 60s and those older and younger. Additionally, subjects in their 70s performed more poorly than those in their 60s. They made more errors and their errors were

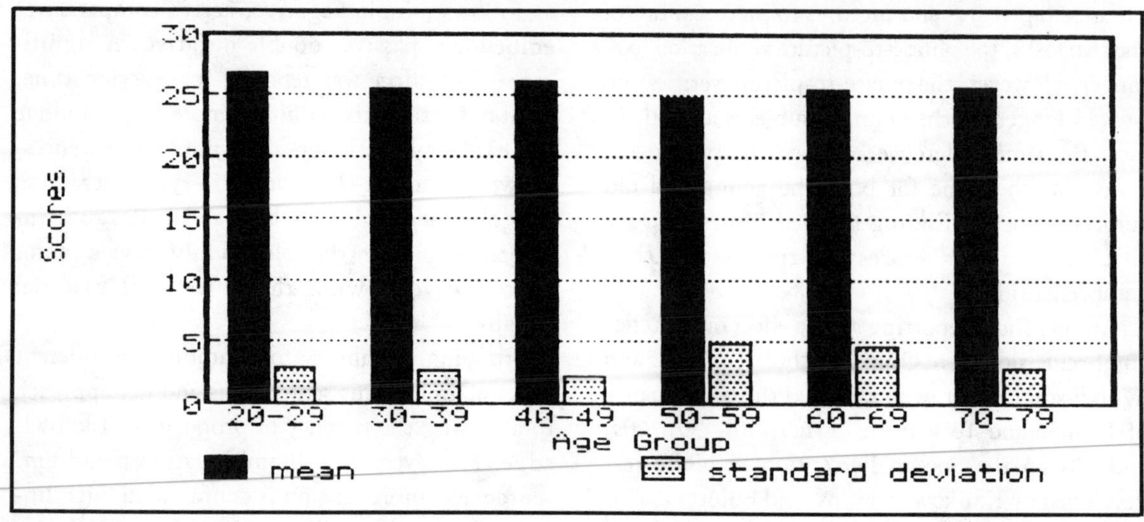

Figure 5-2. *Mean scores and standard deviations on the Sentence Disambiguation Task in Decades Study. (Based on data from Bayles, Tomoeda, and Boone, 1985.)*

more serious; that is, they made more multiple errors within a single sentence enactment and omitted more clause enactments.

Sentence Production

Obler (1980) studied sentence production in the written and oral discourse of 18 normal elderly adults and 18 Parkinson's patients who were in their 50s and 60s. In the written description task, subjects were asked to describe the Cookie-Theft picture from the BDAE. Obler counted the number of words per response, compared them with the number of themes represented, and evaluated whether the sentences were abbreviated or full. Data analysis revealed two different styles of sentence construction: abbreviated and elaborate. Elaborate sentences that had more words per theme were more commonly produced by older adults. Then too, subjects in their 60s were more likely to have fewer nouns per verb.

In a second study, Obler (1980) applied the same analysis to the written descriptions of the Cookie-Theft picture of 106 male subjects ranging in age from 30 to 80. Individuals older than 50 tended to use elaborate sentences rather than the abbreviated style. Yet, subjects in their 30s performed similarly to elderly subjects. Thus, a U-shaped performance curve was obtained. Obler reasoned that the young subjects used a more elaborate style because the task was easy, and the elders used it because of necessity.

In a study of oral narration, 90 subjects were asked to retell a story read to them. Obler (1980) observed an age effect for the incidence of paraphrases and the use of indefinite terms like "something" and "any," with elders using them more frequently.

Summary

The elderly are clearly slower in their ability to perform sentence comprehension tasks. In studies where reaction time was the dependent variable, an age effect was reported. When the dependent variable was the number correct, an age effect was not always reported. Shewan (1979), Nebes (1976), and Bayles and colleagues (1985) did not report age-related comprehension deficits, whereas Feier and Gerstmann (1980) observed a significant decline after age 60 and Obler, Nicholas, Albert and Woodward (1985) reported a linear decline across the decades (see Table 5-1).

In Obler's (1980) study of sentence production, the elderly tended to produce more elaborate sentences, though the tendency was also observed in subjects in their 30s. Then too, the use of indefinite terms increased with age.

Preservation of Schemata

What evidence exists that knowledge of schemata resists the effects of age? Before answering this question, one might ask what would constitute evidence that schemata deteriorate with age. Remember that a schema is a frame of reference, a set of expectations, that individuals learn to apply to particular recurring situations. Schemata exist for going to the dentist, attending a party, and making dinner. Schemata can be distinguished as being linguistic or nonlinguistic. Linguistic schemata are expressions related to each other through their association with certain events, topics, and purposes.

Evidence that knowledge of nonlinguistic schemata deteriorates would be reports of progressive difficulty anticipating events associated with particular contexts, for example, forgetting to leave a tip at the end of a meal, or failing to remember to take a present to the bride and groom at a wedding. Loss of linguistic schemata could be inferred when individuals fail to say the expected in situations where the linguistic script is well known, for example, greeting and saying good-bye, or making introductions. Although no investigator has studied the question of deteriorating schemata in normal healthy aging, clinical experience suggests that schemata remain intact throughout adulthood. If they do deteriorate, the deterioration is insufficient to interfere with daily living.

Preservation of SM Processing Capabilities

After the foregoing discussion of whether the contents of SM are preserved with age, it can now be asked what the literature contains about aging and the processing capabilities of SM. Although the normal elderly person does not exhibit obvious decrements in inferential processing abilities sufficient to interfere with the communicative demands of daily living, studies published in the psychology and linguistics literature suggest that linguistic comprehension diminishes.

Evidence of Age-related Processing Deficits: Discourse Comprehension Studies. Foremost among the studies in the linguistics literature in which an age-related decrease in linguistic comprehension is reported are those of Ulatowska and colleagues, who studied the comprehension of discourse. Their studies have been motivated by the conception of discourse as "representing that level of communicative function wherein the interaction between linguistic and cognitive abilities is most clearly manifested, and where the complexity of language is quite high" (Ulatowska, Cannito, Hayashi, and Fleming, 1985, p. 128). Ulatowska and colleagues focus on information processing in discourse, that is, how information is abstracted and recounted to answer questions, produce stories, summaries, and provide morals.

In a study by Ulatowska, Hayashi, Cannito, and Fleming (1986), age effects on discourse comprehension skills were studied in Catholic nuns living together in the same convent. Individuals in this uniquely homogeneous population were classified as young old (64–76 years) or older old (greater than 76 years) and compared in discourse performance with a middle-aged (27–55 years) control group. Subjects were asked to retell a story and answer probe questions about it. The probe questions were constructed to assess comprehension of explicit and implicit information. The older old nuns exhibited poorer performance on story recall and on the probe questions. The only question for which there was no significant difference between the responses of the old and young was one that required no inferencing.

In a study similar to that of Ulatowska and colleagues, Taub (1979) evaluated discourse comprehension in 30 young (mean age = 27.5) and 30 old (mean age = 67.7) female subjects. Comprehension of discourse was measured by presenting five multiple choice questions simultaneously with half of the prose passages. Memory was measured with the rest of the materials by presenting questions only after the passage had been read and removed from sight. Although an age effect was obtained, it was present only for subjects whose scores on the Vocabulary subtest of the WAIS were average. Older and younger subjects whose scores placed them in the bright range did not differ in their ability to comprehend discourse.

Moenster (1972) and Gordon and Clark (1974) studied text comprehension as a function of age. In both studies, the elderly recalled less information than young adults, and Gordon and Clark found that the performance differences between the young and elderly were greater after a week had elapsed.

Recall of Discourse: Main and Supplemental Ideas. Many investigators have reported an age effect for the recall of narrative stories (Cohen, 1979; Hultsch, Hertzog, and Dixon, 1984; Petros, Tabor, Cooney, and Chabot, 1983; Taub and Klein, 1978; Zelinski, Gilewski, and Thompson, 1980). Others have observed age effects on expository prose (Dixon, Hultsch, Simon, and von Eye, 1984; Dixon, Simon, Nowak, and Hultsch, 1982; Meyer and Rice, 1981; Spilich, 1983; Spilich and Voss, 1982; Surber, Kowalski, and Pena-Paez, 1984; Zelinski et al., 1980; Zelinski, Light, and Gilewski, 1984).

Spilich (1983) investigated discourse processing in young adults, the normal aged, and elderly with memory impairment, using stories designed to be of general and age-cohort interest. Sixteen young adults and 32 elderly subjects participated, equally divided as to normal and memory-impaired. Subjects were informed that they should read the passage aloud and be prepared to recall it later. Immediately following the story reading, subjects were asked to recount the passage. Spilich found an age effect for the mean number of propositions correctly recalled. Young normal subjects recalled 31.1, elderly normal subjects recalled 13.8, and elderly memory-impaired individuals recalled 2.3. While young and old subjects were sensitive to thematic structure, elders were not as efficient as the young at recalling supplemental information.

Mixed results have been obtained from the recall studies in which an account was made of whether the individual recounted main or supplemental information. In some studies elderly adults were found to recall less information at all levels of importance; that is, recall of main points and supplementary detail was equally diminished (Petros et al., 1983; Zelinski et al., 1984). In others, elders were observed to recall less topic information but as much supplemental information as younger individuals (Cohen, 1979; Dixon et al., 1982). In still other investigations, greater age-related differences were reported for the details of the text than for main ideas (Byrd, 1981; Zelinski et al., 1980).

Factors That May Affect Recall of Discourse

Education, Culture, and Verbal Ability Effects. The reasons for the discrepancies between studies may be differences in the educational and verbal abilities of subjects. Dixon and colleagues (1984) examined the relation of verbal ability and text structure effects on adult age differences in text recall. One hundred and eight subjects read and recalled short stories on health and nutrition. Subjects fell in equal numbers into one of three age ranges: 20–39, 40–57, and 60–84. Recall was scored according to the propositional system of Kintsch (1974). Among adults with low verbal ability, age differences were greater at the main idea level than at the detail level. Among adults with high verbal ability, age effects were greater at the detail level.

Zelinski et al. (1984) investigated educational and verbal ability effects on recall in young and aged adults and found no evidence for age-related differences in sensitivity to text thematic structure regardless of educational background and verbal ability. Older people did, however, remember less of what they read than younger individuals.

In a study by Meyer and Rice (1981) in which education was controlled, young and aged college graduates read a story, recalled it, and then had to complete an outline of it. Meyer and Rice reported that by trial three, the young and elderly did not differ in the amount of information recalled or attention to thematic structure.

Decline in Syntactic Knowledge. Kemper (in press–a) examined the effect of syntactic form on elders' recall of main ideas and supplemental information. Twelve elders aged 71 to 89, and a group of middle-aged persons with comparable education, were tested on their recall of 12 prose paragraphs written by Kemper on different topics. In the writing of the paragraphs, only one- and two-clause sentences with predicate infinitives were used. The propositional content of the paragraphs varied as to saliency across 12 levels. Subjects were asked to read each paragraph silently and then, without the paragraph, write as much as they could recall. The written responses of the subjects were parsed into propositions and scored against the propositional structure of the original paragraph. Overall, elderly adults recalled 40 percent of the 127 propositions, whereas middle-aged adults recalled 69 percent. More intriguing, however, was the superior recall by the elders for right-branching sentences and the suppression of recall for left-branching propositions. Left-branching propositions are thought to impose a greater demand on memory. Thus, memory deficits may be more implicated than knowledge of syntax.

Semantic Encoding Deficit. It has been argued that decline in the ability to encode meaning may contribute to poor recall of linguistic information (Belmore, 1981). If a semantic encoding deficit is responsible for poor recall of linguistic information, it would also be the case that those memory tasks on which the elderly have the greatest difficulty are those involving the comprehension of meaningful language. As evidence, Belmore notes that age-related memory impairment is greater for connected prose material than for word lists (Craik, 1977; Craik and Masani, 1967; Gilbert and Levee, 1971). Further, the elderly have been reported to show a greater memory disadvantage in semantic orienting tasks (those requiring processing of meaning) than those which require sensitivity to the physical features of the stimulus material (Craik, 1977; Eysenck, 1974).

Implicit Information May Be Harder than Explicit. Belmore (1981) also explored inferencing capacities using a reading task in which subjects had to verify the truth of statements about a previously read prose passage. The test statements represented either a paraphrase of, or an inference from, the preceding passage. Both accuracy and latency of response were recorded in older (mean age = 67) and younger (mean age = 18) subjects. When the statements were verified immediately after reading the paragraph, and the paragraph was available, no intergroup difference in accuracy was observed. When the verification task was delayed, younger subjects were significantly more accurate. For both groups, response latencies for verification were longer when the test sentence was an inference rather than a paraphrase. Surprisingly, Belmore observed lower accuracy rates for the older subjects when the statements required knowledge of explicitly stated rather than implied information. In this study, evidence for a selective deficit in the processing of implicit information, which in theory would require more inferencing and complex semantic encoding, was lacking. Regardless of the type of statement needing verification, older subjects responded more slowly, and Belmore's findings suggest that an age effect on the ability to draw inferences from linguistic material presented in paragraph form is still debatable.

Cohen (1979) investigated the hypothesis that age-related deficits at the higher level stages of language comprehension affect the understanding of informal conversation. According to Cohen, the popularly held belief that language ability is well preserved in old age may need revision, because the studies from which this conclusion was drawn used single words or word pairs. Cohen argued that comprehension and definition of individual words is a far simpler task than discourse comprehension. Further, other investigators, who have used other than single-word paradigms, have reported age effects. Riegel (1968) reported age-related changes in word association responses. Wetherick (1965) reported an age effect in proverb interpretation and the ability to derive the implication of sets of statements. Thus, Cohen designed an experimental task in which more complex processing was required of subjects, notably (a) the ability to relate different facts presented in the same message and draw the correct inference, (b) the ability to relate new facts to prior knowledge, and (c) the ability to preserve the gist and structure in the recall of a longer message or story.

The results of the study showed that comprehension of spoken language is harder for the elderly because of a diminished ability to simultaneously perform the tasks of grasping the surface meaning and also carrying out integrative, constructive and organizing processes. The observed intersubject differences were not thought to be due to memory deficiencies, since both young and aged subjects performed similarly on questions about information presented in the passages.

A finding similar to Cohen's emerged from a study of Till and Walsh (1980), who used a paradigm in which younger (mean age = 20.4) and older (mean age = 68.4) subjects performed an encoding task on implicational sentences and were given a subsequent recall test. Subjects rated a set of sentences as pleasant or unpleasant and estimated the number of words in each. The rating tasks were followed by a free and cued recall task. Age did not affect free recall, but younger subjects performed better in cued recall when given implicational cues. Each cue was a noun referring to information that might be inferred from the sentence rather than associated with one of its words. Like the subjects in Cohen's study, elders were less able to infer information from stimulus sentences when cued with implied information.

Inferences: Harder than Retrieving Facts. The use of fact retrieval versus inference was studied in young and elderly adults by Camp (1981). According to Camp, two types of retrieval may be used to access one's knowledge: direct retrieval of information stored in memory, and inference, or logical extension of previously stored information. He used a research design in which subjects specified how they arrived at their answers, enabling Camp to ascertain whether inference or direct access was more frequently used. Subjects had to select from among four choices the correct answer to two types of questions: direct access and inferential. Examples of direct access questions are "What man's wife was turned into a pillar of salt?" and "What was the name of the flying horse of mythology?" Questions requiring inferential processing were like the following: "What horror movie character would most probably starve in northern Sweden in the summer?" and "What U.S. president was the first to see an airplane fly?" To control for the effect of intelligence, subjects were given the WAIS Information subtest, after which they were assigned to the high or low group. Elders gave more incorrect answers overall than the younger subjects, but the difference was not statistically significant. Older subjects more frequently felt they had made a wild as opposed to an educated guess in choosing their answers, though the difference was not statistically significant. Camp found that both older and younger subjects were slower in answering the inferential questions. However, the older subjects were not disproportionately slower, and therefore results did not support any age-related deterioration in inferential ability.

Not all investigators report age decrements in inferential abilities. Walsh and Baldwin (1977) studied the ability to infer information from text. In their investigation of stored semantic information, no age differences were found in the ability of young adults (mean = 18.7) and elders (mean = 67.3) to convert partial information statements into complete ideational representation, or in the precision with which semantic information was acquired.

Other Investigations: Other Explanations. Other investigators suggest that the findings of age deficits in comprehension may result from the use of paradigms that measure memory rather than comprehension (Burke and Yee, 1984). They argue that older adults have little trouble understanding language but have difficulty remembering what they have understood. Burke and Yee tested this hypothesis by analyzing the response times of young and old adults in a lexical decision task in which subjects read a sentence and made a lexical decision about a target word presented immediately after the sentence. Then too, subjects were asked to recognize sentences. Three different sentence target conditions were used: in the first, a whole sentence was followed by a word that was either related or unrelated, as in "She gave her hungry dog something to chew: bone, nest"; in the second, a sentence with a word associated with the related target was given, as in "That round table is usually in the kitchen: chair, boat"; and in the last, a sentence implying use of a related target word was presented, as in "The cook cut the meat: knife, key." Additionally, a sentence recognition task was administered. Burke and Yee found no evidence for age-related changes in semantic processing. Both young and old subjects were faster when the word targets were instruments implied by the action of the sentence. However, older adults had more difficulty than younger adults in remembering sentences they had read.

Cerella and Fozard (1984) reported lexical access to be unaffected by age. In this study lexical access was defined as the time required to derive the meaning of a word. Cerella and Fozard measured the time course of lexical access in young and old subjects in three processing conditions: a neutral condition in which subjects were presented with a letter string, a second condition in which portions of the lexicon semantically related to the target were primed, and a third condition in which the stimulus string was embedded in visual noise. Cerella and Fozard found no significant differences as a function of age in the different conditions. A facilitative effect of semantic associations between words was found to be comparable in young and old adults.

Summary

In summary, the results of numerous studies can be interpreted as evidence for an age effect on the comprehension of linguistic information (Table 5-2). Yet, it has not been established whether linguistic comprehension diminishes gradually across adulthood or begins abruptly later in life. In the Ulatowska studies (1985, 1986), the significant differences were primarily between the old old group (older than 76) and individuals in middle age. Further, the cause of the aging effect for linguistic comprehension remains unclear; that is, it is not yet known whether age effects are the result of a semantic encoding deficit, a deficit in inferential processing, or memory failure.

In the psychologic literature, Belmore (1981) reports an age effect when elders had to verify inferences about prose; however, the effect was present only in the delayed condition, implicating memory as a more important factor than a deficit in semantic encoding. Further, Belmore found no evidence of a selective deficit in the processing of implicit information.

Unlike Belmore, Till and Walsh (1980) reported an age effect for inferential ability when subjects had to process implied rather than explicit information. Cohen reported significant differences in the ability of older individuals to simultaneously grasp the "surface meaning" of sentences and carry out integrative and constructive processing. Taub (1979) reported an age effect for discourse comprehension but only for elders whose WAIS Vocabulary scores were average.

Walsh and Baldwin (1977), who studied inferencing from text, observed no age differences. Like Petros and colleagues (1983) and Zelinski and associates (1980; 1984), Kemper (in press-a) observed a decrease in the amount of information elders could recall, and attributed some of the decrement to syntactic processing deficits associated with a high memory load. Even this brief review reveals that much remains to be understood about inferential processing as a function of age, notably the relation of memory to semantic encoding and the relation of memory to the complexity of the information to be comprehended.

Does Ideational Capacity Diminish With Age?

Like comprehension, ideation is a fundamental process of SM. After studies of comprehension are reviewed, the question arises whether ideation diminishes with age, and if so, what the consequences are for communicative functioning. Indeed,

Table 5-2. Summary of Research on Story Comprehension and Aging: Aging and SM Processing Capabilities

Ways Measured	Age Difference	Comments
Story/prose retelling		
Ulatowska et al., 1986	Yes	
Taub, 1979	Yes	But not in subjects with superior vocabulary skills
Moenster, 1972	Yes	
Gordon and Clark, 1974	Yes	Especially with one week delay
Spilich, 1983	Yes	
Kemper (in press–a)	Yes	Also influenced by stimulus syntactic form
Recall of main information		
Petros et al., 1983	Yes	
Zelinski et al., 1984	Yes	
Cohen, 1979	Yes	
Dixon et al., 1982	Yes	
Spilich, 1983	No	
Byrd, 1981	No	
Zelinski et al., 1980	No	
Dixon et al., 1984	Mixed	No effect in high verbal subjects; age effect in low verbal subjects
Meyer and Rice, 1981	No	In high verbal subjects
Recall of supplemental information		
Spilich, 1983	Yes	
Petros et al., 1983	Yes	
Zelinski et al., 1984	Yes	
Byrd, 1981	Yes	
Zelinski et al., 1980	Yes	
Dixon et al., 1984	Yes	In both high and low verbal subjects
Cohen, 1979	No	
Dixon et al., 1982	No	
Meyer and Rice, 1981	No	In high verbal subjects
Explicit or direct linguistic information		
Belmore, 1981	Yes	
Ulatowska et al., 1986	No	Greater age difference than with implicit information
Cohen, 1979	No	
Till and Walsh, 1980	No	
Camp, 1981	No	
Implicit or inferred linguistic information		
Ulatowska et al., 1986	Yes	
Cohen, 1979	Yes	
Till and Walsh, 1980	Yes	
Belmore, 1981	No	
Camp, 1981	No	
Walsh and Baldwin, 1977	No	

some research data imply that the elderly have a diminished capacity to generate ideas, data from studies of discourse production and generative naming.

Data From the Study of Linguistic Discourse. To turn first to the linguistic discourse literature, several reports have been published of production deficits in connected discourse (Gordon, Hutchinson and Allen, 1976; North and Ulatowska, 1981; Obler and Albert, 1981). North, Ulatowska, Macaluso-Haynes, and Bell (in press) observed the production of fewer propositions by the elderly (mean age = 64) in narrative discourse and fewer steps in procedural discourse. Then too, the elderly had more instances of referential ambiguity. The significance of this is that referential ambiguity suggests an inability to specify the participants to which one's predication should be linked, an ideational impairment.

In studies of the discourse of Catholic nuns, Ulatowska et al. (1986) were particularly interested in the quantitative and qualitative characteristics of reference. They observed general impairment of reference associated with all types of discourse tasks, including story retelling, story generation, reconstructing old and new information, and question answering. In spoken texts, the referential deficit was manifested as a reduced variety of noun types and fewer proper names that occurred in association with a general increase in the frequency of pronominal use. Ulatowska and colleagues theorized that the ambiguity of reference in the elderly probably results from physiologic and cognitive decline, stylistic and sociolinguistic alteration, and the pragmatics of compensatory adaptation.

The breakdown of anaphoric reference, reference to things in text, has been noted as a feature of the discourse of Alzheimer's patients (LeDoux, Blum, and Hirst, 1983; Obler, 1983) and schizophrenic patients (Rochester and Martin, 1977) and a sign of cognitive deterioration. Like Ulatowska, Cohen (1979) reported frequent errors in reference to things in text in her study, but she interpreted them as the result of memory limitations. When recounting a story, elderly subjects attributed characteristics or actions to the wrong protagonists and failed to make clear reference, as in the use of pronouns without any preceding proper names or descriptions. Cohen reasons that in the recall of fairly large amounts of information, such as a story, memory is overloaded. Thus, elders adopt the strategy of focusing on the recall of the gist at the expense of less salient details.

Walker, Hardiman, Hedrick, and Holbrook (1981) compared the average number of words contained in clauses and the number of clauses in the natural conversation of old and young adults. Not only did elders use fewer words per clause, they used fewer clauses than younger subjects.

Data From Verbal Description Tasks. Other evidence of possible age-related change in ideational ability comes from a study by Bayles and colleagues (1985) in which ten healthy normal individuals, controlled for intelligence and education, from each decade of life from the third to the eighth, were given a verbal description task. The purpose of the task was to provide as complete a description as possible of an object. The number of information units contained in the sample of descriptive discourse was used to quantify completeness of description. Four common objects were used as stimuli: button, nail, envelope, and marble. Descriptions were tape-recorded and transcribed. One point was awarded for each information unit provided. An information unit was defined as any relevant, truthful, nonredundant piece of information specified in a noun phrase, a noun phrase plus a predicate, or a predicate alone. Although a possible age effect on subject performance was observed, the effect was not in the form of an across-the-decades decline. As can be seen from Figure 5-3, the best performance on the task was given by subjects in their 30s and 40s ($F = 3.35$; $df = 5,54$; $p < .01$). According to Duncan's post hoc contrast test, subjects in their 30s and 40s were significantly better than subjects in their 70s. However, subjects in their 50s and 60s did not perform significantly differently from those in their 20s.

Data from Generative Naming Studies. In a generative naming or verbal fluency task, the subject

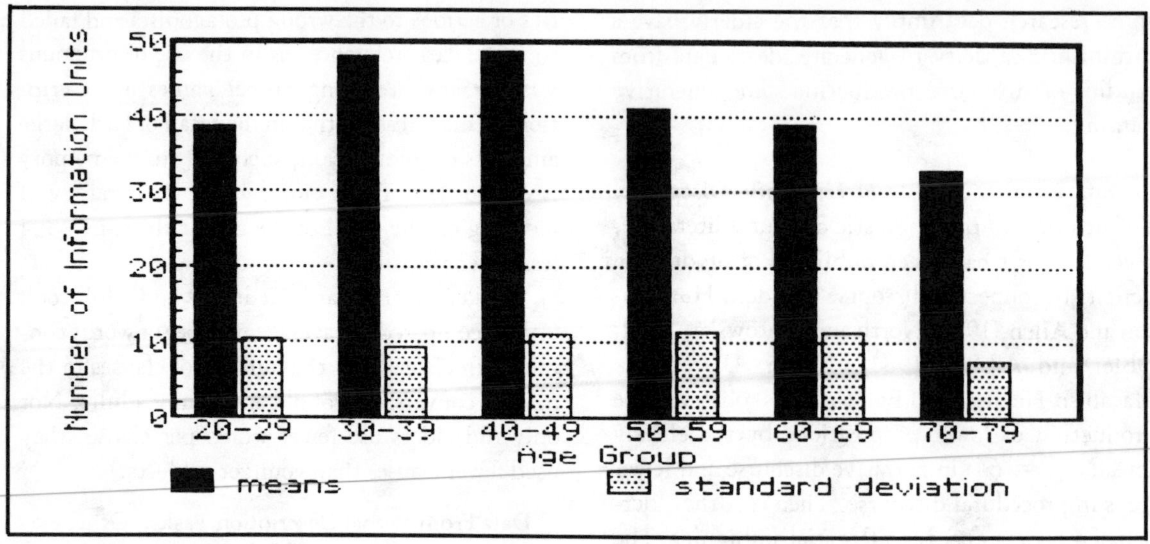

Figure 5-3. *Mean scores and standard deviations on the Verbal Description Task in Decades Study. (Based on data from Bayles, Tomoeda, and Boone, 1985.)*

is asked to name as many examples of a category as possible in a specified period of time. When asked to name words beginning with a particular letter within 1 minute, elders produced significantly fewer words (Obler and Albert, 1981) than younger subjects.

Diminished verbal fluency has also been reported by Spreen and Benton (1969) and Kamin (1957), who compared the verbal fluency of the elderly with high school–aged individuals. Borod and associates (1980) observed a gradual decline across the lifespan in animal generative naming. Adults younger than 40 averaged 26.6 names in 1 minute, whereas adults in their 50s averaged 21.4, and adults in their 70s averaged 18.6.

Other Possible Evidence of Diminished Ideational Capacity. Kogan (1974) studied age effects on the way in which concepts were classified, using an object-sorting task. Fifty cards with black-and-white line drawings of common objects were presented to subjects, who were asked to group the pictures as they wished but to provide a justification. Kogan found that elderly well-educated subjects (N = 168) formed fewer groups, which he interpreted as indicative of a weakening imagination and tendency toward literalness. The younger adults were more inclined to form groups in which each group member was an example of a concept (categorical–inferential) and less inclined to group things according to functional (relational–thematic) or attributive (analytic–descriptive) relations. Although the elderly, like the younger subjects, preferred the categorical–inferential classification system, they used the relational–thematic significantly more frequently. Kogan did not interpret the results as a confirmation of cognitive deterioration with age. Kogan suggests that while the elderly have not lost the capacity for categorical–inferential thinking, they are "more willing to indulge an alternative mode when circumstances permit it" (p. 228).

Cicirelli (1976) studied the logic used by children, young adults, and the elderly in sorting objects. Like Kogan, his results revealed an increase in the use of the relational–thematic basis for classification by the elders, but it was present only after age 60.

The length of time necessary to form verbal associations has been studied by several investigators, and the elderly have been found to take substantially longer than younger subjects to form verbal associations (Birren, Riegel, and Robbin, 1962;

Riegel, 1965; Talland, 1965). Nebes and Andrews-Kulis (1976) were interested in the speed with which individuals of different ages could form verbal mediators. In their task, subjects were asked to form a sentence incorporating a given pair of nouns, and a record was kept of the time needed to form the sentence. Subsequently, subjects were tested to determine the amount of incidental learning that occurred, specifically, how many of the noun pairs they recognized. No significant effects were found for age (young group N = 16, mean age = 20.6; older group N = 16, mean age = 69.9) or sex. However, a main effect for age was observed for incidental learning. Nebes and Andrews-Kulis interpreted the lack of an age effect as evidence against the view that the reported disuse of verbal mediators by the elderly (for example, as reported in paired-associate learning tasks) is due to an inability to rapidly discover meaningful verbal associations between the stimulus words.

Eysenck (1975) studied the ability of young and older subjects to recognize examples of a given category. Subjects were given a category followed by a word (e.g., fruit-ghost) and instructed to decide whether the word belonged to the category. Older subjects were found to be significantly slower on this task. Eysenck held the view that because older subjects could recall examples of a category as swiftly as younger, the difference in performance scores was not due to memory retrieval deficits. Rather, it resulted from slower decision making among the older subjects.

Summary

In summary, ideation and association may diminish with age, but not necessarily gradually (Table 5-3). Processing capacities may be intact in the 50s and 60s, as in early adulthood. But whether the task is inferential, ideational, or associative, the decision-making involved generally takes more time.

Ideational ability, as measured by the number of propositions in connected discourse and the clarity of reference, appears to diminish, just as it does when measured by generative naming ability. However, when ideational ability is measured by a generative task in which individuals are asked to think of as many descriptive ideas about common objects as possible, an across-the-decades decline is not present. Not until the eighth decade is there a significant reduction.

Some evidence exists that associative reasoning, as studied in object sorting tests, declines with age. However, when the measure of associative reason-

Table 5-3. Summary of Research Related to Linguistic Production and Aging: Does Ideational Capacity Diminish with Age?

Discourse production of aged

Fewer propositions in narrative discourse
(North et al., in press)

Fewer steps in procedural discourse
(North et al., in press)

Impairment of reference
(Ulatowska et al., 1986)

Errors in reference when retelling a story
(Cohen, 1979)

Fewer words per clause
(Walker et al., 1981)

Fewer clauses
(Walker et al., 1981)

Fewer information units produced by 70-year-olds
(Bayles et al., 1985)

Generative naming ability

Significantly fewer items generated
(Obler and Albert, 1981; Spreen and Benton, 1969; Kamin, 1957; Borod et al., 1980)

Categorization of items

Concept and functional systems of classification preferred
(Kogan, 1974)

Slower in deciding category membership
(Eysenck, 1975)

Sentence generation

When given a pair of nouns, formed sentences as fast as young subjects
(Nebes and Andrews-Kulis, 1976)

ing was sentence formation from pairs of nouns, no age effect was found. Finally, when the task was the recognition of objects as members of a category, an age effect emerged, which implicated the ability of the elderly to make decisions.

ISSUE 2: AGING AND LINGUISTIC KNOWLEDGE

The second issue of importance, related to the general question whether communication in the normal individual is adversely affected by aging, is whether linguistic knowledge is preserved. Linguistic knowledge can be defined as an individual's knowledge of sounds, grammar, and word meaning, and reference and language use. The discussion of this second issue may be made more manageable if it is first preceded by a discussion of the preservation with age of phonologic and word knowledge.

Is Phonologic and Word Knowledge Preserved with Age?

Age does not appear to adversely affect an individual's phonologic knowledge, or knowledge of the sounds of language and rules for their combination. In fact, phonologic knowledge is preserved even in patients with mild and moderate dementing illnesses. Whitaker (1976) was the first to report the preservation of phonologic knowledge in a severely demented but echolalic woman who no longer produced meaningful speech. When repeating phonologically anomalous sentences presented by the examiner, the woman would spontaneously correct errors. Then too, when this patient produced neologisms, they conformed to the rules of English phonology.

When knowledge of words is discussed, it is necessary to specify whether knowledge of phonemic and orthographic characteristics is meant, or their definition. Vocabulary tests in which individuals are given the word and asked to provide a definition are measures of conceptual knowledge. Tests in which subjects are given the definition, or concept, and asked to produce the word are measures of lexical knowledge. Whereas conceptual knowledge may be maintained until old old age (75+ years), as was discussed earlier in this chapter, evidence exists that the speed of retrieval of lexical knowledge may be decreased.

Bowles, Obler, Albert, and Nicholas (1985) conducted a study in which 18 young individuals, ranging in age from 18 to 33, and 18 older individuals, ranging in age from 65 to 83, were presented with a prime followed by a definition and asked to provide the word defined. Six prime types were used: neutral, the target word itself, orthographically related, semantically related, letter, and unrelated. Both the young and old groups had perfect retrieval in the correct prime condition and in the letters condition, but in all other conditions the older subjects were less proficient. When complete orthographic information was given, as it was when the word itself was the prime, and partial orthographic information in the letters prime, the elderly were significantly benefitted. The authors interpret these data to mean that the elderly have difficulty accessing lexical knowledge. If in fact this is the case, then some information about words is more accessible than other information.

Another type of task that may provide information about the integrity of word knowledge is confrontation naming, in which an individual is given an object or shown a picture of the object for which a name must be provided. Borod and colleagues (1980) studied age effects on a confrontation naming test, the Boston Naming Test (Kaplan, Goodglass, and Weintraub, 1978), and reported a gradual age-related decline in the number of correct responses. However, the decline may have resulted from differences in the educational levels of the subjects for the oldest groups with the lowest naming scores had the fewest years of education.

Is Grammatical Knowledge Preserved with Age?

Knowing how to meaningfully combine words is syntactic knowledge, and age appears to have little effect on it. Even in persons with dementia, this type of linguistic knowledge is well preserved. Halpern, Darley and Brown (1973) studied the syntactic capabilities of patients with diffuse intellectual impairment and observed no impairment of grammatical inflections. Neither did they observe additions, substitutions, or deletions of syntactic words.

In the previously mentioned study by Obler, Fein, Nicholas, and Albert (1985) of the effect of syntax, semantic likelihood, and aging on comprehension, Obler et al. analyzed the types of syntactic forms that were most difficult. The hierarchy from easiest to most difficult was as follows: single negative, active comparative, embedded, passive, double negative. It is important to note that the syntactic forms that were difficult for the elders were also difficult for younger subjects. Therefore, although the elders made more errors overall, they found the same types of items difficult as did younger subjects.

The Token Test (DeRenzi and Vignolo, 1962), especially part five, can be used to assess an individual's knowledge of syntactic relations. When the test was administered to normal adults, education, but not age, was found to be a factor in test performance (DeRenzi, 1979; Orgass and Poeck, 1966; Swisher and Sarno, 1969). Noll and Randolph (1978) gave the test to normal adults ranging in age from 29 to 76 years. No evidence was found of an age effect; however, the sample size was small: 25 subjects in all.

Nebes and Andrews-Kulis (1976) evaluated the grammaticality of sentences produced by subjects in their study of age effects on speed of sentence formation and incidental learning. No significant differences were found in the grammar used by the subject groups. Sentences constructed by the subjects were found to be of ten types, in which the noun pairs were used in the following ways:

1. in two different clauses
2. as subject and direct object
3. as the subject and in an adjective phrase modifying the subject
4. as the subject and in a direct object phrase
5. as the subject and in a prepositional phrase
6. as the subject and in an adverbial phrase
7. as the direct object and in an adverbial phrase
8. as the subject and the complement
9. in a subject phrase and as the complement
10. as compound subjects, objects, or complements

Not all investigators are convinced of the immunity of syntactic ability to age effects. Kynette and Kemper (1986) reported age-related decrements in the degree of syntactic complexity in the spontaneous speech of older adults. Thirty-two English speakers, ranging in age from 50 to 90 years, were interviewed to obtain a 20-minute sample of speech. The language samples were analyzed in terms of five categories: syntax, form class, tense, lexical measures, and dysfluency.

Across the age range of 50 to 90, a reduction in the variability and accuracy of syntactic structures, verb tenses, and form classes was apparent. Performance on lexical measures remained constant, as did dysfluencies.

The 70- and 80-year-olds produced more errors in past tense inflections, subject–verb agreement for person and number, and use of articles and possessive markers. Kynette and Kemper concluded that elderly adults (70s and 80s) did not use grammatical forms and syntactic structures that impose high memory demands, such as sentence-initial relative clauses of noun phrase complements, and structures with multiple embedded clauses. They argued that left-branching grammatical structures may be more difficult for elderly adults to process than right-branching, because the embedded clause interrupts the processing of the main clause.

Kemper (in press-b), in a related study, investigated the ability of elderly adults to imitate complex syntactic constructions. Sixteen elders (70–89 years) and 16 middle-aged adults (30–40 years) were asked to imitate 128 complex sentences involving embedded gerunds, wh-clauses, that-clauses, and relative clauses. Whereas young adults accurately imitated or correctly paraphrased stimulus sentences regardless of length, position, or type of embedded clause, elderly adults could not. They were less able to correctly imitate and paraphrase language constructions with sentence-initial embedded clauses. Kemper concluded that in advanced age, syntactic processing abilities decline to the degree they are associated with increased memory and attentional demands.

In yet another related study by Kemper (1986) of life-span changes in syntactic complexity, diary entries were analyzed. Two sets of diaries provided the data: one set from eight individuals born between 1856 and 1876 who kept a diary for seven or more decades, and the second set from ten adults born between 1820 and 1829. Sentences from the two longest usable entries from each half decade were analyzed for incidence of sentence-initial and sentence-final embedded, coordinate, and subordinate clauses and sentence fragments, as well as average length. Kemper reported an age-related decline in syntactic complexity. Further, the decline was more prominent for sentence-initial constructions than for sentence-final.

Summary

The issue discussed in this section was whether linguistic knowledge is preserved in the normal aging process. Linguistic knowledge was considered to encompass phonologic, lexical, and grammatical knowledge. Of these three types of knowledge, the preservation of phonologic knowledge is least equivocal. Although reports of loss in lexical knowledge are uncommon, some authors report evidence of age-related difficulty accessing lexical knowledge. Most controversial is whether grammatical (that is, syntactic) knowledge deteriorates with age. In some studies, elders have been reported to make more errors in comprehension, imitation, and production of syntactically complex sentences. In other studies, no age effects have been found in the comprehension of complex sentences, the speed of sentence formation, or the complexity of grammar used. Possible differences among these studies may be accounted for by differences in subject age and education. Then too, age effects on linguistic knowledge, if they exist, appear to be subtle and somewhat illusory.

ISSUE 3: AGING AND THE MECHANICS OF COMMUNICATION

What is meant by the mechanics of communication? The basic mechanical aspects of communication involve four processes: (1) the *translation* of ideas into linguistic representations, (2) the *expression* of linguistic representations, (3) the *perception* of linguistic stimuli, and (4) the *derivation* of an idea from a given unit of discourse. Consider that meaningful communication begins with an idea (in SM), which is given a linguistic representation that can be produced orally as spoken discourse or nonorally in writing. Of course, expression is only half the story of the mechanics of communication. The other half is the perception and interpretation of what is perceived, the process whereby an idea is derived from the mental representation of a physical signal. Deterioration in any of these types of mechanical processes (translation, expression, perception, and derivation) can result in a communication disorder.

In old age, mechanical problems are those most likely to affect the ability to communicate. Mechanical problems are more influential than changes in the contents and processes associated with SM or changes in linguistic knowledge. Of the types of mechanical processes, decrements in perception are most common; an abundant literature exists documenting perceptual decrements, the most common of which is loss of hearing (Beasley and Davis, 1981; Corso, 1977a, 1977b; Henoch, 1979; Maurer and Rupp, 1979).

Age-related Hearing Loss. Hearing problems among the aged are pervasive. In the United States hearing loss affects 24 percent of the noninstitutionalized elderly between 65 and 74 years of age and almost 40 percent of those over 75 (Punch, 1983). It is the third most common chronic condition among the noninstitutionalized (Jack, 1981). The institutionalized elderly have an even higher prevalence rate, as much as 90 percent according to Chafee (1967). At present, more than 7 million elders have significant hearing deficits, and by the turn of the century, more than 10 million will be affected.

Presbycusis, or alteration of hearing sensitivity

associated with the normal aging of the auditory system (Corso, 1985), is the most common type of hearing disorder. It is a sensorineural loss resulting from decreased numbers of hair cells or nerve fibers in the cochlea, as well as fibrous changes in the small blood vessels that supply the cochlea. According to Corso (1977b), presbycusis ranks second in prevalence only to arthritis among chronic health conditions. Psychoacoustic investigations of presbycusis substantiate the belief that elderly individuals are increasingly handicapped in oral communication as presbycusis worsens (Bergman, 1971; Corso, 1957, 1963; Jerger, 1973; Konig, 1957; Pestalozza and Shore, 1955; Pickett, Bergman, and Levitt, 1979; Plomp and Mimpen, 1979).

With age, the likelihood of presbycusis increases. Whereas less than 2 percent of the under-17 population are affected, and 12 percent of the 45–64 age group, 39 percent of the over-75 age group are hearing handicapped. Men more than women are susceptible to the condition. Twenty-nine percent of men between the ages of 65 and 74 have presbycusis, compared with 20 percent of the women. Among individuals in the over-75 age group, 44 percent of the men are affected and 35 percent of the women.

The impact of a hearing impairment on communication is hard to overstate. Affected individuals find communication increasingly difficult and tend to withdraw socially. Entertainment options shrink, and victims insidiously lose touch with the world. Additionally, loss of hearing lessens the ability of elderly persons to compensate for other age-related social and physical problems, such as death of a spouse, relocation, or lack of mobility. Finally, it must be mentioned that aged persons with hearing loss are often presumed to be confused or senile (Becker, 1981), and some are misplaced in long-term care facilities. As an aside, an audiologist colleague of the authors was able to motivate an elderly hearing impaired woman to seek audiologic counseling when he told her she might be mistaken as senile because of her unresponsiveness if she refused to wear an aid.

Age-Related Visual Problems. As is the case with hearing, visual problems increase with age. Changes in the visual system may make the perception of linguistic stimuli more difficult, as well as the analysis of lip movements and facial expressions. Between the ages of 35 and 45, most individuals experience deterioration in the lens, which hardens and yellows, causing a change in the spectral distribution of light reaching the retina (Fozard, Wolf, Bell, McFarland, and Podolsky, 1977; Schaie and Geiwitz, 1982; Storandt, 1983). The yellowing of the lens eventuates in greater absorption of blue and green wavelengths, making them harder to discriminate than red and yellow. Between the ages of 55 and 65, changes in the retina and ocular nervous system affect the responsivity of the retina (Schaie and Geiwitz, 1982). Such changes reduce the capacity of the individual to perceive stimuli and transmit perceptual information to the brain for analysis. Then too, the sensitivity of the lens for focusing on close objects becomes impaired. With age the need for increased illumination rises; in fact, the elderly need almost two times as much illumination as younger persons (Cristarella, 1977; Fozard et al., 1977; Schaie and Geiwitz, 1982). Undoubtedly the elderly are frequently hindered in their ability to communicate because of visual problems exacerbated by poor environmental conditions.

Other Age-Related Effects on the Mechanics of Communication. Age-related changes in the musculoskeletal system do not typically result in communication disorders. The effects of musculoskeletal change may be manifested in reduced articulatory proficiency or a change in the fundamental frequency of the voice, making the individual readily identifiable as elderly, but the ability to communicate remains. Changes in muscle, bone, and skin steadily occur throughout adult life. Muscular strength peaks between 25 and 30 years of age, thereafter declining, and older individuals have more fat in proportion to muscle than young adults (Rowe and Besdine, 1982).

Of particular relevance to speech production is the effect of age on the muscles of mastication. Kaplan (1971) reported significant reduction in biting force between young and old adults. Greenfield, Shy, Alvord, and Berg (1957) described weakness of the masticatory musculature secondary to atrophy, and Macmillan (1936) observed a reduction in biochemical efficiency due to changes in muscle attachments. Nonetheless, none of these changes appear to have consequences for normal communication ability (Kahane, 1981), nor does a diminution in the ability of the tongue to make rapid alternating movements, an ability found to be diminished in persons between the ages of 66 and 93 (Ptacek, Sander, Maloney, and Jackson, 1966).

Bone mass diminishes with age. In women, maximum bone loss occurs between the ages of 50 and 65, and in men, between the ages of 70 and 80. In women the loss is accelerated after menopause (Raisz, 1977). Though the loss of bone mass and strength is associated with a higher incidence of fractures, there are no serious consequences to communication ability.

Just as age-related changes are apparent in other body systems, so they are in the respiratory system. Wantz and Gay (1981) reported the occurrence in middle age of a decrease in diaphragm action, vital capacity, maximum breathing capacity, and diffusion and absorption of oxygen. These changes are not handicapping unless the individual is unduly stressed or disease develops.

Before concluding the discussion of the consequences of age on the mechanical aspects of communication, it is important to mention two factors that make it difficult to judge the integrity of the mechanical system, or for that matter, the integrity of any of the other systems in the service of communication. The two factors are behavioral slowing and depression.

Behavioral Slowing. Behavioral slowing is, as Birren, Woods, and Williams (1980) wrote, "perhaps the most ubiquitous and significant change observed in the older organism" (p. 293). Slowness is apparent not only in motor response but in thinking.

Decline in reaction time is one of the most consistent findings in studies of aging The components of reaction time include the time necessary for transmission of sensory information, motor execution, and decision-making (Schaie, 1980). According to Botwinick (1978), the time required in decision making accounts for almost 80 percent of the reaction time. In a study of reaction time differences related to aging for simple and complex tasks, Welford (1977) reported significantly lengthened reaction time for older adults. The magnitude of the increase was 20 percent when the performance tasks were simple and 50 percent when they were complex.

Behavioral slowing in the elderly has been associated with changes in brain electrical activity (Marsh and Thompson, 1977; Woodruff, 1979). The alpha rhythm, the dominant rhythm associated with a relaxed awake state, perceptibly slows by the late 50s and early 60s (Obrist, 1980). Whereas young adults have an alpha rate of 10–11 cycles per second (cps), the rate of the typical 60-year-old is 9 cps, and of 80-year-olds, 8 cps.

Depression. Depression is the most commonly encountered psychiatric illness among the elderly (Georgotas, 1983). Gurland (1976) estimated the prevalence of severe depression after age 65 to be 2–3 percent, and mild depression 3–4 percent. That depression is common among the elderly is not surprising, given the complex social, medical, and economic problems with which they contend.

An in-depth discussion of depression, aging, and dementia is provided in Chapter 14. The point to be emphasized here is that both depression, and age-related behavioral slowing are factors that make judgment of the subsystems of communication challenging.

SUMMARY

The study of possible age effects on the ability to communicate is extremely demanding because effects, when present, are generally subtle, and most tasks are influenced by the subject's intelligence, education, life history, motivation, sensory integrity, mental status, and vigor. Few researchers have been able to control all of these variables in a convincing way. Yet, sufficient research has been done and interstudy comparisons made to say that the ability to communicate diminishes with age. Why?

Because communication ability depends on memory, the ability to process new information and make inferences, and sensory sufficiency. Age effects are most obvious when information to be comprehended is new, complex, and implied and the time allowed for processing is short. In individuals with auditory and visual perceptual problems, impairment is more noticeable.

Of the basic processes that constitute our ability to communicate, specifically comprehension, processing, and production, production is hardest to evaluate. Making inferences about the capability of an individual from performance on a language production task often involves speculation. The researcher does not know if the individual did not produce a particular form, identify a referent, or use certain syntax because he or she could not do so. Nevertheless, sufficient data has been amassed to suggest that the skills enabling people to produce linguistic information decline with age. It is not necessarily the mental lexicon that has deteriorated, but the speed with which the mind works and the ability to access and retrieve information from various memory stores.

A final point needing emphasis is the glaring variability in results from investigations of age effects. This variability is in large part due to marked differences in physical and mental status of the over 60 population. Clinicians must remember that this segment of the population is more heterogeneous than any other and must recognize that their individual patients may be exceptional.

GENERAL SUMMARY AND CLINICAL IMPLICATIONS

1. **The *contents* of semantic memory (SM) are well preserved in normal aging; indeed, vocabulary grows throughout adulthood.**
2. **The *processes* of SM (ideation, inferencing, association) appear to diminish with age. However, changes are subtle and do not dramatically interfere with communicative ability.**
3. **In advanced age, the ability to generate ideas may result in a diminished performance (as compared with young adults) in descriptive discourse or in a naming task.**
4. **An individual's knowledge of grammar is well preserved across the lifespan. Reports of grammatical errors by the aged may result from information processing deficits rather than a loss of grammatical knowledge.**
5. **The most common age-related changes affecting the ability to communicate are perceptual deficits in hearing and vision.**
6. **Age-related behavioral slowing affects the performance of the elderly on timed tests. When time constraints are waived, the performance of the elderly may significantly improve and approximate that of young adults.**
7. **Depression is more common among the elderly than other population segments and can affect cognitive and communicative functioning. In depressed elders, concentration is likely to be poor and test performance inconsistent. Clinicians should screen for depression and refer depressed individuals for treatment.**

REFERENCES

Bayles, K.A., Tomoeda, C.K., and Boone, D.R. (1985). A view of age-related changes in language function. *Developmental Neuropsychology*, *1*, 231-264.

Beasley, D.S., and Davis, G.A. (Eds.) (1981). *Aging: Communication processes and disorders*. New York: Grune and Stratton.

Becker, G. (1981). *The disability experience: Educating health professionals about disabling conditions*. Berkeley, CA: University of California Press.

Belmore, S.M. (1981). Age related changes in processing explicit and implicit language. *Journal of Gerontology, 36*, 316-322.

Bergman, M. (1971). Hearing and aging. *Audiology, 10*, 164-171.

Birren, J.E., Riegel K.F., and Robbin, J.S. (1962). Age differences in continuous word associations measured by speech recording. *Journal of Gerontology, 17*, 95-96.

Birren, J.E., Woods, A.M., and Williams, M.V. (1980). Behavioral slowing with age: Causes, organization, and consequences. In L.W. Poon (Ed.), *Aging in the 1980's: Psychological issues* (pp. 293-308). Washington, DC: American Psychological Association.

Borod, J.C., Goodglass, H., and Kaplan, E. (1980). Normative data on the Boston Diagnostic Aphasia Examination, Parietal Lobe Battery, and the Boston Naming Test. *Journal of Clinical Neuropsychology, 2*, 209-215.

Botwinick, J. (1978) *Aging and behavior* (2nd ed.). New York: Springer.

Botwinick, J., and Storandt, M. (1974). Vocabulary ability in later life. *The Journal of Genetic Psychology, 125*, 303-308.

Bowles, N.L., Obler, L.K., Albert, M.L., and Nicholas, M. (October, 1985). *Naming impairment in the elderly*. Paper presented at the annual meeting of the Academy of Aphasia, Pittsburgh, PA.

Bowles, N.L., and Poon, L.W. (1985). Aging and retrieval of words in semantic memory. *Journal of Gerontology, 40*, 71-77.

Burke, D.M., and Yee, P.L. (1984). Semantic priming during sentence processing by young and older adults. *Developmental Psychology, 20*, 903-910.

Byrd, M. (1981). Age differences in memory for prose passages. Unpublished doctoral dissertation, Department of Psychology, University of Toronto.

Camp, C.J. (1981). The use of fact retrieval vs. inference in young and elderly adults. *Journal of Gerontology, 36*, 715-721.

Cerella, J., and Fozard, J.L. (1984). Lexical access and age. *Developmental Psychology, 20*, 235-243.

Chaffee, C. (1967). Rehabilitation needs of nursing home patients: A report of a survey. *Rehabilitation Literature, 18*, 377-389.

Cicirelli, V.G. (1976). Categorization behavior in aging subjects. *Journal of Gerontology, 31*, 676-680.

Cohen, G. (1979). Language comprehension in old age. *Cognitive Psychology, 11*, 412-429.

Corso, J.F. (1957). Confirmation of the normal threshold for speech on C.I.D. Auditory Test W-2. *Journal of the Acoustical Society of America, 29*, 268-370.

Corso, J.F. (1963). Age and sex differences in pure-tone thresholds. *Archives of Otolaryngology, 77*, 385-405.

Corso, J. (1977a). Auditory perception and communication. In J. Birren and K.W. Schaie (Eds.), *Handbook of the psychology of aging* (pp. 535-553). New York: Van Nostrand Reinhold.

Corso, J. (1977b). Presbycusis, hearing aids, and aging. *Audiology, 16*, 146-163.

Corso, J.F. (1985). Communication, presbycusis, and technological aids. In H.K. Ulatowska (Ed.), *The aging brain: Communication in the elderly* (pp. 33–51). Austin, TX: PRO-ED.

Craik, F.I.M. (1977). Age differences in human memory. In J.E. Birren and K.W. Schaie (Eds.), *Handbook of the psychology of aging* (pp. 384-420). New York: Van Nostrand Reinhold.

Craik, F.I.M., and Masani, P.A. (1967). Age differences in the temporal integration of language. *British Journal of Psychology, 58*, 291-299.

Cristarella, M.C. (1977). Visual function of the elderly. *American Journal of Occupational Therapy, 31*, 432-440.

DeRenzi, E. (1979). A shortened version of the Token Test. In F. Boller and M. Dennis (Eds.), *Auditory comprehension: Clinical and experimental studies with the Token Test* (pp. 33-44). New York: Academic Press.

DeRenzi, E., and Vignolo, L.A. (1962). The Token Test: A sensitive test to detect receptive disturbances in aphasics. *Brain, 85*, 665-678.

Dixon, R.A., Hultsch, D.F., Simon, E.W., and von Eye, A. (1984). Verbal ability and text structure effects on adult age differences in text recall. *Journal of Verbal Learning and Verbal Behavior, 23*, 569-578.

Dixon, R.A., Simon, E.W., Nowak, C.A., and Hultsch, D.F. (1982). Text recall in adulthood as a function of level of information, input modality, and delay interval. *Journal of Gerontology, 37*, 358-364.

Dunn, L.M., and Dunn, L.M. (1981). *Peabody Picture Vocabulary Test-Revised*. Circle Pines, MN: American Guidance Service.

Eysenck, M.W. (1974). Age differences in incidental learning. *Developmental Psychology, 10*, 936-941.

Eysenck, M.W. (1975). Retrieval from semantic memory as a function of age. *Journal of Gerontology, 30*, 174-180.

Feifel, H. (1949). Qualitative differences in the vocabulary responses of normals and abnormals. *Genetic Psychological Monograph, 39*, 151-204.

Feier, C., and Gerstman, L. (1980). Sentence comprehension abilities throughout the adult life span. *Journal of Gerontology, 35*, 722-728.

Fox, C. (1947). Vocabulary ability in later maturity. *Journal of Educational Psychology, 38*, 482-492.

Fozard, J.L., Wolf, E., Bell, B., McFarland, R.A., and

Podolsky, S. (1977). Visual perception and communication. In J.E. Birren and K.W. Schaie (Eds.), *Handbook of the psychology of aging* (pp. 497-528). New York: Van Nostrand Reinhold.

Georgotas, A. (1983). Affective disorders in the elderly: Diagnostic and research considerations. *Age and Ageing, 12*, 1-10.

Gilbert, J.C., and Levee, R.F. (1971). Patterns of declining memory. *Journal of Gerontology, 26*, 70-75.

Goodglass, H., and Kaplan, E. (1972). *The assessment of aphasia and related disorders*. Philadelphia: Lea and Febiger.

Gordon, S.K., and Clark, W.C. (1974). Application of signal detection theory to prose recall and recognition in elderly and young adults. *Journal of Gerontology, 29*, 64-72.

Gordon, S.K., Hutchinson, J.M., and Allen, C.S. (1976). *An evaluation of selected discourse characteristics among the elderly*. Research Laboratory Report, Department of Speech Pathology and Audiology, Idaho State University, Pocatello, ID.

Greenfield, J.C., Shy, G.M., Alvord, E.C., and Berg, L. (1957). *Atlas of muscle pathology in neuromuscular diseases*. Edinburgh: Livingstone.

Gurland, B.J. (1976). The comparative frequency of depression in various adult age groups. *Journal of Gerontology, 31*, 283-292.

Halpern, H., Darley, F.L., and Brown, J.R. (1973). Differential language and neurological characteristics in cerebral involvement. *Journal of Speech and Hearing Disorders, 38*, 162-173.

Henoch, M.A. (Ed.). (1979). *Aural rehabilitation for the elderly*. New York: Grune and Stratton.

Howard, D.V. (1983). The effects of aging and degree of association on the semantic priming of lexical decisions. *Experimental Aging Research, 9*, 145-151.

Hultsch, D.F., Hertzog, C., and Dixon, R.A. (1984). Text recall in adulthood: The role of intellectual abilities. *Developmental Psychology, 20*, 1192-1209.

Jack, S.S. (1981). *Current estimates from the National Health Interview Survey, U.S., 1979*. PHS 81-1564, series 10, no. 136. Hyattsville, MD: Center for Health Statistics.

Jerger, J. (1973). Audiological findings in aging. *Advances in Oto-Rhino-Laryngology, 20*, 115-124.

Kahane, J.C. (1981). Anatomic and physiologic changes in the aging peripheral speech mechanism. In D.S. Beasley and G.A. Davis (Eds.), *Aging: Communication processes and disorders* (pp. 21-45). New York: Grune and Stratton.

Kalikow, D.N., Stevens, K.N., and Elliott, L.L. (1977). Development of a test of speech intelligibility in noise using sentence materials with controlled word predictability. *Journal of the Acoustical Society of America, 61*, 1337-1351.

Kamin, L.J. (1957). Differential changes in mental abilities in old age. *Journal of Gerontology, 12*, 66-70.

Kaplan, H. (1971). The oral cavity in geriatrics. *Geriatrics, 26*, 96-102.

Kaplan, E., Goodglass, H., and Weintraub, S. (1978). *Boston Naming Test* (experimental edition). Boston: Veterans Administration Medical Center.

Kemper, S. (1986). *Life-span changes in syntactic complexity*. Manuscript submitted for publication.

Kemper, S. (in press-a). Syntactic complexity and elderly adult's prose recall. *Experimental Aging Research*.

Kemper, S. (in press-b). Imitation of complex syntactic constructions by elderly adults. *Applied Psycholinguistics*.

Kintsch, W. (1974). *Representation of meaning in memory*. Hillsdale, NJ: Lawrence Erlbaum.

Kogan, N. (1974). Categorizing and conceptualizing styles in younger and older adults. *Human Development, 17*, 218-230.

Konig, E. (1957). Pitch discrimination and age. *Acta Otolaryngologica, 48*, 475-489.

Kramer, N., and Jarvik, L. (1979). Assessment of intellectual changes in the elderly. In A. Raskin and L.F. Jarvik (Eds.), *Psychiatric symptoms and cognitive loss in the elderly* (pp. 221-271). New York: Halsted Press.

Kynette, D., and Kemper, S. (1986). Aging and the loss of grammatical forms: A cross-sectional study of language performance. *Language and Communication, 6*, 65-72.

LeDoux, J.F., Blum, C., and Hirst, W. (1983). Inferential processing of context: Studies of cognitively impaired subjects. *Brain and Language, 19*, 216-224.

Lewinsky, R.J. (1948). Vocabulary and mental measurement: A qualitative investigation and review of research. *Journal of Genetic Psychology, 72*, 247-281.

Macmillan, H.W. (1936). Anatomy of the throat, mylohyoid region and mandible in relation to retention of mandibular artificial dentures. *Journal of the American Dental Association, 23*, 1435-1442.

Marsh, G.R., and Thompson, L.W. (1977). Psychophysiology of aging. In J.E. Birren and K.W. Schaie (Eds.), *Handbook of the psychology of aging* (pp. 219-248). New York: Van Nostrand Reinhold.

Maurer, J.F., and Rupp, R.R. (1979). *Hearing and aging: A guide to rehabilitation*. New York: Grune and Stratton.

Meyer, B., and Rice, G.E. (1981). Information recalled from prose by young, middle, and old adult readers. *Experimental Aging Research, 7*, 253-286.

Moenster, P. (1972). Learning and memory in relation to age. *Journal of Gerontology, 27*, 361-363.

Nebes, R.D. (1976). Verbal-pictorial recoding in the elderly. *Journal of Gerontology, 31*, 421-427.

Nebes, R.D., and Andrews-Kulis, M.S. (1976). The effect of age on the speed of sentence formation and incidental learning. *Experimental Aging Research, 2*, 315-331.

Noll, J.D., and Randolph, S.R. (1978). Auditory semantic, syntactic, and retention errors made by aphasic subjects on the Token Test. *Journal of Communication Disorders, 11*, 543-553.

North, A.J., and Ulatowska, H.K. (1981). Competence in independently living older adults: Assessment and correlates. *Journal of Gerontology, 36*, 576-582.

North, A.J., Ulatowska, H.K., Macaluso-Haynes, S., and Bell, H. (in press). Discourse performance in older adults. *International Journal of Aging and Human Development*.

Obler, L.K. (1980). Narrative discourse style in the elderly. In L.K. Obler and M.L. Albert (Eds.), *Language and communication in the elderly* (pp. 75-90). Lexington, MA: Heath.

Obler, L.K. (1983). Language and brain dysfunction in dementia. In S. Segalowitz (Ed.), *Language functions and brain organization* (pp. 267-282). New York: Academic Press.

Obler, L.K., and Albert, M.L. (1981). Language and aging: A neurobehavioral analysis. In D.S. Beasley and G.A. Davis (Eds.), *Aging: Communication processes and disorders*. (pp. 107-121). New York: Grune and Stratton.

Obler, L.K., Fein, D., Nicholas, M., and Albert, M.L. (October, 1985). *Syntactic comprehension in aging*. Poster presented at the annual meeting of the Academy of Aphasia, Pittsburgh, PA.

Obler, L.K., Nicholas, M., Albert, M.L., and Woodward, S. (1985). On comprehension across the adult life span. *Cortex, 21*, 273-280.

Obrist, W.D. (1980). Cerebral blood flow and EEG changes associated with aging and dementia. In W.W. Busse and D.G. Blazer (Eds.), *Handbook of geriatric psychiatry* (pp. 83-101). New York: Van Nostrand Reinhold.

Orgass, B., and Poeck, K. (1966). Clinical validation of a new test for aphasia: An experimental study of the Token Test. *Cortex, 2*, 222-243.

Owens, N.A. (1953). Age and mental abilities: A longitudinal study. *Genetic Psychology Monographs, 48*, 3-54.

Pestalozza, G., and Shore, I. (1955). Clinical evaluation of presbycusis on the basis of different tests of auditory function. *Laryngoscope, 65*, 1136-1163.

Petros, T., Tabor, L., Cooney, T., and Chabot, R.J. (1983). Adult age differences in sensitivity to semantic structure of prose. *Developmental Psychology, 19*, 907-914.

Pickett, J.M., Bergman, M., and Levitt, M. (1979). Aging and speech understanding. In J.M. Ordy and K. Brizzee (Eds.), *Aging: Vol. 10. Speech systems and communication in the elderly* (pp. 167-186). New York: Raven Press.

Plomp, R., and Mimpen, A.M. (1979). Speech reception threshold for sentences as a function of age and noise level. *Journal of the Acoustical Society of America, 66*, 1333-1342.

Ptacek, P.H., Sander, E.K., Maloney, W.H. and Jackson, C.R. (1966). Phonatory and related changes with advanced age. *Journal of Speech and Hearing Research, 9*, 353-360.

Punch, J. (1983). The prevalence of hearing impairment, *ASHA, 25*, 27.

Raisz, L.G. (19777). Bone metabolism and calcium regulation. In L.V. Avioli and S.M. Krane (Eds.), *Metabolic bone disease* (pp. 1-48). New York: Academic Press.

Ricks, Jr., J.H. (1958). Age and vocabulary test performance: A qualitative analysis of the responses of adults (Doctoral dissertation, Columbia University, 1958). *Dissertation Abstracts International, 19*, 182.

Riegel, K.F. (1965). Speed of verbal performance as a function of age and set: A review of issues and data. In A.T. Welford and J.E. Birren (Eds.), *Behavior, aging and the nervous system* (pp. 150-190). Springfield, IL: Charles C Thomas.

Riegel, K.F. (1968). Changes in psycholinguistic performances with age. In G.A. Talland (Ed.), *Human aging and behavior* (pp. 239-279). New York: Academic Press.

Rochester, S.R., and Martin, J.R. (1977). The art of referring: The speaker's use of noun phrases to instruct the listener. In R.O. Freedle (Ed.), *Discourse processes: advances in research and theory: Vol. 1. Discourse production and comprehension*. Norwood, NJ: Ablex.

Rowe, J.W., and Besdine, R.W. (Eds.) (1982). *Health and disease in old age*. Boston: Little, Brown.

Schaie, K.W. (1980). Intelligence and problem solving. In J.E. Birren and R.B. Sloane (Eds.), *Handbook of mental health and aging* (pp. 262-284). Englewood Cliffs, NJ: Prentice-Hall.

Schaie, K.W., and Geiwitz, J. (1982). *Adult development and aging*. Boston: Little, Brown.

Shakow, D., and Goldman, R. (1938). The effect of age on the Stanford-Binet vocabulary scores of adults. *Journal of Educational Psychology, 29*, 241-256.

Shewan, C.M. (1979). *Auditory Comprehension Test for Sentences*. Chicago: Linguistics Clinical Institutes.

Spilich, G.J. (1983). Life-span components of text processing: Structural and procedural differences. *Journal of Verbal Learning and Verbal Behavior, 22*, 231-244.

Spilich, G.J., and Voss, J.F. (1982). Contextual effects upon text memory for young, aged-normal, and age-impaired individuals. *Experimental Aging Research, 8*, 147-151.

Spreen, O., and Benton, A. (1969). *Neurosensory Center Comprehensive Examination for Aphasia*. Victoria, BC: Neuropsychology Laboratory, Department of Psychology, University of Victoria.

Storandt, M. (1983). Psychologic aspects. In F.V. Steinberg (Ed.), *Care of the geriatric patient* (6th ed.) (pp. 417-428). St. Louis, MO: C.V. Mosby.

Surber, J.R., Kowalski, A.H., and Pena-Paez, A. (1984). Effects of aging on the recall of extended prose. *Experimental Aging Research, 10*, 25-28.

Swisher, L.P., and Sarno, M.T. (1969). Token Test scores of three matched patient groups: Left-brain damaged with aphasia; right-brain damaged with aphasia; non-brain damaged. *Cortex, 5*, 264-273.

Talland, G.A. (1965). Initiation of response, and reaction time in aging, and with brain damage. In A.T. Welford and J.E. Birren (Eds.), *Behavior, aging and the nervous system* (pp. 526-561). Springfield, IL: Charles C Thomas.

Taub, H.A. (1979). Comprehension and memory of prose materials by young and old adults. *Experimental Aging Research, 5*, 3-13.

Taub, H.A., and Klein, G.E. (1978). Recall of prose as a function of age and input modality. *Journal of Gerontology, 33*, 725-730.

Terman, L.M., and Merrill, M.A. (1937). *Stanford Binet Intelligence Scale* (2nd Revision). Iowa City, IA: Houghton Mifflin Company.

Thorndike, R.L. and Gallup G.H. (1944). Verbal intelligence of the American adult. *Journal of General Psychology, 30*, 75-85.

Till, R.E., and Walsh, D.A. (1980). Encoding and retrieval factors in adult memory for implicational sentences. *Journal of Verbal Learning and Verbal Behavior, 19*, 1-16.

Ulatowska, H.K., Cannito, M.P., Hayashi, M.M., and Fleming, S.G. (1985). Language abilities in the elderly. In H.K. Ulatowska (Ed.), *The aging brain: Communication in the elderly* (pp. 125–139). Austin, TX: PRO-ED.

Ulatowska, H.K., Hayashi, M.M., Cannito, M.P., and Fleming, S.G. (1986). Disruption of reference. *Brain and Language, 28*, 24-41.

Walker, V.G., Hardiman, C.J., Hedrick, D.L., and Holbrook, A. (1981). Speech and language characteristics of an aging population. In N.J. Lass (Ed.), *Speech and language: Vol. 6., Advances in basic research and practice* (pp. 144-202). New York: Academic Press.

Walsh, D.A., and Baldwin, M. (1977). Age differences in integrated semantic memory. *Developmental Psychology, 13*, 509-514.

Wantz, M.S., and Gay, J.E. (1981). *The aging process: A health perspective*. Cambridge, MA: Winthrop.

Welford, A.T. (1977). Motor performance. In J.E. Birren and K.W. Schaie (Eds.), *Handbook of the psychology of aging* (pp. 450-496). New York: Van Nostrand Reinhold.

Wetherick, N.E. (1965). Changing an established concept: A comparison of the ability of young, middle-aged and old subjects. *Gerontologia, 11*, 82-95.

Whitaker, H.A. (1976). A case of isolation of the language function. In H. Whitaker and H.A. Whitaker, (Eds.), *Studies in neurolinguistics: Vol. 2* (pp. 1–58). New York. Academic Press.

Woodruff, D.S. (1979). Brain electrical activity and behavior relationship over the life span. In P.B. Baltes (Ed.), *Life-span development and behavior: Vol. 1.* (pp. 111-179). New York: Academic Press.

Zelinski, E.M., Gilewski, M.J., and Thompson, L.W. (1980). Do laboratory tests relate to self-assessment of memory ability in the young and old? In L.W. Poon, J.L. Fozard, L.S. Cermak, D. Arenberg, and L.W. Thompson (Eds.), *New directions in memory and aging: Proceedings of the George Talland Memorial Conference* (pp. 519-544). Hillsdale, NJ: Erlbaum.

Zelinski, E.M., Light, L.L., and Gilewski, M.J. (1984). Adult age differences in memory for prose: The question of sensitivity to passage structure. *Developmental Psychology, 20*, 1181-1192.

Chapter 6

Linguistic Theory and Knowledge, and Dementia

"Paradigms gain their status because they are more successful than their competitors in solving a few problems that the group of practitioners has come to recognize as acute."

Thomas S. Kuhn, 1962
The Structure of Scientific Revolutions

The approach to evaluating the communication disorders experienced by dementia patients is based on information obtained in the last decade about the behavioral consequences of dementing disease and the theoretic conceptualization of what constitutes communication and language. The behavioral consequences of dementing illness have been reviewed; therefore, the focus of this chapter will be on how an understanding of linguistic theory and knowledge enable better understanding and evaluation of the communication disorders of persons with dementia.

PARADIGM SHIFT IN LINGUISTICS: IMPLICATIONS FOR TESTING

The publication of *Syntactic Structures* by Noam Chomsky in 1957 launched a decade in which the focus of linguistic research was on syntax, or the structure of language. In his landmark book, Chomsky argued that the grammar of language consists of a compendium of rules capable of generating an infinite number of acceptable sentences—a view that gave birth to the theory of generative grammar. Chomsky conceptualized the grammar of language as an idealized description of the linguistic competence of native speakers and thus was concerned with defining the rules speakers know rather than accounting for the mistakes they make. These mistakes Chomsky described as performance errors resulting from environmental and physiologic influences such as fatigue, distraction, or forgetfulness. The goal of linguistics was to define the actual competence of the speaker and the features common to all human languages. In Chomsky's theory, humans are biologically endowed with a language acquisition device through which they derive the rules of the grammar. This conceptualization of linguistic knowledge, as learning a set of rules through which an infinite number of sentences could be generated, was a powerful idea and mortally wounded the popular view purveyed by behaviorists that language is a conditioned response learned by imitation. Chomsky challenged the behaviorists to account for the ability of humans to produce unique novel utterances. How, he asked, can the novel utterance be explained if in fact language is learned by imitation and conditioning?—a question behaviorists could not answer.

In Chomsky's approach, language was treated as an abstract device separate from the language user. Chomsky's goal was not to account for how humans use language—a very important fact, for it explains in part why the study of language structure proved so popular. Had Chomsky's goal been to describe how humans use language to communicate, then the effects of context and meaning on structure would have assumed more importance. But Chomsky was addressing a different question, namely, how the grammar could account for all possible sentences in a natural language.

Chomsky's Generative, or Transformational, Grammar

Linguists in the generative grammar school dissociated syntax, semantics, and pragmatics. Their mentalism and formal logic prevented an examination of the sociologic and contextual determinants of language. In generative, or transformational, grammar theory, transformational rules are said to operate upon core sentences generated by a set of phrase structure rules. Phrase structure rules are just as they say, rules for creating linear strings of words, or phrases, and they do so on a word-by-word basis. Chomsky demonstrated that phrase structure rules alone were inadequate to account for the relations between sentences in a natural language and posited the existence of a set of transformational rules to account for the interdependencies among words in a sentence and sets of sentences, as in the following examples:

Phrase structure level: output-core sentence:
Ed drives a pickup truck.
Transformational level: examples of transformations:
Passive transformation:
A pickup truck was driven by Ed.
Question transformation:
Was a pick-up truck driven by Ed?
Relativization transformation:
The truck that was driven by Ed, was it a pick-up?

Simple active declarative sentences are composed at the phrase structure, or base, level and form the basis for all other structures. More complex structures are formulated by transformational rules acting on simple active declarative sentences. At the third level of grammar, morphophonemic, or inflectional, rules are applied. Chomsky argued that transformational rules transformed the deep structure, in which the logical relations of the sentence were marked, to a surface representation, called surface structure.

Reaction Against Generative Grammar Theory

During the period in which the focus of linguistics was on structure, many linguists found the concept of the independence of structure from meaning counterintuitive, as did scholars concerned with accounting for how humans communicate with one another. The idea of the grammar of language being autonomous of meaning was simply unacceptable to a great many language scientists. Thus, in response to the theory proposed in *Syntactic Structures*, an alternative theory developed in which semantics, not syntax, was seen as the generative component of language. This theory became known as the generative semantics theory. Those interested in a detailed review of the debate about the role of structure and semantics in linguistics are referred to Newmeyer's (1980) book *Linguistic Theory in America*. For the purpose of this discussion it is sufficient to recognize that "[in generative semantics] one seems to witness a more faithful reemergence of the time-honored view of language, that it is a correlation of the inner content of meaning and the outer form of sound representation" (Kuroda, 1972, p. 3).

People interested in linguistic communication rejected the automony of syntax because it did not explain how humans use and comprehend language, and many believe that a theory of language ought to account for language use and comprehension. Then too, evidence was mounting from different disciplines that language meaning, use, and context influence the grammar. Thus, a paradigm shift among language researchers occurred. Transformational grammar theory could not provide a full lexical description of language use without making reference to semantics and pragmatics. The authors' interest in characterizing the linguistic communication skills of the dementia patient has coincided with the movement among linguists to include in a theory of language an explanation of linguistic communication.

STUDY OF THE DEMENTIA PATIENT HAS IMPORT FOR DEFINING INTERDEPENDENCIES AMONG LINGUISTIC RULES

The dementia patient presents a particularly interesting case for the study of the relation of linguistic functions to the integrity of the mind and the dependencies between the different types of linguistic knowledge. For example, with dementia patients, the researcher has the unique opportunity to ascertain precisely those aspects of structure and phonology that are influenced by meaning. Through the study of the discourse of dementia patients, it can be seen that not all syntactic (structural) aspects of language are independent of the effects of semantics and pragmatics. Consider the following discourse sample taken from an advanced dementia patient,

> "No, for goodness sake. What is you doing? Coming home from a story, or playing. My parents is a has a present for you. Ah, your parents has the house cleaning, Timmy. We, we, no. Running out at three, then, the car wash, they, uh, fill, four, happy every one, then can come back again."

Structural knowledge, which is independent of semantic and pragmatic effects, is insufficient to enable an individual to meaningfully communicate. It is the performance of the advanced dementia patient that convinces us that knowing the sounds of language, the rules for their combination into words, and word ordering rules is insufficient knowledge to enable communication. It is important that the clinician appreciate the distinction between having certain types of linguistic knowledge and being able to communicate.

Dementia Affects Communication More Than Language Structure

The clinician testing the dementia patient should be concerned with evaluating communication rather than knowledge of language per se. At this juncture, one might logically ask, How does one test communication rather than knowledge of language? Isn't a test of linguistic communication ability necessarily a test of language knowledge? The authors would answer, Not necessarily, just as a test of language knowledge is not necessarily a test of communication ability. In dementia patients, considerable linguistic knowledge is maintained but the ability to communicate, or use that knowledge to share information, is impaired. Tests like the sentence correction test, in which dementia patients spontaneously correct grammar without grasping the meaning of the sentence, demonstrate that language can be tested without testing the ability to use that knowledge to share information. Then too, a test like the verbal description task, on which dementia patients are impoverished in their ability to provide a description of common objects, is a test of the ability to use language. It is not exclusively a test of the knowledge of specific language rules.

To appreciate how to approach the task of evaluating linguistic communication, it is important to discuss more fully the different types of linguistic knowledge and how they interact to make communication possible. What will be discovered is that the types of linguistic knowledge vary in their reliance on conscious processing, the degree to which they can be automatically applied, and the degree to which they are needed to recover meaning. These three variables can guide the clinician in predicting whether a particular type of linguistic knowledge is likely to be preserved in the dementia patient. Rules that require conscious active processing for their application, and are needed to recover meaning, are those less likely to be preserved.

DIFFERENT TYPES OF LINGUISTIC KNOWLEDGE

Phonologic Knowledge

Phonologic knowledge consists of knowledge of not only the sounds of language but the rules that govern their occurrence. Speech sounds, or phonemes, are composed of even smaller units, called phonetic (or distinctive) features, which represent aspects of the articulation of the whole sound. The mastery of these isolatable phonetic features enables speakers to combine sounds and pronounce words with the "correct accent" of the language. During the period of language acquisition, children internally formulate a set of rules that enable them to recognize and produce correctly the sound sequences used in their language. English-speaking children learn that the sequences "pfl" or "sgy" are unacceptable because the order of these phonemes violates the rules they have learned about English. They would, however, accept the sequences "geeot" and "cyrd" because both are consistent with the rules of English phonology.

Phonologic knowledge consists of more than a knowledge of the sounds of language and the rules for their combination. It also consists of knowing how to place stress. For example, in bisyllabic English nouns, stress is usually placed on the first syllable, as in mó-ther, teá-cher, cós-tume, and sín-gle. When a new word is introduced into the language, as is often done by companies manufacturing new products, speakers know where to place stress within the word because they have internalized rules for stress placement based on syllable strength, for example, Klée-nex and Xé-rox.

Phonologic knowledge also is recognized to encompass an understanding of a complex hierarchic structure that organizes English words. These structures are composed of phonemes, syllables, and yet another unit of organization: the foot. The relations between these levels in the phonologic hierarchy are rule-governed, and one consequence of these relations is that they ultimately affect how stress is placed. Stress, tune, and phrasing in English, can be varied in linguistically significant ways because the tonal features can be described independently of their lexical representation (Liberman, 1975).

Stress is, for the most part, determined by the structural properties of English. Tonal and metrical characteristics of sounds and syllables play a role, and semantic and pragmatic knowledge also have an influence. Consider the phrase "Mary had more friends." If the word "Mary" were given extra emphasis, the phrase would imply that a comparison was being made between Mary and one or more individuals. If the word "had" were emphasized, the implication would be that Mary did have more friends, but doesn't now. Finally, if the emphasis were on the word "friends," the implication would be that what Mary had more of was friends, as opposed to something else. Variation of stress at the phrasal level motivated these different interpretations of meaning. Yet, regardless of the stress pattern at the phrasal level, the overall tonal sequence of the phrase would be constant. This is because English declarative sentences normally have a low–high–low tone pattern, regardless of where the main sentential stress is located. The tonal pattern is independent of the sentence stress (Liberman, 1975). However, it is the case in English that prominent stress and high tone generally go together. Providing an account of how stress is assigned in a particular utterance requires the invocation of phonologic, as well as semantic and pragmatic, knowledge and serves as a good example of how different types of linguistic knowledge interact in communication.

Dementia patients retain the ability to produce the sounds of their language and order them appropriately until they are in the advanced stages. Recall that Whitaker's (1976) patient HCEM could repeat sentences that she no longer understood. This ability was not idiosyncratic to HCEM, for other advanced dementia patients have the same ability (Bayles and Boone, 1982). Phonologic knowledge can be applied by dementia patients who are incapable of meaningfully communicating.

Syntactic Knowledge

Syntactic knowledge is knowing how to group words together to form acceptable sentence structure. Such knowledge is implicit, and many speakers cannot formally state syntactic rules; rather, they apply them automatically. Syntactic knowledge also includes understanding the functional relations between different structural elements, for example, whether a noun is behaving as the subject of the utterance, the object of the verb, the indirect object, or the object of a preposition. To understand syntax is to understand the structural mechanisms through which our thoughts are conveyed, but understanding the thoughts themselves requires other kinds of processing, specifically semantic and pragmatic. For example, even though many functional relations are recoverable from the structure of an utterance, some are not recoverable without semantic and pragmatic processing, notably the utterance purpose. Consider the following sentences:

1. Mary is the one to help today.
2. The duck is ready to eat.
3. He hit the man with the stick.

In the first two of these three ambiguous sentences, structural clues are lacking about the intended logical relations, that is, who or what is doing the action and who or what is receiving the action. To derive the speaker's intended meaning in producing these utterances, and to interpret the structure, the listener requires additional information. In the sentence "Mary is the one to help today," it is unclear whether Mary is helping or being helped and whether the word "one" functions as an object or subject. Similarly, in the second sentence, structure does not enable the hearer to know whether the duck is eating or being eaten and whether the word "duck" functions as a subject or object. Although structural clues exist in the third sentence, more than one structure is possible; thus, the sentence is structurally ambiguous. As was true for the other two examples, something more than structural knowledge is necessary to derive the intended interpretation. Speakers of English know that the phrase "with a stick" could modify either "he" or "man." Examples like these provide evidence that linguistic communication results only if the listener uses knowledge *other* than that contained in structure alone.

A thorn in the side of Chomsky's early theory of the independence of grammar (structure) was the fact that syntax does influence meaning, and as the previous examples have demonstrated, meaning can influence the interpretation of syntax. Trying to draw a line between syntax and semantics has been a problematic enterprise for linguists, one that has never been satisfactorily accomplished. Notice how even a minor variation in syntax affects the meaning in the following example:

1. The boy and the girl kissed.
2. The girl kissed the boy.

An analysis of the performance data of the dementia patient may help the linguist better distinguish the dependencies between syntax and semantics. Look at the following sample of language from an advanced dementia patient and try to identify those errors that are strictly syntactic and those that are semantic.

> Well, he went out and got some stuff to bring up this for. That's why the mother was on up here putting out some things that she thought were. And all of us were all running around. This little boy, I know. I was stopped across the building. I kind of slithered. It's kind of unused. And it was already announced that people was to come with their clothes that the young people wear.

In this typical discourse sample of a dementia patient, it can seen that knowledge of word order is well preserved. The point is that to a large extent, syntactic processing is dissociable from semantic and pragmatic processing. Further, the mental mechanism responsible for filling the word slots in the sentence frames has sufficient integrity to put nouns where nouns go, verbs where verbs go, and other parts of speech where they are supposed to go.

Semantic Knowledge

Semantic knowledge is an individual's knowledge of both meaning and reference. Historically, linguists have conceptualized semantics as the study of meaning and attempted to develop a representation system for the interpretation of sentence meaning. Philosophers, on the other hand, have been more concerned with semantics as the study of reference (Akmajian, Demers, and Harnish, 1979; Fodor, 1975) and have worked to define the logic and principles connecting words and sentences with things and events. Both meaning and reference can be shown to constitute semantic knowledge.

Developing an appreciation for the domain of semantic knowledge is a considerably harder task than appreciating phonologic and syntactic knowledge. A tremendous body of literature in both linguistics and philosophy has been published by theorists attempting to specify what it means to have semantic knowledge and how it is used in comprehension. The reader who is unfamiliar with semantic theory may find the concepts in this section challenging; however, the point of including them is to demonstrate why this type of linguistic knowledge is necessarily dependent upon the well-being of conceptual memory and is vulnerable in dementia patients.

Semantics as Meaning. It is knowledge of meaning that enables us to make a host of judgments about language, notably how to distinguish utterances that are synonymous, antonymous, redundant, anomalous, and logically ambiguous.

Synonymous utterances are those which are identical in meaning because they express the same logical relations, as in

1a. Ray gave Sara a compact disc.
1b. Sara was given a compact disc by Ray.
2a. It was Reagan who pressed for prayer in the schools.
2b. Reagan pressed for prayer in the schools.

Antonymous utterances are those expressions opposite in meaning, such as

1a. a small girl
1b. a large boy
1a. an erudite woman
1b. an unschooled man

Redundant utterances are those in which information has been needlessly repeated:

1. the frozen ice
2. the old centenarian
3. the gorgeous beauty queen

Anomalous utterances have illogical meaning, as in

1. round parallelogram
2. a hot ice cream cone
3. easy-going hot-head

Logically ambiguous sentences are those which have more than one interpretation in the logical relations expressed in the sentence, namely, who or what initiated and received the action:

1. Jill was the one to help today.
2. The natives dislike sailing in the harbor.

When the study of semantics is considered to be the study of meaning, a differentiation the theorist must make is between speaker meaning and sentence meaning. They are not necessarily the same. For example, depending upon the situation and speaker, the same string of words, can be used to mean different things. In the following situations the words "I am sorry" can have a variety of interpretations:

Situation 1: Woman apologizing to man for being late.

Situation 2: Pilot refusing to cross picket lines.

Situation 3: Man expressing condolences to bereaved friend at a funeral.

Speaker Meaning and Sentence Meaning. Speaker meaning is what the language user intends to communicate when using a part of the language; and sentence meaning is what the words in an utterance add up to in the language. The derivation of speaker meaning involves a different analysis than the derivation of sentence meaning. Whereas the derivation of speaker meaning requires analysis of context, contextual analysis is unnecessary in the derivation of sentence meaning.

An appraisal of the nature of "semantic" judgments, that is, speaker meaning, synonymy, anomaly, and so on, makes it apparent that they require the most fundamental thought process, namely categorization, or seeing a relation as a result of comparison. Thus, the authors agree with Jackendoff (1983), who wrote, "When we are studying semantics of a natural language, we are by necessity studying the structure of thought" (p. *x*). The ability to categorize deteriorates in persons with dementia, and thus the semantic content of their utterances vividly reveals their disordered thinking.

Semantics as Reference. The referential theory of semantics conceptualizes the meaning of a word or expression as that to which the word or expression refers. A problem for the theory, however, has been that not all words refer to things, for example, words like "could," "so," "beauty," and "mystery." Another problem for the referential theory is that expressions that do refer to the same thing do not necessarily have the same meaning. Consider that the words "Napoleon," "the king of France," "the vanquished at Waterloo," and "Josephine's lover" all refer to the same man, yet do not have the same meaning. Referential theorists have trouble distinguishing between a language user's knowledge of language and knowledge of the world. Nevertheless, people understand words with no tangible referent, and indeed, most reference is variable depending on the context in which the word or expression is used. A way of surmounting this problem has been to distinguish between sense and reference. The sense of a word is one's concept of the referent, whereas the reference is the set of all real or imaginary things that fit the concept.

A semantic theory must account for an individual's knowledge of what is being referred to when language is used, that is, referred to by both the speaker and the sentence. Just as sentence meaning was distinguished from speaker meaning, sentence (or linguistic) reference must be distinguished from speaker reference.

Sentence Reference and Speaker Reference. Sentence reference is what the expression, as part of the language, refers to and can be further specified as singular or general (Akmajian et al., 1979). Singular linguistic reference, a somewhat misleading term, includes proper names, pronouns, and phrases such as "This year's winner of the Nobel prize for medicine" or "the milk in the refrigerator," which refer to definite things, irrespective of whether they are singular or plural. General linguistic reference includes common nouns, verbs, and adjectives. The following are examples of singular and general reference:

1. The first man to walk on the moon was Armstrong. (singular expression)
2. Each man who walked on the moon was an astronaut. (general expression).

Speaker reference is what the speaker refers to in producing an utterance and may be the same as what the words refer to. However, speaker reference is often different from word reference, as when a mother says "my little doll" to refer to her baby daughter, or "this old rag" when talking about last year's dress.

So far it has been said that semantic knowledge includes knowledge of meaning and reference, but that is not the sum total of semantic knowledge. It also consists of being able to recognize linguistic truth, truth that depends not on word knowledge but rather on linguistic facts. For example, knowledge of the world is not required to determine that the following types of sentences are true:

1. Either X or not X. Either the cheese is tainted, or it is not tainted.
2. If X and X′, then X. If the dog is lost and the cat is lost, then the dog is lost.
3. All X's that are Y's are X's. All flowers that have thorns are flowers.
4. If every X is Y, then it is not true that no X is Y. If every Grand Prix driver is a woman, then it is not true that no Grand Prix driver is a woman.

Each of these examples expresses a property of language that, if adhered to, makes a sentence true in a logical sense. This is not an exhaustive list of the types of sentences in which it is possible to establish the truth value of the sentence without invoking knowledge of the state of the world. In addition to truth properties, there are truth relations, the most important of which is entailment. One sentence is said to entail another sentence when the truth of the first guarantees the truth of the second, and the falsity of the second guarantees the falsity of the first, as in the following examples:

1. "The man is short" entails that the man has a height.
2. "The test is hard" entails that the test is not easy.

Summary. Semantic knowledge is our knowledge of meaning properties and relations, referential properties and relations, and truth properties and relations. An adequate semantic theory must attribute to each expression "in the language the semantic properties and relations it has and should define those properties and relations" (Akmajian et al., 1979, p. 240). To have intact semantic knowledge is to be able to derive the sense and reference of the expressions of the language.

Pragmatic Knowledge

As the definition of linguistic knowledge moves to pragmatics, it is important to emphasize that the boundary between semantics and pragmatics is hard to demarcate. A principal reason for the territoriality dispute is that in order to give a full account of speaker meaning, reference must be made to to context, and contextual effects on meaning have traditionally been assigned to the domain of pragmatics.

The modern use of the term "pragmatics" is attributable to the philosopher Morris, who was concerned with the science of semiotics, or signs. Morris (1938) delineated three branches of inquiry in the science of semiotics: syntactics, semantics, and pragmatics. Syntactics was described as the study of the "formal relations of signs to one another." Semantics was described as the "study of the relations of signs to the objects to which signs are applicable," and pragmatics was the study of "the relation of signs to interpreters." The definition of the term "pragmatics" has undergone some revision since 1938 and, according to Levinson (1983), refers to "those linguistic investigations that make necessary reference to aspects of the context" (p. 9). The term "context" is used by Levinson to refer to the identities of the participants in a verbal exchange and their beliefs, knowledge, and intentions, as well as the temporal and spatial dimensions of the communicative event.

Bar-Hillel (1971) defines pragmatics as that which is left over after semantics is taken out. Hurford and Heasley (1983) conceive of it as the rules that account for interpersonal meaning. Jackendoff (1983) argues that semantic and pragmatic rules are rules for the manipulation of conceptual structures and that if there is a distinction between semantic and pragmatic rules, then it lies only in the formal manipulations the rules perform on conceptual structures.

Today, pragmatic theorists are interested in the relation between language structure and principles of language use. According to Dascal (1983), pragmatics designates a cluster of problems rather than a well-established discipline. He suggested the following criteria for the demarcation: an aspect of meaning is pragmatic if

1. It has to do with the nature of the speech act performed by the utterance of a sentence.
2. It has to do with the meaning the utterance has in excess of (or distinct from) the sense of the sentence uttered.
3. It cannot be predicted from the sentence uttered alone, but requires, for its specification, information about the context of the utterance (Dascal, 1983, p. 24).

Dascal's criteria are helpful in specifying the domain of pragmatics in a general way. The specific phenomena to which these criteria make reference are deixis, implicature, presupposition, and speech acts.

Deixis. Deixis is a Greek word meaning "indicating." Deictic terms are those which indicate person, place, or time and can be said to belong in the domain of pragmatics because they relate context and language structure. The study of deixis concerns the grammatical representation of the features of a context. Because deixis refers to the ways in which contextual features are specified grammatically, it also concerns the relation between utterance interpretation and contextual analysis. All languages have a subset of deictic words whose meaning varies according to the conditions of use. To appreciate the contribution to meaning of deictic information, consider a sample of discourse in which it is absent:

1. I'm not here about *that*, but *he* must see me about *this*. (what, who, which)
2. I left 15 minutes ago. (from when)

The pronouns "I" and "you" are common deictic words, as are the words "here," "today," and "you." Deixis is a part of the pragmatic domain because pragmatics concerns contextual effects on meaning.

Conversational Implicature. Conversational implicature is that which is implied by the context and content of a conversation. The concept of conversational implicature provides an account of how it is possible to mean more than is said. In the following example, the words expressed do not, by themselves, convey the full meaning, which also depends on the speaker's intent and the way in which language is used.

Mother: Are these all that are left of the cookies I made for Mrs. Martin?
Child: Yes, I am afraid so.

Notice that the mother has asked a question about the amount of cookies remaining; yet we know that she is implying disapproval and frustration. Conversational implicature provides a bridge between what is literally said and what is conveyed. These bridges are girded by social knowledge, and in this case, we know that it is a violation of a social convention to take the cookies destined for someone else.

The key ideas in implicature were proposed by Grice (1975; 1978), who argued that conversation is governed by the following set of logical rules, referred to as conversational maxims:

1. maxim of cooperation
2. maxim of quality
3. maxim of quantity
4. maxim of relevance
5. maxim of manner

The cooperation maxim is a tacit agreement among conversationalists that they will contribute to the conversation in an orderly and polite way. The maxim of quality is the understanding that participants will be truthful and have appropriate substantiation for the information reported. The maxim of quantity prescribes that conversants will say neither too much or too little; and the relevance maxim prescribes that what is said will be pertinent to the situation and topic. Finally, the maxim of manner calls for speakers to be perspicuous, that is, plain to the understanding.

Conversants use these maxims to understand the speakers' meaning, or comprehend. Their existence allows conversants to generate inferences beyond the interpretation of literal semantic content, and the inferences they generate are referred to as conversational implicature. Some evidence that the maxims of conversation exist is that they can be violated, and in so doing, conversants can communicate specific messages. For example, all of you have undoubtedly experienced being with someone all evening who was furious at you, a fact he or she did not wish to admit linguistically; yet, the anger was communicated through an evening's worth of monosyllabic responses.

A crucial point in understanding the relations obtaining between pragmatics and semantics is that conversational implicature affects meaning. Meaning is derived from the way in which language is used in a particular context, as well as the degree to which the conversational participants adhere to the maxims of conversation. Thus, when we attempt to explain communication, reference must be made both to pragmatic and semantic knowledge.

Presupposition. Another pragmatic phenomenon is presupposition. Presuppositions are the background assumptions against which the main import of an utterance is assessed (Levinson, 1983). Consider the following:

1a. She didn't realize the plane had been hijacked.
1b. Presupposition: The plane had been hijacked.
2a. Zendejas managed to kick the extra point.
2b. Presupposition: Zendejas tried to score the extra point.

3a. While Mt. St. Helens was erupting, the seismologists were asleep.
3b. Presupposition: Mt. St. Helens was erupting.
4a. Julie is a better swimmer than Sara.
4b. Presupposition: Sara is a swimmer.

Presupposition is a special species of pragmatic inference that is derived from conventions about the use of referring expressions (Strawson, 1950). Strawson argued that statements such as those in 1a–4a presuppose statements 1b–4b if, and only if, the "a" statements are a precondition on the truth or falsity of the "b" statements.

Speech Act Theory. Traditionally, speech act theory has been considered part of pragmatic theory. Speech act theorists attempt to identify social meaning in terms of the activity performed by a speaker in the act of speaking.

The genesis of speech act theory was Austin's (1962) observation that while sentences can often be used to report states of affairs, the utterance of some sentences must be treated as the performance of a particular act. For example, when the minister utters the sentence,"I now pronounce you man and wife," a marriage has been accomplished. When a jury spokesman declares "We find the defendent guilty," the defendant is subject to punishment. Austin described such utterances as performatives, and the circumstances required to obtain for their success, a set of "felicity conditions."

As Austin's theory was extended, it became clear that in uttering any sentence, a speaker can be said to have performed some act. When the act had an effect on the hearer (i.e., the hearer was persuaded when the speaker's intention was to persuade), the act was said to be perlocutionary. Utterances that did not have an effect on the hearer, but represented the performance of an act, were called illocutionary acts. As speech act theory has developed, distinctions have been drawn between the types of acts in which we engage and the conditions that must exist for their occurrence. The problem for speech act theorists continues to be that as it is presently formulated, speech act theory does not offer a way of specifying how a particular set of linguistic elements uttered in a particular conversational context comes to receive a particular interpretation. Nonetheless, speech act theorists have increased our understanding of why *communication* must encompass more than linguistic structure, indeed involves all types of linguistic knowledge. Take, for example, the following:

> A mother and her young son arrive home from the store with a car full of groceries. The son rushes in the house empty-handed, and the mother calls after him, "What's the matter; have you broken your arms?"

The mother does not think her son has broken his arms, nor is she requesting an answer to her question, but she is directing him to help her carry in the groceries. How do we know that? We cannot glean that meaning from a literal interpretation of the words she uttered. It is knowledge of context and the social principles of how language is used that enables us to comprehend her meaning. According to Hurford and Heasley (1983), "Illocutionary acts form a kind of social coinage, a complicated currency with specific values, by means of which speakers manipulate, negotiate and interact with other speakers" (p. 246).

One aspect of illocutions that has received attention is directness. A direct illocution is one interpreted literally, as in

The moon is full. (when the moon is full)
The Chateau St. Jean wine is gone. (when the wine is gone)
Will you lend me your car? (when the speaker wants to be lent a car)

But frequently we do not mean our utterances to be interpreted literally, as in the following:

Can you pass the salt?
Am I the only one who is freezing in here?
Didn't you know this seat is reserved?

A simple yes-or-no answer is not expected to these questions; rather, we expect the salt to be passed, the heat to be turned up, and a seat to be vacated. Part of speech act theory is to account for how individuals know whether an utterance is to be interpreted literally and whether it is a direct or an indirect illocution.

Summary

Linguistic communication results from the interaction of syntactic, semantic, phonologic, and pragmatic knowledge. The boundaries defining these different linguistic domains are elusive, particularly if one is reviewing them in relation to the question of how humans communicate. How can pragmatics, which is concerned with contextual effects on meaning, be separated from semantics, the study of meaning? The fact that they have been treated as separable domains is the result of the types of questions linguists have addressed. The value of separating them for those interested in explaining human communication is unclear.

A way of classifying linguistic knowledge that may have more educational value for clinicians caring for dementia patients is to subdivide linguistic knowledge according to psychologic or physiologic criteria. For example, if we were to subdivide linguistic knowledge according to psychologic criteria, we might make a distinction between those aspects of the process of linguistic communication that require conscious processing (self-knowing) and those that do not, or those dependent on the integrity of semantic memory and those that are not. If either of these criteria were used for the classification of communicative processes, then semantic and pragmatic phenomena would be classified together, for they both involve conscious processing and the integrity of semantic memory.

Semantic and pragmatic analyses are complex, more so than structural and phonologic. The predictability of the latter makes automatic, nonconscious processing more feasible. Because the possible number of utterances in a natural language is infinite, no formula exists to enable humans to verify meaning automatically and unconsciously.

TESTING LINGUISTIC KNOWLEDGE

Testing Phonologic Knowledge of Dementia Patients

The clinician interested in testing phonologic knowledge can have patients judge phonologically aberrant sentences, correct phonologic errors, and attempt to pronounce newly created words. Testing phonologic knowledge is not likely to provide the clinician with the best type of information for discriminating the dementia patient from normal individuals, because in mild and moderate dementia, phonologic knowledge is well maintained.

Testing Syntactic Knowledge of Dementia Patients

Using knowledge of syntax as a measure of the communication ability of dementia patients is a questionable idea (except possibly for Pick's disease and multi-infarct dementia patients). Because knowledge of structure is preserved, measures of syntactic knowledge and structural analysis of discourse will not enable the clinician to make an early diagnosis. Syntactic judgment and correction tests have been given to dementia patients, but statistically significant differences between the performance of mild AD patients and the normal elderly typically are not obtained (Bayles, 1982).

Kempler, Curtiss, and Jackson (1986) compared syntactic and lexical semantic knowledge in the speech and writing of 20 AD patients and 20 normal individuals who were matched for age and education. They reported that the speech output of AD patients contained a normal range and frequency of syntactic constructions but poor lexical use. Writing to dictation showed a similar pattern, and the ability to use syntactic cues was significantly more intact than the ability to use semantic cues.

Testing Semantic Knowledge of Dementia Patients

As yet, no one has comprehensively studied the dementia patient's knowledge of meaning, reference, and truth properties and relations, to our knowledge. Because the study of semantics is the study of thought, and because in dementing disease, thought inherently deteriorates, it necessarily follows that all types of semantic knowledge will be affected in the demented individual. What is yet to be reported is the precise nature of that dissolution process.

The authors recommend the development of tests in which assessment is made of the ability of dementia patients to make semantic judgments, and to interpret both sentence and speaker meaning, and sentence and speaker reference. Further, tests should be developed of the ability to judge linguistic truth properties and relations.

Testing Pragmatic Knowledge of Dementia Patients

To test pragmatic knowledge, clinicians will have to consider deixis, conversational implicature, presupposition, and speech act knowledge.

Testing Deixis in Dementia Patients. A good way to evaluate deixis is in discourse analysis. For example, when the discourse of the severely demented individual is analyzed, deictic information is notably disturbed, as in the following:

> "Why it's, it's been pretty good. We haven't had any, any, uh, uh, let me see this is Thur-, this is Wednesday, isn't it? And we didn't have anything but just a mere handful of 'em. And, uh, we got through there and, and did the best we could. Because so many of them were off, you know, getting things and they were all off. And then, the next thing was, uh . . . oh, I've forgotten."

The patient's disorientation for time, place, or person is obvious from the absence of deictic information. The utterances have no meaningful relation to context.

Testing Conversational Implicature in Dementia Patients. To our knowledge, no one has yet reported a study in which an account was made of the ability of dementia patients to systematically violate the rules of conversation. From clinical experience, it appears dementia patients violate conversational rules, but not purposefully. For example, dementia patients frequently say things that have no basis in reality, but they are not unrealistic by design. Obler and Albert (1981) reported that mild dementia patients often say too much, exhibiting logorrhea, but again not intentionally.

Testing Presupposition in Dementia Patients. Linguistic presupposition ability has not been well studied in normal adults or dementia patients. As a special case of inference, presupposition can be expected to be disordered in the dementia syndrome because of the extensive deterioration in inferential abilities of demented individuals.

Testing Speech Act Knowledge and Use in Dementia Patients. A standardized test for assessing an adult speaker's knowledge of different speech acts, and the ability to derive contextual effects on speech act interpretation, is unavailable. Tests could be devised for assessing knowledge of illocutions and ability to use language meaningfully. In the Tucson study (Bayles, 1985) dementia patients were asked to define common illocutions, such as promising, denying, greeting, and so on. Mild dementia patients performed similarly to elderly control subjects, but moderate dements were significantly impaired. A significant difference was found between mild AD patients and normal subjects in the ability to judge whether an utterance in a particular context was intended literally. This finding suggests that development of assessment techniques for evaluating the ability to judge literality may be clinically useful.

Testing Semantic AND Pragmatic Knowledge of Dementia Patients

Another unit, larger than the word or sentence, that must be considered in evaluating dementia patients is discourse, in both text and conversation. Certainly the exclusive consideration of the word or sentence alone will not tell us the whole story of what was communicated and, in the case of the dementia patient, the whole story of what is impaired. Full understanding of communication requires consideration of the relations between speakers, speakers and the context, and speakers and the utterances they produce in context. The medium for studying these relations is the conversation or the text.

Consideration of a unit larger than the sentence, be it conversation or a text, is an important and relevant linguistic development for those interested in characterizing the linguistic communication problems associated with dementia. It is in these larger units of language that the problems of the dementia patient become apparent. Demented individuals frequently produce sentences that in isolation seem meaningful; it is only when intersentential relations are analyzed that the inappropriateness of the individual sentences becomes apparent, as in the following example:

Meaningful-sounding sentences:
Look at that, that's where it goes.
Did you see that?
Do you know what that is up there?
Actual text:
EXAMINER: What does it mean to thank someone?
DEMENTIA PATIENT: Well, according to what you want to do, not me. Look at that, that, that's where it goes. Did you see that? How it's going . . . ? Do you know what that is up there?

For transformational grammarians, the sentence was the primary object of concern; indeed, language was conceptualized as a set of sentences. The goal of transformational theory was to specify which sentences were categorically possible without regard for their occurrence in context. But for many scholars, the study of the sentence became meaningful only if there was acknowledgement of the context in which the sentence was used, and of the motivation of the speaker in producing the sentence, as well as knowledge of other sentences in the communicative event.

The favorable reception given to discourse and textual analysis has resulted, in part, from the difficulty linguists and psychologists have had in accounting for a host of linguistic communication phenomena when the sentence alone is the level of analysis and the objective is to describe human communication. A necessary strategy for adequately evaluating the linguistic communication skills of the dementia patient is to evaluate units of language larger than the sentence, most notably text and conversation.

Text Defined

A text is a unified, hierarchically ordered network in which concepts interrelate to form propositions that are themselves related. Linguists studying discourse have focused on the relations between sentences, and the degree to which a set of concatenation, or linking, rules can be derived that will define a text. Clinicians can conduct a structural analysis of text, a conceptual analysis, or both. Those who use a structural approach argue that it promises to integrate linguistic findings about relations between sentences. In the conceptual approach, the text itself, as a thematically homogeneous unit, is the object of analysis. Considerable attention by linguists has been given to defining the structural and semantic devices by which the propositions in the text are related to each other in a coherent way.

Cohesion. Coherence is a necessary condition for text. Cohesive devices are those that relate the propositions to each other to form a coherent whole. Cohesive relationships exist when the interpretation of some aspect of the text is dependent on the interpretation of another. An example of a cohesive relation is the following:

> *Amadeus* was the best motion picture in 1985.
> It was based on the Broadway play about Mozart.

The word "it" is dependent for meaning upon the interpretation of the previous sentence and refers back to *Amadeus*. The most complete account of cohesion is the one by Halliday and Hasan (1976), who specify in detail the structural and logical devices by which propositions and concepts are related.

Cohesive Devices. The basic types of cohesive devices are reference, substitution, ellipsis, and lexical relations. *Referential devices* refer to things in or out of text, or to things that have happened or will happen. If the reference is to something that is outside of the text, the reference is said to be exophoric. Exophoric reference is not cohesive because it does not bind together textual elements (Halliday and Hasan, 1976). If reference is to something within text, it is endophoric. Endophoric references can be subdivided into two groups: those referring to preceding text, or anaphoric references, and those referring to things that will follow, or cataphoric references. The essential point about reference, from the point of view of Halliday and Hasan, is that every instance of reference has a presupposition that must be satisfied; that is, the "thing referred to has to be identifiable somehow" (p. 33).

When the cohesive device is *substitution*, the hearer/reader is forced to find another expression for which the one in question is a paraphrase: "George Washington was our first President. As Father of our country, he holds a special place in American history." "Father of our country" is a substitution for "George Washington."

In the case of *ellipsis*, the hearer/reader must find a previous expression to substitute, as in the following examples:

1. Ursula and Adam were seriously thinking of visiting Europe. Ursula is likely to. (visit Europe)
2. Sara will always remember the senior prom. Kurt will too. (always remember the senior prom)

Lexical Relations, or lexical cohesion, are established through the structure of the vocabulary used. Two separate, though related, aspects constitute lexical cohesion: reiteration and collocation. According to Halliday and Hasan (1976), reiteration is simply the repetition of a lexical item usually marked by a reference word such as "the" or a demonstrative, or the occurrence of a synonym within the text. Collocation is the use of lexical items that tend to appear in similar contexts, for example, cactus—spine—sticker—sharp, and dessert—chocolate—cake—pie.

The study of text or discourse has gone through three phases. In the 1950s it received its first serious notice as an important object of linguistic analysis (Coseriu, 1955; Harris, 1952; Karlsen, 1959; Uldall, 1957), and although important work was done, text analysis was not in the mainstream of linguistic inquiry. About 1968, several linguists independently recommended that linguistic analysis expand beyond the sentence level (Crymes, 1968; Dik, 1968; Hasan, 1968; Heidolph, 1966; Koch, 1971; Palek, 1968). The impetus for this movement was in part the aforementioned growing dissatisfaction with the transformational grammar paradigm in which the focus was on the sentence. By 1972, because of the influence of a number of alternative theories to transformational grammar (van Dijk, 1972; Dressler, 1972; Kuno, 1972; Petofi, 1971; Schmidt, 1973), the linguistic community was more receptive to the concept of text analysis.

Whereas the linguistic approach to text analysis was to apply to the text those principles that had been popular for sentence analysis, sociologists of the same period were studying the text, or discourse, as a form of social interaction (Gumperz and Hymes, 1972; Labov, 1972a, 1972b). Adding to the momentum of text analysis research was the interest of psychologists who viewed it as a better medium for understanding human information processing and memory. As deBeaugrande (1980) wrote, "This interdisciplinary demand for theories and models has been a major impetus in the development of text linguistics" (p. xiii).

More recently, text researchers have been concerned with issues like the mental representation of text, the structural and logical elements that lead to the coherence that defines a text, and the nature of the inferential processes involved in text comprehension.

Text Analysis of Dementia Patients. Shekim and LaPointe (1984) studied the ability of dementia patients to produce narrative and procedural discourse. An analysis of the textual material produced by subjects in their study revealed significantly more exophoric references, (references to things outside of the text), more sentence deviations, more pauses greater than 5 seconds, and fewer cohesive ties.

Analysis of the text produced by mild and moderate dementia patients talking and writing about

Norman Rockwell pictures, in a study conducted by the authors, (Bayles, Boone, Tomoeda and Slauson, 1986) revealed a significantly diminished ability even among mild dementia patients in idea production and explaining the moral or gist. Further, significantly more sentence deviations and fragments were present and vocabulary was less diverse, though total output did not always diminish.

Conversational Analysis

Another language unit, larger than the sentence, that has been the object of study by researchers in several disciplines, is conversation. Thus far, conversational analysis has been primarily an inductive process, that is, a search for the common features of conversations. Analysts have reviewed voluminous transcriptions of naturally occurring conversation, searching for recurrent patterns. Proponents of conversational analysis emphasize that it has yielded most of the substantial insights about the organization of text. Opponents have argued that it is based on vague theoretic underpinnings. Much of the important work in conversational analysis has been done by sociologists known as ethnomethodologists, people who study the ethnic methods of the production and interpretation of social interaction (Garfinkel, 1972; Turner, 1976).

The rationale for the use of conversational analysis for utterance interpretation is that linguistic analysis alone "renders an account that is propositionally ambiguous, functionally equivocal, and interactionally indeterminate" (Dore and McDermott, 1982, p. 374). Most words have several meanings, many sentences are ambiguous, and speech acts are multifunctional; thus, without well-specified contexts, utterance interpretation is impossible.

More recently the focus of research has turned from general constructional features of conversation to the analysis of specific routines such as conversational repair and requests for information. A central topic in conversational analysis, one discussed earlier in the chapter in relation to pragmatics, is implicature. Some utterances can be understood only by relating the logical relations

Table 6-1. Responses of Severe AD Patients to a Structured Conversational Interaction

Behavior	% Occurrences	% Non-occurrences
Responded with extended hand when offered handshake	45.0%	55.0%
Requested more information to clarify an ambiguous question	14.6%	85.4%
Corrected an incorrect statement made by the examiner	49.2%	50.8%
Verbally interrupted the examiner	52.9%	47.1%
Maintained eye contact during interaction	85.7%	14.3%
Relevant verbal response when complimented	33.3%	66.7%
Complimented examiner after receiving a compliment	4.8%	95.2%
Provided information about the complimented object	9.5%	90.5%
Clarified a response when asked by the examiner	26.7%	73.3%
Took a gift when handed to them	46.7%	53.3%
Unwrapped the gift	0.0%	100.0%
Made a relevant response when thanked for their time	64.7%	35.3%
Replied appropriately in response to "I enjoyed meeting you."	40.0%	60.0%

expressed in the utterance to social convention (McCawley, 1978; Sadock, 1978).

Conversational analysts are also interested in topic development and maintenance. The topic of a conversation is not always obvious without consideration of a sequence of utterances. From the study of conversational sequences, analysts hope to learn how people know when to talk and what to say to elicit responses from other conversants. Related to understanding this is understanding how speaker turns are allocated.

Conversational Ability of Dementia Patients. Reports of systematic study of the conversational ability of dementia patients would be important contributions because loss of conversational skill is likely to be an early marker of the dementia syndrome. The increased interest of sociologists and psychologists in conversational analysis in the last decade has provided language analysts with a variety of methods for quantifying conversational ability. Undoubtedly, in the next decade, several enterprising researchers will study the dissolution of this skill in dementia.

In an ongoing study supported by the National Institute of Mental Health, the authors have attempted to engage severely demented AD patients in conversation, using a standardized approach. To date, 20 severely demented patients have been studied who have exhibited the interesting behaviors summarized in Table 6-1.

RECOMMENDATIONS FOR EVALUATING THE COMMUNICATION DEFICITS OF DEMENTIA PATIENTS

The background information about the linguistic communication problems of dementia patients and the paradigm shift in linguistics provides a perspective for understanding the authors' recommendations about evaluating the communication of the dementia patient. As yet, no battery is available that has been demonstrated to be valid and reliable for evaluating the breadth of the communication deficits associated with dementia. However, many tests have been given to dementia patients that appear quite sensitive to early changes. Rather than attempt to review all the tests that have been given, it would seem more instructive to present a set of basic clinical principles to guide clinicians in the composition of a test battery.

Assess the Integrity of the Contents of SM. The first and very important principle is to select measures that assess the preservation of the contents of semantic memory: the concept, proposition, and schema. To validly test conceptual knowledge, the patient must be required to do more than access the mental dictionary. Naming a picture or object does not, by itself, constitute proof of the preservation of conceptual knowledge. Appropriate tests include expressive vocabulary measures, expressive pantomime, sentence creation, and production of coordinate, superordindate, and subordinate concepts.

When assessing a patient's propositional knowledge, the goal is to ascertain whether the patient perceives the relation between two or more concepts. Examples of appropriate tests of propositional knowledge are linguistic disambiguation tasks, explaining and creating sentences, and reading comprehension tests.

Assessing a patient's knowledge of schemata may be accomplished by observation of the individual in everyday situations. Observe patients as they do things, like make a doctor's appointment or plan a birthday party. Then too, see if they can recognize common situations described by the examiner.

Assess the Integrity of the Processes of SM. The second principle to be recommended in the linguistic evaluation of dementia patients is to incorporate tasks that will assess the processing capabilities associated with semantic memory, namely, the ability to make inferences and generate ideas. Inferencing is the ability to form a conclusion. Linguistically oriented tasks that can be used to evaluate inferential processes are these: identifying similarities and differences between linguistically presented stimuli, deriving the correct sequence of linguistically presented information, and explaining metaphor and ambiguity.

Analyze Communication Beyond the Sentence Level. The third basic principle in testing the dementia patient is to include an analysis of a unit of language larger than the sentence, namely, discourse. Discourse is the most natural and common type of communication and requires the integration of all types of linguistic knowledge. It is a medium through which the social, psychologic, and linguistic aspects of communication can be studied. With discourse analysis, the clinician can quantify the emptiness of language associated with dementia, the fragmentation of thought, and anomia. The methodology for analyzing discourse has been refined in the last decade (Labov and Franshel, 1977; van Dijk, 1977; deBeaugrande, 1980; Brown and Yule 1983). Clinicians now have models for quantifying the structural and logical components of discourse. An important technique through which the relation of cognition to communication can be examined is the study of coherence and cohesive devices. Coherence is a general cognitive concept definable in terms of plausibility, conventionality, and conclusiveness of text (Ulatowska, North, and Macaluso-Haynes, 1981). The clinician can study the structural and semantic devices that make the discourse cohesive.

The many anecdotal reports of dementia patients having difficulty maintaining the topic, taking turns, being insensitive to others in the conversation, saying either too much or too little, and failing to repair misunderstandings suggest that many aspects of conversational ability are affected.

Adopt Ecologically Valid Test Paradigms. The fourth basic principle in evaluating the patient with dementia is to adopt ecologically valid test paradigms, to obtain information about how people behave in everyday life. Both the study of discourse and the study of conversation have good ecologic validity because they are the most naturally occurring linguistic activities. Certainly the spouses of patients are interested in what the patient understands from that which is heard or read.

Test Communication Processes That Are Nonautomatic. The fifth basic test principle is to test processes that are nonautomatic. Automatic processes are carried on without conscious monitoring and are those most likely to be maintained in early dementia. As pharmacologic therapy is developed for dementing disorders, the primary clinical objective will be to identify dementia early, and the most logical way to approach early definition is to evaluate those processes most vulnerable to dementing disease effects. Semantic and pragmatic processing are generally not automatic, whereas phonologic and syntactic processes are.

Assess Generative and Creative Communication Abilities. The sixth test principle is to use tests that require the patient to actively participate. A task in which the patient must use language creatively is more likely to be sensitive to early dementia than one in which the patient can be passive. When patients must generate the answer, they are actively participating.

SUMMARY

The study of the communication disorder of dementia patients has coincided with a surge of interest in the semantic and pragmatic aspects of language and a deemphasis on the structural. Semantic and pragmatic types of linguistic knowledge are those most adversely affected in dementing illness. In this chapter, the shift in the focus of language study was reviewed and the types of linguistic knowledge specified. Recommendations were made about evaluating the different types of linguistic knowledge in dementia patients. Finally, principles for defining the communication disorder of dementia were recommended.

GENERAL SUMMARY AND CLINICAL IMPLICATIONS

1. The interest of language scholars in describing how humans use language to communicate, in addition to explaining how the grammar of a natural language can generate all possible sentences, has resulted in the development of new techniques for describing communicative performance.
2. In the last decade, considerable attention has been given to explicating semantic and pragmatic linguistic knowledge, and techniques for analyzing text, conversation, and language use offer clinicians a productive way to study the effects of dementing illness on communicative functioning.
3. For theoreticians, dementia patients are a fascinating experiment of nature, for it is through them that brain–language scientists can study intralinguistic relationships between different kinds of linguistic knowledge (phonologic, syntactic, semantic, and pragmatic) and interrelationships between linguistic knowledge and cognitive processes (memory, conscious attention, perception, and so on).
4. To date, it appears that the deterioration of SM affects semantic and pragmatic knowledge more than phonologic and syntactic. In fact, to a large extent, semantic and pragmatic knowledge appear to be dissociable from phonologic and syntactic knowledge.
5. Semantic and pragmatic linguistic rules, which are applied in the recovery of meaning, require conscious active processing for their application and are those most likely to be affected in dementing illness. Clinicians desirous of differentiating the mild dementia patient from normal subjects should use tasks designed to test these rules.
6. Phonologic knowledge is knowledge of the the sounds of language, the rules that govern their occurrence, and the rules for applying stress. Dementia patients retain phonologic knowledge until the advanced stages of dementia.
7. Syntactic knowledge is understanding the structural mechanisms through which our thoughts are conveyed, but understanding the thoughts themselves requires semantic and pragmatic knowledge. Semantic and pragmatic rules are rules for the manipulation of conceptual structures.
8. Semantic knowledge is knowledge of word meaning and reference.
9. An aspect of meaning is pragmatic if it concerns the nature of the speech act performed by uttering a sentence, and the meaning of the utterance distinct from its sense, and if it can not be predicted from the sentence in isolation but requires contextual reference.
10. Analysis of the discourse and conversation of dementia patients offers clinicians a rich medium in which to study vocabulary diversity, language output, sentence structure, development of theme, and cohesion.
11. Guidelines for clinical evaluation of communicative functioning of dementia patients, which have evolved from new directions in psychology, linguistics, philosophy, and speech and hearing sciences, are to (a) assess the integrity of the contents of SM, (b) assess the processes of SM, (c) analyze communicative skill beyond the sentence level, (d) adopt ecologically valid test paradigms, and (e) assess generative and creative communicative abilities.

REFERENCES

Akmajian, A., Demers, R.A., and Harnish, R.M. (1979). *Linguistics: An introduction to language and communication*. Cambridge, MA: The MIT Press.

Austin, J.L. (1962). *How to do things with words*. Oxford: Claredon Press.

Bar-Hillel, Y. (1971). Out of the pragmatic wastebasket. *Linguistic Inquiry, 2*, 401-407.

Bayles, K.A. (1982). Language function in senile dementia. *Brain and Language, 16*, 265-280.

Bayles, K.A. (1985, February). *Effects of dementing illnesses on communicative function*. Paper presented as part of a symposium at the International Neuropsychological Society Meeting, San Diego, CA.

Bayles, K.A., and Boone, D.R. (1982). The potential of language tasks for identifying senile dementia. *Journal of Speech and Hearing Disorders, 47*, 210-217.

Bayles, K.A., Boone, D.R., Tomoeda, C.K., and Slauson, T.J. (1986). [Neurogenic communication disorders in adults: Andrus study.] Unpublished raw data.

Beaugrande, R. de (1980). *Advances in discourse processes: Vol. 4. Text, discourse, and process*. Norwood, NJ: Ablex.

Brown, G., and Yule, G. (1983). *Discourse analysis*. Cambridge: Cambridge University Press.

Chomsky, N. (1957). *Syntactic structures*. The Hague: Mouton.

Coseriu, E. (1955-1956). Determinacion y entorno. *Romanistisches Jahrbuch, 7*, 29-54.

Crymes, R. (1968). *Some systems of substitution correlations in modern American English*. The Hague: Mouton.

Dascal, M. (1983). *Pragmatics and the philosophy of the mind 1: Thought in language*. Philadelphia: John Benjamin.

Dijk, T.A. van (1972). *Some aspects of text grammars*. The Hague: Mouton.

Dijk, T.A. van (1977). *Text and context explorations in the semantics and pragmatics of discourse*. New York: Longman.

Dik, S. (1968). *Coordination*. Amsterdam: North Holland.

Dore, J., and McDermott, R.P. (1982). Linguistic indeterminacy and social context in utterance interpretation. *Language, 58*, 374-398.

Dressler, W. (1972). *Einfuhrung in die Testlinguistik*. Tubingen: Niemeyer.

Fodor, J. (1975). *The language of thought*. New York: Thomas Y. Crowell.

Garfinkel, H. (1972). Remarks on ethnomethodology. In J. Gumperz and D. Hymes (Eds.), *Directions in sociolinguistics: The ethnography of communication* (pp. 301-324). New York: Holt, Rinehart, and Winston.

Grice, H.P. (1975). Logic and conversation. In P. Cole and J. Morgan (Ed.), *Syntax and semantics: Vol. 3. Speech acts* (pp. 41-58). New York: Seminar Press.

Grice, H.P. (1978). Further notes on logic and conversation. In P. Cole (Eds.), *Pragmatics* (pp. 113-127). New York: Academic Press.

Gumperz, J., and Hymes, D. (Eds.) (1972). *Directions in sociolinguistics: The ethnography of communication*. New York: Holt, Rinehart, and Winston.

Halliday, M., and Hasan, R. (1976). *Cohesion in English*. London: Longman.

Harris, Z. (1952). Discourse analysis. *Language, 28*, 1-30 and 474-494.

Hasan, R. (1968). *Grammatical cohesion in spoken English*. London: Longman.

Heidolph, K-E. (1966). Kontextbeziehungen zwischen Sätzen in einer generativen grammatik. *Kybernetika, 2*, 274-281.

Hurford, J.R., and Heasley, B. (1983). *Semantics: A coursebook*. Cambridge, England: Cambridge University Press.

Jackendoff, R. (1983). *Semantics and cognition*. Cambridge, MA: The MIT Press.

Karlsen, R. (1959). *Studies in the connection of clauses in current English: Zero, ellipsis, and explicit form*. Bergen: Eides Boktrykkeri.

Kempler, D., Curtiss, S., and Jackson, C. (1986). *Syntactic preservation in Alzheimer's disease*. Manuscript submitted for publication.

Koch, W. (1971). *Taxologie des Engischen*. Munich: Fink.

Kuno, S. (1972). Functional sentence perspective. A case study from Japanese and English. *Linguistic Inquiry, 3*, 269-320.

Kuroda, S.Y. (1972). Anton Marty and the transformational theory of grammar. *Foundations of Language, 9*, 1-37.

Labov, W. (1972a). *Language and the inner city: Studies in the black English vernacular*. Philadelphia: University of Pennsylvania Press.

Labov, W. (1972b). *Sociolinguistic patterns*. Philadelphia: Univeristy of Pennsylvania Press.

Labov, W., and Franshel, D. (1977). *Therapeutic discourse*. New York: Academic Press.

Levinson, S.C. (1983). *Pragmatics*. Cambridge, England: Cambridge University Press.

Liberman, M.Y. (1975). *The intonational systems of English*.

Unpublished doctoral dissertation. Massachusetts Institute of Technology, Cambridge, MA.

McCawley, J. (1978). Conversational implicature and the lexicon. In P. Cole (Ed.), *Pragmatics* (pp. 245-259). New York: Academic Press.

Morris, C.W. (1938). Foundations of the theory of signs. In O. Neurath, R. Carnap, and C. Morris (Eds.), *International encyclopedia of unified science* (pp. 77-138). Chicago: University of Chicago Press.

Newmeyer, F.J. (1980). *Linguistic theory in America*. New York: Academic Press.

Obler, L.K., and Albert, M.L. (1981). Language and aging: A neurobehavioral analysis. In D.S. Beasley and G.A. Davis (Eds.), *Aging: Communication processes and disorders* (pp. 107-121). New York: Grune and Stratton.

Palek, B. (1968). *Cross-reference: A study from hypersyntax*. Prague: Charles University Press.

Petofi, J. (1971). *Transformationsgrammatiken und eine kotextuelle Texttheorie*. Frankfurt: Athenaum.

Sadock, J. (1978). On testing for conversational implicature. In P. Cole (Ed.), *Pragmatics* (pp. 281-297). New York: Academic Press.

Schmidt, S. (1973). *Texttheorie*. Munich: Fink.

Shekim, L.O., and LaPointe, L.L. (1984). *Production of discourse in individuals with Alzheimer's disease.* Paper presented at the 12th annual meeting of the International Neuropsychological Society, Houston, TX.

Strawson, P.F. (1950). On referring. *Mind, 59*, 320-344.

Turner, R. (Ed.) (1976). *Ethnomethodology: Selected readings*. Harmondsworth: Penguin.

Ulatowska, H.K., North, A.J., and Macaluso-Haynes, S. (1981). Production of narrative and procedural discourse in aphasia. *Brain and Language, 13*, 345-371.

Uldall, H.J. (1957). *Outline of glossemantics*. Copenhagen: Nordisk Sprog-og Kulturforlag.

Whitaker, H.A. (1976). A case of isolation of the language function. In H. Whitaker and H.A. Whitaker (Eds.), *Studies in neurolinguistics: Vol. 2* (pp. 1-58). New York: Academic Press.

Chapter 7

Differentiating Dementia and Aphasia

APHASIA AND DEMENTIA—COMING TO TERMS

Many medical professionals, particularly neurologists, define the term "aphasia" as "the loss of expression or understanding caused by brain damage" (Rose, 1984). For these individuals the definition of aphasia does not connote etiology, or information about the onset of language dysfunction, nor the degree of linguistic impairment relative to general cognitive impairment. Aphasia is considered a general condition with many subtypes, one of which is the aphasia of dementia.

Some of our most distinguished neurology colleagues and expert aphasiologists apply the term "aphasia" to the language problems of dementia patients, among them Kertesz, Benson, and Cummings. Cummings, Benson, Hill, and Read (1985) note that "aphasia is a consistent manifestation of DAT (dementia of the Alzheimer's type) . . . " (p. 396). Kertesz (1985) reported that "when language function in Alzheimer's disease was reviewed in a hospitalized population, aphasia was found in all the patients" (p. 322). Not only do these individuals call the language impairment of dementia patients "aphasia," they describe their communication problems in terms of the classic aphasia syndromes. Both Kertesz (1985) and Cummings and colleagues (1985) have written that the evolution of language dissolution in dementia begins with anomic aphasia and evolves into transcortical sensory aphasia, which may evolve to Wernicke's aphasia. Likening the communication dissolution pattern in dementia to the classic aphasia syndromes may help clinicians conceptualize certain aspects of the communication impairment in dementia. However, it is important to realize that although dementia patients have some behaviors associated with transcortical sensory aphasia or Wernicke's aphasia, these labels do not completely, or in the opinion of the authors, adequately define their communication deficits. Cummings and associates (1985) make this point: "DAT (dementia of Alzheimer's type) produces a unique pattern of language alteration. For most of its course, the language disorder resembles, but is not identical to, transcortical sensory aphasia; as the disease progresses, the language disorder resembles Wernicke's aphasia" (p. 396).

What Criteria Apply?

Most speech–language pathologists are uncomfortable calling the communication problems of dementia patients "aphasia," if the authors' personal survey techniques are reliable. To them, "aphasia" has a narrower meaning. In addition to denoting a loss of language due to central nervous system damage, it connotes that (a) language loss is disproportionate to other types of cognitive impairment, (b) language loss is due to focal brain damage, and (c) the damage occurred suddenly. Although it is true that dementia patients typically have more widespread damage, which occurred insidiously and is generally proportional to other cognitive deficits, these conditions may not necessarily exist. For example, consider the distinction of focal damage versus diffuse. Improved imaging techniques show that many aphasic stroke patients have multiple lesions (Alavi, et al., 1986), raising the question as to how many lesions must exist before the damage is considered to be diffuse and the patient suffering from multi-infarct dementia.

If the feature of suddenness of onset is used as the criterion for differentiating these two groups, the multi-infarct patient again poses a problem. Most multi-infarct patients with dementia have one or more large areas of infarction, and if a large infarct occurs in a brain area specialized for language, they appear to suffer a "sudden" loss of language.

Finally, the criterion that linguistic communication skills in aphasia are more severely compromised than other cognitive skills may also be inappropriate in some instances. Some dementia patients initially have communication problems that are disproportionately larger than intellectual problems (Assal, Favre, and Regli, 1984; Kirshner, Webb, Kelly, and Wells, 1984; Mesulam, 1982; Wechsler, 1977).

Prominent Aphasia May Define a Subgroup of AD Patients

Evidence is mounting that a subset of dementia patients may have aphasia that is more prominent than cognitive dysfunction. Wechsler (1977) reported that a "focal aphasic syndrome was the first and outstanding manifestation of a degenerative presenile dementia in a 67-year-old man" (p. 303). The patient had a strikingly dilated left sylvian fissure in the presence of moderately diffuse cortical atrophy. The presenting signs were incorrect use of words in conversation and repetitiousness. Gradually, word-order problems appeared, as did problems in the comprehension of spoken language. Handwriting continuously deteriorated, and perseverations proliferated, as did paraphasia. On occasion, he was echolalic and used verbal stereotypy.

More recently Kirshner and colleagues (1984) reported six dementia patients, in whom language disturbance was an isolated initial symptom or prominent part of more general cognitive deterioration, in the absence of stroke or transient ischemic attack (TIA). Then too, Mesulam (1982) reported six cases of progressive "aphasia" who had left perisylvian atrophy. Two of these patients ultimately became fully demented. Finally, Foster and colleagues (1982) described decreased glucose metabolic activity in the temporoparietal area of the left hemisphere in a dementia patient with severe aphasia. Thus, it is clear that the criterion that dementia patients always have language disturbance proportionate to cognitive disturbance is sometimes inappropriate.

A further complication of the use of the criterion of the proportion of linguistic to cognitive deficit as a way of distinguishing dementia and aphasia is the presence of intellectual deficit in aphasia patients. While it is true that language generally is disproportionately more affected in aphasia, many aphasic patients have prominent intellectual deficits. In these patients, quantification of intellectual dysfunction is difficult because of coexisting language deficits. Kertesz (1979) reminds us that "any statement one makes about impaired or retained intelligence depends on how one tests for it" (p. 254), and testing the intelligence of aphasic patients with expressive language deficits is problematic. Using the Raven's Colored Progressive Matrices (Raven, 1965), Kertesz and McCabe (1975) found that all aphasic patients differed in intellectual performance from non–brain-damaged age-matched controls, but the numerical differences were much greater in the aphasic patients with impaired comprehension. Orgass, Hartje, Kerschensteiner, and Poeck (1972) gave the Wechsler performance scale to patients with right hemisphere-damage only, patients with left hemisphere-damage only, and non–brain-damaged patients. Patients with left hemisphere damage and aphasia were worse than patients with left hemisphere damage and no aphasia, and patients with right hemisphere damage. The single test for which this performance pattern was exceptional was Block Design, on which patients with right hemisphere-damage performed more poorly. Weisenberg and McBride (1935) tested aphasia patients on a wide range of verbal and nonverbal intelligence tests and concluded that intelligence is affected in aphasia.

Thus, because intellectual functioning is sometimes affected in aphasia patients with focal brain damage, and certain dementia patients may exhibit language impairment disproportionate to intellectual impairment, clinicians can not always use the relation of linguistic to cognitive impairment as the criterion for differential diagnosis.

Summary

In summary, an increased understanding of the behavioral problems of dementia patients and the advent of new neuroimaging techniques, such as magnetic resonance imaging and positron emission tomography, lead us to ask what terminology should be used to describe the linguistic communication problems associated with dementing illness. Currently, some professionals refer to the linguistic communication problems of dementia as "aphasia," some even describe the language of dementia in terms of the classic aphasia syndromes, and still others believe the term "aphasia" to be totally inappropriate for use with dementia patients.

OPPOSITION TO CALLING THE COMMUNICATION IMPAIRMENT OF DEMENTIA PATIENTS "APHASIA"

Wertz (1978) writes that "when both hemispheres have been damaged, the interaction among these different deficits creates an extremely confusing clinical picture, and labeling the result APHASIA is not useful" (p. 20). Gustafson, Hagberg, and Ingvar (1978), after studying the degree to which regional cerebral blood flow changes in dementia patients correlate with aphasic symptoms, write, "It should be emphasized that the present ten patients did not show signs of classical 'focal' aphasia of clearcut expressive (Broca), receptive (Wernicke), or other types" (p. 116). De Ajuriaguerra and Tissot (1975) specify that a pitfall to be avoided in studying the language problems of dementia is "reducing all language disturbances to instrumental disorders by seeking to group them with those found in aphasia due to circumscribed lesions" (p. 324). Reinvang (1984) writes, "Although we may be well advised not to speak of the disorder of communication in diffuse afflictions of the brain as 'aphasia', a more open attitude to comparative study of language behavior in different neurologic diseases would be fruitful" (p. 14). Thus, in 1986 we are in the same quandry Critchley (1964a) described 22 years ago, when he remarked, "The question which is constantly cropping up, and which will do so more in the future is, what are we going to name or term the type of speech disorder which we meet with in a patient with brain atrophy . . . the patient showing clinically a mild dementia" (p. 327).

WHAT SHOULD WE CALL THE COMMUNICATION PROBLEMS OF THE DEMENTIA PATIENT?

One possibility is to consider the communicative impairment of AD patients a new type of aphasia and refer to it as "Alzheimer's aphasia." Similarly, the language problems associated with Parkinson's, Pick's, and Huntington's diseases could be referred to as "Parkinson's," "Pick's," and "Huntington's aphasia," respectively. Proponents of this suggestion argue that calling the linguistic communication impairment associated with AD "Alzheimer's aphasia" is as appropriate as calling the linguistic communication impairment associated with AD "transcortical sensory aphasia," "anomic aphasia," or "Wernicke's aphasia." They argue that the use of the names of these aphasic syndromes with dementia patients seems counterproductive because it implies that dementia patients have patterns of brain damage similar to those associated with the various aphasia syndromes. In fact, however, Alzheimer's and other dementia patients have linguistic communication deficits that are fundamentally different from the classic aphasia syndromes.

A strong argument against calling the communication disorders of AD patients "Alzheimer's aphasia" is the variability in communicative performance that may exist among patients with the disease. As was emphasized earlier, several investigators have reported the existence of a subgroup in whom language disturbance is considerably greater than intellectual disturbance.

Another possibility is to use the suggestions of Critchley (1964b) and call the language of dementia "dyslogia." The motivation for this term is the inherent existence of cognitive impairment in the dementia syndrome. Halpern, Darley and Brown (1973) use the phrase "the language of generalized intellectual deterioration" to describe the linguistic communication problems associated with AD. The length of this label probably accounts for its infrequent use.

Emery (1985) suggests the term "regressive aphasia" for use with AD patients. She argues that none of the eight recognized patterns of aphasia can be accurately applied to the pattern of communicative change that characterizes AD patients. The term "regressive aphasia" is meant to imply a process of linguistic dissolution in which occurs a "linguistic reversion to earlier and less advanced or complex forms" (p. 47). Emery emphasizes that the best known patterns of aphasia were delineated on populations that included no AD patients, and thus "it is understandable that there is a *lack of goodness of fit* between the language decrement found in SDAT (senile dementia of the Alzheimer's type) and the established categories of language disturbance" (p. 47).

The issue of what to call the linguistic communication problems associated with dementing illness is complex and likely to challenge the assumptions most of us have about the terminology used to describe neurogenic communication disorders. With the burgeoning clinical population of dementia patients, it is an issue that will become more prominent in the next few years. In this book, the term "aphasia" is used to refer to communicatively disordered patients with focal brain damage due to trauma or vascular disease. The basis for this decision is that the term "aphasia" is considered an inappropriate descriptor for the communication deficits of dementia patients by most speech–language pathologists. However, the authors support Reinvang's (1984) view that a more open attitude to the comparative study of language behavior in different neurologic diseases would be constructive.

DIFFERENTIAL DIAGNOSIS

What Type of Aphasic Patient is Likely to be Confused with a Dementia Patient?

Aphasia is the primary neurogenic communication disorder of adulthood (Davis and Baggs, 1984). Most patients with aphasia have suffered a cerebrovascular accident (Wertz, 1978) or trauma. In terms of fluency, most stroke patients are nonfluent (Brust, Shafer, Richter, and Bruun, 1976), the ratio of nonfluent to fluent being two to one. A common difference between Broca's (nonfluent) and Wernicke's (fluent) aphasia patients is age. Davis and Holland (1981) report the average age of Broca's aphasia patients to be 52, an average of 10 to 12 years younger than those with Wernicke's aphasia (Harasymiw, Halper, and Sutherland, 1981; Holland, 1980; Kertesz and Sheppard, 1981, Reinvang, 1983).

To answer the question of which type of aphasia patient is most likely to be confused with a dementia patient, consideration must be given to both the causes and the severity of dementia and aphasia (Table 7-1). For example, dementia patients with primarily subcortical pathologic changes and extrapyramidal signs are not likely to be confused with

Table 7-1. Types of Aphasia and Dementia Patients Not Likely to Be Confused

Mildly aphasic	with	Advanced dementia
Severely aphasic	with	Mild dementia
Anterior aphasic	with	Mild/moderate AD dementia

patients having any of the aphasia syndromes in which fluency is preserved: Wernicke's, transcortical sensory, and conduction. Dementia patients with subcortical pathologic changes have motor control problems that interfere with fluent effortless speech. Additionally, Alzheimer's patients, whose speech is typically fluent, are not likely to be confused with Broca's or transcortical motor aphasia patients, who have nonfluent speech. Then too, advanced dementia patients, with their prominent intellec-

Table 7-2. The Best Dimensions for Differentiating Dementia Patients from Aphasia Patients

Aphasia Type	Alzheimer's	Parkinson's	Huntington's
Broca's			
Agrammatism Telegraphic speech Some deficit in comprehension Nonfluent	Fluency	Agrammatism	Cognitive deficits
Wernicke's			
Fluent speech Paraphasias Impaired comprehension Syntax and prosody largely intact Impaired naming Deficits in reading and writing	Verbal and visual memory History	Fluency History	Cognitive deficits Fluency History
Conduction			
Poor repetition Relatively fluent Good comprehension Phonemic paraphasias	Comprehension Repetition	Comprehension Repetition	Comprehension Repetition
Transcortical Sensory			
Preserved repetition Poor comprehension Fluent speech	Memory Repetition History	History Fluency	History Cognitive deficits Fluency
Transcortical Motor			
Preserved repetition Agrammatism Poor speech output Good comprehension	Fluency Comprehension	History Agrammatism	History Cognitive deficits
Anomic			
Markedly impaired naming Good comprehension Fluent but empty speech Circumlocutory paraphasia	Memory Comprehension	Motor signs Cognitive deficits	Motor signs Cognitive deficits
Global			
Severe expressive deficits Severe receptive deficits Stereotypic, repetitive utterances	History	History	History

tual deficits, are not likely to be confused with any mild aphasia patient, who is oriented and without memory deficits. With this mention of the differential diagnoses that are not likely to be confusing, the task of specifying those that are has been simplified.

The differential diagnoses likely to be confusing are those in which the clinician must differentiate fluent aphasia from the communication disorder(s) of AD. Mild AD patients are verbally fluent and produce speech with subtly disordered content, much like that of a mild fluent aphasic. Consider the following samples of discourse, one produced by an Alzheimer's patient and the other by a patient with Wernicke's aphasia. Which is which?

Aphasia-Dementia Comparison

Patient 1 (describing a nail): Nail, and, and, and they and then ah, the, the, and the nails, or the nail, are, oh, by, are four, are oh, a nail, and the nail is one and a half inches long. And the, and the tip of this is, is, is, apered.

Patient 2 (describing a button): Right, yet, on a button, very pretty. Well a man, I used to when I, uh, but nobody would hardly that. This has four, two things. Very much. This you mean that hold that back. Well, it is a the first day of a child's doesn't carry it very good. And uh, but, as time goes on it becomes a very (unintelligible word).

As these examples demonstrate, a factor other than language, is necessary to distinguish these patients. To satisfy curious readers, Patient 1 is the aphasia patient and Patient 2 the dementia patient. In Table 7-2 the best dimension for distinguishing the different types of mild dementia patients from patients with the classic aphasia syndromes has been specified.

Because AD patients are verbally fluent, they are not easily confused with Broca's and transcortical motor aphasia patients, who have fluency problems. On the other hand, AD patients can be confused with Wernicke's, anomic, and transcortical sensory aphasia patients because all are typically fluent. Memory testing, a review of the patient's medical and psychologic history, and performance on a repetition task will differentiate the memory impairment and behavioral disturbances that accompany Alzheimer's disease.

Individuals with prominent subcortical pathologic changes, notably those with Parkinson's and Huntington's diseases, are not easily confused with fluent aphasia patients. Rather, Parkinson's and Huntington's patients, with subcortical pathology and speech motor disorders, may be confused with Broca's or transcortical motor aphasia patients, whose halting effortful speech is suggestive of motor dysfunction.

Another type of dementia patient that may be confused with an aphasia patient, specifically a nonfluent aphasia patient, is one with hereditary dysphasic dementia (Morris, Cole, Banker, and Wright, 1984). Patients with this syndrome have been reported to have reduced speech output, decreased verbal fluency, increased hesitancy, and dysnomia.

Right Hemisphere Involvement Versus Dementia

Yet another type of focally brain-injured patient, who can be confused with the dementia patient, is the individual with right hemisphere injury. These patients routinely experience spatial disorientation, deficits in the recognition and expression of emotion in speech, and reduced appreciation of prosody (Table 7-3). Such deficits can affect the language user's sensitivity to context and ability to use language meaningfully (Joynt and Goldstein, 1975; Foldi, Cicone, and Gardner, 1983; Gardner, Brownell, Wapner, and Michelow, 1983; Millar and Whitaker, 1983). Like dementia patients, those

Table 7-3. Right Hemisphere Specialized Processes That Directly and Indirectly Affect Communication

Processes That Directly Affect Communication	Processes That Indirectly Affect Communication
Recognition of emotionally intoned speech	Facial recognition
	Holistic processing
Production of emotionally intoned speech	Visuospatial reasoning
	Gross musical processing
Cadence	Copying figures
Affective gesturing	Nonverbal memory

with right hemisphere damage may make literal interpretations of metaphor, be unable to derive the gist of a discourse, and be insensitive to humor. According to Myers (1984) they may give poorly thought out answers to questions, have difficulty distinguishing between explicit and implied information, have a tendency to be literal, overpersonalize external events, and be unable to tell a story—all problems observable in dementia patients. However, right-hemisphere stroke patients, like left-hemisphere stroke patients, generally have sensory and motor signs of unilateral brain damage and do not exhibit the auditory comprehension problems typical of dementia patients.

Table 7-4. Arizona Battery for Communication Disorders (ABC) of Dementia

Mode of Response		Task
Oral	Nonoral	
		Sensory perception
X		Auditory Discrimination
		Receptive language
X	X	Peabody Picture Vocabulary Test
		Reading Comprehension
	X	• Words
	X	• Sentences
	X	• Paragraphs
		Sentence Disambiguation
	X	• Nonoral
		Expressive language
X	X	Oral Description of Objects
	X	Pantomime Expression
	X	Drawing
X		FAS Verbal Fluency
		Sentence Disambiguation
X		• Oral
X		Oral Discourse
	X	Written Discourse
		Receptive/expressive
X		Repetition
		Orientation and memory
X	X	Mental Status Test (MST)
		Story Retelling
X	X	• Immediate
X	X	• Delayed
	X	Recognition Memory
	X	• Spatial
	X	• Verbal

To differentially diagnose dementia and aphasia patients, a unique testing strategy is required, one that will enable the clinician to observe critical intergroup differences. Over the past decade, with the support of the National Institute of Aging, the authors have attempted to develop such a strategy, which is exemplified in what we will call the Arizona Battery for Communication Disorders (ABC) of Dementia (Table 7-4). Through the support of the American Association of Retired Persons, Andrus Foundation, considerable normative data have been obtained, and although more are needed before the battery is ready for clinical use, an introduction to the types of subtests, their associated response mode, and the performance data of dementia and aphasia patients may prove instructive.

Auditory Discrimination Task

An auditory discrimination test is included to test hearing acuity for conversational speech and assess the examinee's understanding of the concepts "same" and "different." Word pairs are presented orally, with equal emphasis and identical intonation contours. The examinee must identify whether the two spoken words are the same word repeated or different words. Each stimulus pair of words differs by a single feature, for example, gear/beer and lame/tame. A trial item is presented to teach the task. Those who no longer understand the concepts of "same" and "different" are simply asked to repeat each word. Patients who do not discriminate same or different with 80 percent or better accuracy, or who cannot repeat the words with 80 percent or better accuracy, are suspected of having a hearing loss sufficient to make the administration of most of the test battery unreliable.

Mental Status Examination

Mental status examination is an integral part of the communication evaluation of the dementia patient, because progressive disorientation is a well documented cardinal feature. Further, performance on mental status examinations correlates strongly with severity of dementia (Folstein, Folstein, and

McHugh, 1975; Kahn, Goldfarb, Pollack, and Peck, 1960; Mattis, 1976). The mental status examination in the Arizona battery consists of 9 questions that yield 13 pieces of information about the patient's general knowledge and orientation to time, place, and person.

To discriminate well-oriented but expressively impaired patients, an alternative mode of responding has been developed. The orally unresponsive patient is given a board on which are printed names of numbers, months, seasons, cities, and presidents. By pointing to the correct item, the patient can construct answers to all the questions.

The mean performance scores on the Mental Status Test of normal subjects, mild and moderate AD patients, and fluent and nonfluent aphasia patients who participated in the Andrus Foundation study are presented in Table 7-5. Dementia and nonfluent aphasia patients both performed significantly more poorly than normal subjects.

Story-Retelling Task

A story-retelling task is included to assess immediate and delayed verbal memory and articulatory proficiency. In previous studies, the Story-Retelling task emerged as sensitive to mild dementia in Alzheimer's, Parkinson's, and Huntington's patients. Since it was first used, the task has undergone revision, most notably in how it is scored. In its original form, differentiation was not made for the type of information remembered or for main or secondary ideas. Now, three types of scores are recorded, one for the number of main ideas recounted, one for the amount of supplemental information, and one for whether the recounted events are correctly sequenced.

The following short story is told to the examinees, who have been instructed that they will be asked to recount it immediately and at the end of the test session:

> While a lady was shopping, her wallet fell out of her purse. But, she did not see it fall. When she got to the check-out counter, she had no way to pay for her groceries. So she put the groceries away and went home. Just as she opened the door to her house, the phone rang and a small child told her that she had found her wallet. The lady was very relieved.

For expressively impaired patients, the events of the story have been illustrated on nine cards, which they can arrange in the correct sequence. Thus, the examiners can distinguish the individual who remembers the story, but is expressively impaired, from the individual who forgot it.

In Table 7-6 are presented the mean performance scores for immediate and delayed story-retelling of normal subjects, Alzheimer's patients, and fluent and nonfluent aphasia patients who participated in the Andrus Foundation study. Notice the sharp decline in the amount of information remembered in the delayed condition by Alzheimer's patients. Memory problems and forgetting were more prominent in the AD patients.

Delayed Recognition Span Test

With this task, the clinician can compare verbal and nonverbal memory (Moss, Albert, Butters, and Payne, 1986). Subjects must discriminate a newly placed disc on a board on which a six-by-five dot matrix is imprinted. After each newly placed disc is discriminated, the board is covered, and another disc is placed on the board while a 10-second delay is imposed. Discs are added to the

Table 7-5. Mean Performance (and SD) on Mental Status Test (MST)

	Groups				
Task	Elderly Controls	Mild AD	Moderate AD	Nonfluent Aphasia	Fluent Aphasia
MST	12.8	7.1*	1.8†	8.8*	10.2
	(0.7)	(3.2)	(2.4)	(5.5)	(4.2)

*Performance differed significantly from that of the elderly control group at $p < .05$.
†Performance differed significantly from those of all other subject groups at $p < .05$.

Table 7-6. Mean Performance (and SD) on Story-Retelling Immediate (SR-1) and Delayed (SR-2) Condition

	Groups				
Task	Elderly Controls	Mild AD	Moderate AD	Nonfluent Aphasia	Fluent Aphasia
SR-1	19.7	8.8†	2.9*	14.1‡	15.2‡
	(3.1)	(4.4)	(3.7)	(4.7)	(3.1)
SR-2	18.7	0.3†	0.5†	9.0‡	13.9‡
	(3.3)	(1.1)	(1.8)	(6.3)	(6.0)

*Performance differed significantly from those of all other subject groups at $p < .05$.
†Performance differed significantly from those of the elderly control, nonfluent aphasia, and fluent aphasia groups at $p < .05$.
‡Performances differed significantly from those of the elderly control, mild AD, and moderate AD groups at $p < .05$.

board until the subject makes an error in identifying the newly placed disc, or completes the task. Fourteen discs are used. Words are printed on the back of the discs, and in the second part of the task, subjects are asked to recognize newly placed words. To eliminate position as a cue, when the test is of verbal memory, the position of previously placed words is varied each time the board is covered and a new word is placed.

Patients with focal lesions and aphasia performed considerably better than AD patients on both the nonverbal and verbal portions of the delayed recognition task, although the performance of nonfluent aphasics was significantly inferior to that of normal subjects (Table 7-7). Patients with dysfluent aphasia scored lower on the verbal memory portions, whereas fluent aphasic subjects scored more poorly on spatial or nonverbal memory. Normal subjects performed slightly better on the verbal memory portion, as did mild AD patients and fluent aphasia patients. Moderate AD and nonfluent aphasia patients performed slightly better on the spatial memory task. Overall, moderate AD patients performed worst, followed by mild AD. Nonfluent and fluent aphasic patients performed similarly.

Verbal Description Task

One task that reliably differentiates mild dementia patients from normal subjects is the verbal description task, in which subjects are given common objects to describe. After the examiner demonstrates the task by providing a complete description of a pencil, subjects are given two items individually and asked to tell everything they can about them. In earlier versions of this task, four items were used,

Table 7-7. Mean Performance and (SD) on Verbal and Spatial Recognition Memory Tasks

	Groups				
Task	Elderly Controls	Mild AD	Moderate AD	Nonfluent Aphasia	Fluent Aphasia
Verbal recognition	11.5	3.1*	1.5*	7.6†	9.3
	(2.5)	(2.0)	(1.8)	(5.1)	(3.2)
Spatial recognition	10.3	2.9*	1.8*	9.1	8.0
	(2.4)	(1.7)	(2.3)	(3.4)	(3.0)

*Performances differed significantly from those of the elderly control group, nonfluent aphasia group, and fluent aphasia group at $p < .05$.
†Performance differed significantly from that of the elderly control group at $p < .05$.

Table 7-8. Mean Performance (and SD) on Verbal Description Task (Total Information Units)

	Groups				
Task	Elderly Controls	Mild AD	Moderate AD	Nonfluent Aphasia	Fluent Aphasia
Verbal description	44.2	17.5*	6.2*	8.3*	26.6†
	(18.2)	(9.7)	(7.8)	(9.1)	(7.7)

*Performances differed significantly from that of the elderly control group at p < .05.
†Performance differed significantly from those of the elderly control group and moderate AD group at p < .05.

but equally good intergroup discrimination has been demonstrated with two.

Each subject's responses are taped and later transcribed. During testing, the examiner records as many of the patient's responses as possible to aid in tape transcription. A point is awarded for each relevant piece of information given by the subject. The discourse elicited in this task also can be analyzed for instances of perseveration.

To distinguish expressively impaired aphasic individuals, in whom reading skill is intact, from dementia patients, who are ideationally impoverished, an alternative response option was added that does not require speech. Expressively impaired subjects are given a board on which are specified 100 descriptive words, half of which apply to the test stimuli and half of which are unrelated. Expressively impaired patients can select appropriate descriptors using a pointer. Although a point is awarded for each appropriate descriptor designated, the score is not analogous to the score obtained when the response is verbal. The purpose of the alternative mode of response is to identify individuals with expressive language problems who nevertheless recognize how to describe the objects.

The mean performance scores of normal subjects, Alzheimer's patients, and individuals with left hemisphere damage who participated in the comparative study are presented in Table 7-8. Nonfluent aphasia patients and individuals with moderate AD performed most poorly on this task. Nonfluent aphasia patients were not confused with the AD patients, however, because they typically could pick out appropriate descriptors for the test stimulus items when shown the communication board. Significantly less information was provided by mild AD (mean = 17.5) patients than normal subjects (mean = 44.2).

Reading Comprehension Task

The Arizona Battery contains a three-part reading comprehension task designed to evaluate silent reading comprehension of words, sentences, and paragraphs. Eight words, printed in large letters on white cards, are presented individually to exam-

Table 7-9. Mean Performance (and SD) on Silent Reading Comprehension Task

	Groups				
Task	Elderly Controls	Mild AD	Moderate AD	Nonfluent Aphasia	Fluent Aphasia
Reading comprehension	17.3	10.9*	4.0†	12.6*	14.2
	(1.3)	(3.4)	(4.2)	(2.9)	(3.0)

*Performances differed significantly from that of the elderly control group at p = .05 level.
†Performance differed significantly from those of all other subject groups (the elderly control group, mild AD group, nonfluent aphasia group, and fluent aphasia group) at p < .05.

inees, who must identify the correct picture corresponding to the printed word from among four line drawings.

In the second part of the task, subjects are asked to silently read seven sentences and answer a written question about each by selecting the correct answer from among four choices. The eight stimulus words used in the word reading portion are used to form the seven stimulus sentences. The sentences are controlled for length, vocabulary, and syntactic complexity and are presented in large print on white cards.

Finally, subjects are asked to read a four sentence paragraph, which is constructed from the same core vocabulary used in the sentence portions. Because the vocabulary is controlled, the examiner can determine at what point reading comprehension breaks down: at the word, sentence, or paragraph level.

The overall performance scores on the reading comprehension task of normal subjects, Alzheimer's patients and those with and left hemisphere damage are presented in Table 7-9. Moderate AD patients performed worst, significantly more poorly than normal subjects and both fluent and nonfluent aphasia patients. However, the nonfluent aphasia patients performed significantly more poorly than normal subjects. Dementia patients had modest difficulty at the word level and prominent difficulty at the sentence and paragraph levels.

Sentence Disambiguation Task

To evaluate the ability of individuals to reason linguistically, subjects are asked to paraphrase ambiguous sentences, or select two correct illustrations of sentence meaning from among eight. Five sentences require an oral response; five require a picture identification.

Of the ten sentences presented, two have structural ambiguities in which the ambiguous elements are adjacent to each other, two are structurally ambiguous with nonadjacent elements, two are lexically ambiguous, two are logically ambiguous with a syntactic clue, and two are logically ambiguous with no syntactic clue. Each set of five sentences is composed of one sentence from each of the aforementioned types of ambiguous sentence pairs. Sentences are read aloud by the examiner as the subject reads along from a card on which the sentence is printed in large letters. The examiner reads the sentences in a neutral tone, with equal stress on each word and no chunking.

Identification can be made of the type of ambiguity most difficult for patients with different etiologies. Resolution of the ambiguity in the lexically

Table 7-10. Mean Performance (and SD) on Sentence Disambiguation Test: Oral Form and Nonoral Form

	Groups				
Task	Elderly Controls	Mild AD	Moderate AD	Nonfluent Aphasia	Fluent Aphasia
Sentence Disambiguation (Oral)	3.5	0.7*	0.3*	0.9*	1.5*
	(1.4)	(1.4)	(0.5)	(1.7)	(1.8)
Sentence Disambiguation (Nonoral)	4.1	2.0*	0.9†	2.2	3.6
	(1.0)	(1.6)	(1.7)	(1.5)	(0.9)

*Performances differed significantly from that of the elderly control group at $p < .05$.

†Performance differed significantly from those of the elderly control group and fluent aphasia group at $p < .05$.

ambiguous sentences requires word analysis, whereas resolution of sentences with logical ambiguity requires the analysis of subject–verb–object relations. Structurally ambiguous sentences require a structural, as well as lexical and logical, analysis for disambiguation.

The average performance of normal subjects, Alzheimer's patients, and those with left-hemisphere damage, subjects in the Andrus Foundation study, is presented in Table 7-10. Moderate AD patients performed the worst. The aphasia patient groups were not significantly different in performance. Mild AD patients were significantly poorer than normal subjects, but not aphasia patients. Notice that the picture identification portion of the task was easier for all subjects. The motivation for presenting illustrations of the different sentence interpretations was to provide a means whereby expressively

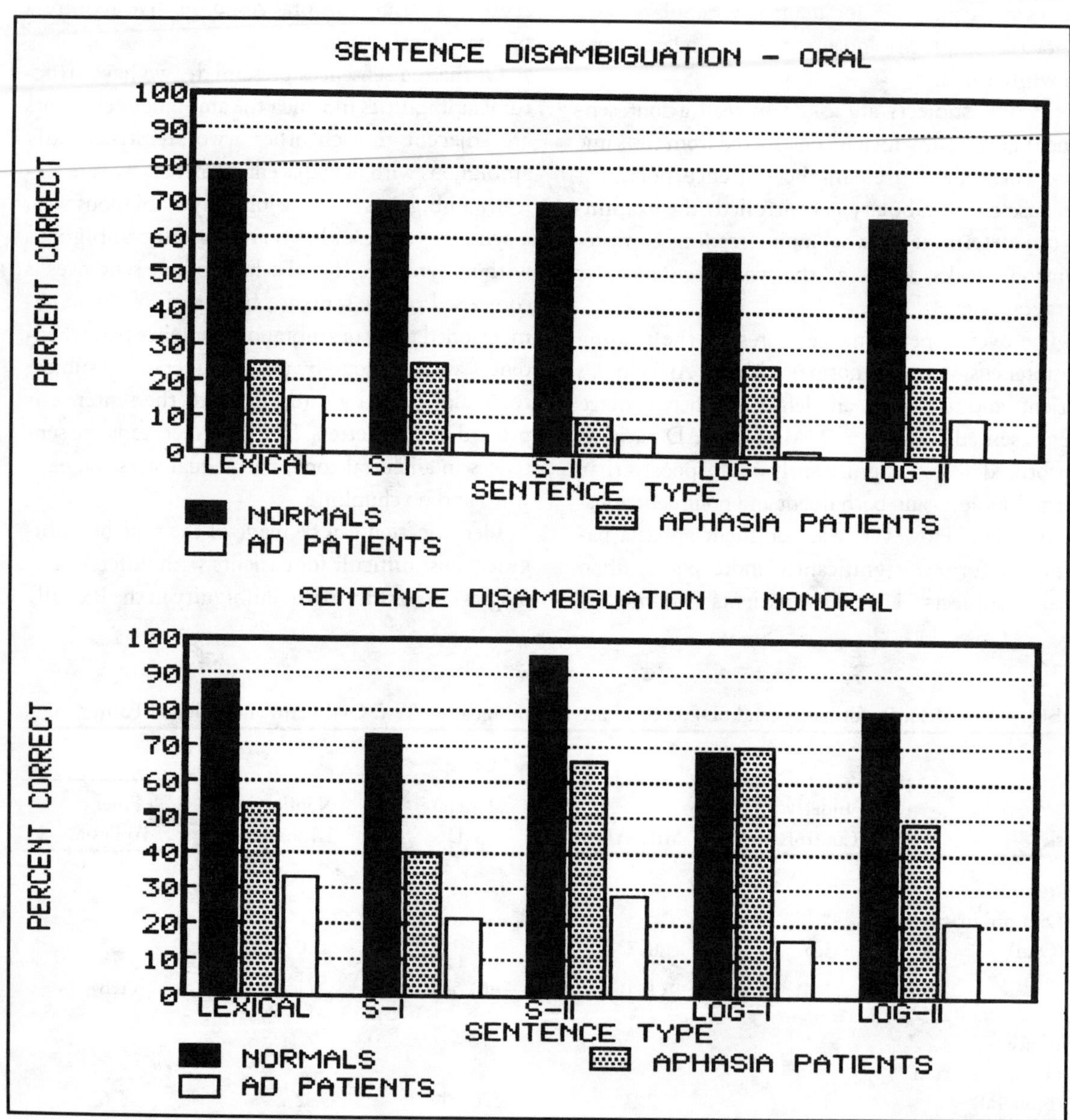

Figure 7-1. *Mean percentage correct of Alzheimer's and aphasia patients and normal subjects, according to type of judgments of linguistically ambiguous sentences.*

Table 7-11. Mean Performance and (SD) on Pantomime Expression Task

	Groups				
Task	Elderly Controls	Mild AD	Moderate AD	Nonfluent Aphasia	Fluent Aphasia
Pantomime expression	39.7	17.3*	8.0†	29.2	30.7
	(9.9)	(9.5)	(10.2)	(12.6)	(12.3)

*Performance differed significantly from those of the elderly control group and moderate AD group at $p < .05$.
†Performance differed significantly from those of the elderly control group, nonfluent aphasia group, and fluent aphasia group at $p < .05$.

impaired aphasic individuals could demonstrate their linguistic reasoning ability.

Performance on Sentence Disambiguation Test: Oral and Nonoral

The average accuracy rates of each subject group, according to type of linguistically ambiguous sentence, are presented in Figure 7-1. In normal subjects and AD patients, the shape of the profile was generally the same, a fact indicating that they found the same sentence types difficult. The profile least similar in pattern to that of normal subjects was that of the aphasia patients. Overall, the two easiest sentence types were lexically ambiguous, as in "The fans were noisy that night," and structurally ambiguous in which the ambiguous elements were nonadjacent, as in "He hit the man with the stick."

Pantomimic Expression Task

Langhans (1985) and Kempler (1984) recently demonstrated the sensitivity of the New England Pantomime Test (NEPT) (Duffy and Duffy, 1985) to mild Alzheimer's type dementia. Langhans observed that of the receptive and expressive portions of the test, the expressive was more sensitive to dementing illness effects. Thus, ten expressive items were selected for inclusion in the Arizona Battery: book, saw, needle, telephone, spoon, teapot, toothbrush, banana, hat, and stamp.

Patients are shown a picture of each item and asked to demonstrate its use. The examiner watches the subject's complete pantomime before scoring it. Scoring consists of simply checking on a checklist each of the actions the subject provides. When the components of the pantomime are produced in an appropriate sequence, the individual receives an additional point. If a sequence error occurs, one point is subtracted. For example, the relevant actions listed for book are these:

+1 opens book
+1 flips pages
+1 reads or scans page
+1 closes book

Table 7-12. Mean Performance (and SD) on Drawing Task

	Groups				
Task	Elderly Controls	Mild AD	Moderate AD	Nonfluent Aphasia	Fluent Aphasia
Drawing	18.93	10.39*	2.04†	12.61	14.82
	(3.60)	(4.53)	(3.84)	(3.97)	(4.43)

*Performance differed significantly from that of the elderly control group at $p < .05$.
†Performance differed significantly from those of all other subject groups at $p < .05$.

+1 puts book down
+1 other appropriate action (e.g., marking his place in book)
+1 appropriate sequence
−1 error in sequence

The scoring procedures of the NEPT are not used. Rather than rating of responses on a 16-point scale, one point is awarded for each relevant action. Three speech–language pathologists predetermined the most common relevant actions involved in pantomiming the use of each object. If, however, the subject uses an appropriate but unlisted action, a point is awarded.

The Alzheimer's patients in the Andrus Foundation study had marked difficulty with expressive pantomime (Table 7-11), as they did in the studies of Kempler (1984) and Langhans (1985). Fluent and nonfluent aphasia patients performed similarly to each other and poorer than normal subjects.

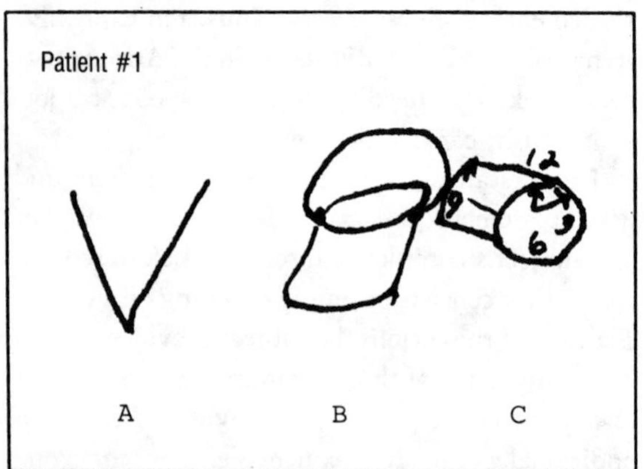

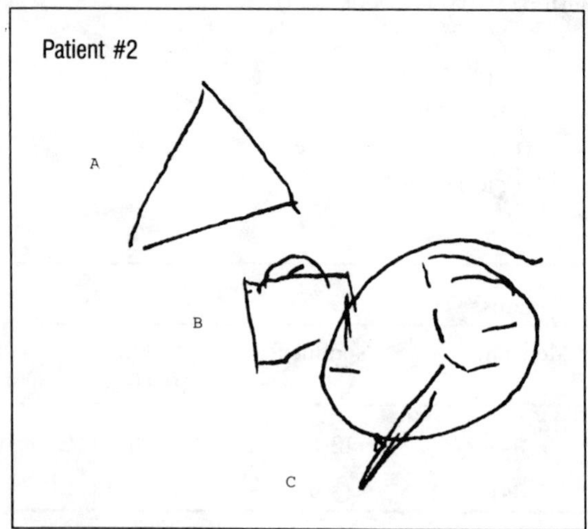

Figure 7-2. *Drawings by mildly demented Alzheimer's patients:* **(A)**, *triangle,* **(B)**, *bucket,* **(C)**, *clock.*

Drawing Task

Visuospatial problems are a well-documented sequela of Alzheimer's (Adams and Victor, 1977; McKhann et al., 1984; Sim and Sussman, 1962, Sjögren, Sjögren, and Lindgren, 1952) and Parkinson's diseases (Bowen, Hoehn, Yahr, 1972; Levita, Riklan, and Cooper, 1964; Loranger, Goodell, McDowell, Lee, and Sweet, 1972; Pirozzolo, Hansch, Mortimer, Webster, and Kuskowski, 1982). Thus, a visuospatial construction task was included, in which subjects were asked to draw three increasingly complex figures: triangle, pail (bucket), and clock. Performance scores were based on the number of features included in the drawings. The highest possible score was 21, and as can be seen in Table 7-12, moderate AD patients in the Andrus Foundation study performed the worst, much worse than all other groups including mild AD. Mild AD patients, however, were significantly poorer in figure drawing than the normal elderly.

In Figures 7-2 and 7-3 are drawings made by mild and moderately demented patients. Notice the added difficulty they had drawing the clock, the hardest of the three figures.

Generative Naming Task

The FAS Verbal Fluency Test (Borkowski, Benton, and Spreen, 1967) is included in the Arizona Battery because verbal fluency, or generative naming, measures have demonstrated sensitivity to mild dementia (Bayles and Tomoeda, 1983; Benson, 1979; Borkowski et al., 1967; Eslinger, Damasio, Benton, and Van Allen, 1985; Wertz, 1979) In this test, patients are asked to produce as many words as possible beginning with each of three letters: F, A, and S. One minute is allotted for generating the words for each letter. Credit is not given for proper nouns or derivatives of words previously given. Neither are numbers credited. Performance on this test depends upon verbal expressive

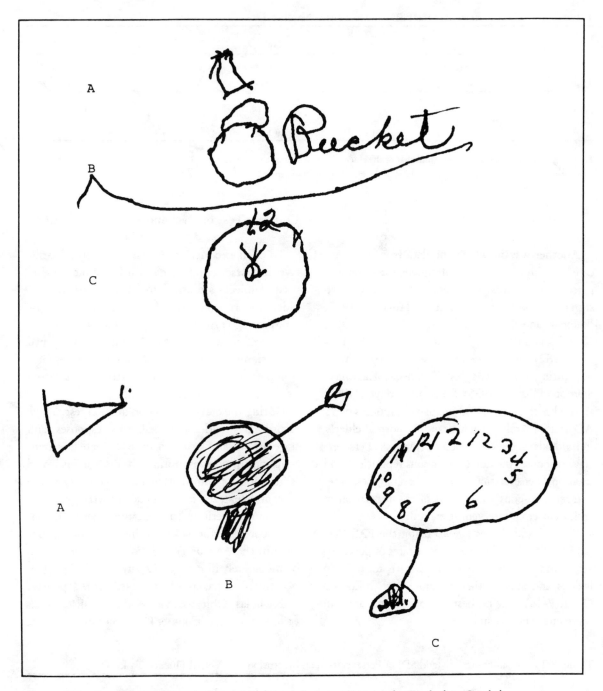

Figure 7-3. *Drawings by moderately demented Alzheimer's patients:* (A), *triangle,* (B), *bucket,* (C), *clock.*

skill and the ability to switch sets and attention; therefore, no alternative mode of response was developed.

In the Andrus Foundation study, the average number of words generated by normal subjects was 39.8, as can be seen in Table 7-13, an average significantly better than that produced by either aphasia patients or Alzheimer's patients. Not surprisingly, nonfluent aphasia patients performed poorly, and similarly to moderate AD patients. Then too, fluent aphasia patients scored lower than mild AD patients, making this test inappropriate for dif-

Table 7-13. Mean Performance (and SD) on Generative Naming Task

	Groups				
Task	Elderly Controls	Mild AD	Moderate AD	Nonfluent Aphasia	Fluent Aphasia
FAS	39.8	17.2*	4.1†	5.8*	15.2*
	(12.6)	(12.0)	(5.2)	(4.4)	(8.5)

*Performances differed significantly from that of the elderly control group at $p < .05$.
†Performance differed significantly from those of the elderly control group and mild AD group at $p < .05$.

ferentiating aphasia stroke patients from mild and moderate AD patients.

Another way in which the data from this task can be analyzed is for the frequency and type of perseverative errors. Perseveration is a well-known sign of brain damage (Allison and Hurwitz, 1967; Freeman and Gathercole, 1966; Halpern, 1965; Helmick and Berg, 1976; Santo Pietro and Rigrodsky, 1982) and has been reported to increase with dementia severity (Bayles, Tomoeda, Kaszniak, Stern, and Eagans, 1985). Slauson and Bayles (1985) studied perseverative and intrusive responses of 35 AD and 24 stroke patients, and 29 normal elderly individuals on the verbal description task. Perseverative responses included continuous repetitions and ideational perseveration after an intervening response. Intrusive responses consisted of the repetition of an idea after an intervening stimulus.

Slauson and Bayles (1985) using the FAS Verbal Fluency Test observed higher rates of perseveration and intrusion in patients with focal brain lesions and aphasia than in those with mild AD (Table 7-14). The highest rate of both occurred in moderate AD patients.

Contrast Test of Oral and Written Discourse

To elicit production of oral and written narrative discourse, two Norman Rockwell pictures are used. Subjects are asked to write, or orally provide, a description of the "Homecoming" and "Easter Morning" prints. These two prints were selected from the Rockwell collection because they had equal elicitation potential in a pilot study of the elicitation potential of ten Rockwell pictures preselected by the authors for consideration.

During the oral discourse production test, a tape recording is made of the subject's responses, and the examiner also writes them to facilitate tape transcription. After transcription, the discourse is scored for number of information units, coherence, and gist, and analyzed for frequency of carrier phrases, continuous repetitions, and ideational perseveration. The poorest performance on this task, among subjects in the Andrus Foundation study, was given by moderately impaired AD patients (Table 7-15). Nonfluent aphasia patients also scored poorly.

Nicholas, Obler, Albert, and Helm-Estabrooks (1985) used the Cookie-Theft picture from the

Table 7-14. Mean Frequency (and SD) of Perseveration and Intrusion in a Verbal Fluency Task

	Groups			
Response Type	Elderly Controls	Mild AD	Moderate AD	Focal/Aphasia
Perseverations %	1.23	6.11	9.78	7.45
	(2.02)	(8.71)	(27.39)	(8.54)
Intrusions %	0.0	1.39	12.5	9.45
	(0.0)	(3.67)	(29.76)	(28.66)

Table 7-15. Mean Performance (and SD) on Oral Description Task, Norman Rockwell Picture (Total Information Units)

	Groups				
Task	Elderly Controls	Mild AD	Moderate AD	Nonfluent Aphasia	Fluent Aphasia
Oral description	76.6	33.1*	11.3†	17.4†	52.7
	(29.7)	(20.2)	(9.8)	(10.7)	(29.6)

*Performance differed significantly from that of the elderly control group at $p < .05$.
†Performances differed significantly from those of the elderly control group and fluent aphasia group at $p < .05$.

BDAE to elicit oral discourse samples from 19 AD patients, 16 with Wernicke's aphasia, eight with anomic aphasia, and 30 normal individuals. The discourse samples were analyzed to determine the amount of "empty speech" defined as "words or phrases that either detracted from or did not contribute to a coherent description of the target picture" (p. 405). The group with the least informative speech was the Wernicke's aphasia group, followed by AD and then anomic aphasia. The only significant differences between AD and Wernicke's patients were in the production of neologisms and occurrence of literal and unrelated verbal paraphasias; in both cases, Wernicke's aphasia patients produced more. No significant differences were found between AD patients and anomic patients.

Peabody Picture Vocabulary Test

A linguistic communication test battery would be incomplete without a test of receptive vocabulary. Thus, the PPVT (Dunn, 1959) is included in the Arizona Battery. Subjects must select the correct line drawing, from among four, corresponding to a word spoken by the examiner. The words are graduated in difficulty. Historically, interpretation of scores as a measure of receptive vocabulary has been complicated by the possibility that errors were due to visual–perceptual defects. To ascertain the degree to which error responses, in the normative study resulted from visual–perceptual deficits, subjects were asked to orally define those words missed during the test administration. The examiner represented the easiest missed word and asked the subject to orally define it. If definitions of the first three represented words were wrong, the assumption was made that the error response resulted from unfamiliarity with the word and not from a visual–perceptual defect. In only 1 percent of the cases did subjects know the word definition and missed the item because of apparent perceptual problems.

Moderate AD patients performed significantly poorer than patients with fluent or nonfluent aphasia (Table 7-16), and severity of dementia correlated strongly with PPVT performance. In-

Table 7-16. Mean Performance (and SD) on the Peabody Picture Vocabulary Test (PPVT)

	Groups				
Task	Elderly Controls	Mild AD	Moderate AD	Nonfluent Aphasia	Fluent Aphasia
PPVT	138.1	103.4*	58.8†	116.8	117.2
	(10.9)	(25.6)	(40.1)	(33.0)	(20.9)

*Performance differed significantly from that of the elderly control group at $p < .05$.
†Performance differed significantly from those of all other subject groups at $p < .05$.

terestingly, a significant difference in the performance of fluent and nonfluent aphasia patients was not observed.

Repetition Task

A repetition task was not originally included in the communication evaluation of dementia patients. In the early stages, repetition deficits, if present, are mild and poorly differentiate dementia patients from normal subjects. When the differential diagnosis is between dementia and aphasia, however, repetition becomes important. In this case, patients are asked to repeat a set of ten words and eight sentences from the Western Aphasia Battery (Kertesz, 1982). Four of the sentences are high probability, and four low. Subjects receive two points per word if they are able to repeat the item after the first presentation. One point per word is awarded for correct repetition after the second stimulus presentation. Thus, subscores are obtained for word repetition, and low- and high-probability sentence repetition. These are summed to a total score. An example of a low-probability sentence is "The Chinese fan had a rare emerald"; a high-probability sentence is "We heard him speak on the radio last night."

Performance Profiles of Aphasia Patients on the Arizona Battery for Communication Disorders of Dementia

The Arizona Battery has been given to 26 stroke patients with aphasia, and unique performance profiles were obtained for the different types of aphasia patients. Aphasia type was determined by subject performance on the Western Aphasia Battery (Kertesz, 1982). Of the aphasia patients, six performed as Broca's aphasia, five as Wernicke's, three as transcortical motor, four as conduction, and eight as anomic. Because of the small sample size, firm conclusions cannot be formed about differences in performance profiles between the various types of aphasia patients. The aphasia patient group most similar in performance to the AD patients was Wernicke's, and the aphasia patient group least similar in performance was conduction.

Differentiating Aphasia Patients from Each Other

Having reviewed the performance typical of AD, fluent, and nonfluent aphasia patients, the question arises as to the efficacy of the test battery for differentiating the fluent and nonfluent aphasia patients from each other. Analyses of variance were calculated to determine whether significant differences existed in the performance of the fluent and nonfluent aphasia patients. Significant performance differences were observed on the following tasks. On the Verbal Description Task, Story-Retelling Delayed Condition, and Oral Description Task, fluent aphasia patients were better. On the Sentence Disambiguation Task with pictures, nonfluent aphasia patients were better.

Summary

The Arizona Battery for Communication Disorders of Dementia differs from many aphasia batteries in that its design permits clinicians to examine verbal and nonverbal memory, visuospatial construction, orientation, and linguistic reasoning in addition to fluency, auditory comprehension, reading, writing, naming, repetition, and spontaneous language, dimensions explored by most aphasia tests (Kertesz, 1979). It is the relation of performance on these nonlinguistic tests to linguistic test performance that enables the clinician to make the differential diagnosis, an important point to be emphasized. The purpose of this battery is not to quantify the communication deficit of the patient with focal brain damage, but to quantify the communication deficits of individuals with dementia.

Aphasia batteries have not been designed to differentiate aphasia patients from persons with dementia, so although they provide considerable information about the communication ability of the dementia patient, they do not always include measures that will enable the clinician to make the critical contrasts necessary for differential diagnosis. Nevertheless, to the degree that the clinician recognizes the inherent limitations of aphasia batteries, their administration to dementia patients will provide clinically useful information. Therefore, the performance of dementia patients on some well-known aphasia batteries has been reported in the succeed-

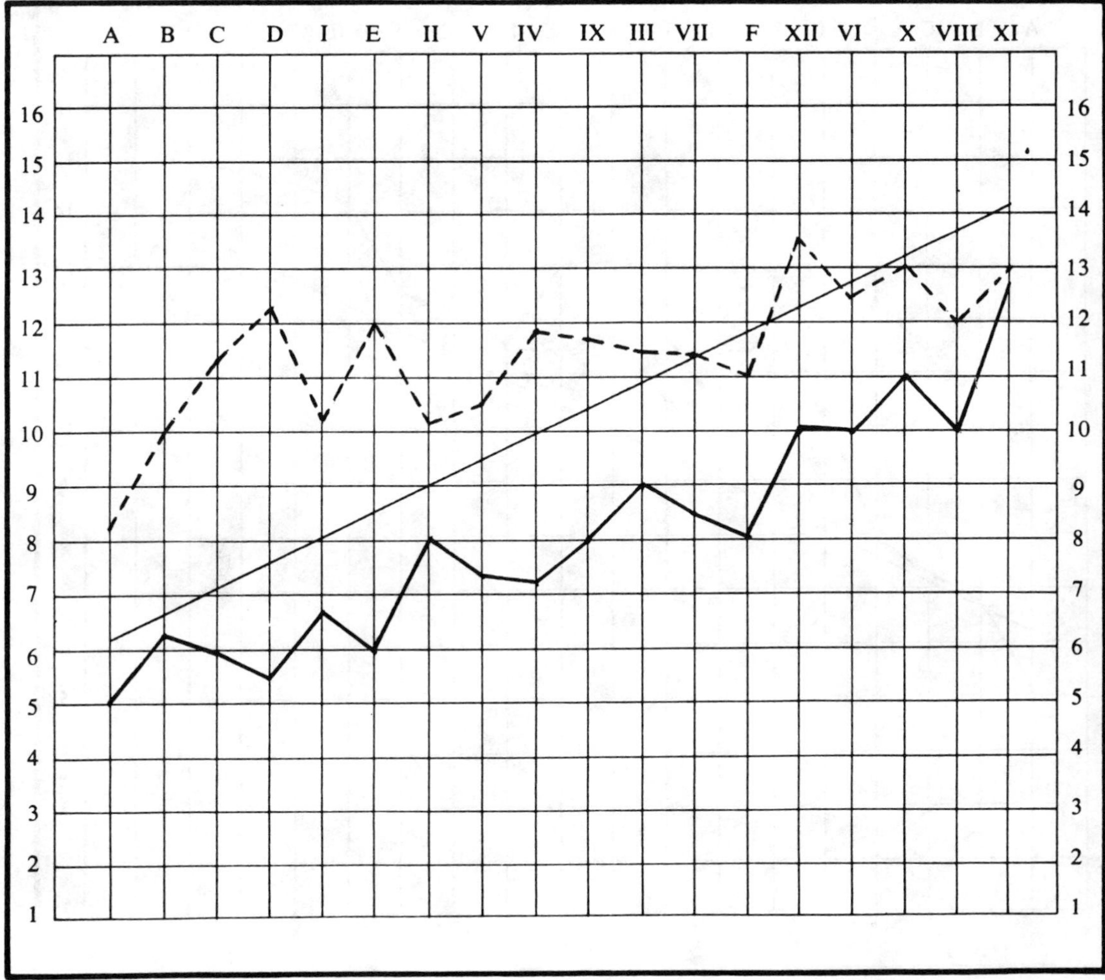

Figure 7-4. *Comparison of mean performance of aphasia (solid line) and dementia (dotted line) patients on the PICA Ranked Response Summary. (Adapted from Wertz, 1982, with permission. © 1982 by BRK Publishers.)*

ing section. (Note: at this writing, published reports of the performance of dementia patients are unavailable for all the well-known aphasia batteries).

PERFORMANCE OF DEMENTIA PATIENTS ON APHASIA TESTS

Performance of Dementia Patients on the PICA

The Porch Index of Communicative Ability (PICA) was devised by Porch (1967a, 1967b, 1973) and is composed of 18 subtests. Eight subtests evaluate the gestural modality, four test the verbal, and six the graphic. Subject responses are scored on a 16-point scale in terms of accuracy, responsiveness, completeness, promptness, and efficiency.

Watson and Records (1978) administered the Porch Index of Communicative Ability (1973) to 12 patients who had suffered bilateral brain damage and 12 with left cerebral vascular accident (CVA). When performance comparisons were made, the dementia patients performed better on all subtests (Figure 7-4). Scores within the dementia group ranged from 8.4 to 13.5, and within the CVA group, the range was 5.2 to 12.8.

In the second part of the Watson and Records study, the effectiveness of the PICA in identifying and assessing behaviors of patients with AD, in contrast to patients with left cerebral vascular accidents, was investigated. The PICA was administered to 20 AD and 20 left CVA patients. A reversal was observed of the relation between auditory and visu-

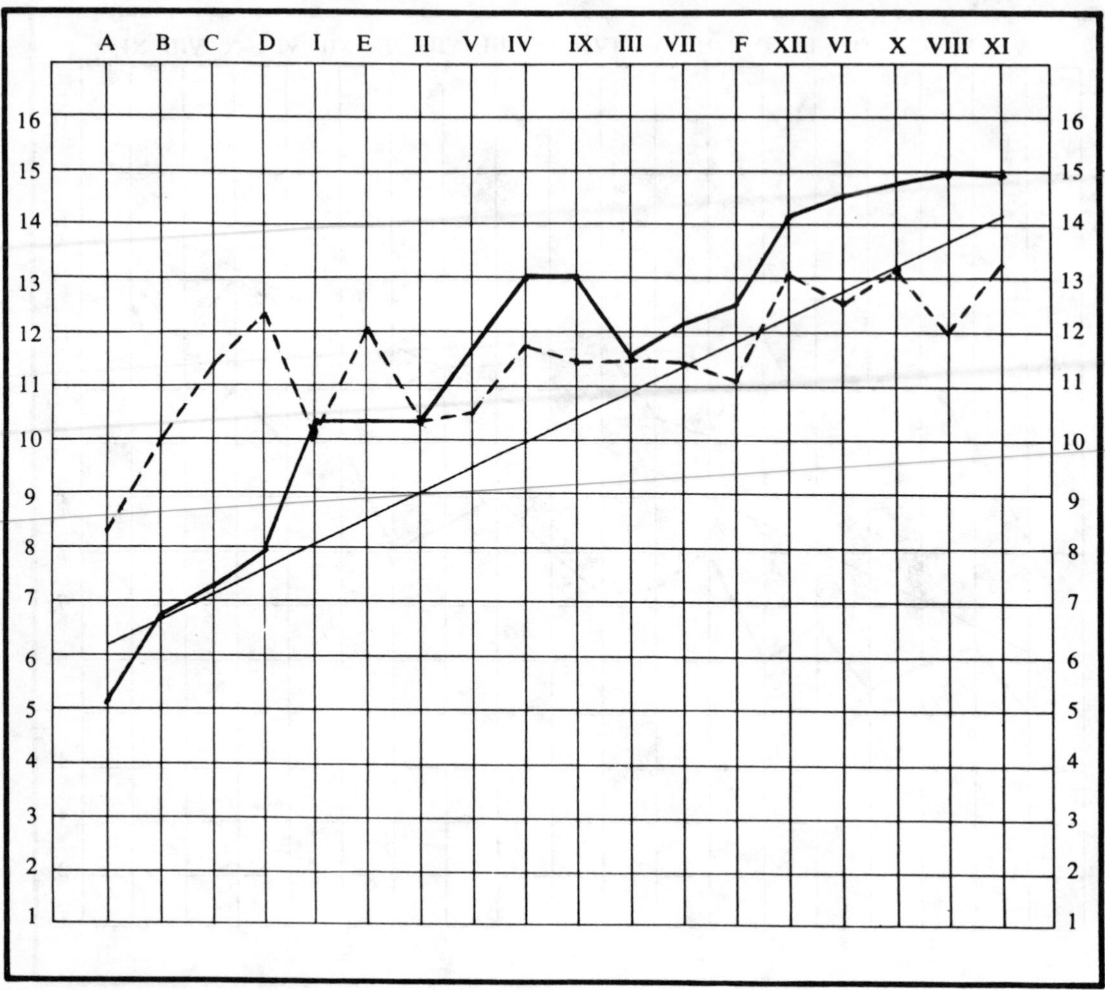

Figure 7-5. *Comparison of PICA 60th percentile performance by demented patients with 60th percentile performance by aphasic patients. Solid line represents performance of aphasia patients and the dotted line, the performance of dementia patients. (Adapted from Wertz, 1982, with permission. © 1982 by BRK Publishers.)*

al tasks that typifies the performance of aphasia patients. Whereas patients with unilateral damage perform more poorly on auditory tasks, as compared with visual, the converse was true for patients with bilateral/diffuse damage. Dementia patients did less well gesturally and graphically than verbally.

Using the data of Watson and Records (1978), Wertz (1982) attempted to answer the question whether the performance profiles on the PICA of dementia and aphasia patients, equated for severity, would still look different. The dementia patients in the Watson and Records study performed at the 60th percentile overall. Because Porch (1973) provides 60th percentile performance data for aphasia patients in the normative sample, Wertz was able to answer his question (Figure 7-5). Differences between the performances of the two patient groups remained. Dementia patients performed *better* than aphasia patients on the harder writing tasks (Subtests A, B, and C), but *worse* on reading tasks (Subtests V and VII), verbal tasks of naming, sentence completion, and repetition (Subtests IV, IX, and XII), auditory tasks (Subtests VI and X), and visual tasks (Subtests VIII and XI).

Bollinger (1970) compared the performance of patients with chronic brain syndrome (an earlier term used for dementia patients) and arteriosclerosis to that of normal subjects on the PICA (Porch, 1967a, 1967b) and the Raven's Colored Progressive Matrices (Raven, 1956), a nonverbal reasoning test. Both groups of brain-damaged patients performed similarly on the Raven's test, suggesting comparability in terms of cognitive ability. When compared with normal subjects, arteriosclerotic and chronic brain syndrome patients were significantly impaired in performance on all PICA subtests. Of the two brain-injured groups, the chronic brain syndrome patients performed more poorly, though not significantly so. The graphic modality was the one most affected in both patient groups, significantly more so than either the gestural or verbal.

Performance of Dementia Patients on the BDAE

The Boston Diagnostic Aphasia Examination (BDAE) was developed by Goodglass and Kaplan (1972) and is designed to identify patients according to the classic aphasia syndromes: Wernicke's, Broca's, transcortical sensory, transcortical motor, global, anomic, and conduction. Examination is made of expository speech, auditory comprehension, oral expression, understanding of written language, and writing. Kaszniak and Wilson (1985) administered parts of the BDAE to 62 AD patients in the Chicago study and analyzed performance using one-way analysis of variance. Significant group main effects were obtained on all dependent variables between the AD patients and normal subjects matched for age and education (see Chapter 4).

When the performance of mild Alzheimer's dementia patients was compared with that of aphasia patients, the AD subjects performed better than patients with global or Wernicke's aphasia. Conversational speech was relatively normal, and articulation, phrase length, and grammar were initially

Table 7-17. Performance Comparisons of Alzheimer's, Aphasic Stroke Patients and Non-Brain Damaged Subjects on the Oral Language Subtests of the Western Aphasia Battery (WAB)

		Groups				
WAB Subtest		AD	Stroke	t	Non–BD	t
Fluency						
	X̄	6.8	5.4	2.45*	10.0	6.67†
	SD	2.5	3.1		0.0	
Information						
	X̄	4.3	4.8	0.85	10.0	10.96†
	SD	2.6	3.4		0.0	
Comprehension						
	X̄	4.6	6.2	2.58*	9.9	8.55†
	SD	3.1	2.9		0.2	
Repetition						
	X̄	5.7	5.8	0.13	9.8	5.86†
	SD	3.5	3.7		0.3	
Naming						
	X̄	3.6	4.5	1.34	9.5	9.52†
	SD	3.1	3.3		0.3	
Aphasia quotient						
	X̄	50.1	53.5	0.58		
	SD	27.0	29.9			

Adapted from Appell, J., Kertesz, A., and Fisman, M. (1982). A study of language functioning in Alzheimer patients. *Brain and Language, 17*, 73–91.

*Significant difference in performance relative to Alzheimer's disease patient group at $p < .02$.

†Significant difference in performance relative to Alzheimer's disease patient group at $p < .001$.

only mildly impaired. Moderate impairment was noted on auditory comprehension as measured by word discrimination, body part identification, and verbal commands. Severely impaired performance of AD patients was observed in the comprehension of complex material and the ability to answer logical questions. Responsive naming was not as affected as body part naming, visual confrontation naming, and animal naming (the latter is a generative naming task). Phrase repetition for high-probability phrases was less impaired than repetition of low-probability phrases. In general, the AD patients were less impaired than the average aphasia patient included in the BDAE standardization sample.

Performance of Dementia Patients on the WAB

The Western Aphasia Battery (WAB) developed by Kertesz (1982) is the newest major aphasia battery, and is designed similarly to the BDAE. Its expressed purpose is to evaluate the main clinical aspects of language function: content, fluency, auditory comprehension, repetition, and naming, as well as reading, writing, and calculation. Further, nonverbal skills such as drawing, praxis, and visuospatial construction ability are also tested. The battery is designed for research and clinical use. On the basis of scaled scores of subtests, clinicians can calculate an overall "aphasia quotient" (AQ), which is derived as a percentage of a hypothetic normal score of 100. As a summary score, the aphasia quotient is a reliable measure of language impairment (Kertesz, 1979; Kertesz and Poole, 1974), and the cortical quotient is a summary score of the cognitive functions measured.

Appell, Kertesz, and Fisman (1982) administered the WAB to 24 Alzheimer's patients and reported significant differences in their performance from that of normal subjects on all language variables (Table 7-17). When compared with aphasic stroke patients (N = 141), the AD patients had higher fluency and lower comprehension scores. The spontaneous speech of AD patients had a high incidence of circumlocutions and semantic paraphasias, though no phonemic paraphasias were observed. The performance of the AD patients was more similar to that of stroke patients with transcortical sensory, Wernicke's, anomic, or global aphasia than to that of patients with Broca's and transcortical motor aphasia (Table 7-18).

Tikofsky (1985) administered the WAB to 34 patients referred to the Memory Disorders Clinic of the Milwaukee Veterans Administration Medical Center. Tikofsky hypothesized that the primary language deficit presented by the dementing patients would be in the area of word retrieval and would be manifested in low scores on the word fluency and naming tasks.

Six of the 34 subjects obtained aphasia quotients in the normal nonaphasic range (AQ > 93.8). Of those scoring in the aphasia range, 23 performed as though anomic aphasia patients, 2 as though Wernicke's, and 1 as though conduction; 2 were unclassifiable. The poorest performance was consistently observed on the generative naming, or word fluency, task, a task that has a .77 correlation with the AQ. Tikofsky concluded that dementia patients typically generate WAB AQs in the aphasia range, but the performance characteristics of the dementia patients are unlike those observed in aphasia patients after stroke, the reason being that the primary deficit of dementia patients is cognitive.

Table 7-18. Percentage Frequency of Different Aphasic Syndromes in Alzheimer's Patients, Stroke Patients, and All Aphasic Types

Aphasia Type	Alzheimer's (n = 25)	Stroke (n = 141)	Aphasic (n = 365)
Global	24	14	16
Broca's	0	19	17
Isolation	8	2	3
Wernicke's	28	11	15
Transcortical motor	0	5	4
Transcortical Sensory	16	9	7
Conduction	4	9	9
Anomic	20	31	29

From Appell, J., Kertesz, A., and Fisman, M. (1982). A study of language functioning in Alzheimer patients. *Brain and Language, 17*, 73-91. By permission.

Summary

An approach to the differential diagnosis of dementia from aphasia patients was explained in this chapter. Fourteen measures were described as being appropriate for inclusion in a communication test battery for dementia. Together they constitute the Arizona Battery for Communication Disorders of Dementia, which is in the process of being standardized. In general, the measures included in the battery have a demonstrated sensitivity to mild dementia. The procedures for their use have evolved through many years of research. On the basis of currently available data, both mild and moderate dementia patients have performance profiles that are unique and significantly different from those obtained by aphasia patients.

GENERAL SUMMARY AND CLINICAL IMPLICATIONS

1. Use of the term "aphasia" to describe the communication disorders of dementia patients is controversial. For many speech–language pathologists, the term "aphasia" should be reserved for patients with language loss due to focal brain damage.

2. Of the patients with classic aphasia syndromes, those with fluent aphasias and preserved repetition are more likely to be confused with AD patients. The most common type of fluent aphasia is Wernicke's, which is twice as common as Broca's (a nonfluent type).

4. Not only are Wernicke's aphasia patients more common than Broca's, they are, on the average, older by 10 to 12 years.

5. Dementia patients with primarily subcortical pathologic changes and extrapyramidal signs are not likely to be confused with fluent aphasia patients.

6. Differentiating the aphasia patient from the dementia patient may not be as simple as previously believed, because some aphasia patients demonstrate cognitive impairment and some dementia patients exhibit language impairment disproportionate to their cognitive functioning.

7. Clinicians desirous of differentiating aphasia due to focal brain damage from dementia should test the following: verbal and nonverbal memory, visuospatial construction, orientation, and linguistic reasoning, as well as fluency, auditory comprehension, repetition, reading, writing, praxis, naming, and spontaneous language.

8. Aphasia test batteries administered to dementia patients can provide valuable information about communicative functioning, though they were not necessarily designed for the differential diagnosis of aphasia and dementia.

9. When evaluating the communicative and cognitive abilities of elderly individuals, inquire about drug regimen and history. Many routinely prescribed medications alter intellectual and motor functioning and therefore can confound test results.

REFERENCES

Adams, R.D., and Victor, M. (1977). *Principles of neurology*. New York: McGraw-Hill.

de Ajuriaguerra, J., and Tissot, R. (1975). Some aspects of language in various forms of senile dementia (some comparisons with language in childhood). In E.H. Lenneberg and E. Lenneberg (Eds.), *Foundations of language development: Vol. 1.* (pp. 323-339). New York: Academic Press.

Alavi, A., Dann, R., Chawluk, J., Alavi, J., Kushner, M., and Reivich, M. (1986). Positron emission tomography imaging of regional cerebral glucose metabolism. *Seminars in Nuclear Medicine, 16*, 2-34.

Allison, R.S., and Hurwitz, L.J. (1967). On perseveration in aphasics. *Brain, 90*, 429-448.

Appell, J., Kertesz, A., and Fisman, M. (1982). A study of language functioning in Alzheimer patients. *Brain and Language, 17*, 73-91.

Assal, G., Favre, C., and Regli, F. (1984). Aphasia as a first sign of dementia. In J. Wertheimer and M. Marois (Eds.), *Senile dementia: Outlook for the future* (pp. 279-282). New York: Alan R. Liss.

Bayles, K.A., and Tomoeda, C.K. (1983). Confrontation and generative naming abilities of dementia patients. In R.H. Brookshire (Ed.), *Clinical Aphasiology Conference Proceedings* (pp. 304-315). Minneapolis, MN: BRK Publishers.

Bayles, K.A., Tomoeda, C.K., Kaszniak, A.W., Stern, L.Z., and Eagans, K.K. (1985). Verbal perseveration of dementia patients. *Brain and Language, 25*, 102-116.

Benson, D.F. (1979). Neurologic correlates of anomia. In H. Whitaker and H.A. Whitaker (Eds.), *Studies in neurolinguistics* (pp. 293-328). New York: Academic Press.

Bollinger, R.L. (1970). *Communication abilities of "chronic brain syndrome" patients*. Unpublished doctoral dissertation, University of Washington, Seattle.

Borkowski, J.G., Benton, A.L., and Spreen, O. (1967). Word fluency and brain damage. *Neuropsychologia, 5*, 135-140.

Bowen, F.P., Hoehn, M.M, and Yahr, M.O. (1972). Parkinsonism: Alterations in spatial orientation as determined by a route-walking test. *Neuropsychologia, 10*, 355-361.

Brust, J.C.M., Shafer, S., Richter, R., and Bruun, B. (1976). Aphasia in acute stroke. *Stroke, 7*, 167-174.

Critchley, M. (1964a). Commentary. In A.V.S. deReuck and M. O'Connor (Eds.), *Disorders of language* (p. 327). Boston: Little, Brown.

Critchley, M. (1964b). The neurology of psychotic speech. *British Journal of Psychiatry, 110*, 353-364.

Cummings, J.L., Benson, D.F., Hill, M.A., and Read, S. (1985). Aphasia and dementia of the Alzheimer type. *Neurology, 35*, 394-397.

Davis, G.A., and Baggs, T.W. (1984). Rehabilitation of speech and language disorders. In L. Jacobs-Condit (Ed.), *Gerontology and communication disorders* (pp. 185-243). Rockville, MD: American Speech-Language-Hearing Association.

Davis, G.A., and Holland, A.L. (1981). Age in understanding and treating aphasia. In D.S. Beasley and G.A. Davis (Eds.), *Aging: Communication processes and disorders* (pp. 207-228). New York: Grune and Stratton.

Duffy, R.J., and Duffy, J.R. (1985). *The New England Pantomime Tests.* Austin, TX: PRO-ED.

Dunn, L.M. (1959). *Peabody Picture Vocabulary Test*. Circle Pines, MN: American Guidance Service.

Emery, O.B. (1985). Language and aging. *Experimental Aging Research, 11*, 3-60.

Eslinger, P.J., Damasio, A.R., Benton, A.L., and Van Allen, M. (1985). Neuropsychologic detection of abnormal mental decline in older persons. *Journal of the American Medical Association, 253*, 670-674.

Foldi, N.S., Cicone, M., and Gardner, H. (1983). Pragmatic aspects of communication in brain-damaged patients. In S.J. Segalowitz (Ed.), *Language functions and brain organization* (pp. 51-86). New York: Academic Press.

Folstein, M.F., Folstein, S.E., and McHugh, P.R. (1975). "Mini-mental state": A practical method for grading the mental state of patients for the clinician. *Journal of Psychiatric Research, 12*, 189-198.

Foster, N.L., Patronas, N.J., De La Paz, R., DiChiro, G., Brooks, R., Chase, T., Fedio, P., Denaro, A., and Durso, A. (1982). PET studies of Alzheimer's disease. *Neurology, 32*, A167.

Freeman, T., and Gathercole, C.E. (1966). Perseveration—the clinical symptoms—in chronic schizophrenia and organic dementia. *British Journal of Psychiatry, 112*, 27-32.

Gardner, H., Brownell, H.H., Wapner, W., and Michelow, D. (1983). Missing the point: The role of the right hemisphere in the processing of complex linguistic materials. In E. Perecman (Ed.), *Cognitive processing in the right hemisphere* (pp. 169-191). New York: Academic Press.

Goodglass, H., and Kaplan, E. (1972). *Assessment of aphasia and related disorders*. Philadelphia: Lea and Febiger.

Gustafson, L., Hagberg, B., and Ingvar, D.H. (1978). Speech disturbances in presenile dementia related to local cerebral blood flow abnormalities in the dominant hemisphere. *Brain and Language, 5*, 103-118.

Halpern, H. (1965). Effect of stimulus variables on verbal perseveration of dysphasic subjects. *Perceptual and Motor Skills, 20*, 421-429.

Halpern, H., Darley, F.L., and Brown, J.R. (1973). Differential language and neurological characteristics in cerebral involvement. *Journal of Speech and Hearing Disorders, 38*, 162-173.

Harasymiw, S.J., Halper, A., and Sutherland, B. (1981). Sex, age, and aphasia type. *Brain and Language, 12*, 190-198.

Helmick, J.W., and Berg, C.B. (1976). Perseveration

in brain-injured adults. *Journal of Communication Disorders, 9*, 141–156.

Holland, A.L. (1980). *Communicative Abilities in Daily Living.* Austin, TX: PRO-ED.

Joynt, R., and Goldstein, M. (1975). The minor hemisphere. *Advances in Neurology, 7*, 147-183.

Kahn, R.L., Goldfarb, A.I., Pollack, M., and Peck, A. (1960). Brief objective measures for the determination of mental status in the aged. *American Journal of Psychiatry, 117*, 326-328.

Kaszniak, A.W., and Wilson, R.S. (1985, February). *Longitudinal deterioration of language and cognition in dementia of the Alzheimer's type.* Paper presented as part of a symposium entitled, "Communication and cognition in dementia: Longitudinal perspectives." International Neuropsychological Society, San Diego, CA.

Kempler, D. (1984). *Syntactic and symbolic abilities in Alzheimer's disease.* Unpublished doctoral dissertation, University of California, Los Angeles.

Kertesz, A. (1979). *Aphasia and associated disorders.* New York: Grune and Stratton.

Kertesz, A. (1982). *The Western Aphasia Battery.* New York: Grune and Stratton.

Kertesz, A. (1985). Aphasia. In P.J. Vinken, G.W. Bruyn, and H.L. Klawans (Eds.), *Handbook of clinical neurology: Vol. 1 (45). Clinical neuropsychology* (pp. 287-331). New York: Elsevier Science.

Kertesz, A., and McCabe, P. (1975). Intelligence and aphasia: Performance of aphasics on Raven's Coloured Progressive Matrices. *Brain and Language, 2*, 387-395.

Kertesz, A., and Poole, E (1974). The Aphasia Quotient: The taxonomic approach to the measurement of aphasic disability. *Canadian Journal of Neurological Sciences, 1*, 7-16.

Kertesz, A., and Sheppard, A. (1981). The epidemiology of cognitive and aphasic impairment in stroke. *Brain, 104*, 117-128.

Kirshner, H.S., Webb, W.G., Kelly, M.P., and Wells, C.E. (1984). Language disturbance: An initial symptom of cortical degeneration and dementia. *Archives of Neurology, 41*, 491-496.

Langhans, J.J. (1985). *Pantomime recognition and expression in persons with Alzheimer's disease.* Unpublished doctoral dissertation, University of Arizona.

Levita, E., Riklan, M., and Cooper, I.S. (1964). Cognitive and perceptual performance in parkinsonism as a function of age and neurological impairment. *Journal of Nervous and Mental Disorders, 139*, 516-520.

Loranger, A.W., Goodell, H., McDowell, F.H., Lee, J.E., and Sweet, R.D. (1972). Intellectual impairment in Parkinson's syndrome. *Brain, 95*, 405-412.

Mattis, S. (1976). Mental status examination for organic mental syndrome in the elderly patient. In L. Bellak and T.B. Karasu (Eds.), *Geriatric psychiatry* (pp. 77-121). New York: Grune and Stratton.

McKhann, G., Drachman, D., Folstein, M., Katzman, R., Price, D., and Stadlan, E.M. (1984). Clinical diagnosis of Alzheimer's disease: Report of the NINCDS-ADRDA work group under the auspices of Department of Health and Human Services Task Force on Alzheimer's disease. *Neurology, 34*, 939-944.

Mesulam, M-M (1982). Slowly progressive aphasia without generalized dementia. *Annals of Neurology, 11*, 592-598.

Millar, J.M., and Whitaker, H.A. (1983). The right hemisphere's contribution to language: A review of the evidence from brain-damaged subjects. In S.J. Segalowitz (Ed.), *Language function and brain organization* (pp. 87-113). New York: Academic Press.

Morris, J.C., Cole, M., Banker, B.Q., and Wright, D. (1984). Hereditary dysphasic dementia and the Pick-Alzheimer spectrum. *Annals of Neurology, 16*, 455-466.

Moss, M.B., Albert, M.S., Butters, N., and Payne, M. (1986). Differential patterns of memory loss among patients with Alzheimer's disease, Huntington's disease, and alcoholic Korsakoff's syndrome. *Archives of Neurology, 43*, 239-246.

Myers, P.S. (1984). Right hemisphere impairment. In A. Holland (Ed.), *Language disorders in adults* (pp. 177–208). Austin, TX: PRO-ED.

Nicholas, M., Obler, L.K., Albert, M.L. and Helm-Estabrook, N. (1985). Empty speech in Alzheimer's disease and fluent aphasia. *Journal of Speech and Hearing Research, 28*, 405-410.

Orgass, B., Hartje, W., Kerschensteiner, M., and Poeck, K. (1972). Aphasic und nichtsprachliche intelligenz. *Nervenarzt, 43*, 623-627.

Pirozzolo, F.J., Hansch, E.C., Mortimer, J.A., Webster, D.D., and Kuskowski, M.A. (1982). Dementia in Parkinson disease: A neuropsychological analysis. *Brain and Cognition, 1*, 71-83.

Porch, B.E. (1967a). *Porch Index of Communicative Ability: Vol. 1. Theory and development.* Palo Alto, CA: Consulting Psychologists Press.

Porch, B.E. (1967b). *Porch Index of Communicative Ability: Vol. 2. Administration, scoring and interpretation.* Palo Alto, CA: Consulting Psychologists Press.

Porch, B.E. (1973). *Porch Index of Communicative Ability.* Palo Alto, CA: Consulting Psychologists Press.

Raven, J. (1965). *Coloured progressive matrices.* London: Lewis.

Reinvang, I. (1983). *Aphasia and brain organization*. Oslo: University of Oslo.

Reinvang, I. (1984). The natural history of aphasia. In F.C. Rose (Ed.), *Advances in neurology: Vol. 42. Progress in aphasiology* (pp. 13-22). New York: Raven Press.

Rose, F.C. (1984). Introduction. In F.C. Rose (Ed.), *Advances in neurology: Vol. 42. Progress in aphasiology* (pp. 1-8). New York: Raven Press.

Santo Pietro, M.J., and Rigrodsky, S. (1982). The effect of temporal and semantic conditions on the occurrence of the error response of perseveration in adult aphasics. *Journal of Speech and Hearing Research, 25*, 184-192.

Sim, M., and Sussman, I. (1962). Alzheimer's disease: Its natural history and differential diagnosis. *Journal of Nervous and Mental Diseases, 135*, 489-499.

Sjögren, T., Sjögren, H., and Lindgren, A.G.H. (1952). Morbus Alzheimer and morbus Pick. *Acta Psychiatrica et Neurologica Scandinavica, (Suppl. 82)*, 1-152.

Slauson, T.J., and Bayles, K.A. (1985). *Intrusive and perseverative responses of aphasia and dementia patients*. Paper presented at the national meeting of the American Speech-Language-Hearing Association, Washington, DC.

Slauson, T.J., and Bayles, K.A. (1986). *The effect of presentation modality on the intrusive and perseverative responses of Alzheimer's disease patients and the normal elderly*. Paper presented to the International Neuropsychological Society Meeting, Denver, CO.

Tikofsky, R.S. (1985, June). *Performance characteristics of demented patients on the Western Aphasia Battery and Boston Naming Test*. Paper presented to the 9th European Conference of the International Neuropsychological Society, Veldhoven, The Netherlands.

Watson, J.M., and Records, L.E. (1978). The effectiveness of the Porch Index of Communicative Ability as a diagostic tool in assessing specific behaviors of senile dementia. In R.H. Brookshire (Ed.), *Proceedings of the clinical aphasiology conference* (pp. 93-105). Minneapolis, MN: BRK Publishers.

Wechsler, A.F. (1977). Presenile dementia presenting as aphasia. *Journal of Neurology, Neurosurgery, and Psychiatry, 40*, 303-305.

Weisenberg, T., and McBride, K.E. (1935). *Aphasia: A clinical and psychological study*. London: Oxford University Press.

Wertz, R.T. (1978). Neuropathologies of speech and language: An introduction to patient management. In D.F. Johns (Ed.), *Clinical management of neurogenic communication disorders* (pp. 1–101). Austin, TX: PRO-ED.

Wertz, R.T. (1979). Word fluency measure (WF). In F.L. Darley (Ed.), *Evaluation of appraisal techniques in speech and language pathology* (pp. 243-246). Reading, MA: Addison-Wesley.

Wertz, R.T. (1982). Language deficit in aphasia and dementia: The same as, different from, or both. In R. Brookshire (Ed.), *Proceedings of the Clinical Aphasiology Conference* (pp. 350-359). Minneapolis, MN: BRK Publishers.

Yahr, M.D. (1978). Overview of present day treatment of Parkinson's disease. *Journal of Neural Transmission, 43*, 227-238.

Chapter 8

Case Histories

The history of six individuals with dementing illness will be described in this chapter to illustrate the impact of dementia on their lives and their families. Included in the case histories are the patients' performance scores on a variety of communication tests. The tests administered to each patient were not always the same. Test performance scores have been included to help the clinician appreciate the relation between functional status and psychometric test performance. To provide a frame of reference for interpreting scores on the measures of communication, the mean scores of other dementia subjects and the normal elderly control subjects also are presented. Additionally, to familiarize the reader with the relative difficulty of the tests given, the test scores of the individual patients have been transformed to standard scores and plotted on a graph on which are the standardized mean scores of other dementia patients.

JIM: A MILDLY DEMENTED PATIENT WITH PRESUMPTIVE ALZHEIMER'S DISEASE

The research team became acquainted with Jim when his wife, Edith, called the clinic after reading about the team's Alzheimer's research project in the Alzheimer's Disease and Related Disorders Association—Tucson chapter's newsletter. Edith wanted to learn more about the communication problems of her husband, Jim, who had been diagnosed as having Alzheimer's disease 18 months earlier. Jim was 76 years old at the time of diagnosis, but Edith suspected the disease had begun as much as 2 years earlier.

Before retiring for the first time at age 60, Jim had managed a large resort in California, a job he had held for 30 years. After retirement, he and Edith moved to Tucson to be close to their youngest child and her family, but within a short time, Jim retired from retirement. He returned to work as manager of a local country club, a job he found so enjoyable that he worked for another 10 years. However, in the last 2 years of employment, Jim easily became tired and often stayed home. Encouraged by his wife and daughter, he permanently retired at 72.

Within a year Jim recognized that he was having difficulty remembering the names of good friends, a problem that embarrassed him. To compensate for his poor memory, he began rehearsing the names of people he expected to meet. In conversations with friends at the country club, Jim concealed his fear and joked about losing his mind. In weaker moments, though, he confided his concerns to Edith. Jim was worried that the progressive mental deterioration that assailed both of his parents was beginning in him. Still, he continued to handle the family's financial affairs and a busy social schedule, and he almost never missed a morning swim.

At first Edith was not overly concerned about Jim's failing memory. She remembers frequently having to supply him with words and names for which he appeared to be searching. Because Jim's forgetfulness increased gradually, Edith did not realize how serious it had become until an old out-of-town friend came to visit. After a few days of sightseeing with Jim and Edith, she questioned Edith about Jim's memory. From the moment of her first question, Edith's concern grew, though months went by before she arranged to consult with a physician. During this period, Edith recalls consciously avoiding situations likely to cause Jim embarrassment. She learned how to supply him with information indirectly by saying things like "Do you mean Mary and Paul Jones, the couple we visited two summers ago?" or "Here is Doris; I know she will want your opinion on the new Buick she bought." Although sometimes frustrated by the lack of specific information in Jim's verbal communication, Edith was good at inferring his intent from contextual clues.

Finally, after Jim described himself as having "breezed through" a physical examination, she asked her personal physician about his growing memory problem. The physician told Edith that Jim's memory problem could result from many causes and that he should be examined by a neurologist. Later her physician admitted his keen concern about the possibility of Alzheimer's disease. A few days later, while reading the morning paper, Edith noticed an article on Alzheimer's disease and by the time she finished reading it, she had broken into a cold sweat. "The behaviors described fit Jim perfectly," she later said, and that same day she made an appointment for Jim with a neurologist.

The neurologist ordered a CT scan, laboratory tests, audiologic and visual examinations, and mental status screening. No evidence of pathologic change was seen on the CT scan. The only abnormal result of the laboratory tests was an elevated cholesterol level. Jim's uncorrected vision for his right and left eyes was 20/100 and 20/80, respectively. He passed an audiometric examination, having only a slightly raised threshold in the left ear at 4000 Hz. What was abnormal was Jim's performance on the mental status test. He was unable to name a few common objects, count backwards by seven, recall more than few items in a delayed recall task, and remember the day of the week and date. Thus, a complete neuropsychologic evaluation was scheduled.

According to a full neuropsychologic evaluation, Jim performed like an individual with mild dementia. Attention, memory, reasoning, orientation, visuospatial construction ability, and learning were all impaired. Edith was devastated. The neuropsychologist recommended she join an Alzheimer's support group, and she did. Before attending a group meeting, she read about the authors' research project in the ADRDA newsletter. She was extremely interested in asking us about the disease process and its effects on Jim's behavior. Most of all, Edith wanted to know what she could do to help Jim communicate better.

Jim missed his first clinic appointment. Edith assumed he could locate the clinic using the map she provided because he had been to the medical center alone on several occasions. However, on the day of his appointment, he became confused and drove around for an hour, lost. Fortunately Jim found his way home safely. When Edith learned what had happened, she called to make arrangements for him to be tested again, but this time at their home.

Jim greeted the examiner at the door. Seemingly alert, well-dressed, and cordial, he did not remember why the examiner was there, though Edith had reminded him just moments before. Jim willingly took the tests in the communication battery, at times apologizing for his performance. Midway through the tests, Jim pointed to his forehead and said, "You know the meanest part of this thing is that sometimes they're there and then they're not." Four times during the evaluation he asked where Edith had gone. Each time the examiner assured him that Edith was in the next room. At the conclusion of the evaluation, Jim spoke further of his impairment: "I don't read books anymore. I can't remember . . . the words . . . the thoughts are gone before they reach my mind."

Jim's Performance on the Arizona Communication Test Battery

Jim's performance on the subtests in the communication test battery has been graphed in Figure 8-1. The configuration of his performance is very similar to that of other mild Alzheimer's patients.

Jim's worst performance among measures of communication was on the delayed Story-Retelling task. Of the possible 16 information units that could be recounted, he remembered 8 in the immediate recall condition and only 2 in the delayed condition. His second worst performance was on the Reading Comprehension task. A score of 18 was possible on this task, and Jim scored 12. Jim's best performance was on the Pantomime Expression task, in which subjects must demonstrate the use of pictured common objects.

The communication problems experienced by Jim are apparent in the following excerpt of verbal descriptive discourse.

E: Tell me everything	
you can about this.	
(marble)	
Jim: This is . . . this is a	FALSE STARTS
. . . well, un . . . round	
ball, has to be round, I	REVISIONS
guess. And, uh, there is	
something that belongs	INDEFINITE
to it that's inside. I can	REFERENCE
see it, but I don't know	INTACT SYNTAX
what it is. But uh, it's	VAGUE
something. I suppose	TANGENTIAL
you drop it every once in	
a while you have to look	LOGICAL FUNCTOR
for it and pick it up	ABSENT
again. This thing doesn't	
float in water so you have	
to watch it pretty closely	
if you have it around the	ILLOGICAL
house. Uh, I think it's	FEW IDEAS
quite pretty. Hum, I can't	EXPRESSED
see anything else about	
that.	
E: Do you know what it	
is called?	

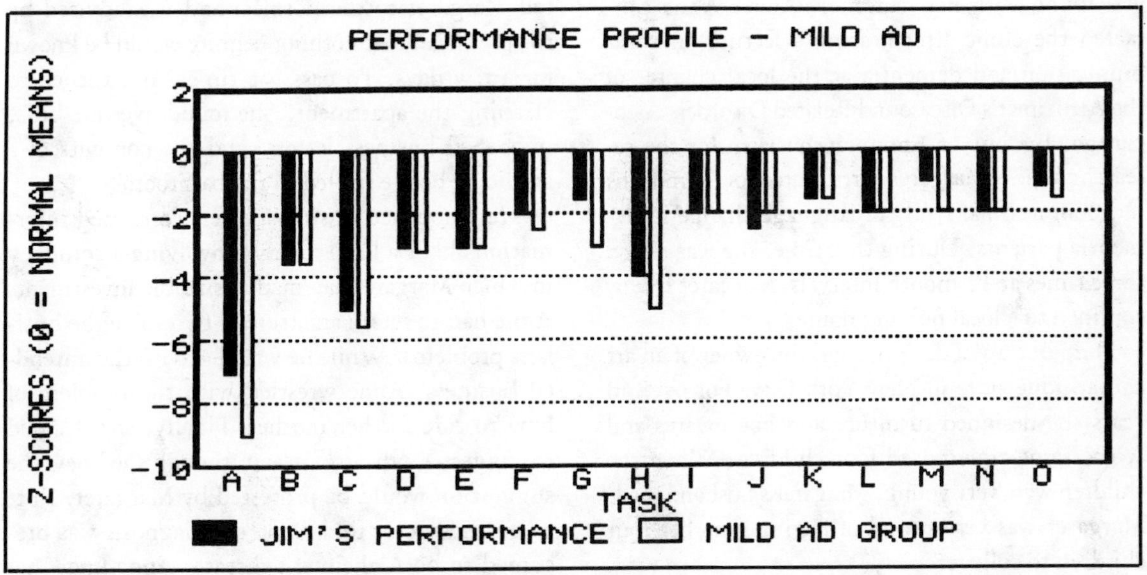

Figure 8-1. *Jim's performance on the Arizona communication battery. A Mental Status Questionnaire: B Story-Retelling—Immediate; C Story-Retelling—Delayed; D Delayed Recognition Memory—Verbal; Delayed Recognition Memory— Spatial; F Drawing; G Peabody Picture Vocabulary Test; H Reading Comprehension; I, Verbal Description; J, FAS Verbal Fluency Measure; K, Oral Description—Picture; L, Written Description—Picture; M, Pantomime Expression; N, Sentence Disambiguation—Oral; O, Sentence Disambiguation—Nonoral.*

Jim: Haven't any idea. What is it?	KNOWS WHEN TO RESPOND TO QUESTIONS ANOMIA
E: It's a marble.	
Jim: Oh, I suppose so. I haven't had anything to do with marbles for so long.	RECOGNITION OF NAME

After the examination, Jim's communication deficits were explained to Edith, and she was counseled about the changes she could expect as the disease progressed. To teach her how to control environmental and linguistic variables that might help Jim communicate, she was scheduled for two appointments in the clinic.

MARGARET: A MODERATELY DEMENTED PATIENT WITH PRESUMPTIVE ALZHEIMER'S DISEASE

The research team first met Margaret when she was living with her daughter, Anne. Anne contacted the clinic after hearing a lecture on communication and dementia at the local chapter of the Alzheimer's Disease and Related Disorders Association. Because of Anne's enthusiasm for the research project, Margaret participated for 24 months in a longitudinal study of language change in dementia patients. During that time, she was tested three times at 12-month intervals. Margaret is now confined to a local nursing home.

Margaret was a designer and the owner of an art and antique store in New York City. For over 40 years she designed furniture and housewares and at the same time raised four children. When the children were very young, Margaret's husband died. Margaret was very proud of having sent her four children to college.

In 1975 Margaret decided to sell her business and retire. Even though her children had moved from New York, she planned to stay and did so until 1979, when her daughter, Anne, realized her mother needed supervision.

Anne could not pinpoint exactly when her mother's functioning had declined. She remembers noticing, on her visit to New York in 1979, that Margaret's housekeeping was poor. Anne also recalled having seen many recent unopened newspapers piled near the fireplace, though she did not ask Margaret about them at the time. Anne attributed her own lack of concern about the poor housekeeping and unread papers to her mother's physical robustness. The fact that Margaret had had trouble remembering the name of someone from the old neighborhood did not seem serious in someone so spry. Thus, Anne returned to Tucson believing her mother to be forgetful, but not atypical of other old people she had known.

Six months after her visit, Anne received a phone call from her mother's neighbor, who explained that Margaret was sick in bed and would not admit friends to her apartment. In fact, Margaret had not invited anyone into the apartment for over a month, a behavior totally unlike her.

The following morning Anne flew to New York and found her mother sick in bed in an apartment littered with unopened mail and garbage, and reeking from the smell of decaying food. Anne admitted Margaret to the hospital and was advised by the physician that nothing definite would be known for a few days. To pass the time, Ann turned to cleaning the apartment. She found overdue bills, unopened business letters, and the contents of a medicine bottle spilled in the bathroom.

The unopened business letters contained information about a legal dispute involving a company in which Margaret had made a sizeable investment. Anne had to retain an attorney to resolve the business problems. While he wrestled with the untended business, Anne wrestled with the problem of how to care for her mother. Finally, she decided to suggest a move to Tucson, though she knew the suggestion would be protested by Margaret. But, when the doctor told Anne the diagnosis was presumed to be Alzheimer's disease, Anne knew her mother would have to move.

Anne joined the ADRDA when she returned to Tucson, and it was through this organization that she learned of the authors' program. She was particularly interested in knowing if her mother comprehended what she read and heard on television.

Margaret's Performance on a Communication Test Battery

When Margaret was first tested in the longitudinal study, she exhibited marked communication problems typical of moderately demented patients (Figure 8-2). Among the measures of communication, Margaret's poorest performance, in relation to normal elderly subjects, was on the Confrontation Naming task. Although she correctly named 17 of 20, normal subjects exhibited virtually no variance in performance on the task. The second most discriminating test was the Semantic Judgment and Correction portion of the Sentence Correction task. In this test patients have to judge whether a sentence makes sense and must correct those sentences with semantic errors.

Like other mild AD patients, Margaret's best performance was on Digit Span, an ability known to hold until advanced dementia. In the following sample of Margaret's discourse, the anomia and perseveration typical of AD patients is apparent.

E: Tell me everything	
you can about this ob-	
ject. (nail)	
Margaret: A nail I think	
is what that would be	SEMANTIC
listed as. I don't know.	PARAPHASIA
It's a very simple and	VAGUE
easy one. It'd be a nice	DESCRIPTORS
type one to have if you	
were going to do any work	SYNTAX INTACT
with it. They could be	
made in any length. And	
it's nice, a nice one.	IDEATIONAL
	PERSEVERATION
E: Anything else?	
Margaret: Oh, there's	
probably a lot of things I	
could tell you about it or	IDEATIONAL
should. This one's nice. It	PERSEVERATION
could be made shorter	
and it could be made also	
to have a. . . . What do	DYSNOMIA
you call them? The other	FRAGMENT
end of the thing. I can't	INDEFINITE
think of what they call it.	REFERENCE
A little square with a hole	IRRELEVANT
in the middle that this	INFORMATION
would fit into. I don't know	VAGUE
what it would be. But	SUBJECT-VERB
there's lots of nice	AGREEMENT ERROR
things in them.	PERSEVERATION

Over the course of 36 months, Anne reported many changes in Margaret's behavior. During the first year of living with Anne, Margaret was able to help with household chores and feed herself. She could get dressed if Anne helped her pick out the right clothes. She appeared to enjoy Anne's children, making cookies and watching television. In the second year, Margaret experienced difficulty dressing and cooking. Though she had been an accomplished seamstress, Margaret could no longer operate a sewing machine, or the washing machine, the microwave oven, the television, or the electric can opener. More and more of the time, Margaret seemed dazed. Her patience with the children diminished markedly. By the third year, Margaret had forgotten the names of Anne's children and husband and frequently raised her voice at the family. She began to have difficulty with bathing and toileting. Daily she asked to go home and appeared continuously confused about her surroundings.

At the time of her final communication evaluation, Margaret was unable to complete many of the tasks. Her third test performance can also be seen in Figure 8-2. In comparison with the first test performance, Margaret had dramatically changed. Her best performance was on Forward Digit Span, on which she scored similarly to normal control subjects. When her verbal discourse at this stage is compared with the earlier sample, the impact of the disease is obvious.

E: Tell me everything you	
can this object. (nail)	
Margaret: Oh, my, well,	
this. It's a nice one before	VAGUE
you can have something	
more than the mailman,	NONSENSICAL
jailman. Do you have	UTTERANCE
one like this?	INTACT QUESTION
Funny, that one can be	FORM
placed over this when	ABSENCE OF DEICTIC
they're ready. I want to	INFORMATION
give this to you.	ACCEPTABLE
Can I give this back	SENTENCE
to you?	INTACT QUESTION
E: Can you tell me	FORM
anything else about it?	
Margaret: It has a nice	CORRECT SYNTAX BUT
movement to it.	IRRELEVANT CONTENT

After the test session, the examiner talked with Anne, who was visibly tired. Anne said she had been agonizing about how to continue caring for her mother at home. The most upsetting problem was Margaret's incontinence, which the children found disgusting. Anne said that her children and friends felt uncomfortable being at home because of Margaret's aimless wandering and bizarre mean-

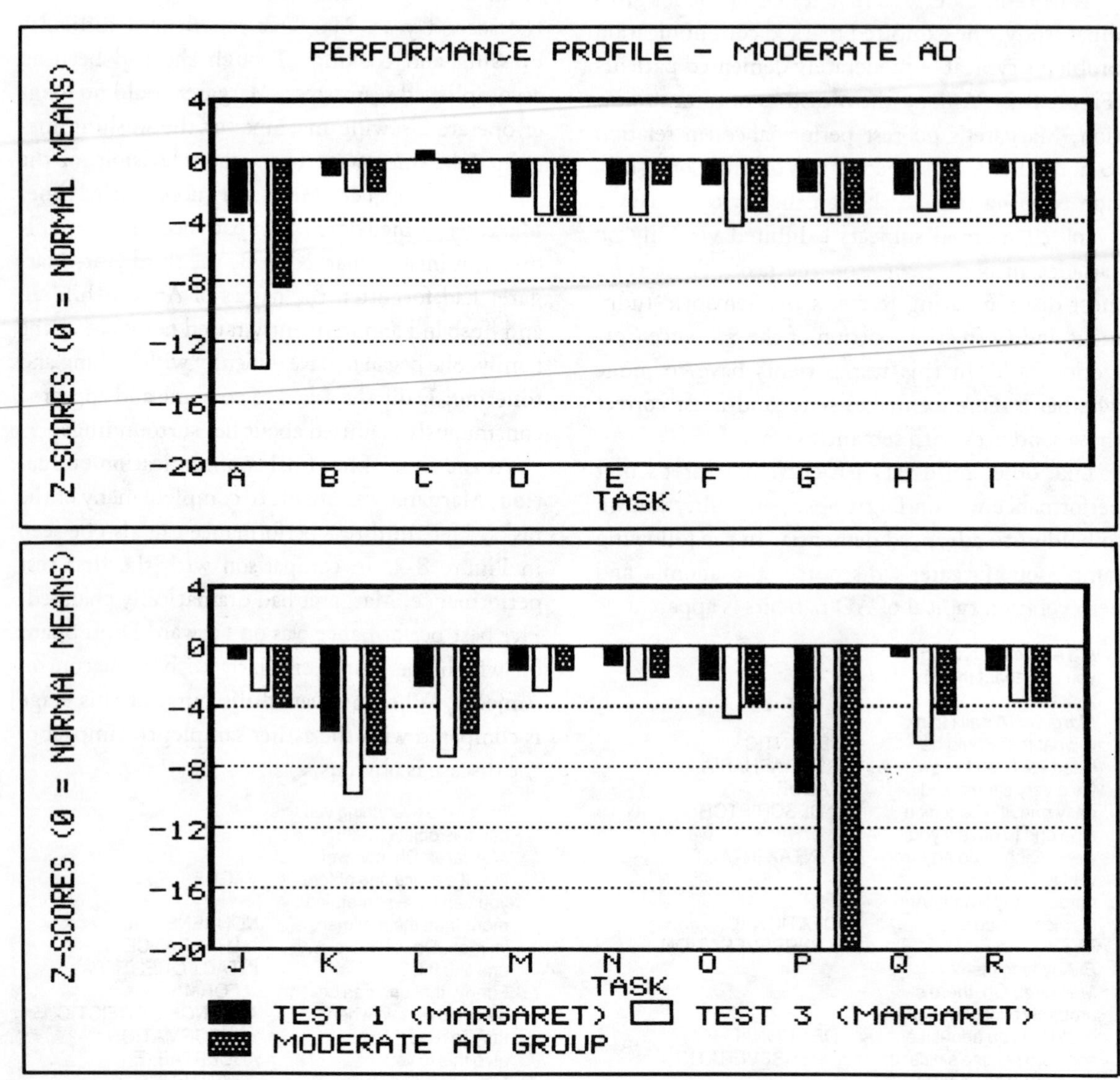

Figure 8-2. *Margaret's performance on a communication test battery. A, Mental Status Questionnaire; B, Nonsense Syllable Learning Test; C, Forward Digit Span—WAIS; D, Block Design—WAIS; E, Similarities—WAIS; F, Story Retelling—Immediate; G, Story Retelling—Delayed; H, Peabody Picture Vocabulary Test; I, Sentence Correction Syntactic Judgment; J, Sentence Correction Syntactic Correction; K, Sentence Correction Semantic Judgment; L, Sentence Correction Semantic Correction; M, Verbal Description; N, FAS Verbal Fluency Measure; O, Vocabulary—WAIS; P, Confrontation Naming; Q, Pragmatics; R, Disambiguation.*

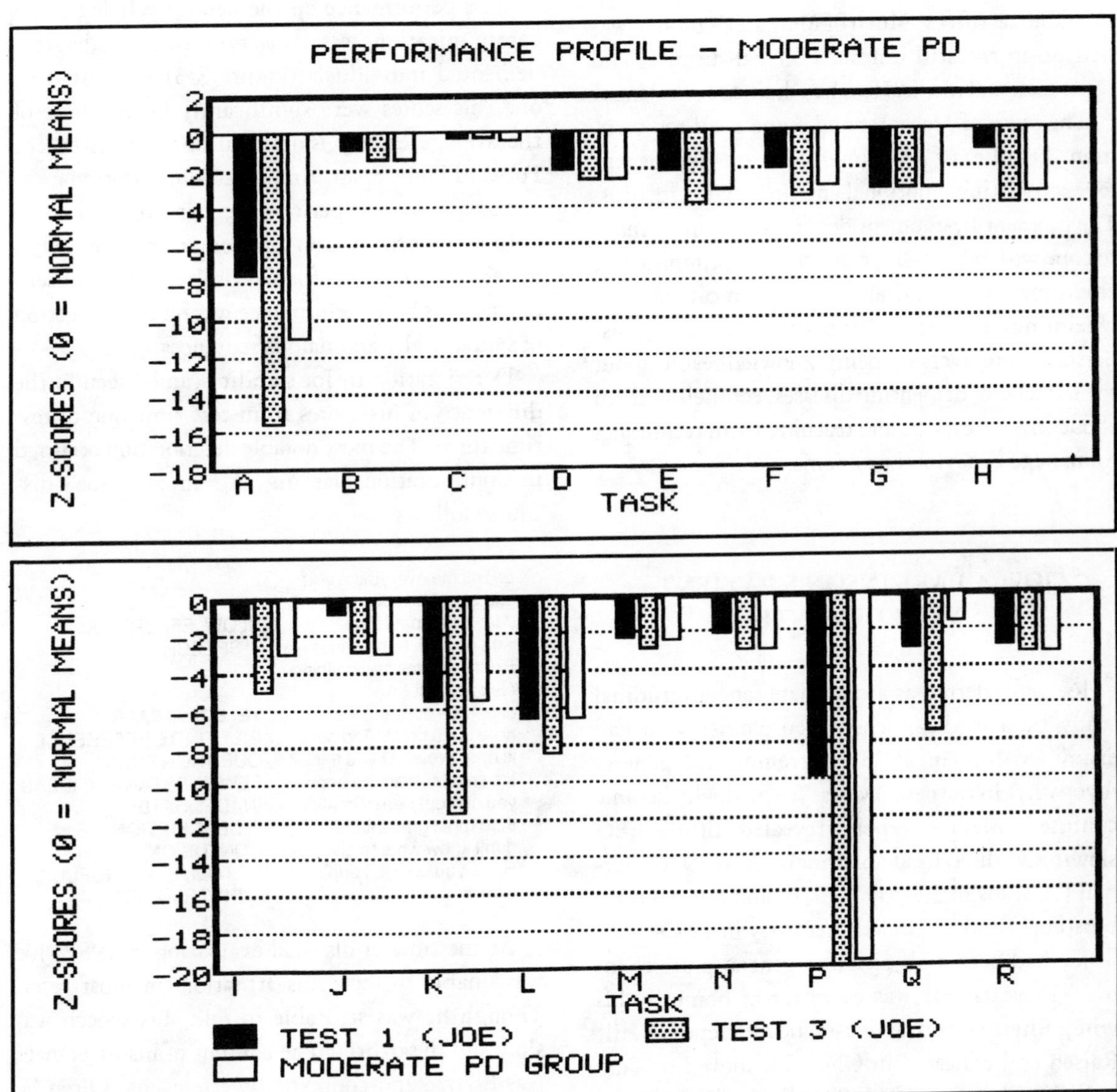

Figure 8-3. *Joe's performance on a communication test battery. A, Mental Status Questionnaire; B, Nonsense Syllable Learning Test; C, Forward Digit Span—WAIS; D, Block Design—WAIS; E, Similarities—WAIS; F, Story Retelling—Immediate; G, Story Retelling—Delayed; H, Peabody Picture Vocabulary test; I, Sentence Correction Syntactic Judgment; J, Sentence Correction Syntactic Correction; K, Sentence Correction Semantic Judgment; L, Sentence Correction Semantic Correction; M, Verbal Description; N, FAS Verbal Fluency Measure; O, Vocabulary—WAIS; P, Confrontation Naming; Q, Pragmatics; R, Disambiguation.*

ingless chatter. A nursing home seemed to be the only alternative, but the cost of nursing home care would mean the family would have to make considerable sacrifices. Much of Margaret's money was tied up in the still unresolved legal dispute, and court costs and medical fees had drained her savings.

The story of Margaret and Anne is all too common. Families of Alzheimer's disease victims suffer excruciating emotional and financial hardships. The moment-by-moment decisions they must make to cope with progressive cognitive, communicative, emotional, and physical deterioration can be overwhelming. Professional caregivers can best assist personal caregivers by being knowledgeable about the sequelae of dementing diseases, counseling them about what to expect, and teaching them techniques to manage behavioral problems.

JOE: A PARKINSON'S PATIENT WITH DEMENTIA

Joe was referred as a candidate for longitudinal study by a medical school neurologist who had examined him in 1973 for tremor and general myopathy. In the next 3 years, Joe gradually became confused. Medical reports revealed diffuse EEG slowing with no focal abnormalities in 1976, normal CT scans in 1975 and 1976, and normal cerebrospinal fluid and blood chemistry in 1979.

Joe had been a physician in general practice for over 35 years. He was cared for at home by his wife, Phyllis, and a live-in housekeeper, Gail. Raised and educated in Ohio, Joe moved to Tucson with Phyllis in 1934. The diagnosis of PD was made in 1974, and progressive intellectual impairment was evident by 1977.

At the time of his first examination, Joe was disoriented for time and, because of his motor control problems, needed assistance to eat and dress. Phyllis reported that his slowness to respond was the most frustrating part of caregiving. In fact, she had stopped giving him a daily bath because it took 2 hours. Indeed, getting him up, dressed, and fed filled the entire morning.

Joe's Performance on a Communication Test Battery

Joe's performance on the neuropsychologic and communication tests was typical of moderately demented individuals (Figure 8-3). At test time one, his scores were significantly below those of the average elderly individual on all tests except Forward Digit Span. Among communication measures, his poorest performance, in comparison to normal subjects, was on Confrontation Naming followed by correction of semantically anomalous sentences. His best performance was on the correction of syntactically anomalous sentences.

Deterioration in Joe's ability can be seen in the difference in his scores from test time one to test time three. The most notable deterioration occurred in Confrontation Naming. A sample of Joe's discourse follows.

E: Tell me everything you can about this object. (nail)	
Joe: It's a small nail, with a head. (long pause)	SLOW, EFFORTFUL SPEECH
E: Can you tell me anything else about it?	
Joe: It's a nail, and it's . . . here . . . a point. And here is one. Wouldn't you think? It's smaller than the ones you can get here. Smaller than most gray things. I don't know what to give you. Here, you take it. I don't want it.	TELEGRAMMATIC INDEFINITE REFERENCE QUESTION FORM FEW SUBSTANTIVE IDEAS INADEQUATE DESCRIPTION CONFUSION LITTLE MEANGINGFUL INFORMATION

At the time of his final evaluation in 1982, Joe was unable to focus his attention on most tests. Though he was still able to talk, his speech was slow and dysarthric. The content of his utterances was bizarre and contextually irrelevant. Often he would begin to answer a question, but stop before expressing a meaningful thought. His wife, Phyllis, had decided to place him in a nursing home because even with the housekeeper's help, she felt she could no longer adequately care for him. And, in the last 6 months, her own health had deteriorated.

KATE: A PATIENT WITH HUNTINGTON'S DISEASE

Kate was 36 years old when first examined in the clinic. She had been diagnosed as having Hunt-

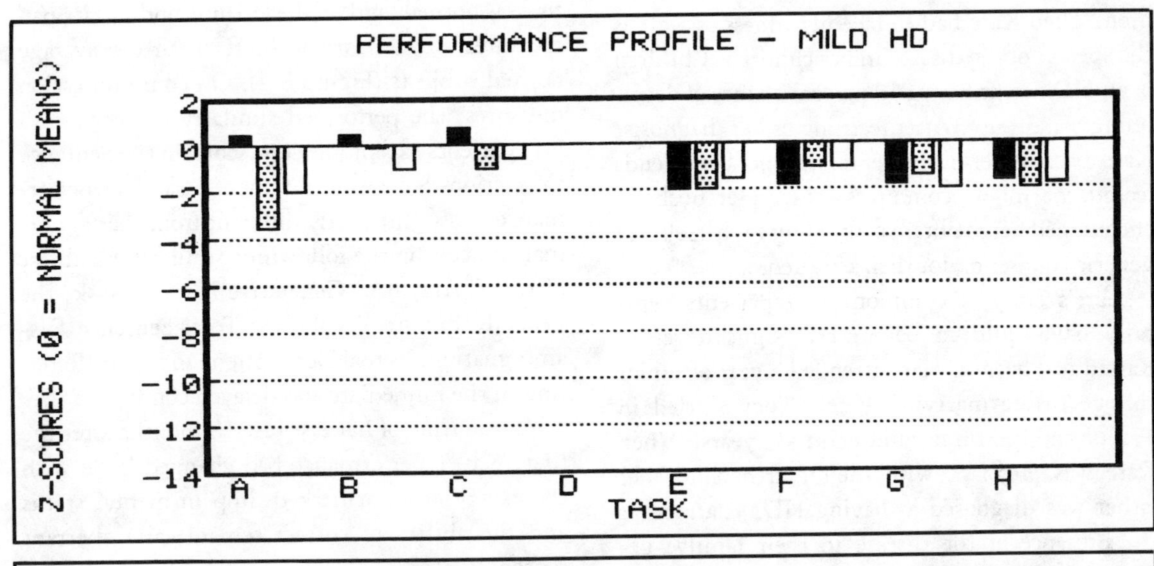

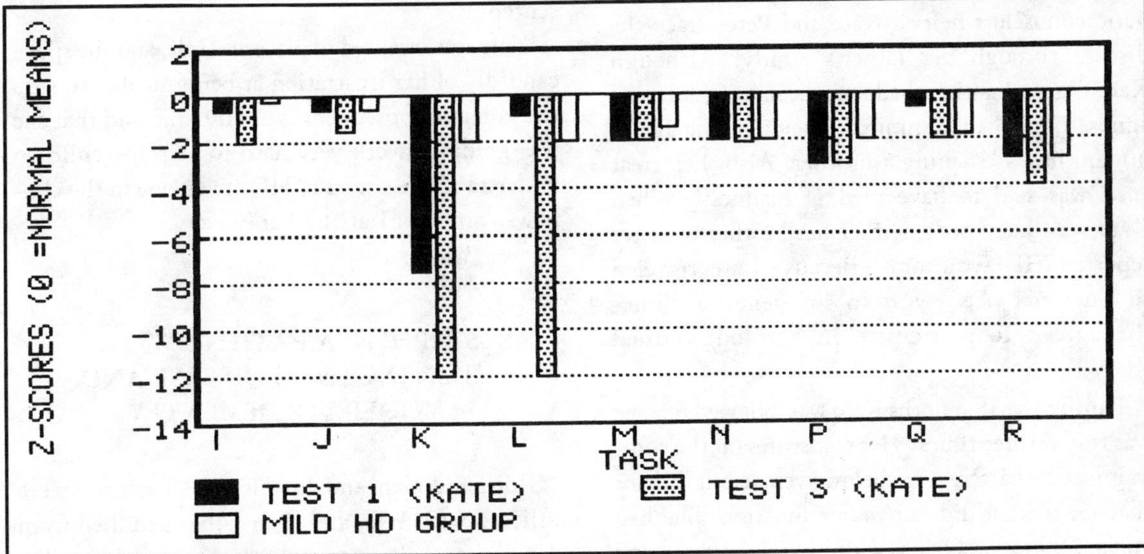

Figure 8-4. *Kate's performance on a communication test battery. A, Mental Status Questionnaire; B, Nonsense Syllable Learning Test; C, Forward Digit Span—WAIS; D, Block Design—WAIS; E, Similarities—WAIS; F, Story Retelling—Immediate; G, Story Retelling—Delayed; H, Peabody Picture Vocabulary Test; I, Sentence Correction Syntactic Judgment; J, Sentence Correction Syntactic Correction; K, Sentence Correction Semantic Judgment; L, Sentence Correction Semantic Correction; M, Verbal Description; N, FAS Verbal Fluency Measure; O, Vocabulary—WAIS; P, Confrontation Naming; Q, Pragmatics; R, Disambiguation.*

ington's disease (HD) in 1977 when she was 33 years old. Although Kate's father and grandmother were HD victims, she did not know it or realize her risk until after she had had four children. Then Kate had to face her illness as well as the specter of the disease in her children. Children of an HD parent have a 50 percent chance of developing the disease. After learning of her diagnosis, Kate became seriously depressed and her friends feared she might commit suicide. Her husband encouraged her to obtain counseling for herself and genetic counseling for their children.

Kate's story is common. HD patients typically have children before HD signs develop. Raised in Phoenix, Kate attended a year of junior college before marrying Peter. They settled in Tempe and had three children in 4½ years. When Kate was pregnant with their fourth child, her father was diagnosed as having HD. Alarmed at the presence of the disease in their family, genetic counselors helped Kate and Peter trace the disease through her father's family. Although Kate's grandmother had not been officially diagnosed, she had commited suicide at the age of 40 and had a "shaking" disorder. Also, her great aunt was said to have died of madness. When Kate was diagnosed, neither her brother or sister reported HD symptoms. Because Kate traveled to Tucson twice a year to the genetics clinic, she agreed to participate in our longitudinal study.

During the 18 months Kate was followed up, she was tested three times. Her test scores on the communication battery were below average but did not change; neither did her motor function. She had obvious motor problems, with intention tremor and jerky hand movements. She struggled to sign her name on the consent form, and because of poor fine motor control, she was unable to complete the writing task or manipulate the blocks on the WAIS Block Design test. Kate's speech was abnormally slow, averaging 100 words per minute (normal speaking rate is 160 to 170 words per minute), and low in volume, though she varied intonation and stress.

Kate's Performance on a Communication Test Battery

At the time of her first test, Kate's mental status was normal, and on the learning and Digit Span measures, she performed better than the average normal subjects (Figure 8-4). On communication measures, she performed similarly to other mild HD patients except for a low score on the Sentence Correction–Semantic Judgment task. Her performance was significantly different from that of normal subjects on the following: Similarities subtest of the WAIS, FAS Generative Naming task, the Peabody Picture Vocabulary Test, Sentence Disambiguation, Verbal Description, and Story-Retelling in the immediate and delayed conditions.

At the time of her last test 18 months after the first, Kate's performance had changed little with the exception of a marked drop in mental status and the ability to correct semantically aberrant sentences.

Kate was oriented to place and self, and she spoke candidly of her frustration at being unable to stop the horrible consequences of HD. She said that she was going to work very hard to help her children understand the effects of HD. Everyone in the clinic was proud of Kate for her bravery.

STEPHEN: A PATIENT WITH HUNTINGTON'S DISEASE AND MODERATE DEMENTIA

Both Stephen and his sister, Charlene, were afflicted with HD, and their father had died from the disease. Charlene, who had suffered the disease since 1968, was severely demented and was cared for in a nursing home in northern Arizona. Stephen was diagnosed in 1972, although the onset was traced back to 1970. Stephen was cared for by his wife in their trailer home. Two years after entering the study, he was admitted to a skilled nursing facility.

Stephen exhibited the signs of HD at age 40. His wife described him as awkward at first, and

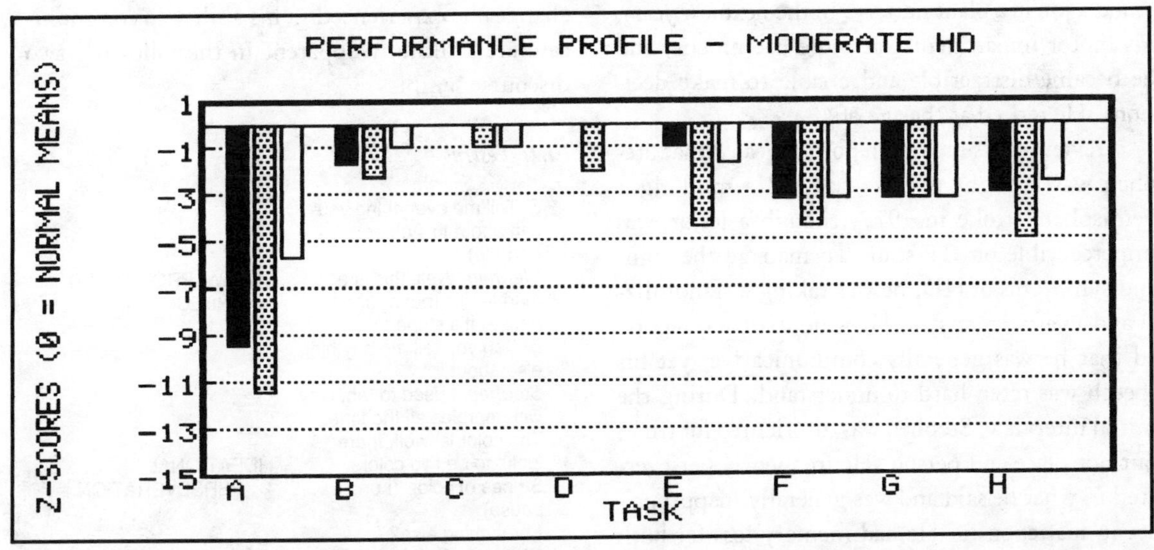

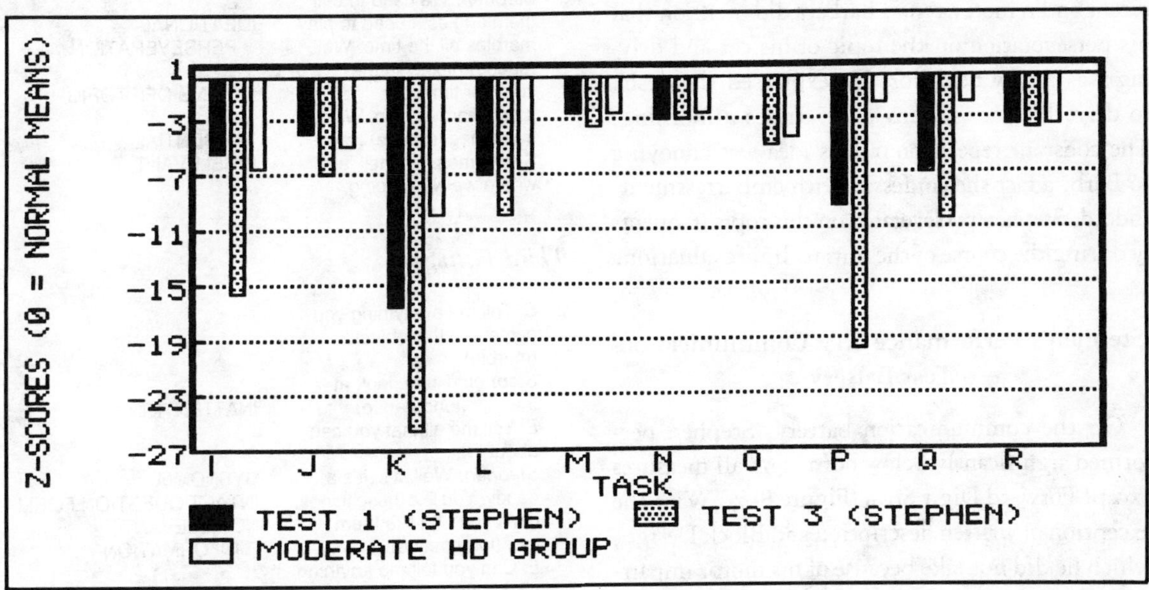

Figure 8-5. *Stephen's performance on a communication test battery. A, Mental Status Questionnaire; B, Nonsense Syllable Learning Test; C, Forward Digit Span—WAIS; D, Block Design—WAIS; E, Similarities—WAIS; F, Story Retelling—Immediate; G, Story Retelling—Delayed; H, Peabody Picture Vocabulary Test; I, Sentence Correction Syntactic Judgment; J, Sentence Correction Syntactic Correction; K, Sentence Correction Semantic Judgment; L, Sentence Correction Semantic Correction; M, Verbal Description; N, FAS Verbal Fluency Measure; O, Vocabulary—WAIS; P, Confrontation Naming; Q, Pragmatics; R, Disambiguation.*

the awkwardness worsened. When his motor problems did not improve, he was forced to quit his job as an electrician. To support the family, he found a job in a plant nursery. In the next few years, his motor impairment was more prominent, and he became distractible and unable to make decisions. He retired at the age of 48.

A review of his medical reports revealed that Stephen was thought to have suffered a mild right hemisphere stroke in 1977, though a lesion was imperceptible on CT scan. To manage the signs and symptoms of HD, he was taking a tranquilizer and an antidepressant. His wife, Barbara, reported that he was generally communicative, yet his speech was often hard to understand. During the initial interview, Stephen was disoriented for time, but not place and person. He frequently perseverated in what he said and was generally inappropriate in his reponses. He had memory loss for both recent and remote events. Barbara did mention that his perseveration on the topic of his car and driving was a new behavior. He expressed the desire to drive his car as many as 15 times a morning. The constant repetition of this idea was annoying to Barb, a fact she confessed with embarrassment. Indeed, Stephen perseverated on this topic frequently during the course of the initial clinic evaluation.

Stephen's Performance on a Communication Test Battery

On the communication battery, Stephen performed significantly below normal on all measures except Forward Digit Span (Figure 8-5). With the exception of written description and Block Design, which he did not take because of his motor impairment, he completed all the tests.

Stephen's best performance, among the neuropsychologic measures, was on the Forward Digit Span test; his worst was on the mental status test. Among the communication measures, Stephen performed worst on the Sentence Correction task, in which he had to identify and correct semantically anomalous sentences. He performed best on the Similarities subtest of the WAIS, a test of verbal associative reasoning.

During the 36 months of his participation in the research program, Stephen's cognitive and communicative functioning markedly deteriorated. The changes he experienced in his ability to communicate are strikingly apparent in the following two discourse samples.

First Testing

E: Tell me everything you can about this object. (marble)	
Stephen: Well, this is a marble. It's round. (long pause) It's striped.	SLOW, PROLONGED SPEECH
E: Can you tell me anything else about it?	
Stephen: I used to, ah, play with marbles all the time. The color is, well, there looks to be two colors. Stripes of color. (Long pause)	IDEATIONAL PERSEVERATION
E: Anything else?	
Stephen: We used to call them aggies. I used to play marbles all the time. Well,	IDEATIONAL PERSEVERATION
(pause) mostly in the summer time 'cuz	MOVING OFF TOPIC
it was warmer then. We'd go swimming. (pause) Sometimes we'd tell 'em where we were going.	TANGENTIAL IRRELEVANT

Third Testing

E: Tell me everything you can about this object. (marble)	
Stephen: Hmm, look at that . . . (long pause)	INATTENTION
E: Tell me all that you can about that.	
Stephen: Well, it's, it's a dandy. You like those things, don't you? I, I like them too. (long pause)	DYSNOMIA INTACT QUESTION FORM NO RELEVANT INFORMATION
E: Can you tell me anything else about this?	
Stephen: Just dandy, that's all. I like 'em all.	PERSEVERATION LACK OF CONTENT

DORIS: A PATIENT WITH MULTI-INFARCT DEMENTIA

Patients with the diagnosis of multi-infarct dementia, or MID, are behaviorally heterogeneous. Their cognitive and linguistic profiles differ by virture of differences in the distribution of their infarcts. Although their behavioral deficits differ, there are common features among these patients, notably sudden onset of behavioral problems, stepwise deterioration in function, focal neurologic signs, and a history of hypertension. Nevertheless, the reader should be aware that remarkably different deficits are observable from patient to patient.

Doris was tested in the spring of 1985. At that time she was being cared for by her stepson, Mark, and her daughter-in-law, Karen. Doris had recently moved in with them after maintaining an apartment in Tucson by herself for several years. After her husband died during World War II, Doris had become a court reporter and was active in numerous civic organizations. In 1972, at the age of 60, she decided to retire. Her service to the community did not stop with retirement. In fact, she transformed a volunteer weekend position into a 5-days-a-week unpaid job. The source of her greatest pleasure was her four grandchildren, to whom she was devoted.

Early in 1983, Doris complained of being absent-minded. On the day after telling Karen about her memory problem, Karen noticed that Doris forgot to take home her sweater, her glasses, and a plant cutting. In spite of her forgetfulness, Doris remained cheerful and energetic, and Karen was not seriously concerned until 2 months later when Doris complained of feeling dizzy and weak after returning home from her volunteer job. When she tried to walk to the sofa, her legs buckled and she fell. She was unconscious for a few minutes. When she regained consciousness and spoke to Karen, her speech was slurred and her voice was inadequately loud.

Terrified, Karen and Mark rushed Doris to the nearest hospital. Doris remained conscious the rest of the evening, but the next day she had another stroke. After 3 days of observation and tests, the doctors informed Mark and Karen that they suspected Doris of having vascular dementia because the CT scan showed that Doris had experienced many small strokes. Doris had a history of hypertension, though Mark and Karen thought it was being controlled with medication. The physicians believed Doris may have been negligent in taking her medication.

The bedside neuropsychologic screening examination revealed that Doris was confused and had poor memory for recent events, and her speech contained semantic paraphasias. When Mark and Karen visited her, she recognized them and asked about each of the grandchildren by name. But as she talked about the children, it became obvious that she was confusing the boys and referred to the eldest as if he were the youngest. Mark and Karen hoped that Doris would regain her memory after leaving the hospital, and she did improve somewhat in the familiar surroundings of Mark and Karen's home. Nonetheless, after a week of convalescence, it became clear that Doris could no longer live independently. She would turn on the stove and forget to turn it off. She confused her medications, and tried to wash the clothes in the dryer. Thus, the decision was made that Doris would live with Mark and Karen. Shortly thereafter, Doris was evaluated by the research team.

Performance on a Communication Test Battery

Among the neuropsychologic tests, Doris performed most poorly in her first examination on the Vocabulary subtest of the WAIS (Figure 8-6). Her best performance was on the Digit Span test. Among the measures of communication, Doris's best performance was on the Sentence Correction Task, in which she was asked to correct syntactically erroneous sentences. On this task her performance was better than that of the average normal subject. Her worst performance was on the Vocabulary subtest of the WAIS.

Over the 18 months Doris was followed up in the research program, her mental status markedly deteriorated, a finding corroborated by her family's report of increasing disorientation. Also dropping markedly was her ability to correct semantically anomalous sentences. On the delayed Story-Retelling task, Doris recalled nothing of the story she had been asked to remember an hour earlier.

The following is a sample of discourse from a conversation with Doris at the time of her last evaluation. The numerous semantic paraphasias, anomia, and poverty of expression portray her aphasia.

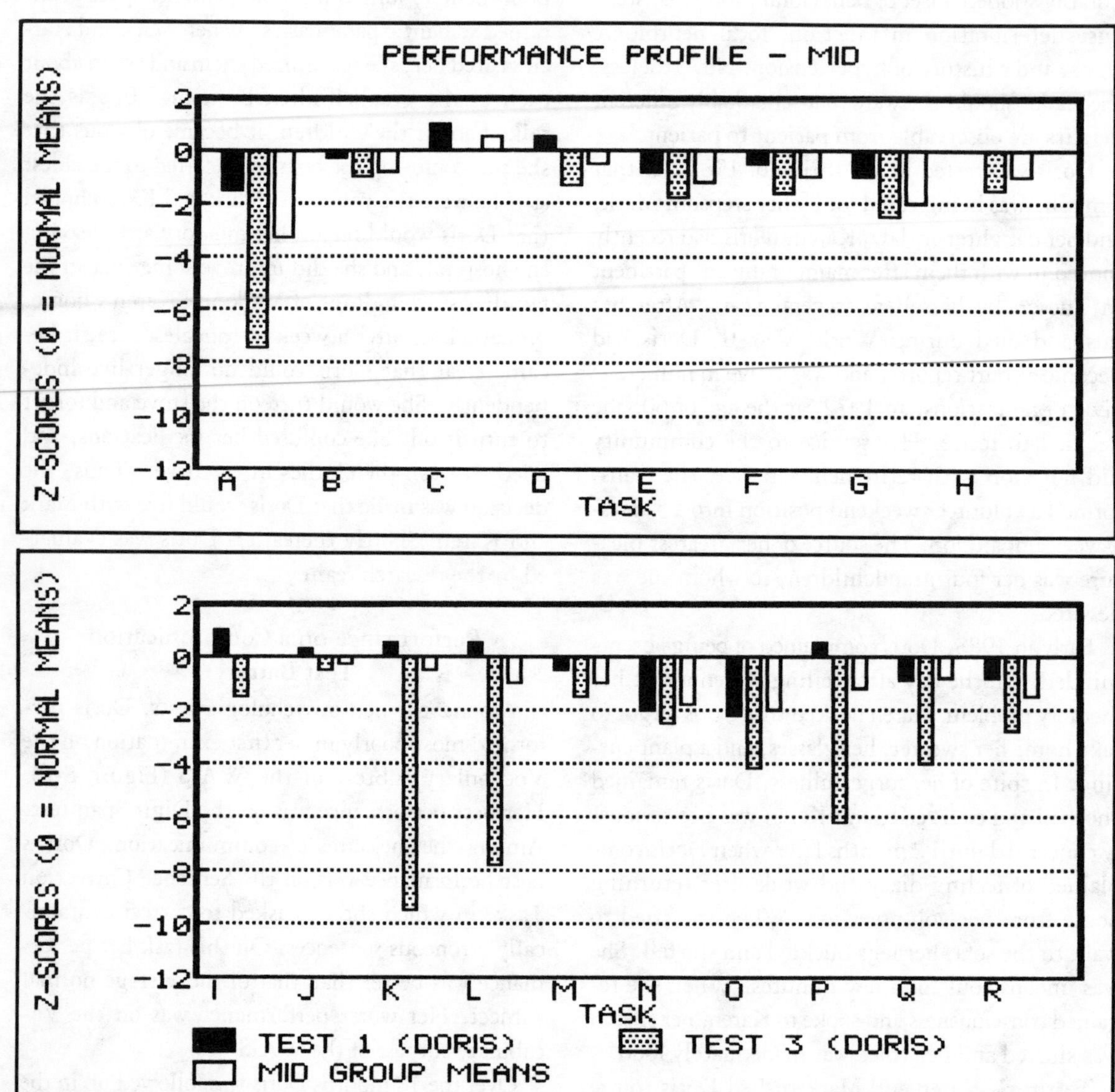

Figure 8-6. *Doris's performance on a communication test battery. A, Mental Status Questionnaire; B, Nonsense Syllable Learning Test; C, Forward Digit Span—WAIS; D, Block Design—WAIS; E, Similarities—WAIS; F, Story Retelling—Immediate; G, Story Retelling—Delayed; H, Peabody Picture Vocabulary Test; I, Sentence Correction Syntactic Judgment; J, Sentence Correction Syntactic Correction; K, Sentence Correction Semantic Judgment; L, Sentence Correction Semantic Correction; M, Verbal Description; N, FAS Verbal Fluency Measure; O, Vocabulary—WAIS; P, Confrontation Naming; Q, Pragmatics; R, Disambiguation.*

E: Tell me everything you can about this object. (Marble)	
Doris: This is a. . . one of a kind thing. It's a. . . it's pretty.	FALSE START VAGUE ANOMIA
E: Pretty?	
Doris: Yes, and it's kind of a circle. From the center to the outside and back again, all around. And in the center, the round and out.	SEMANTIC PARAPHASIA FRAGMENT IDEATIONAL PERSEVERATION
E: Can you tell me anything else about this?	
Doris: Well, it's a pretty one, and nice.	PERSEVERATION
E: Anything else?	
Doris: Well, no, I don't believe that I can give you that one. Not that one at all. Not at all.	INDEFINITE REFERENCE LIMITED VOCABULARY DIVERSITY

Doris lived with Mark and Karen for 2 years, during which time she gradually worsened. For most of that time, however, with constant supervision, Doris could help Karen with simple household chores. Mark and Karen enrolled her in an adult day care program 2 days a week to give Karen respite. Ultimately, though, Doris had to be moved to a nursing home.

Chapter 9

Methodology in Normal Aging and Dementia Research

"Ultimately, research designs become orchestrations of ideal arrangements, on the one hand, and constraints and limitations, on the other . . ."

Nesselroade and Labouvie (1985, p. 35)

The interpretation and clinical application of research findings concerning both normal aging and dementia rest upon the assumption that the findings are valid. In various of the previous and following chapters, the conclusions drawn from particular studies are questioned because of research methodologic problems. It is the purpose of this chapter to systematically explore research design and other methodologic issues that affect validity. It is the authors' hope that consideration of these issues will result in the reader being a more informed and cautious "consumer" of the research literature in aging and dementia.

METHODOLOGIC ISSUES IN NORMAL AGING RESEARCH

If one wishes to determine how a particular cognitive process changes across the adult life span, several issues concerning research method and design must be addressed. The type of research design employed can substantially constrain interpretation of research observations. Differences between research designs employed in various studies often account for lack of consensus in obtained results. The complexity of methodologic issues in gerontologic research sometimes necessitates that investigators (and authors of research reviews!) remain tentative in drawing conclusions.

Cross-Sectional Research Designs

The great majority of studies concerned with communication or cognition and aging have employed a *cross-sectional* research design, in which individuals of different ages are compared at the same point in time. Indeed, a survey of publications appearing in the *Journal of Gerontology* over a 12-year period revealed studies with cross-sectional designs to be reported seven times more frequently than studies in which a single group of individuals is longitudinally followed up over time (Abrahams, Hoyer, Elias, and Bradigan, 1975). Cross-sectional designs have the advantage of permitting reasonably rapid collection of data that would, at first glance, appear to adequately answer questions concerning adult development and aging.

However, cross-sectional designs also have several disadvantages. The greatest of these is that persons of different ages vary from each other along many dimensions besides chronologic age. Schaie (1965) first introduced the term *cohort effects* to describe these nonmaturational variables, and has defined them (Schaie, 1972) as "a temporally unique generalized input from the environment." Cohort effects can include differences between age groups in the type and average number of years of formal education, and mass media characteristics. Cohort effects can also include age group differences in health and medical care trends (e.g., antibiotics and most immunizations were unavailable when today's elderly were children), nutrition habits, exposure to environmental toxins, and prevailing social customs. Brief consideration of these possible contributors to cohort effects will reveal that each can have a marked effect upon behavior in general, and performance on cognitive tasks in particular. Thus, because such cohort effects are inextricably *confounded* with chronologic age in cross-sectional studies, it is not possible to differentiate *ontogenetic* (having to do with the developmental evolution of individuals) from cohort contributions to obtained research results. It has sometimes been assumed that cohort effects have greater relevance for behavioral than for biologic research. However, consider the example of a hypothetic cross-sectional study of brain weight across adult age groups. In order to estimate the extent of loss of brain cells with aging, an investigator might compare autopsy brain weights of persons who died of accidental causes in their 20s, 30s, 40s, 50s, 60s, and 70s. Suppose the investigator finds that autopsy brain weight decreases with older age at death, and concludes that a given percent of brain mass is lost with each successive decade of life. The validity of this conclusion rests on the assumption that individual ("ontogenetic") changes, with increasing age, are resulting in cell loss and consequently smaller brain mass. However, an equally tenable explanation for the observed brain weight differences might be that childhood nutrition and other cohort differences resulted in the older age groups' being of generally smaller body size in adulthood. Since brain weight is correlated with body size, the observed age group differences might thus reflect cohort differences and not the consequences of individual aging.

A second problem with cross-sectional studies, as discussed by Salthouse (1982), is that it is frequently difficult to obtain equally representative samples of persons within each age group. For example, an investigator interested in studying a particular aspect of semantic memory and aging might construct a cross-sectional study in which men and women in the 20- to 30-year age range would be compared with those who were 70 to 80 years old. The investigator could solicit research volunteers by placing an advertisement in local newspapers or other public sources. Older and younger persons responding to this solicitation might be quite different in terms of how well they represent the general population of their age. Members of the younger aged population are generally accustomed to frequent standardized testing during their school years, and may well have previously participated as a volunteer in psychologic research (e.g., as part of a college psychology course experience). Presuming that such previous experience would make it more likely for a person to volunteer to participate in the investigator's study, and given that such previous experience is fairly common within the younger aged population, those who volunteer for the project might be expected to be reasonably representative of the general population of 20- to 30-year-olds.

In contrast, members of the general population of 70- to 80-year-olds have had considerably less experience with standardized testing during their school years, and the majority have probably never participated in a previous psychologic research project. Many, perhaps because of biases and stereotypes about psychology and psychologists acquired during earlier adulthood, may be afraid of what volunteering to participate might entail. Therefore, those older persons who do volunteer to participate in the investigator's study are likely to be relatively unique and not generally representative of the general population of 70-to 80-year-old persons. Differences in representativeness are thus confounded with age in the study, creating problems in interpretation of obtained results and in making judgments about the *generalizability* of such results.

Longitudinal Research Designs

Longitudinal research designs, in which the same individuals are tested repeatedly over a period of time, have several distinct advantages, as detailed by Schaie (1983a). Salthouse (1982) points out that the two most important of these are that individual aging trends can be investigated, and greater statistical power is provided, allowing for greater sensitivity in assessing small age influences. In addition, longitudinal studies enable identification of interindividual variability in intraindividual change (degree of variability shown by different individuals in their behavioral change over time). Longitudinal studies also allow an examination of interrelationships among intraindividual changes (i.e., constancy and change for the entire organism), and inferences concerning determinants of intraindividual change (causal inferences) (Schaie, 1983a).

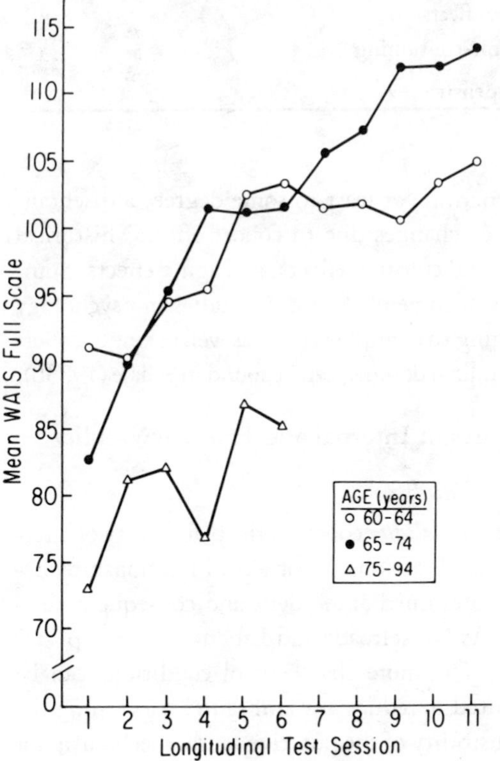

Figure 9-1. *Mean intelligence test scores at the time of first testing as a function of the number of longitudinal test sessions. Only subjects who were tested on all test sessions, up to and including the abscissa test number, are represented. (From Siegler, I. C., and Botwinick, J. {1979}. A long term longitudinal study of intellectual ability of older adults: The matter of selective attrition.* Journal of Gerontology, 34, *242–245 by permission. Copyright 1979 by the Gerontological Society.)*

Despite these significant strengths, longitudinal research designs do have drawbacks and limitations, among which Salthouse (1982, pp. 21–24) includes the following. First, human aging research employing this approach may be impractical because of the enormous time period involved (the study may have approximately the same lifespan as the investigator!). Related to this are the significant problems of the expense and inflexibility of longitudinal studies. Once the study begins, the original procedures must be continued, even though they may become outmoded or obsolete. As with cross-sectional designs, obtained samples of individuals may not be representative of their parent populations. It is obviously difficult to obtain volunteers willing to participate in a long-term project. Even when it can be assumed that the initial sample is representative, some individuals may drop out of the study over time, and those continuing may thus no longer be representative.

Another disadvantage involves the confounding of age and test sophistication. As subjects grow older, they also receive more testing experience, and thus changes may represent "practice effects" rather than age itself. The impact of repeated participation is illustrated by data collected on intelligence test scores within the Duke Longitudinal Studies (see Siegler, 1983), as shown in Figure 9-1, taken from Siegler and Botwinick (1979).

Finally, longitudinal designs share with cross-sectional designs the problem of separating the effects of age from the effects of the historical time period in which the data are collected. Thus, observed intraindividual change over time in longitudinal investigations may be due to the impact of cultural and social changes intervening between the times of data collection, rather than individual aging effects.

Summary

In summary, neither cross-sectional nor longitudinal research designs are without their respective drawbacks, and each has unique strengths.

Table 9-1. Advantages and Disadvantages of Longitudinal Versus Cross-Sectional Research Designs

	Advantages	Disadvantages
Cross-sectional research designs	Economical data collection	Different environmental exposures at various ages may produce cohort effects
		Difficult to obtain equally representative samples in all age groups
Longitudinal research designs	Increased statistical power	Selective attrition may bias results
	Individual age trends can be investigated	Participants may not be representative of population
		Procedures may become obsolete
		Increased test experience may affect results (practice effect)
		Cultural and social changes may confound age effects
		Time-consuming
		Expensive

Advantages and disadvantages of each have been summarized in Table 9-1. What is important to recognize is that substantially different results may be given by these two different research designs, even though all other aspects of the research are similar. Differences between the two approaches are worth remembering when apparently contradictory findings are reported in the literature concerned with some particular aspect of communication, cognition, and aging.

Sequential Research Strategies

It should be pointed out that several alternative strategies have been suggested to reduce the limitations inherent in both cross-sectional and single-cohort longitudinal designs (e.g., Baltes, 1968; Schaie, 1965). These are generally referred to as "sequential" strategies, implying that a sequence of samples (i.e., different cohorts obtained at the same or at different time periods) is taken across several measurement occasions (Schaie, 1983a). The issues involved in different types of these kinds of research designs are complex, highly technical, and beyond the scope of the present chapter. However, the reader should be aware that these designs often permit, at least to some degree, a disentangling of changes due to cohort effects, historical (social and cultural) effects, and aging effects. Summaries of some of the major studies in psychology and aging that employ these, as well as single-cohort longitudinal designs, can be found in Schaie (1983b).

Issues in Internal and External Validity

Internal Validity

Internal validity concerns the plausibility of alternative explanations for observed relationships between presumed antecedent and consequent variables. As Nesselroade and Labouvie (1985, p. 41) state, "The more that control conditions can be instituted to reduce any ambiguity concerning the responsibility of the putative causal mechanism for the observed effect, the more internally valid the design." In this light, it can be seen that many of the issues concerning advantages and disadvantages of cross-sectional and longitudinal research designs, as discussed earlier, affect the internal validity of conclusions concerning age effects on behavior.

Nesselroade and Labouvie (1985) outline several potential threats to internal validity. The first concerns the presence versus absence of experimental manipulation of the putative causal variable. While strong inference of causality can be made when subjects are assigned randomly to treatment conditions in which a presumed causal variable is manipulated, aging is not a causal variable that lends itself to such manipulation. When experimental manipulation and random subject assignment are not possible, appropriately designed studies, particularly those employing longitudinal or sequential designs, may permit alternative models of causal relationships to be compared for goodness of fit to the obtained data. While it is beyond the scope of the present chapter to discuss such data analytic procedures, they typically involve covariance structure analysis and its variations (see Bentler, 1980). Cross-sectional designs, as discussed earlier, would typically have relatively low internal validity as indicators of ontogenetic age changes. Thus, the second threat to internal validity involves the dimension of simultaneity versus succession of observations.

The third dimension of threat to internal validity discussed by Nesselroade and Labouvie (1985) concerns the degree of situational background control. Situational background control involves attending "to those environmental variables that compete with 'target' causal variables in the sense that their effects might plausibly include those reflected in the measurement variables to be explained." (Nesselroade and Labouvie, 1985, p. 43). Cohort confounds are an example of this type of threat to internal validity.

The final dimension involves issues concerning the representativeness of subjects. Again, this was discussed earlier in the present chapter, regarding both cross-sectional and longitudinal research designs.

External Validity

External validity refers to the degree that observed relationships are generalizable to other observations and to populations of interest. The confounding of aging and effects of repeated testing, and of aging and selective participation or attrition or both, represent types of threats to external validity. In general, the best assurance of external validity is obtained through random selection of research participants, a goal that is simply not possible to obtain in human aging research.

In addition to concerns about the representativeness of subject samples, the investigator must also be concerned about the representativeness of measurement approaches selected. If a selected measure is not adequately representative of the hypothetic construct it is presumed to assess, it is said to have poor *construct validity*. If the measure does not sufficiently sample the full range of dimensions thought to be contained within the construct, it is said to have poor *content validity*.

Even in the most carefully designed of sequential research approaches, where subjects are reasonably representative of their parent populations, subject attrition low and not systematic, and measures representative of their construct domains, problems in interpretation of results may still exist. One variable notorious for creating such problems is health status. If only the most healthy of older adults are selected to participate in a particular study, then the sample will not be representative of the broader population of older adults, who are at higher risk for health problems, and show greater illness prevalence, than younger adults. On the other hand, when older subjects in ill health (or with health problems unknown to the investigator) are participants in studies of "normal aging," then observed cross-sectional age group differences may be due to poor health and not "normal aging" (Salthouse, 1982). What appear to be "normal aging" changes in longitudinal studies may similarly be reflecting the increasing incidence of health problems as participants grow older. Numerous studies have shown various aspects of health status to have a marked impact upon cognitive measures in studies of adult aging (see review by Siegler and Costa, 1985).

Summary

Given this range of methodologic problems, involving issues in selection of research design and considerations of internal and external validity, contradictory results and a lack of consensus are not surprising in many areas of normal aging research. Determining whether conclusions have been drawn from cross-sectional, longitudinal, or sequential research designs can often help in reconciling such disagreement. Even when the particular research design adopted appears optimal for answering the specific question being asked, various threats to internal and external validity must be considered. These considerations have important implications for the relative confidence that can be placed in obtained results, as well as their generalizability.

METHODOLOGIC ISSUES IN DEMENTIA RESEARCH

Since most dementia patients are older adults, investigations of cognitive and communicative functioning in dementia share with other gerontologic research those problems in research design and threats to validity discussed earlier. In addition, dementia research poses several relatively unique measurement and other methodologic problems. The following provides a brief review of those issues unique to studies of dementia. Further discussion can be found in Kaszniak (1986) and in Kaszniak and Davis (1986).

Cross-Sectional versus Longitudinal Research Designs

All of those issues just described, concerning the relative advantages and disadvantages of cross-sectional versus longitudinal research designs in normal aging, apply equally to research in dementia, with some slight modification. First, because cognitive change in dementing illness occurs more rapidly than in normal aging, longitudinal research in dementia is not quite as time-consuming. Typical recent longitudinal studies of AD (e.g., Kaszniak, Wilson, Fox and Stebbins, in press; Wilson and Kaszniak, 1986; Storandt, Botwinick and Danziger, (1986) have followed up patients and normal control subjects over 3 years of repeated evaluation and documented significant cognitive deterioration.

For this same reason, there is likely to be less confounding between cohort effects and duration of dementia, than between cohort effects and age in normal aging studies. That is, since dementia progresses relatively rapidly over a short number of years, patients at different stages of their disorders are likely to represent the same cohort, in terms of variables such as education, mass media exposure, health and medical care history, and nutrition habits. Consequently, interpretation of results based upon cross-sectional samples of dementia patients, when appropriately compared with normal individuals matched on age, education, and other demographic variables, is somewhat less ambiguous than interpretation of normal aging cross-sectional studies.

It would thus appear that cross-sectional designs for the study of dementia might be preferable, given the additional cost, time, and effort of longitudinal studies. However, cross-sectional dementia studies pose unique problems in the definition of stage or severity of illness. The majority of cognitive and linguistic investigations of dementia contrast a normal control group with a group of patients varying in dementia severity and presumed duration of illness. This is problematic, since dementia is a progressive syndrome, with the type and severity of deficits shown by patients at one stage of the disorder different from those shown by patients at another stage. It is therefore not surprising that most cross-sectional comparisons of dementia patients and normal control subjects find the dementia group to have greater variability on dependent measures than control subjects. This difference in variability between groups creates problems in the application of various statistical procedures, and the interpretation of average score differences between groups (e.g., several parametric statistical tests assume *homogeneity* or equivalence of variance between groups being contrasted). Unfortunately, most investigators have paid insufficient attention to this issue in their published research.

Issues in Internal and External Validity

As discribed earlier, *internal validity* refers to the plausibility of alternative explanations for observed relationships between presumed antecedent and consequent variables. As with normal aging research, dementia studies are liable to several threats to internal validity. The presence or absence of dementia cannot be experimentally manipulated, and therefore caution must be exercised in concluding that the disease itself has caused the cognitive deficits observed. Because clinical diagnosis of a particular dementing illness is fallible, one needs to be concerned with the *reliability* of diagnosis. At present, there are no absolute proven biologic markers of AD, and clinical diagnosis relies heavily upon the process of elimination, in which other possible diagnoses are systematically ruled out. Much early research concerned with cognition in dementia did not employ extensive diagnostic protocols to eliminate other diagnostic possibilities, and the results of such research cannot therefore be unambiguously interpreted. As will be discussed in subsequent chapters, the problems associated with differentiating the contributions of progressive brain disease from depression in this type of research are particularly salient.

Applying longitudinal research designs can increase the validity of causal inferences concerning the effects of a dementing illness upon cognition, since the patterning of change over time can be examined and statistically modeled. However, longitudinal studies of dementia suffer from greater external validity problems than comparable studies of normal aging, as will be discussed, because of selective subject attrition.

Issues concerning the representativeness of subject selection can pose a particular threat to internal validity (as well as to external validity) in dementia research. If the subjects selected for the study (e.g., AD patients) are not reasonably representative of the full range of severity of the illness (e.g., either all very severely impaired or all very mildly impaired), then this *truncation of range* will affect the magnitude of any relationship that can be observed between cognitive measures and any other variable. In other words, when the severity of dementia is limited in a particular sample of patients, there will simply be too little variability on any particular cognitive measure to relate to any other measure. The investigator might therefore be misled into the interpretation that two measures are not related, when the apparent lack of relationship is really an artifact of sampling bias.

Research on dementia also shares with normal aging studies various threats to *external validity* (degree that observed relationships are generalizable to other observations and populations of interest). A particular threat to external validity concerns selective subject attrition. For example, AD patients have shortened life expectancy compared with age-matched healthy older persons (Katzman, 1976), and the likelihood of death increases with greater dementia severity (Kaszniak, Fox, Gandell, Garron, Huckman and Ramsey, 1978). Those AD patients who are more severely demented at the beginning of a longitudinal study are therefore at greater risk of dying before the study is completed. Similarly, patients who agree to participate in a longitudinal study may, as their dementia severity increases, refuse to continue to participate and thus be lost to follow-up. Similarly, as dementia severity increases, the patient may no longer be able to comprehend the nature of instructions on some particular cognitive task. Therefore, longitudinal data on such a task is limited to only those patients whose dementia progressed more slowly, and the resulting inferences are not generalizable to the entire population of dementia patients. These sources of selective attrition in longitudinal studies of dementia can seriously bias results, and investigators must exercise great caution in assessing whether attrition is selective and in accounting for the effects of such attrition in data analysis.

A related threat to external validity is posed by issues concerning the representativeness with which tests sample the hypothetic construct they are designed to operationalize. If, for example, a task samples only a limited range of variability of a construct (e.g., the task difficulty is either very high or very low), then the potential magnitude of any observable relationship between the task and any other variable will be limited.

Dementia research can present with unique difficulties in the *construct validity* of measures employed. Construct validation is typically conceptualized as an ongoing effort to identify the meaning of particular hypothetic constructs, and their operationally defining measures, usually through factor analytic approaches. The factorial complexity of a measure limits its construct validity. This is particularly problematic for dementia research, as the factor structure of measures may be progressively altered in the course of disorders such as AD. As an increasing range of cognitive functions become more severely impaired over time in AD, the construct validity of a measure may change, being "contaminated" by other hypothetic processes, increasingly impaired in AD, but not contributing to performance on the measure by healthy control subjects. This can be illustrated by a study reported by Wilson, Bacon, Fox and Kaszniak (1983a). In this study, measures of verbal primary and secondary memory were shown not to be correlated with each other, and were differentially related to EEG measures in a healthy control sample. However, these two measures were significantly correlated in the AD patient sample, with one possible interpretation being that primary memory deficit in AD was making an increasing contribution to secondary memory deficit in these patients. The measure of secondary memory thus cannot be considered as a "pure" measure of this construct in AD, as it appears to be contaminated with primary memory. The measure of secondary memory has lost some of the construct validity that it possessed when employed with normally aged individuals. Although for much research concerned with cognition in dementia, no solution may exist for such difficulties, both investigators and those who wish to apply research results must be aware of the limitations these problems place on our confidence in the external validity of research data.

Research concerning communication and cognition in dementia is beset by several very difficult methodologic problems, not all of which can ever be entirely resolved in any particular investigation. Confidence in the validity of conclusions therefore often depends upon the convergence and agreement of results reported from studies employing different research designs, subject sampling procedures, and measurement approaches. For this reason, the present book has often included studies that if examined alone contain sufficient methodologic problems to prevent unambiguous interpretation, but produce results that converge with those of other studies.

Summary

It has been the purpose of this chapter to provide the reader with a general introduction to research design and validity issues particular to aging and dementia research. Cross-sectional and longitudinal research designs were contrasted, and the related issues of internal and external validity explored.

Studies of dementia share several of the methodologic and validity issues common to research in normal aging. Cross-sectional research designs would appear to be advantageous in dementia research, given the fewer problems as compared with normal aging studies, with cohort by age (or length of illness) confounding. However, cross-sectional dementia research suffers from particular difficulties in defining severity of dementia or length of illness. Particular threats to validity include problems caused by the limited range of variability for certain measures (due to the interaction of task difficulty and the severity of dementia), and changes, with increasing dementia severity, in the construct validity of measures. Longitudinal studies involving dementia patients experience more severe problems with selective attrition than are typically found in normal aging studies.

CLINICAL IMPLICATIONS

1. Issues concerning research design and validity have distinct implications for our clinical expectations regarding older persons. Observed differences between older and younger persons may reflect, often to a large degree, cohort, rather than developmental, phenomena. It should therefore not be expected that such apparent differences are necessarily predictors of how any given individual will "age."
2. As a corollary, contributors to age-cohort differences, such as educational background and prior health history, that can differ among both younger and older individuals need to be taken into account in the attempt to understand the cognitive or communicative behavior of the older adult. The expectations for performance consistent with normal aging will, for example, differ greatly between the individual with a fourth-grade education and the person who was involved in a profession requiring a doctoral degree.
3. Research design and validity problems in dementia research must be noted in any attempt to apply the results of such research. For example, the apparent lack of relationship between a particular psychologic or communication assessment instrument and some external criterion (e.g., radiologic brain imaging, neuropathologic changes) may reflect limited measurement range within the sample under study, rather than lack of external validity of measurement.

REFERENCES

Abrahams, J.P., Hoyer, W.J., Elias, M.F., and Bradigan, B.(1975). Gerontological research in psychology published in the Journal of Gerontology 1963-74: Perspectives and progress. *Journal of Gerontology*, *30*, 668-673.

Baltes, P.B.(1968). Longitudinal and cross-sectional sequences in the study of age and generation effects. *Human Development*, *11*, 145-171.

Bentler, P.M.(1980). Multivariate analysis with latent variables. *Annual Review of Psychology*, *31*, 419-456.

Kaszniak, A.W. (1986). Clinical memory testing: External validations. In G. Maddox (Ed.),*Encyclopedia of aging*. New York: Springer.

Kaszniak, A.W., and Davis, K. (1986). Instrument and data review: The quest for external validators. In L.W. Poon, B.J. Gurland, C. Eisdorfer, T. Crook, L.W. Thompson, A.W. Kaszniak, and K. Davis (Eds.), *The handbook of clinical memory assessment of older adults*. Washington, DC: American Psychological Association.

Kaszniak, A.W., Fox, J., Gandell, D.L., Garron, D.C., Huckman, M.S., and Ramsey, R.G. (1978). Predictors of mortality in presenile and senile dementia. *Annals of Neurology*, *3*, 246-252.

Kaszniak, A.W., Wilson, R.S., Fox, J.H., and Stebbins, G.T. (in press). Cognitive assessment in Alzheimer's disease: Cross-sectional and longitudinal perspectives. *Canadian Journal of Neurological Sciences*.

Katzman, R. (1976). The prevalence and malignancy of Alzheimer's disease. *Archives of Neurology*, *33*, 217-218.

Nesselroade, J.R., and Labouvie, E.W.(1985). Experimental design in research on aging. In J.E.Birren and K.W.Schaie (Eds.), *Handbook of the psychology of aging (2nd ed.)* (pp.35-60).New York: Van Nostrand Reinhold.

Salthouse, T.A.(1982). *Adult cognition: An experimental psychology of human aging*. New York: Springer-Verlag.

Schaie, K.W.(1965). A general model for the study of developmental problems. *Psychological Bulletin*, *64*, 92-107.

Schaie, K.W.(1972). Limitations on the generalizability of growth curves on intelligence. *Human Development*, *15*, 141-152.

Schaie, K.W.(1983a). What can we learn from the longitudinal study of adult psychological development? In K.W. Schaie (Ed.), *Longitudinal studies of adult psychological development* (pp. 1-19). New York: Guilford.

Schaie, K.W. (Ed.) (1983b). *Longitudinal studies of adult psychological development*. New York: Guilford.

Siegler, I.C. (1983). Psychological aspects of the Duke

Longitudinal Studies. In K.W. Schaie (Ed.), *Longitudinal studies of adult psychological development* (pp. 136-190). New York: Guilford.

Siegler, I.C., and Botwinick, J. (1979). A long-term longitudinal study of intellectual ability of older adults: The matter of selective attrition. *Journal of Gerontology, 34*, 242-245.

Siegler, I.C., and Costa, P.T. (1985). Health behavior relationships. In J.E.Birren and K.W. Schaie (Eds.), *Handbook of the psychology of aging (2nd ed.)* (pp. 144-166). New York: Van Nostrand Reinhold.

Storandt, M., Botwinick, J., and Danziger, W.L. (1986). Longitudinal changes: Mild SDAT and matched healthy controls. In L. Poon, B.J. Gurland, C. Eisdorfer, T. Crook, L.W. Thompson, A.W. Kaszniak, and K. Davis (Eds.), *The handbook of clinical memory assessment of older adults*. Washington, DC: American Psychological Association.

Wilson, R.S., Bacon, L.D., Fox, J.H., and Kaszniak, A.W. (1983). Primary memory and secondary memory in dementia of the Alzheimer type. *Journal of Clinical Neuropsychology*, *5*, 337-344.

Wilson, R.S. and Kaszniak, A.W. (1986). Longitudinal changes: Progressive idiopathic dementia. In L.W. Poon, B.J. Gurland, C. Eisdorfer, T. Crook, L.W. Thompson, A.W. Kaszniak, and K. Davis (Eds.), *The handbook of clinical memory assessment of older adults*. Washington, DC: American Psychological Association.

Chapter 10

Intelligence and Information Processing Speed in Normal Aging and Dementia

"Old age takes away from us what we have inherited and gives us what we have earned."

Gerald Brennan

Assume that a 76-year-old woman has sought consultation with her physician because she fears that she is becoming "senile." Upon arriving for her appointment, she complains that her memory has been failing, and provides several examples of losing keys, misplacing her eye glasses, and forgetting appointments. She is unable to state exactly when this memory difficulty began, but estimates that it has been developing over the past several years. During the interview, her physician notes that she responds to questions rather slowly, and occasionally has trouble expressing herself. While attempting to respond to the physician's questions, she is easily distracted by noise in an adjacent room. Her face remains fairly expressionless during the interview, although she appears on the brink of tearfulness while describing a particularly embarrassing incident of forgetfulness. The physician conducts a routine physical examination, the results of which are unremarkable, except for moderately elevated blood pressure.

This example illustrates the kind of diagnostic dilemma frequently faced by clinicians whose practice includes older persons. What is the appropriate diagnosis for this woman's complaint? Are her memory changes a normal manifestation of aging? Could this reflect the early stage of a degenerative brain disorder such as Alzheimer's disease? Might her general lack of emotional expression, except for near tearfulness, be indicative of a depression that is causing her forgetfulness? Given her high blood pressure, could her memory difficulty reflect small cerebral infarctions? All of these are legitimate questions, the answers to which require additional diagnostic assessment. In order for the clinician to be adequately alert to the range of diagnostic possibilities, a knowledge of the typical symptoms and course of dementing illness is necessary. Further, because most dementias are age-associated, a knowledge of the psychologic aspects of normal aging is also necessary.

The present section of the book has been written to provide the reader a familiarity with the cognitive and emotional features of dementia, as contrasted with those of normal aging. Where the features of dementia overlap with those of other syndromes, such as depression, these are also contrasted. In the present and following chapters, a detailed examination of the research literature concerned with cognitive functioning in normal aging and dementia is presented. Knowledge of this literature contributes importantly to accuracy in clinical assessment, since the choice of assessment approaches and instruments is informed by research results. Separate chapters contrast normal aging and dementia changes in intelligence and information processing speed, perception and attention, and memory for events. These are followed by a review of neuropsychologic approaches and instruments that are appropriate for the assessment of older persons suspected of having dementia. For the reader less familiar with research approaches in gerontologic psychology and human neuropsychology, the material of these chapters may be rather difficult. However, it is the authors' belief that the effort of digesting this material will be rewarded by a deeper understanding of important clinical phenomena.

WHY STUDY INTELLIGENCE AND INFORMATION PROCESSING SPEED?

Most persons think of intellectual deterioration as synonymous with dementia. Indeed, evidence of intellectual deterioration is necessary for a DSM-III diagnosis of dementia to be made. As demonstrated in previous chapters, dementia patients show deterioration in abstract thinking, reasoning, and understanding of logical relationships. All of these abilities are generally considered to be aspects of intelligence. However, a range of other cognitive functions have also traditionally been included within the construct of intelligence. In fact, it is difficult to find a human cognitive process that has not been included, at one time or another, within the definition of intelligence. There continues to be considerable debate among psychologists and other cognitive scientists as to the most appropriate definition (Sternberg, 1985). Despite this debate, the use of intelligence tests remains widespread. Psychometric measures of intelligence typically consist of several different cognitive tasks, each designed to assess a somewhat different aspect or functional domain. Because of the historically important role intelligence testing has played in clinical research and assessment in dementia, the present chapter will review the relevant literature.

A common cultural stereotype is that intelligence also declines somewhat with normal aging. Research designed to examine the question whether intelligence declines with aging has indicated that the answer must be more complex than a simple "yes" or "no." The clinical application of intelligence testing in the diagnosis of dementia is dependent upon a knowledge of normal age changes in intelligence test performance. For this reason, the chapter begins with a brief review of both cross-sectional and longitudinal studies of intelligence test performance and aging.

Finally, the importance of considering speed of performance and information processing will be emphasized. Slowing of response and processing speed has been shown to make a major contribution to changes in intelligence test performance with aging. In addition, recent research suggests that a slowing of information processing speed can account for the normal aging effects on the semantic memory tasks reviewed earlier in the book. Behavioral slowing is also a major feature of dementia and other disorders from which dementia must be differentiated. Research concerned with the measurement of motor and processing speed will be reviewed, along with its implications for understanding both normal aging and dementia-related changes in cognition.

PSYCHOMETRIC MEASURES OF INTELLIGENCE IN NORMAL AGING

The relationship of adult age to psychometric measures of intelligence was one of the earliest concerns in gerontologic psychology. Though a great deal of data has accumulated, this remains a controversial area. Part of the controversy grows out of the lack of consensus about how the construct of intelligence is to be defined and measured. Despite definitional and measurement problems, the employment of "intelligence tests" has played a historically important role in generating current hypotheses in cognition and aging, and continues to play a useful function in clinical assessment.

Intellectual deterioration has long been a part of our cultural stereotype of growing old. Both cross-sectional and longitudinal studies have supported the conclusion that some decline in psychometric measures of intelligence does occur with normal aging. However, this decline is less general, smaller in magnitude, and begins later in life than either cultural stereotype or early research in this area suggests.

Most intelligence tests, such as the Wechsler Adult Intelligence Scale (WAIS) (Wechsler, 1958), are composed of an aggregation of multiple subtests, each presumably assessing some hypothetically different aspect of the broader construct of intelligence. Typically, observed scores on these subtests are combined to provide a summary measure, usually expressed as an intelligence quotient (IQ). When early investigators examined such summary measures in relationship to adult age in cross-sectional studies (e.g., Jones and Conrad, 1933; Miles and Miles, 1932; Wechsler, 1939), they concluded that intelligence did indeed decline with increasing age.

The conclusions from early studies have been criticized on several different grounds. First, many of the component subtests in intelligence batteries are timed, and the subject receives a higher score for solving a problem more quickly. Since speed of performance and information processing appear to reliably slow with age, the speed component may confound measures of intellectual ability. Second, many of these early studies employed intelligence test batteries that were child-oriented. Some contained stimulus items that an older adult might perceive as silly and therefore unworthy of much response effort. Third, in combining scores from various subtests, differences between subtests in their relationship to age were masked. As later studies demonstrated, age is differentially related to the various subtests of the WAIS, as well as to different subportions of other intelligence assessment instruments. Fourth, these studies were criticized for not taking into account age group differences in education, interests, and motivation in the interpretion of results.

Cohort versus Aging Effects on Intelligence

The marked relationship between education and intelligence test scores is illustrated in the results of Green (1969), who employed the WAIS in a cross-sectional design. When WAIS full-scale IQ, the summary measure across all subtests, and average number of years of formal education were both plotted on the same graph, against age of the subject groups, a striking correspondence was observed between educational level and IQ. Further, when age groups were equated for educational level, by randomly selecting and deselecting subjects, older subjects no longer showed lower IQ scores. Thus, what had appeared to be an age-related deterioration in measured intelligence was better explained as a cohort confound between chronologic age and education. Older individuals had, on the average, less formal education.

When Green (1969) separated the WAIS full-scale IQ into its component verbal IQ and performance IQ scores, verbal IQ actually showed an increase with older age, among the educationally matched age groups, whereas performance IQ showed a slight decline. Differences between the age relationships of these various component parts of intelligence tests will be discussed in greater detail later. Of importance for the present discussion is that cohort effects in early cross-sectional studies appear to be responsible for a substantial portion of the "age deterioration" in intelligence test scores.

When results of large-scale longitudinal/ sequential studies of psychometric intelligence, such as the 21-year Seattle Longitudinal Study (Schaie, 1983), became available, even less age-related decline was observed than had been suggested by cross-sectional studies. For at least those measures concerned with the recall and use of previously acquired knowledge, little evidence of deterioration was apparent until after 70 years of age. For those tasks involving more active and novel problem-solving, a somewhat greater age decline was observed. This decline, although more gradual across the adult age span, is again most marked in older old age.

Components of Psychometric Intelligence

It has thus become increasingly clear that "general intelligence" cannot be said to deteriorate with age. Some abilities measured by intelligence tests appear to remain essentially invariant across most of the adult age span, while others show clear change. Although, as yet, no generally accepted explanation exists for such differential declines, many authors have attempted to summarize and describe the differential decline pattern (see Salthouse, 1982, pp. 55–70). Most of these descriptions suggest that aging is associated with an impairment of the ability to acquire or use new information, while culturally dependent information, obtained by the individual from prior interactions with the environment, remains unchanged.

The best known and most frequently cited description of the differential decline pattern with age is that proposed by Horn and colleagues (e.g., Horn and Cattell, 1967; Horn and Donaldson, 1976). They suggested that adult age relationships can be understood if two types of intelligence are distinguished. The first, called *fluid intelligence*, is reflected in tests of memory span, figural relations, inductive reasoning, and most processes involved in acquiring new information. Fluid intelligence is that type which decreases with older age. The second type, called *crystallized intelligence*, is the cumulative product of information previously acquired by the activity of fluid intelligence, and thus represents the store of culturally transmitted information. Crystallized intelligence is measured by tests like vocabulary definition, general information knowledge, comprehension, arithmetic ability, and reasoning with familiar material. Crystallized intelligence is that type which remains stable throughout most of adult life.

This distinction between fluid and crystallized intelligence does provide a reasonably good description of the pattern of intelligence test scores across adult age. However, it remains a description, rather than an explanation. Horn (1975) has speculated that fluid intelligence might be based upon diffuse neural activity, whereas crystallized intelligence is derivable from focused, specific neural activity. However, such speculations would require considerable elaboration of mechanisms before neurophysiologic correlates could be fruitfully explored and hence a theoretical position further developed.

Summary

What has emerged from studies of aging and psychometric intelligence is that no general statements can be confidently made. Different component abilities show different age relationships, and cohort confounds can contribute considerably to obtained results. What appears needed is a focus upon specific areas of cognitive functioning, employing content-valid and construct-valid measurement approaches and sophisticated research designs. Such an approach would yield a data base allowing greater specificity and greater confidence in determining how normal aging and cognition are related. The beginnings of such a data base are outlined here and in the chapters that follow.

SPEED OF BEHAVIOR AND INFORMATION PROCESSING

A general slowing of behavior with increased age is one of the most reliable observations emerging from the literature on psychology and aging. As Salthouse (1985, p. 400) stated in his recent review of this topic, "Seldom in psychology is a researcher at a loss for new adjectives to describe the reliability of a particular behavioral phenomenon." Across 50 published studies, employing various timed psychometric measures, the median correlation between the psychomotor measure and age was 0.45, with a range of 0.15 to 0.64 (Salthouse, 1985). As Salthouse points out, these results are even more impressive when it is remembered that most of the timed tasks used in these studies are of uncertain reliability. Low reliability of any measure necessarily attenuates its possible magnitude of correlation with any other variable, such as age.

Despite the impressive consistency of the age–behavioral speed relationship, there are some exceptions. Older adults in very good cardiovascular health have faster reaction times than less healthy older adults (e.g., Light, 1978; Spirduso and Clifford, 1978). When selected samples of all healthy physically fit older adults are compared with inactive younger adults, differences in speed may not be observed. The second exception appears to occur when vocal, rather than manual, responses are required in timed tasks (e.g., Nebes, 1978; Salthouse and Somberg, 1982): older adults are slower in manual, but not vocal, reaction time. However, some investigators have found that younger adults are faster than older adults in vocal reaction time (e.g., Waugh, Fozard, and Thomas, 1978). It thus remains unclear whether this is a true exception to the relationship of general behavioral slowing and age.

The Locus of Behavioral Slowing with Age

Despite the generally high agreement between studies, the specific locus for this slowing is debatable. The available research (see review by Salthouse, 1985) has made it clear that slowing cannot be accounted for by slowed sensory processes or slowed motor response alone. Indeed, on tasks that allow an assessment of the speed of a mental process, apart from any general slowing in sensory processing or motor response, age differences in favor of young adults continue to be found (Berg, Hertzog, and Hunt, 1982; Gaylord and Marsh, 1975; Cerella, Poon, and Fozard, 1981). Processing of both linguistic (e.g., Howard, Shaw, and Heisey, 1986) and nonlinguistic material (e.g., Gaylord and Marsh, 1975) appear to slow in older age.

Various investigators have attempted to determine whether the aging and behavior slowing relationship is due to slowing in one particular component of information processing. For example, stimulus encoding versus central decision processes versus response selection or execution have been experimentally examined. Research has been unsuccessful at eliminating any of these processes as candidates (Cerella, Poon, and Williams, 1980; Salthouse, 1985). Age differences appear in every component considered, and within every processing stage.

The Complexity Hypothesis

The proposal that all central processes are slowed by approximately the same degree has been termed the "complexity hypothesis" (Cerella et al., 1980). According to this hypothesis, the absolute difference in response time for old and young persons should vary according to the complexity of the task. However, the rate of slowing, as indicated by the ratio of old persons' response times to young persons' response times, should be constant across tasks. This hypothesis has gained support in recently published research (e.g., Puglisi, 1986).

One important prediction from this hypothesis is that the magnitude of correlations across both timed and untimed measures should be larger with older age. This prediction follows the logic that both the speed and the probability of successful completion of many activities should be affected by the general slowing, and thus, persons with a slow "cycle time" should be slower and less accurate across a wide variety of measures than persons with a fast cycle time (Salthouse, 1985, pp. 417–418). As employed in this context, cycle time is an analogy to the time taken by a digital computer to complete one program instruction cycle. Some recent research has confirmed this prediction of greater correlation across timed and untimed tasks for older than for younger adults (e.g., Berg et al., 1982).

Can Slowed Processing Account for Age Differences in Semantic Memory?

One very intriguing possibility is that a generalized slowing in cycle time might account for age differences observed in other higher cognitive processes. For example, there is evidence from studies employing the semantic priming methodology, and varying the prime-target onset asynchrony, of a slowing with age in one or more aspects of semantic activation. In a study reported by Howard and colleagues (1986), 54 young (mean age = 20.2 years) and 54 older (mean age = 68.4 years) adults completed a task in which the priming word was followed by a "target" word, or nonword set of letters. Subjects were to respond "yes" if the target was a word and "no" otherwise. On word-target trials, three different kinds of primes were presented: (1) associated (e.g., the prime-target pair "dog/cat"); (2) unassociated (e.g., the prime-target pair "sew/cat"); and (3) neutral (e.g., the prime-target pair "blank/cat"). The stimulus onset asynchrony (SOA), the time between the onset of the prime and the target, was varied, between 150, 450, and 1000 ms. The most important finding of this study was an age difference in the minimum SOA at which "priming" was observed. The minimum SOA was longer for the older adults. Howard and colleagues argued that this age difference in onset of priming reflects a slowing with age in one or more aspects of semantic activation. This slowing could be in the rate at which seeing a dog activates the lexical or conceptual "node" for dog, the rate at which activation spreads from node to node in the semantic network, or both. As stated by Howard and associates (1986), "Regardless of the locus of this slowing, it is of some importance because it would contribute to the difficulties some elderly people experience in understanding language under certain circumstances" (p. 201).

Madden (1985) has recently reported results arguing that this slowing may be general to all processes involved in semantic memory activation. The study reported by Madden compared 16 younger (mean age = 18.6 years) and 16 older (mean age = 67.5 years) adults in a task requiring a decision regarding the synonymy of two visually presented words. On the "yes-response" trials, the two words either were identical, differed only in case, or were synonyms that differed in case. Age differences in decision time were greater for the synonyms than for the other word pair classes. However, the proportional slowing of decision time shown by the older subjects was constant across word-pair type. This finding is consistent with the complexity hypothesis of Cerella and colleagues (1980). Madden concluded that a generalized age-related slowing in the speed of information processing could account for age differences in the retrieval of letter identity and semantic information from long-term memory.

Summary

Available evidence indicates that the slowing of information processing with older age is a pervasive and general phenomenon, affecting all types of stimulus materials and all processing stages. The complexity hypothesis predicts that age-related slowing should increase with greater processing complexity. It also predicts that the rate of slowing, as measured by the ratio of older to younger persons' response times, should remain constant across tasks. This hypothesis has gained considerable recent support. Some theorists have argued that this general slowing of information processing may be sufficient to explain a great many observations of change in cognitive processes with aging. While slowing may not prove to have such powerful and broad explanatory power, it is clearly a major contributor to age differences in cognition and communication.

PSYCHOMETRIC MEASURES OF INTELLIGENCE IN DEMENTIA

The DSM-III criteria for the diagnosis of dementia state that intellectual deterioration is the essential feature of this syndrome. Certainly, those studies which have employed standardized "intelligence tests" are in good agreement that dementia patients show lower mean IQ scores than groups of age-matched healthy control subjects (see review by Miller, 1977). Chapter 14 will discuss the diagnostic utility of intelligence testing. The present focus is upon gaining an understanding of what test performance tells us about the nature of dementia.

Intelligence Test Patterns in Dementing Illness

Intelligence tests, like the Wechsler Adult Intelligence Scale (WAIS) (Wechsler, 1958; Matarazzo, 1972) are composed of several distinct subtests. Each subtest is designed to assess a different aspect of linguistic and nonlinguistic knowledge, problem-solving ability, or both. Studies of normal aging, as reviewed earlier, have indicated different age sensitivities of these various subtests. Familiar, well-learned, and over-practiced knowledge and skill (such as that generally represented by the WAIS Verbal IQ) remain intact with aging. The ability to solve novel, unfamiliar problems (such as that generally represented by the WAIS Performance IQ) somewhat deteriorates. In AD, deterioration occurs in both types of intellectual ability (Larrabee, Largen, and Levin, 1985), although Performance IQ is almost always lower than Verbal IQ (Miller, 1977). For highly educated AD patients, in the early stages of their dementia, only Performance, and not Verbal, IQ may be below that of age- and education-matched healthy control subjects (Weingartner et al., 1981). Some investigators (Brinkman and Braun, 1984; Fuld, 1982) have found the pattern of WAIS subtest scores to be useful in the differential diagnosis of dementing illnesses. Chapter 14 contains additional discussion of WAIS subtest patterns in neuropsychologic assessment. Examples of the WAIS subtest score pattern of two groups of AD patients examined by the present authors, one with mild dementia and the other with moderate dementia, are presented in Figures 10-1 and 10-2. AD patients with severe dementia are typically too impaired to be formally testable on measures such as the WAIS.

Patients with dementia associated with PD and with HD demonstrate a similar greater impairment in Performance, compared with Verbal, IQ (e.g., Loranger, Goodell, McDowell, Lee, and Sweet, 1972; Brouwers, Cox, Martin, Chase, and Fedio, 1984). The pattern of WAIS subtest scores obtained by a group of HD patients examined by the present authors is presented in Figure 10-3.

Patients with MID have a less predictable pattern of WAIS subtest scores, apparently corresponding to the variability in location of their multiple infarcts (see Brust, 1983). Examples of the WAIS subtest patterns obtained by two different MID patients are presented in Figure 10-4.

Are Intelligence Tests Sensitive Indicators of Mild Dementia?

Intelligence test batteries such as the WAIS, although demonstrating clear impairment with more advanced AD, are not the most sensitive indicators of dementia. Storandt, Botwinick, Danziger, Berg, and Hughes (1984), comparing a group of mildly demented AD patients with age-matched healthy persons, found specific tests of episodic memory, concentration, and generative naming to be better discriminators than various of the WAIS subtests. These results are consistent with the claim of this book: that semantic and episodic memory are particularly impaired in dementia. It is important to include tests designed to examine various aspects of episodic and semantic memory in any diagnostic evaluation battery for dementia.

Even in the examination of patients who show clear deficit on the WAIS, it is not clear exactly how to interpret the nature of their difficulties on various subtests. As discussed earlier, part of the problem is the lack of agreement on how to define the construct of intelligence. A second problem is that each intelligence scale subtest involves multiple information-processing components. A more productive approach to understanding the nature of cognitive deficit in dementia is an examination of the performance of AD and other dementia patients on tasks designed to specifically isolate these different components. Data emerging from this approach are reviewed in the remaining portion of the present and subsequent chapters.

Summary

Early in the course of AD, patients demonstrate deficits in those intelligence test subtests contributing to Performance IQ. Intelligence tests are not, however, the best procedures for distinguishing normal older persons from AD patients. Specific measures of episodic and semantic memory more accurately differentiate AD patient and healthy elderly groups. While AD has its greatest effect upon WAIS performance subtest scores, all subtests reveal deterioration as the disease progresses.

SPEED OF BEHAVIOR AND INFORMATION PROCESSING IN DEMENTIA

The behavioral and cognitive slowing that characterizes normal aging is exaggerated in dementia. While clinical observers frequently note this

Scaled Score	RAW SCORE											Scaled Score
	VERBAL TESTS						PERFORMANCE TESTS					
	Information	Digit Span	Vocabulary	Arithmetic	Comprehension	Similarities	Picture Completion	Picture Arrangement	Block Design	Object Assembly	Digit Symbol	
19	—	28	70	—	32	—	—	—	51	—	93	**19**
18	29	27	69	—	31	28	—	—	—	41	91-92	**18**
17	—	26	68	19	—	—	20	20	50	—	89-90	**17**
16	28	25	66-67	—	30	27	—	—	49	40	84-88	**16**
15	27	24	65	18	29	26	—	19	47-48	39	79-83	**15**
14	26	22-23	63-64	17	27-28	25	19	—	44-46	38	75-78	**14**
13	25	20-21	60-62	16	26	24	—	18	42-43	37	70-74	**13**
12	23-24	18-19	55-59	15	25	23	18	17	38-41	35-36	66-69	**12**
11	22	17	52-54	13-14	23-24	22	17	15-16	35-37	34	62-65	**11**
10	19-21	15-16	47-51	12	21-22	20-21	16	14	31-34	32-33	57-61	**10**
9	17-18	14	43-46	11	19-20	18-19	15	13	27-30	30-31	53-56	**9**
8	15-16	12-13	37-42	10	17-18	16-17	[illegible]	11-12	23-26	28-29	48-52	**8**
7	13-14	11	29-36	8-9	14-16	14-15	13	8-10	20-22	24-27	44-47	**7**
6	9-12	9-10	20-28	6-7	11-13	11-13	11-12	5-7	14-19	21-23	37-43	**6**
5	6-8	8	14-19	[illegible]	8-10	7-10	8-10	3-4	8-13	16-20	30-36	**5**
4	5	7	11-13	4	6-7	5-6	5-7	2	3-7	13-15	23-29	**4**
3	4	6	9-10	3	4-5	2-4	3-4	—	2	9-12	16-22	**3**
2	3	3-5	6-8	1-2	2-3	1	2	1	1	6-8	8-15	**2**
1	0-2	0-2	0-5	0	0-1	0	0-1	0	0	0-5	0-7	**1**

Figure 10-1. *Average WAIS-R profile of ten mildly demented AD patients.*

Scaled Score	RAW SCORE											Scaled Score
	VERBAL TESTS						PERFORMANCE TESTS					
	Information	Digit Span	Vocabulary	Arithmetic	Comprehension	Similarities	Picture Completion	Picture Arrangement	Block Design	Object Assembly	Digit Symbol	
19	—	28	70	—	32	—	—	—	51	—	93	**19**
18	29	27	69	—	31	28	—	—	—	41	91-92	**18**
17	—	26	68	19	—	—	20	20	50	—	89-90	**17**
16	28	25	66-67	—	30	27	—	—	49	40	84-88	**16**
15	27	24	65	18	29	26	—	19	47-48	39	79-83	**15**
14	26	22-23	63-64	17	27-28	25	19	—	44-46	38	75-78	**14**
13	25	20-21	60-62	16	26	24	—	18	42-43	37	70-74	**13**
12	23-24	18-19	55-59	15	25	23	18	17	38-41	35-36	66-69	**12**
11	22	17	52-54	13-14	23-24	22	17	15-16	35-37	34	62-65	**11**
10	19-21	15-16	47-51	12	21-22	20-21	16	14	31-34	32-33	57-61	**10**
9	17-18	14	43-46	11	19-20	18-19	15	13	27-30	30-31	53-56	**9**
8	15-16	12-13	37-42	10	17-18	16-17	14	11-12	23-26	28-29	48-52	**8**
7	13-14	11	29-36	8-9	14-16	14-15	13	8-10	20-22	24-27	44-47	**7**
6	9-12	9-10	20-28	6-7	11-13	11-13	11-12	5-7	14-19	21-23	37-43	**6**
5	6-8	8	14-19	5	8-10	7-10	8-10	3-4	8-13	16-20	30-36	**5**
4	5	7	11-13	4	6-7	5-6	5-7	2	3-7	13-15	23-29	**4**
3	4	[illegible]	9-10	3	4-5	2-4	3-4	—	2	9-12	16-22	**3**
2	3	3-5	6-8	1-2	2-3	1	2	[illegible]	[illegible]	6-8	8-15	**2**
1	0-2	0-2	0-5	0	0-1	0	0-1	0	0	0-5	0-7	**1**

Figure 10-2. *Average WAIS-R profile of ten moderately demented AD patients.*

Scaled Score	RAW SCORE											Scaled Score
	VERBAL TESTS						PERFORMANCE TESTS					
	Information	Digit Span	Vocabulary	Arithmetic	Comprehension	Similarities	Picture Completion	Picture Arrangement	Block Design	Object Assembly	Digit Symbol	
19	—	28	70	—	32	—	—	—	51	—	93	**19**
18	29	27	69	—	31	28	—	—	—	41	91-92	**18**
17	—	26	68	19	—	—	20	20	50	—	89-90	**17**
16	28	25	66-67	—	30	27	—	—	49	40	84-88	**16**
15	27	24	65	18	29	26	—	19	47-48	39	79-83	**15**
14	26	22-23	63-64	17	27-28	25	19	—	44-46	38	75-78	**14**
13	25	20-21	60-62	16	26	24	—	18	42-43	37	70-74	**13**
12	23-24	18-19	55-59	15	25	23	18	17	38-41	35-36	66-69	**12**
11	22	17	52-54	13-14	23-24	22	17	15-16	35-37	34	62-65	**11**
10	19-21	15-16	47-51	12	21-22	20-21	16	14	31-34	32-33	57-61	**10**
9	17-18	14	43-46	11	19-20	18-19	15	13	27-30	30-31	53-56	**9**
8	15-16	12-13	37-42	10	17-18	16-17	14	11-12	23-26	28-29	48-52	**8**
7	13-14	11	29-36	8-9	14-16	14-15	13	8-10	20-22	24-27	44-47	**7**
6	9-12	9-10	20-28	6-7	11-13	11-13	11-12	5-7	14-19	21-23	37-43	**6**
5	6-8	8	14-19	5	8-10	7-10	8-10	3-4	8-13	16-20	30-36	**5**
4	5	7	11-13	4	6-7	5-6	5-7	2	3-7	13-15	23-29	**4**
3	4	6	9-10	3	4-5	2-4	3-4	—	2	9-12	16-22	**3**
2	3	3-5	6-8	1-2	2-3	1	2	1	1	6-8	8-15	**2**
1	0-2	0-2	0-5	0	0-1	0	0-1	0	0	0-5	0-7	**1**

Figure 10-3. *Average WAIS-R profile of 14 HD patients.*

Scaled Score	Information	Digit Span	Vocabulary	Arithmetic	Comprehension	Similarities	Picture Completion	Picture Arrangement	Block Design	Object Assembly	Digit Symbol	Scaled Score
	RAW SCORE											
	VERBAL TESTS						PERFORMANCE TESTS					
19	—	28	70	—	32	—	—	—	51	—	93	**19**
18	29	27	69	—	31	28	—	—	—	41	91-92	**18**
17	—	26	68	19	—	—	20	20	50	—	89-90	**17**
16	28	25	66-67	—	30	27	—	—	49	40	84-88	**16**
15	27	24	65	18	29	26	—	19	47-48	39	79-83	**15**
14	26	22-23	63-64	17	27-28	25	19	—	44-46	38	75-78	**14**
13	25	20-21	60-62	16	26	24	—	18	42-43	37	70-74	**13**
12	23-24	18-19	55-59	15	25	23	18	17	38-41	35-36	66-69	**12**
11	22	17	52-54	13-14	23-24	22	17	15-16	35-37	34	62-65	**11**
10	19-21	15-16	47-51	12	21-22	20-21	[illegible]	14	31-34	32-33	57-61	**10**
9	17-18	[illegible]	43-46	11	19-20	18-19	15	[illegible]	27-30	30-31	53-56	**9**
8	15-16	12-13	37-42	[illegible]	17-18	16-17	14	11-12	23-26	28-29	48-52	**8**
7	13-14	11	29-36	8-9	14-16	14-15	[illegible]	8-10	20-22	24-27	44-47	**7**
6	9-12	9-10	20-28	6-7	11-13	11-13	11-12	5-7	14-19	21-23	37-43	**6**
5	6-8	8	14-19	[illegible]	8-10	7-10	8-10	3-4	8-13	16-20	30-36	**5**
4	5	7	11-13	4	6-7	5-6	5-7	2	3-7	13-15	23-29	**4**
3	4	6	9-10	3	4-5	2-4	3-4	—	2	9-12	16-22	**3**
2	3	3-5	6-8	1-2	2-3	1	2	1	1	6-8	8-15	**2**
1	0-2	0-2	0-5	0	0-1	0	0-1	0	0	0-5	0-7	**1**

Figure 10-4. *WAIS-R profile of two different MID patients (Patient A, solid line; Patient B, dashed line.)*

slowing, few systematic attempts have been made to prospectively document and explore slowed response and information processing in persons with dementia.

Alzheimer's Disease

Birren and Botwinick (1951) reported an early attempt to document slowing in dementia, in which they showed patients with "senile psychosis" to be slower in writing than age-matched healthy older persons. However, they interpreted this decreased writing speed to reflect aphasic disturbance rather than more basic and generalized response slowing.

Miller (1974) was among the first to systematically investigate the nature of response slowing in dementia. Examining a group of presenile AD patients and age-matched normal control subjects, Miller showed the patient group to be much slower on a simple task requiring subjects to move ten pegs from one set of holes to another. Miller then went on to compare the patient and control groups on a task designed by Singleton (1954) to study motor speed in normal aging. The task involved an apparatus in which five grooves or channels were set in a horizontal board, radiating from a central point. When cued by lights in a separate display, the subject was to move a stylus from the center, down one of the channels, and back to the center, to start a new trial. A record was made of the time spent at the central point after the cue onset. This was presumed to reflect the time taken by the subject in deciding where to move. The time taken to execute the movement was also recorded. The dementia patients were much slower than control subjects in execution of movements, with the difference in decision times being less marked. This result differed from those obtained in studies of the effects of normal aging on this task, where the most marked differences had been in decision times.

In contrast, the results of more recent studies, employing both simple and choice reaction time (RT) tasks, have suggested that it is primarily decision time that is slowed in AD. In simple reaction time tasks, the participant must respond as quickly as possible whenever a signal occurs. In choice reaction time tasks, the response is made to only one stimulus, and not to other stimuli that may occur. These studies (Ferris, Crook, Sathananthan, and Gershon, 1976; Pirozzolo, Christensen, Ogle, Hansch, and Thompson, 1981) found a disproportionately greater reaction time with choice than with simple RT procedures, when senile-onset AD patients were compared with age-matched healthy control subjects. Such differential group effects, with choice RT affected more than simple RT, are typically interpreted as evidence for greater slowing in decision processes, as compared with sensory and motor. It is important to consider this slowing when interacting with AD patients. The rate of presentation of information should be relatively slow, and sufficient time must be allowed for the patient response.

In a more recent study, Vrtunski, Patterson, Mack, and Hill (1983) compared 13 senile-onset AD patients and 34 age- and education-matched healthy control subjects on a two-choice reaction time procedure. However, the standard response key switches were replaced by pressure transducers, allowing for continuous recording of movement components. These movement components are assumed to reflect various aspects of psychomotor organization. As expected, AD patients were slower than control subjects in all movement components. However, the most striking finding was that the AD patients' psychomotor organization, as inferred from movement component relationships, appeared to be disintegrated.

Taken as a whole, the available research on behavioral slowing in AD suggests that sensory, cognitive, and motor components of response speed are slowed in comparison with healthy control subjects. Further, motor response in AD, within a choice RT paradigm, lacks the organized relationships normally seen. The observation of slowed performance across a variety of tasks can contribute to the diagnosis of AD, though it is important to evaluate slowing in comparison with appropriate age expectation. Further, the clinician must be aware of those other disorders, such as Parkinson's disease, depression, and chronic physical illness, in which slowing is also a prominent feature.

Parkinson's Disease

Bradykinesia

Response slowing has received considerable attention in PD. Slowness of movement, termed "bradykinesia," has long been recognized as a classic sign of this disorder (Klawans, 1973). Clinical observers (and neuroscientists) have variously attributed bradykinesia to a slowing of motor planning (Marsden, 1982), a slowing of motor initiation (Denny-Brown and Yanagisawa, 1976), and a slowing of response execution (Anderson and Horak, 1984).

Bradyphrenia

In addition to bradykinesia, "bradyphrenia," a slowing of cognition, is present in some Parkinson's patients. One of the first systematic attempts to study cognitive slowing in parkinsonism was published by Garron, Klawans, and Narin (1972). These investigators constructed a computer-administered set of cognitive tasks, based upon Guilford's (1967) model of intellectual functioning, which allowed measures of both speed and accuracy. Garron and colleagues found a bimodal distribution of timed scores for PD patients, but not for control subjects. Further, the intellectual performance of the faster PD patients, as shown by task accuracy, was similar to that of age-matched control subjects, while the intellectual performance of slower patients was significantly impaired. In light of other variables assessed in this study, the authors interpreted their results as consistent with the existence of two groups of PD patients: the first characterized by normal intellectual ability and cognitive speed, and the second by a greater degree of bradykinesia, slowed cognition, intellectual impairment, and later age of onset. More recently, Cummings and Benson (1984) have noted the association between cognitive slowing, forgetfulness, and difficulty in manipulation of acquired information in parkinsonism, and have discussed this within the context of the concept of "subcortical dementia."

Can Bradyphrenia be Distinguished from Bradykinesia in PD?

Given the well-documented existence of motor slowing in PD, it would seem possible that bradyphrenia might reflect a slowing of those motor behaviors by which thought is expressed (e.g., speech motor acts and writing), rather than any primary slowing of thought processes themselves. Wilson, Kaszniak, Klawans, and Garron (1980) attempted to address this issue in their comparison of nondemented PD patients and matched healthy individuals. They employed the Sternberg (1969) character classification paradigm to determine whether cognitive slowing was characteristic of PD. Within this paradigm, choice RT is measured under conditions of varying short-term memory demands. Subjects are given a variable memory set of one to four digits to remember. After a brief rehearsal time, the subject is presented with a probe digit. He or she must quickly respond with a button press or lever movement to indicate whether the probe digit is or is not a member of the memory set. Sternberg (1969) found normal subjects to show RTs that linearly increased with greater memory set size. That is, the larger the set of digits that had to be remembered, the incrementally longer it took subjects to "scan" the memory set and decide whether the probe digit was a member of the set. This linear increase in response latency held true both for correct "positive" responses (when the probe was a member of the set) and for correct "negative" responses (when the probe was not a member). The slopes of the corresponding positive and negative RT by set size functions were also found to be parallel. Sternberg (1969) interpreted the slope of the RT by set size function to represent the speed of memory scanning. The "zero intercept" (point at which the RT by set size function would intercept with the hypothetic set size of zero) was interpreted as representative of basic sensory and motor response time.

Applying this procedure to PD patients, Wilson and colleagues (1980) found memory scanning speed to be significantly slower for the older, but not the younger, PD patients. This is shown in Figure 10-5. The authors interpreted the results to support the existence of cognitive slowing, or bradyphrenia, in a subgroup of Parkinson's patients defined by age.

More recently, Rafal, Posner, Walker, and Fried-

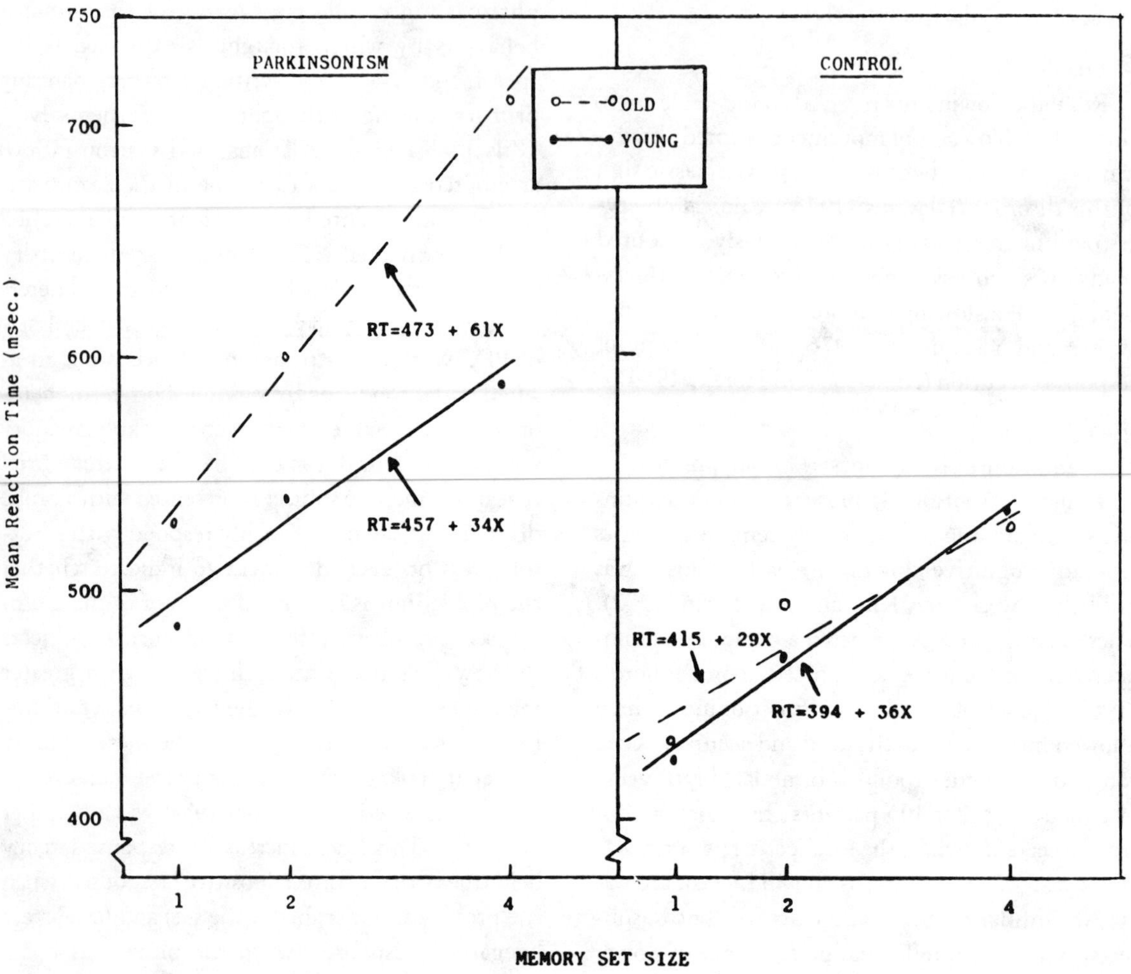

Figure 10-5. *Reaction time (RT) by memory set size slopes of performance by older and younger Parkinson's disease patients and healthy control subjects on Sternberg Character Classification Task. (From Wilson, Kaszniak, Klawans, and Garron, (1980). High speed memory scanning in Parkinsonism.* Cortex, 16, 67–72. *With permission of Masson Italia Periodici S.r.l.)*

rich (1984) examined rate of information processing in PD, employing the Sternberg paradigm. Rafal and colleagues also used two other tasks that assessed speed of shifting visual attention and duration of preparation for manual movements, respectively. For a group of ten nondemented PD patients, they found that changes in motor functioning, in response to L-DOPA, were not accompanied by changes in information processing speed. From this they argued that bradyphrenia can not be attributed to the same basal ganglia mechanisms that cause slowing of movement. Rafal and colleagues went on to suggest that bradyphrenia may be a feature characteristic of only a subgroup of Parkinson's patients.

Wilson and colleagues (1980) found slowed memory scanning only in their older PD patients, who also had a later age of disease onset. Some investigators (e.g., Lieberman et al., 1979) have found dementia in PD to be associated with older age of disease onset. It is therefore possible that bradyphrenia is an early feature of incipient dementia, occurring in patients with later age of onset. Further research is needed to test this hypothesis. Since depression can be associated with PD, and since slowed thinking is a clinical feature of depression, such research will need to disentangle the contributions of age at disease onset and depression (e.g., Swanda and Kaszniak, 1984).

Behavioral Slowing in Depression and Chronic Illness

A major depressive episode, as defined by the DSM-III (American Psychiatric Association, 1980), is often marked by slowness of movement and thought. This slowness is typically referred to as "*psychomotor retardation*." While psychomotor retardation is more common, some depressed patients may show an increase in motor activity and restlessness, referred to as "*psychomotor agitation*." As described in Chapter 14, several rating scales are available that permit the quantification of clinical observations of psychomotor retardation or agitation. Employing one such rating scale, Sarteschi, Cassano, Castrogiovanni, and Conti (1973) found psychomotor retardation or agitation to be more common in older depressed patients. Thus, the clinician must be vigilant for indications of depression when attempting to evaluate the diagnostic significance of slowing in patients suspected of dementia.

Behavioral slowing is also common in older persons with chronic physical illness. Other symptoms common in chronic illness, such as fatigue, poor appetite, weight loss, and sleep difficulty, can make differentiation from depression difficult. This symptom overlap argues for the necessity of thorough medical examination of any older individual suspected of having dementia or depression. Recent research (Okimoto et al., 1982) has also argued for the necessity of evaluating older medical patients for possible psychologic symptoms of depression. Okimoto and colleagues found psychologic symptoms, such as feeling sad, hopeless, and irritable, to be more discriminating of depression in elderly medical outpatients than somatic symptoms, such as fatigue, weight loss, and sleep difficulty. The chapter on management in this volume provides some guidance concerning interview protocols useful in screening for depression in older persons. More detailed guidance in the assessment of depression in older adults, as well as a review of relevant literature, can be found in Kaszniak and Allender (1985).

Summary

Patients with AD demonstrate slower response in motor tasks than age-matched healthy individuals, but it is not yet clear whether this is most attributable to motor or cognitive slowing. AD patients also demonstrate a disorganization of the normal relationships among various movement components. Slowing in the initiation of movement, termed bradykinesia, is a major feature of PD. While some research supports the presence of additional cognitive slowing, termed bradyphrenia, it appears to be associated primarily with a subgroup of PD patients with later age of disease onset. Psychomotor retardation or agitation is a common feature of depression, particularly in the elderly. Behavioral slowing and fatigue are also common symptoms of chronic illness in older age. The present authors are not aware of any published research specifically concerned with information processing speed in other dementias. However, speed of performance on various motor and perceptual-motor tasks has been reported to be decreased in HD (Caine, Bamford, Schiffer, Shoulson and Levy, 1986). Given the important role that the study of information processing speed has played in research and theory on normal aging and cognition, it is obvious that this topic deserves greater research effort.

CLINICAL IMPLICATIONS

1. The available research on psychometric intelligence and aging argues strongly against expecting a general decline in intelligence in normal aging. Indeed, those aspects of intelligence test performance dependent upon previously well-learned skills and knowledge are very little affected by age. Ability to solve novel problems, particularly when such problem solving requires the learning/remembering of new information, and fast performance, can be expected to decrease in normal aging. Even here, the most marked change does not occur until older old age.
2. The older adult can be expected to behave and process information more slowly than the younger person. Consequently, the experienced clinician will develop comfortable and "natural" ways of slowing the rate of questions and presentations of information to the older adult, in order to minimize the consequences of slowed processing rate.
3. Although psychometric measures of intelligence are useful in clinical assessment, the clinician must be cautious in inferring the nature of a particular patient's cognitive deficit from the pattern of subtest scores. Psychometric measures of intelligence cannot be relied upon as sensitive indicators of mild dementia.
4. Dementia patients can be expected to be considerably slower in task performance and response to instructions than healthy older persons. This necessitates that sufficient time is allowed, during both assessment and other clinical interaction, for the dementia patient to process information and respond. Dementia patients will be at a particular disadvantage when under time pressure or when stimuli are changing rapidly.
5. Task performance that is slower than age expectation raises the index of suspicion of AD. However, it must be remembered that other disorders, such as PD, depression, and chronic physical illness, can all manifest with behavioral slowing.
6. While further research is needed, RT-based measures of cognitive slowing in PD might eventually provide a means for predicting those patients who will later demonstrate dementia.

REFERENCES

American Psychiatric Association (1980). *Diagnostic and statistical manual of mental disorders (3rd ed.).* Washington, DC: American Psychiatric Association.

Anderson, M.E., and Horak, F.B. (1984). Motor effects produced by disruption of basal ganglia output to the thalamus. In J.S. McKenzie, Q.E. Kemm, and L.N. Wilcock (Eds.), *The basal ganglia: Structure and function* (pp.355-371). New York: Plenum.

Berg, C., Hertzog, C., and Hunt, E. (1982). Age differences in the speed of mental rotation. *Developmental Psychology*, *18*, 95-107.

Birren, J.E., and Botwinick, J. (1951). The relation of writing speed to age and to the senile psychoses. *Journal of Consulting Psychology*, *15*, 243-249.

Brinkman, S.D., and Braun, P. (1984). Classification of dementia patients by WAIS profile related to cholinergic deficiencies. *Journal of Clinical Neuropsychology*, 6, 393-400.

Brouwers, P., Cox, C., Martin, A., Chase, T., and Fedio, P. (1984). Differential perceptual-spatial impairment in Huntington's and Alzheimer's diseases. *Archives of Neurology*, *41*, 1073-1076.

Brust, J.C.M. (1983). Dementia and cerebrovascular disease. In R. Mayeux and W.G. Rosen (Eds.), *The dementias* (pp. 131-147). New York: Raven Press.

Caine, E.D., Bamford, K.A., Schiffer, R.B., Shoulson, I., and Levy, S. (1986). A controlled neuropsychological comparison of Huntington's disease and multiple sclerosis. *Archives of Neurology*, *43*, 249-254.

Cerella, J., Poon, L.W., and Fozard, J.L. (1981). Mental rotation and age reconsidered. *Journal of Gerontology*, *36*, 620-624.

Cerella, J., Poon, L.W., and Williams, D.M. (1980). Age and the complexity hypothesis. In L. Poon (Ed.), *Aging in the 1980's: Psychological issues* (pp. 332-342). Washington, DC: American Psychological Association.

Cummings, J.L. and Benson, F. (1984). Subcortical dementia: Review of an emerging concept. *Archives of Neurology, 14*, 874-879.

Denny-Brown, D., and Yanagisawa, N. (1976). The role of the basal ganglia in the initiation of movement. In M.D. Yahr (Ed.), *The basal ganglia* (pp. 115-149). New York: Raven Press.

Ferris, S., Crook, T., Sathananthan, G., and Gershon, S. (1976). Reaction time as a diagnostic measure in senility. *Journal of the American Geriatric Society, 12*, 529-533.

Fuld, P.A. (1982). Behavioral signs of cholinergic deficiency in Alzheimer dementia. In S. Corkin, K.L. Davis, J.H. Growdon, E. Usdin, and R.L. Wurtman (Eds.), *Aging: Vol. 19. Alzheimer's disease: A report of progress* (pp. 193-196). New York: Raven Press.

Garron, D.C., Klawans, H.L., and Narin, F. (1972). Intellectual functioning of persons with idiopathic parkinsonism. *The Journal of Nervous and Mental Disease, 154*, 445-452.

Gaylord, S.A., and Marsh, G.R. (1975). Age differences in the speed of a spatial cognitive process. *Journal of Gerontology, 30*, 674-678.

Green, R.F. (1969). Age-intelligence relationships between ages sixteen and sixty-four: A rising trend. *Developmental Psychology, 1*, 618-627.

Guilford, J.P. (1967). *The nature of human intelligence.* New York: McGraw-Hill.

Horn, J.L. (1975). Psychometric studies of aging and intelligence. In S. Gershon and A. Raskin (Eds.), *Aging: Vol. 2. Genesis and treatment of psychological disorders in the elderly* (pp. 19-43). New York: Raven Press.

Horn, J.L., and Cattell, R.B. (1967). Age differences in fluid and crystallized intelligence. *Acta Psychologica, 26*, 107-129.

Horn, J.L., and Donaldson, G. (1976). On the myth of intellectual decline in adulthood. *American Psychologist, 31*, 701-709.

Howard, D.V., Shaw, R.J., and Heisey, J.G. (1986). Aging and the time course of semantic activation. *Journal of Gerontology, 41*, 195-203.

Jones, H.E., and Conrad, H.S. (1933). The growth and decline of intelligence: A study of a homogenous group between the ages of ten and sixty. *Genetic Psychology Monographs, 13*, 223-298.

Kaszniak, A.W. and Allender, J. (1985). Psychological assessment of depression in older adults. In G.M. Chaisson-Stewart (Ed.), *Depression in the elderly: An interdisciplinary approach* (pp. 107-160). New York: John Wiley.

Klawans, H.L. (1973). *The pharmacology of extrapyramidal movement disorders.* New York: S. Karger.

Larabee, G.J., Largen, J.W., and Levin, H.S. (1985). Sensitivity of age-decline resistant ("Hold") WAIS subtests to Alzheimer's disease. *Journal of Clinical and Experimental Neuropsychology*, 7, 497-504.

Lieberman, A., Dziatolowski, M., Kupersmith, M., Serby, M., Goodgold, A., Korein, J., and Goldstein, M. (1979). Dementia in Parkinson disease. *Annals of Neurology*, 6, 335-359.

Light, K.C. (1978). Effects of mild cardiovascular and cerebrovascular disorders on serial reaction time performance. *Experimental Aging Research, 4*, 3-22.

Loranger, A.W., Goodell, H., McDowell, F.H., Lee, J.E., and Sweet, R.D. (1972). Intellectual impairment in Parkinson's syndrome. *Brain, 95*, 405-412.

Marsden, C.D. (1982). The mysterious motor function of the basal ganglia: The Robert Wartenberg Lecture. *Neurology (NY), 32*, 514-539.

Matarazzo, J.D. (1972). *Wechsler's measurement and appraisal of adult intelligence.* Baltimore: Williams and Wilkins.

Madden, D.J. (1985). Age-related slowing in the retrieval of information from long-term memory. *Journal of Gerontology, 40*, 208-210.

Miles, C.C., and Miles, W.R. (1932). The correlation of intelligence scores and chronological age from early to late maturity. *American Journal of Psychology, 44*, 44-78.

Miller, E. (1974). Psychomotor performance in presenile dementia. *Psychological Medicine, 4*, 65-68.

Miller, E. (1977). *Abnormal aging: The psychology of senile and presenile dementia.* New York: John Wiley.

Nebes, R.D. (1978). Vocal versus manual response as a determinant of age differences in simple reaction time. *Journal of Gerontology, 33*, 884-889.

Okimoto, J.T., Barnes, R.F., Veith, R.C., Raskind, M.A., Inui, T.S., and Carter, W.B. (1982). Screening for depression in geriatric medical patients. *American Journal of Psychiatry, 139*, 799-804.

Pirozzolo, F.J., Christensen, K.J., Ogle, K.M., Hansch, E.C., and Thompson, W.G. (1981). Simple and choice reaction time in dementia: Clinical implications. *Neurobiology of Aging, 2*, 113-117.

Puglisi, J.T. (1986). Age-related slowing in memory search for three-dimensional objects. *Journal of Gerontology, 41*, 72-78.

Rafal, R.D., Posner, M.J., Walker, J.A., and Friedrich,

F.J. (1984). Cognition and the basal ganglia: Separating mental and motor components of performance in Parkinson's disease. *Brain*, *107*, 1083-1094.

Salthouse, T.A. (1982). *Adult cognition: An experimental psychology of human aging*. New York: Springer-Verlag.

Salthouse, T.A. (1985). Speed of behavior and its implications for cognition. In J.E. Birren and K.W. Schaie (Eds.), *Handbook of the psychology of aging (2nd ed.)* (pp. 400-426). New York: Van Nostrand Reinhold.

Salthouse, T.A., and Somberg, B.L. (1982). Skilled performance: The effects of adult age and experience on elementary processes. *Journal of Experimental Psychology: General*, *111*, 176-207.

Sarteschi, P., Cassano, G.B., Castrogiovanni, P. and Conti, L. (1973). The use of rating scales for computer analysis of the affective symptoms in old age. *Comprehensive Psychiatry*, *14*, 371-378.

Schaie, K.W. (1983). The Seattle longitudinal study: A 21-year exploration of psychometric intelligence in adulthood. In K.W. Schaie (Ed.), *Longitudinal studies of adult psychological development* (pp. 64-135). New York: Guilford.

Singleton, W.T. (1954). The change in movement timing with age. *British Journal of Psychology*, *45*, 166-172.

Spirduso, W.W., and Clifford, P. (1978). Neuromuscular speed and consistency of performance as a function of age, physical activity level and type of physical activity. *Journal of Gerontology*, *33*, 26-30.

Sternberg, R.J. (1985). Human intelligence: The model is the message. *Science*, *230*, 1111-1118.

Sternberg, S. (1969). Memory scanning: Mental processes revealed by reaction-time experiments. *American Scientist*, *57*, 421-457.

Storandt, M., Botwinick, J., Danziger, W.L., Berg, L., and Hughes, C.P. (1984). Psychometric differentiation of mild senile dementia of the Alzheimer type. *Archives of Neurology*, *41*, 497-499.

Swanda, R.M., and Kaszniak, A.W. (1984, November). Differential effects of age of onset and depression in Parkinson's disease. *The INS Bulletin*, 40-41.

Vrtunski, P.B., Patterson, M.B., Mack, J.L., and Hill, G.O. (1983). Microbehavioral analysis of the choice reaction time response in senile dementia. *Brain*, *106*, 929-947.

Waugh, N.C., Fozard, J.L., and Thomas, J.C. (1978). Age-related differences in serial binary classification. *Experimental Aging Research*, *4*, 433-441.

Wechsler, D. (1939). *Measurement of adult intelligence*. Baltimore: Williams and Wilkins.

Wechsler, D. (1958). *The measurement and appraisal of adult intelligence*. Baltimore: Williams and Wilkins.

Weingartner, H., Kaye, W., Smalling, S.A., Ebert, M.H., Gillin, J.C., and Sitaram, N. (1981). Memory failure in progressive idiopathic dementia. *Journal of Abnormal Psychology*, *90*, 187-196.

Wilson, R.S., Kaszniak, A.W., Klawans, H.L., and Garron, D.C. (1980). High speed memory scanning in Parkinsonism. *Cortex*, *16*, 67-72.

Chapter 11

Perception and Attention in Normal Aging and Dementia

"It is because something of exterior objects penetrates in us that we see forms and that we think."

Epicurus, letter to Herodotus

Six years ago, Mr. N was diagnosed as having probable Alzheimer's disease. Since then, he has retired from his job and has continued to experience increasingly severe memory, communication, and other cognitive problems. Two years ago, his night wandering and incontinence became so frequent that his wife could no longer care for him at home. He entered a nursing home, where she continued to visit him daily. Mr. N always seemed happy to see her, and the nursing staff reported that her visits had a calming effect upon him. Yet, over the past 6 months, he often has failed to recognize his wife, and is agitated during her visits. Nurses report that he has had similar difficulty recognizing familiar staff members, and is unable to focus on a task or conversation for more than a few seconds. During a particularly painful recent visit for Mrs. N, he acted as though she were a stranger, making repeated requests that she let him see his wife.

What is the nature of Mr. N's failure to recognize his wife and other familiar persons? This type of difficulty is generally considered to indicate a failure in perceptual recognition. That is, a particular sensory stimulus fails to elicit the mental representation of its meaning.

WHY STUDY PERCEPTION AND ATTENTION?

Most clinicians who work with AD and other dementia patients are familiar with the occurrence of perceptual problems in the moderate to severe stages. Perceptual problems are manifest not only in failure to recognize familiar individuals, but also in the misperception of objects. For example, a moderate to severe AD patient may attempt to use a screwdriver as a pencil, or a comb as an eating utensil.

While the majority of such obvious perceptual problems, collectively termed "agnosias," occur in more advanced dementia, some AD patients show dramatic visuospatial deficits early in the disease course. As noted earlier in the book, this has led some writers (e.g., Albert and Moss, 1984) to conclude that there are three distinguishable subtypes of AD patients. The first, and most common, type of AD patient has memory impairment as the most striking early symptom. This memory deficit is accompanied by difficulties in abstract reasoning, in communication, and in shifting and maintaining attention. A second type of AD patient shows early symptoms of aphasia, which progressively worsen over time. Memory, abstraction, and attentional deficits become evident as the disease progresses, but are much less striking than the aphasic disorder. The third type of AD patient has marked visuospatial problems early, which are more striking than the other cognitive deficits.

Thus, clinical observation has suggested that there is a subgroup of AD patients who show visual-perceptual problems quite early in their course of dementia. It is speculated that this subgroup of patients may have a particularly severe accumulation of neuritic plaques and neurofibrillary tangles in focal brain areas that are primarily responsible for the disrupted perceptual processing. For example, Crystal, Horoupian, Katzman, and Jotkowitz (1982) reported on a patient who initially had tactual perceptual recognition problems and decreased position sense in the left hand, but no apparent memory difficulties. An isotope brain scan, electroencephalogram (EEG), and skull radiograph were all normal. Four years later, she also showed abnormal movements of the left arm, as well as memory deficit and communication difficulty. At that time, an EEG documented mild diffuse slowing, and a later CT scan showed mild cortical atrophy, somewhat greater on the right side than on the left. Biopsy of her right frontal cerebral cortex revealed numerous neuritic plaques and scattered neurofibrillary tangles, prompting a diagnosis of AD. Over the subsequent 3 years, the patient became progressively demented. Crystal and colleagues concluded that this patient's initial left-sided perceptual symptoms were due to a right hemisphere focal accentuation of the neuritic plaques and neurofibrillary tangles of AD.

The striking perceptual deficits seen late in the course of dementia for most AD patients, and early for a small subgroup, are clinically obvious. However, as this chapter will demonstrate, more subtle perceptual processing deficits are common relatively early in the disease course. In addition, problems in attentional focusing and capacity are also pervasive. These perceptual and attentional deficits limit the efficiency of all other cognitive processing, and are important considerations in clinical assessment. As Albert and Moss (1984) point out, problems in perception and attention can significantly contaminate the measurement of other processes, such as memory.

The purpose of this chapter is to review research on visual perception and on attention in normal aging and dementia. Research concerned with AD will be the focus, although other dementing illnesses will be discussed where research evidence is available. These data are of clinical utility only within the contexts of knowledge concerning the role of perception and attention in cognition.

THE ROLE OF PERCEPTION AND ATTENTION IN HUMAN INFORMATION PROCESSING

Understanding the role of perception and attention requires an examination of how environmental events are transformed into mental representations. Most conceptualizations of human information processing hypothesize that information flows through a series of stages or processes from the sensory receptors to some "higher" level of representation (c.f. Reed, 1982; Rumelhart, 1977; Wickelgren, 1979).

Traditionally, the relevant mental structures and processes responsible for this transformation have been described by the hypothetic constructs of sensation, perception and attention. Admittedly, the distinctions between these are rather arbitrary. Further, it is likely, as Fodor (1983) argues, that the characteristic operations of transformations differ between the various sensory modalities. The use of terms such as sensation, perception, and attention would seem to suggest relatively discrete processing stages. However, information processing is more appropriately conceptualized as a continuous operation, with at least some degree of parallel processing. Traditional conceptions hypothesize that transformations of sensory input occur in a "bottom– up" direction, from sensory receptor to higher levels of processing. Research evidence also argues for the existence of processing in a "top–down" manner, with higher order mechanisms exerting control upon sensory and perceptual transformations. Rumelhart (1977) provides a detailed discussion of this research.

A general schema for conceptualizing the relationships between sensory systems, perception or pattern recognition systems, attention, and other cognitive processes is presented in Figure 11-1, taken from Rumelhart (1977). The terms employed and relationships indicated in this figure will be clarified in what follows within the present chapter. For the moment, it is important to note that environmental stimuli are conceived of as eventuating in mental representations through the activities of a number of distinguishable processes. Theoretically, age group differences and dementia patient deficits could result from change in any or all of these processes. It must be emphasized that changes in the early aspects of information processing, such as sensory receptor functioning or perceptual pattern detection, can have significant effects upon "higher" cognitive processes. For example, limitations in visual acuity and failure to extract critical features from visual-perceptual representations would result in a degraded mental representation of a stimulus. If this representation is sufficiently degraded, it may fail to activate appropriate concepts or schema in semantic memory. The result would be an individual who fails to think about or respond to the visual environment in expected ways.

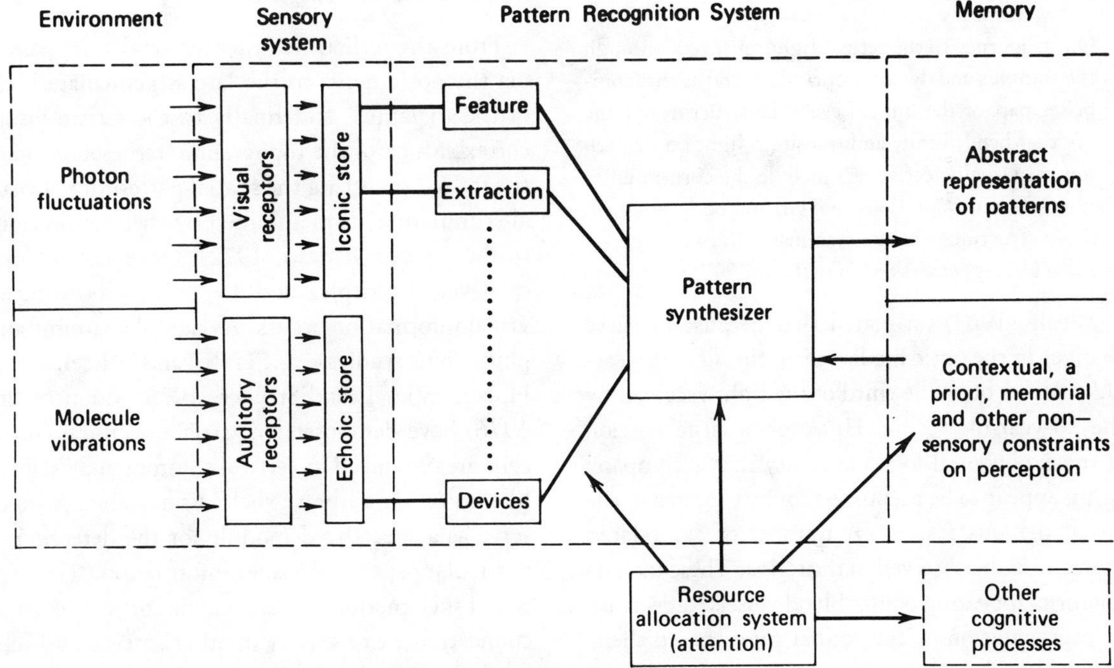

Figure 11-1. *Schematic illustration of relationships among sensory systems, perception, attention, and other cognitive processes. (From Rumelhart, D. E. {1977}.* Introduction to human information processing. *New York: John Wiley, by permission. Copyright 1977 by John Wiley).*

VISUAL PERCEPTION IN NORMAL AGING

In the examination of perception presented in the present chapter, only visual perception will be discussed. The decision to limit discussion to the visual system is based on three considerations. First, auditory perception, a critical function for human communication, was already briefly reviewed in a previous chapter. Second, the most striking perceptual problems in AD involve visuospatial processing. Third, considerably more is known about visual processing in normal aging (c.f. Hoyer and Plude, 1980) and AD.

Sensory Receptors and Aging

Age-related changes in visual information processing can be found within the most peripheral aspects of the visual system, the optic media. As Kline and Schieber (1985) state, in their recent review of this area:

> On its journey to the retina, light must pass through the complex and dynamic optical apparatus that comprises part of the human eye. The structures of the eye that bend, limit, and transform light on its path toward visual effectiveness include the cornea, anterior chamber, pupil, lens, and vitreous body. . . . All these structures change systematically with age — some greatly, others only a little. (p. 297)

Weale (1963) estimated that because of these changes in the optic media, the retina of a 60-year-old receives only one third of the light received by the 20-year-old retina. However, a large portion of the exponential losses in acuity that accompany aging appear to be accounted for by changes in the visual nervous system. A number of age-related changes can be observed in the retina. These include sclerotic-appearing ocular blood vessels, a decrease in pigmentation of the retinal pigment epithelium, a loss of photoreceptors, and atrophy of bipolar and ganglia cells (Kline and Schieber, 1985). These structural changes in the retina contribute to age-related alteration in amplitude and latency of the summated electroretinogram (see Fozard, Wolf, Bell, McFarland and Podolsky, 1977), an indicator of the physiologic activity of retinal cells.

It must also be pointed out that a number of pathologic changes of the visual system increase in incidence with older age. Those most significant age-related changes include glaucoma, cataract, diabetic retinopathy and senile macular degeneration (Kline and Schieber, 1985). While these disorders do not affect all older persons, when present they markedly impair the quality of visual information processing.

Aging and Perceptual Processing

In addition to changes with age in sensory receptor structure and function, age-related postsensory information processing changes impose further limitations. As will be seen, these limitations are particularly salient for stimuli that are brief or that change rapidly.

Anatomic and Physiologic Changes

From the retina, neurosensory codes are passed via the optic nerve to the lateral geniculate body of the thalamus, and finally to the striate visual cortex. Much of the topographic representation of the retina, reflecting the spatial patterning of visual stimulation, is maintained by these projections to the cortex (Geldard, 1972). Once at the cortical level, a complex and hierarchic processing of visual information occurs. As careful anatomic and physiologic studies (e.g., Hubel and Wiesel, 1968; Hubel, Wiesel, and Stryker, 1978; Mountcastle, 1976) have demonstrated, striate occipital cortex cells are organized in vertical columns and "slabs," like books on a library shelf. Each slab appears to serve as a specialized module for the detection of particular aspects of visual information. The output of such modules is carried, via cortical–cortical connections, to a variety of other cortical and subcortical areas, for further information processing (see Changeux, 1985, pp. 52–66, for a highly readable further discussion).

Cortical structural and chemical changes with aging contribute to the variety of visual-perceptual changes described here. Structural changes include a decrease in visual cortex neuronal population (Devaney and Johnson, 1980), and a decrease in the number of dendritic spines, critical for synaptic communication between neurons (Cotman and Holets, 1985; Scheibel, Lindsay, Tomiyasu, and Scheibel, 1975). Chemical changes include an alteration in the synthesis and breakdown of neurotransmitters employed within the visual cortex (Rogers and Bloom, 1985).

Perceptual Psychologic Phenomena and Aging

As Hoyer and Plude (1980) point out, "All perceptual processes take time, and therefore *time* constitutes one type of limitation to perceptual processing. A second type of limit to processing is *space*, which has to do with how much information can be handled at any one moment" (p. 228). Most of the available evidence concerning perceptual processing and aging has focused on time limitations.

Information processing models have typically hypothesized the existence of modality-specific postsensory mechanisms that enable brief storage of information for further processing. These mechanisms are collectively referred to as "sensory memory." The sensory memory system specific to visual information processing has been labeled "iconic memory" (Neisser, 1967), whereas that specific to the auditory system is termed "echoic memory" (Crowder, 1980; Neisser, 1967).

Iconic Memory: A Stage of Visual Information Processing

Iconic memory has commonly been measured by the *backward masking technique*. Hoyer and Plude (1980) explain the nature of masking phenomena as follows:

> When two visual stimuli are flashed in rapid succession, their visual traces interact. When the first stimulus obscures the second, the phenomenon is called forward masking; when the second stimulus obscures the first, it is called backward masking. In either case the interference results because the visual system takes some amount of time to clear or to recover from stimulation. The longer this signal processing takes, the greater is the opportunity for masking to occur. Susceptibility to masking . . . is usually indexed by the critical period required to escape masking effects. (p. 229)

In a typical backward masking experiment, a target letter or number is presented for a short duration (usually varying from about 10 to 150 ms), followed by a masking stimulus, which effectively terminates the display. The duration of exposure necessary for successful target identification is recorded. Walsh, Till, and Williams (1978) employed this technique in a series of studies, and found a constant though small increase with age in the time required to escape masking. Another method used to study iconic memory and aging presents multiple letters followed by a mask. Speed, accuracy, and identification rate for the letters are evaluated. Using this approach, Cerella, Poon, and Fozard (1982) found a slowing in the rate of older adults' correct letter identification, which was similar in magnitude to the slowing found by Walsh and colleagues (1978).

Most recently, Gilmore, Allan, and Royer (1986) have assessed iconic memory in aging, using the partial report paradigm designed by Sperling (1960). Within this paradigm, visual displays consist of nine letters, arranged in either three rows or three columns, defined by physical proximity. After a warning signal, the letter display is presented for a brief duration, followed by an auditory signal indicating which row or column the participant is to report. Application of this paradigm with younger adults (Sperling, 1960) had shown such partial report (in contrast to full report of the visual display) to suggest that iconic memory preserves, very briefly, the entire display. Gilmore and colleagues replicated this result with both their younger (mean age = 22.1 years) and older (mean age = 68.6 years) adult samples. However, accuracy decreased more for the older adults, with increasing duration between onset of the visual display and onset of the auditory cue. These results are consistent with somewhat more rapid decay of the icon for older persons.

Older persons thus appear to require longer visual stimulus exposure than younger adults, and may also be characterized by a more rapid decay of iconic memory. In addition, recent research suggests that older persons may have a deficit in perceptual organization.

Evidence of Perceptual Organization Deficit with Aging

One approach to the study of perceptual organization employs a visual search task, requiring the participant to find a target stimulus within a visual array. On the basis of results generated by this approach, Farkas and Hoyer (1980) concluded that older adults experience smaller "perceptual units" than younger adults. The concept of perceptual units comes from studies demonstrating that various aspects of spatial organization determine how stimuli are grouped into organized units (e.g., Prinzmetal and Banks, 1977). Organization into perceptual units aids in locating target elements within a display, presumably by reducing the information processing load. The work of Farkas and Hoyer (1980) suggests that older adults differ from younger adults in their initial segregation of an array into perceptual units. The presumed consequence is that elderly adults have a greater burden in making decisions about the content of the display.

Recently, Gilmore, Tobias, and Royer (1985) compared younger (mean age = 20 years) and older (mean age = 68.8 years) adults in the extent to which perceptual grouping by proximity and similarity predicts the formation of perceptual units. In this study, the dependent variable was the time taken to determine the presence or absence of a target letter in visual arrays of one, five, or nine elements. Relationships among the elements were varied in terms of proximity and similarity. Both age groups were able to take advantage of organization by proximity or similarity for smaller (i.e., four) numbers of nontarget elements. However, the older adults were not able to benefit from such organization when the array consisted of eight nontarget elements. Gilmore and colleagues (1985) concluded that older persons have a reduction in the size of perceived visual units. Discussing the implications of this observation, Gilmore and colleagues (1985) state:

> A reduction in the size of the unit that can be effective in the early stage of image analysis can have a profound impact on higher stages of processing. . . . The chunking or grouping of similar visual information permits the isolation and analysis of more unique information by the processor. If the visual unit is reduced, then the total amount of visual information that is captured by this limited capacity system must also be reduced. The lower levels of information made available by the initial stage of processing can have a ripple effect on the system resulting in slower and less efficient processing at each successive stage. (p. 592).

Summary

Available evidence indicates that the representation of visual information within iconic memory decays more rapidly for older than for younger adults. Older adults therefore require longer stimulus exposure in order to maintain comparable accuracy of stimulus identification. This age-related change places the elderly at a perceptual disadvantage when visual stimuli are very brief or rapidly changing. Further, older adults have a reduced size of the perceived visual unit. This results in a reduction in the total amount of visual information that can be initially captured and further analyzed. A less complete or elaborate mental representation would thus be available to "higher" cognitive processes, such as concept or schema activation. Beyond a certain point, a mental representation may be so degraded that it no longer activates the appropriate concept or schema.

ATTENTION AND AGING

The concept of attention has a long history within psychology. William James (1890) conceived of attention as that mental process whereby focus was placed upon one out of several possible objects or trains of thought, and through which concentration of consciousness occurred. Thus, two aspects of attention were hypothesized: (1) a selective property through which a particular feature of perception or thought is made the focus of awareness, and (2) a concentration (capacity) property through which mental effort amplifies or enhances a mental representation. These two aspects continue to be studied by cognitive psychologists (see Kahneman, 1973; Reed, 1982, pp. 38–61).

Selective Attention

Several authors (e.g., Layton, 1975; Schonfield, 1974) suggest that aging is associated with a deficit in the ability to extract relevant from irrelevant information. This suggestion is derived from the results of several experiments in which older and younger persons are compared in paradigms requiring them to ignore irrelevant information. In some of these paradigms (e.g., Rabbitt, 1965), participants are required to detect a target that changes position in a visual display as the number of nontarget items is increased. Within this type of task, participants find it increasingly difficult to detect a target as the number of nontarget items increases. Rabbitt (1965) found the magnitude of the display size effect to be larger for older than for younger adults. Rabbitt concluded that older persons have more difficulty ignoring irrelevant stimuli.

This conclusion has been questioned by Wright and Elias (1979). They point out that nontargets in visual-search tasks must first be discriminated from targets. Hence, obtained age differences may reflect difficulty in *discriminating* relevant from irrelevant stimuli, rather than in *ignoring* irrelevant information. Wright and Elias employed a different experimental paradigm, in which younger and older adults were required to respond, as quickly as possible, to a target presented at the center of a display. On some trials, other items bordered the target stimulus. The target responses of both age groups were slowed by the presence of irrelevant stimuli. Further, the magnitude of this effect was comparable for the two age groups.

More recently, Nissen and Corkin (1985) reported on a comparison of younger (mean age = 19.4 years) and older (mean age = 63.6 years) adults on a visual reaction time task. In this task, a warning cue appeared at the beginning of each trial indicating the probable location of a target signal. The reaction times of both groups were shortest when the stimulus appeared at the expected (that is, the cued) location. Reaction times were longest when the target appeared at an unexpected location. Both groups were faster on trials preceded by a 3 second warning interval than on those with a 2 second warning interval. These effects of spatial and temporal expectancy were as large in the older group as in the younger group. Thus, the selective function of attentional processes, as measured in this study, appears to be maintained in older people.

Other recent studies have also failed to find older persons to be more affected by irrelevant stimuli than younger persons. Nebes and Madden (1983) found no age effect on the ability to detect a target presented in a color different from nontargets. Similarly, Gilmore and colleagues (1985) found both younger and older adults equally able to take advantage of the organization of spatial arrays in finding a target among nontarget elements.

In summary, early studies had suggested an age-associated deficit in the ability to extract relevant from irrelevant information. However, the results obtained in these studies more likely reflected perceptual than attentional factors. More recent research has failed to find age differences in the ability to segment and select visual information on the basis of precued spatial location, color, and small areas of spatial similarity. The selective function of attentional processes, at least within the visual information processing system, thus appears to be maintained with aging.

Attentional Capacity

In addition to the selective aspects of attention just described, recent formulations of attention (e.g., Hoyer and Plude, 1980; Kahneman, 1973) have emphasized *capacity limitations*. In an influential paper, Hasher and Zacks (1979) pointed out that information processing operations vary in their attentional capacity requirements. Some operations, termed "automatic," use little of the person's limited capacity for attention. Other operations, termed "effortful," require much attentional capacity. Examples of automatic operations include the discrimination of basic sensory features of stimuli, and the execution of familiar and well-practiced skills. Examples of effortful processes include the active rehearsal of information the person wishes to remember, and the comprehension of information conveyed in complex sentence structures. Similar distinctions were previously drawn between *automatic* and *controlled* processes (Schneider and Schiffrin, 1977), and between *conscious* and *unconscious* processes (Posner and Snyder, 1974). Effortful, controlled, or conscious processes are presumed to make greater demands upon limited processing resources. Automatic or unconscious processes make fewer demands.

The influence of the Hasher and Zacks (1979) formulation on research in gerontologic psychology resulted from their hypothesizing of a specific age relationship in automatic and effortful processing. They reasoned that if there is an age-related decrease in the capacity of attention, then those tasks that require effortful processing are likely to be more difficult for older persons than tasks that can be performed automatically. A variety of tasks have been employed in recent research attempting to test the prediction of differential age effects in automatic versus effortful processing. A frequently employed paradigm involves examining age differences in the ability of young and old individuals to perform two tasks simultaneously. In this paradigm, the amount of practice, or other task dimensions, are varied in order to manipulate the degree to which one or both tasks can be automatically versus effortfully processed. The literature based upon this paradigm is large and complex, and no attempt will be made to review studies in detail here.

There are several reports of "divided attention" tasks presenting particular problems for older adults (e.g., Wright, 1981). Other studies (e.g., Somberg and Salthouse, 1982) find no age differences in single versus dual task performance. These mixed results may be due in part to a range of methodologic and conceptual problems inherent in all of the published studies (see Salthouse, 1982, pp. 177–198 for review).

However, recent research suggests that the automatic versus effortful processing distinction may also explain discrepancies between the findings of earlier divided attention and aging studies. Somberg and Salthouse (1982) failed to find any marked age differences in a dual-task paradigm that required only sensory processing. A subsequent study (Salthouse, Rogan and Prill, 1984), using more complex divided attention tasks, revealed large age differences. If it is assumed that the sensory tasks can be performed more automatically, whereas more complex tasks require greater effort, then these results are consistent with the Hasher and Zacks (1979) hypothesis.

Despite the attractiveness of the Hasher and Zacks hypothesis, it must be pointed out that distinguishing between what is automatic and effortful is not always clear-cut. Applying the distinction to explain the effects of task complexity may seem circular. Nonetheless, the idea that tasks vary in the demand they place upon a limited capacity processing system, and that older adults have decreased capacity, remains intriguing. In terms of practical implications, these ideas suggest that the performance of older adults is facilitated when tasks are designed to maximize reliance upon familiar and well-practiced skills. As will be discussed in the subsequent chapter, the distinction between automatic and effortful processing has also been invoked to explain age group differences in memory for events.

Summary

Age-related changes are seen in anatomic and functional aspects of visual sensory reception. Other aspects of early visual information processing, affecting the quality of visual perception, also change with aging. These include a faster decay in iconic memory, despite apparently unchanged capacity of this brief visual storage process, and a reduction in size of the perceptual unit. Both of these changes likely have "ripple effects" upon later aspects of the processing of visual information.

Selective aspects of visual attention do not change significantly with older age, and attentional capacity is reduced in older age only when multiple complex tasks must be simultaneously performed. It has been proposed that age group differences in the performance of complex dual tasks reflect an age related decrease in the capacity of effortful processing resources. However, the general status of proposed age-relationships between effortful and automatic information processing remains controversial.

PERCEPTION AND ATTENTION IN DEMENTIA

Perception and attention have not been as fully studied in dementia as in normal aging. Given the relative paucity of empirical data, the studies reviewed here must be interpreted with caution until sufficient replication and extension of findings are available.

Visual-Perceptual and Visual-Constructive Deficits in Dementia

Visual-Perceptual Deficits

Severe visual-perceptual deficits, referred to as visual agnosia in the clinical literature, have been noted by clinical observers of dementia patients. Ernst, Dalby, and Dalby (1970) were among the earliest of investigators to empirically study visual perception in presenile dementia patients. They documented a range of visual recognition problems in a group of nine patients, but found no single characteristic impairment pattern.

More recently, Eslinger and Benton (1983) investigated spatial and nonspatial visual perceptual abilities in a group of 40 older dementia patients (of mixed etiology) and a group of age-matched healthy control subjects. The spatial and nonspatial tasks employed were, respectively, the Benton Line Orientation Test (Benton, Varney and Hamsher, 1978) and the Benton Facial Recognition Test (Benton and Van Allen, 1968). The Line Orientation Test requires the participant to select from an array of different angled lines the one that matches the angle of a target line. The Facial Recognition Test requires the selection from a set of six pictured faces, varying in person, angle, and lighting, those that match a target face. The dementia patients, as a group, were significantly impaired on both of these tasks. In a study specifically comparing mild to moderate AD patients with age-matched healthy control subjects, Wilson, Kaszniak, Bacon, Fox, and Kelly (1982) found the patients to be significantly impaired on the Benton Facial Recognition Test.

Visual-Constructive Deficits

In addition to visual-perceptual deficits, related difficulties with visual-constructive tasks also are observed in dementia patients. Typical tasks involve asking the patient to copy a pattern of blocks arranged by the examiner, or the copying of geometric drawings. Examples of attempts made

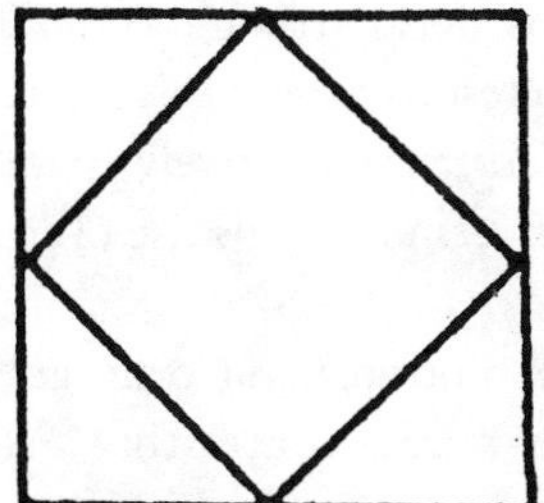

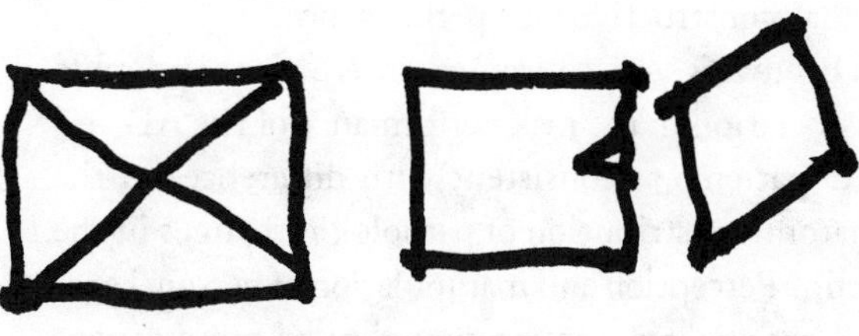

Figure 11-2. *Geometric example (*left*) and attempts of a moderately demented AD patient (*right*) to copy example.*

by a moderately demented AD patient to copy drawings are presented in Figure 11-2. Visual-constructive deficits appear common in even mildly demented AD patients. Storandt, Botwinick, Danziger, Berg, and Hughes (1984) found mild AD patients to make significantly more errors than age-matched healthy control subjects on a geometric design copy task. Further, this same group of investigators found that the number of these errors was predictive of the rate of dementia progression. Those mild AD patients who progressed to moderate or severe dementia over 1 year committed a greater number of geometric design copying errors at initial examination (Berg et al., 1984).

Visual-Perceptual and Visual-Constructive Deficits in AD versus HD

Brouwers, Cox, Martin, Chase, and Fedio (1984) reported a study in which they compared mild AD and HD patients with healthy control subjects on a variety of visuospatial and visual-constructive tasks. The AD and HD patient groups were comparable in WAIS Full-Scale IQ and in scores on a commonly employed psychometric measure of memory abilities. The results demonstrated significant visuospatial and visual-constructive impairment, relative to healthy control subjects, for both the AD and HD patients. However, each patient group exhibited a different pattern of impairment. The AD group demonstrated greatest impairment in extrapersonal visuospatial perception and visual-constructive ability, but were unimpaired on tasks assessing perception of egocentric (personal) spatial coordinates. The HD patients showed their greatest impairment when manipulation of personal space was required by a task, but were not impaired in visual-constructive task performance.

Brouwers and colleagues interpret this double dissociation in the task performance of the AD and HD patients as consistent with differences in the anatomic distribution of pathologic changes in the brain. Perception and manipulation of personal spatial coordinates were presumed to be more dependent upon the integrity of frontal lobe cerebral structures, which are more damaged in HD. Extrapersonal visuospatial and visual-constructive task performance was presumed to be more dependent upon parietal lobe structures, which are more damaged in AD. Differences between dementia patient groups in various aspects of visuospatial and visual-constructive ability, as demonstrated by Brouwers and colleagues, could be of potential diagnostic and clinical management value. Replication of these observations, and extension to other dementia patient groups, would thus be of considerable interest.

Specifying the Locus of Visual-Perceptual Deficit in AD

While visual-perceptual impairment thus is well documented in AD, the studies just described do not clarify the locus of impairment in visual information processing. Schlotterer, Moscovitch, and Crapper-McLachlan (1983) have investigated visual acuity and spatial frequency contrast sensitivity in AD patients and healthy age-matched control subjects. Spatial frequency contrast sensitivity is a basic perceptual capacity of the visual system, presumed to be at the basis of all spatial perception. It is measured by the number of alternating pairs of black and white regions, termed "sinusoidal gratings," that can be perceived per degree of visual angle. AD patients who ranged from mild to moderate dementia severity did not differ from age-matched healthy control subjects in either visual acuity or spatial frequency contrast sensitivity. However, both groups were impaired on these measures, relative to younger adult subjects. Thus, AD does not involve any greater change than that seen in normal aging, in more peripheral aspects of visual sensory and perceptual functioning. Spatial frequency contrast sensitivity has been observed to be impaired in patients with focal striate (occipital) cortex lesions. It is of interest to note in this respect that in AD, the striate cortex is relatively spared from the degenerative effects of the disease (Terry and Katzman, 1983).

In the same paper, Schlotterer and colleagues (1983) also reported a study contrasting AD patients, healthy age-matched control subjects, and healthy younger adult control subjects on a visual pattern backward masking task. Schlotterer and associates found, as would be predicted from the normal aging research, that the older healthy adults required more time to escape the effects of the mask than did the younger adults. The AD patient group was not different from the healthy older adult control subjects when the backward masking stimulus was a homogeneous light flash, the effects of which are assumed to involve relatively peripheral visual factors. However, when the backward masking stimulus was a visual pattern, the AD patients required significantly more processing time to escape the effects of the patterned backward mask. This argues that AD patients, who experience only normal aging changes in the more peripheral processes contributing to iconic memory, are more impaired than age-matched control subjects in higher-order central contributors to this early visual information process.

Thus, AD patients show only normal aging limitations in visual acuity and frequency contrast sensitivity. However, AD patients do demonstrate greater than age-expected slowing in the preattentive visual information process labeled as iconic memory. This suggests that at least one contributor to the visual-perceptual impairment of AD patients involves a slowing of post–striate cortex processing of visual information. While longitudinal studies of these visual processing phenomena are not yet available, it is likely that such slowing begins early in the disease course. Except for that small subgroup of AD patients with dramatic early visuospatial deficit, progression to severe impairment does not occur until the moderate to severe dementia stages.

Attention in Dementia

Selective Attention Deficit in AD

In an early study of selective attention, employing a sample of presenile dementia patients, Lawson, McGhie, and Chapman (1967) required subjects to report sets of visual or auditory digits. Some of the stimulus trials were presented against a background of auditory or visual distracting stimuli. Compared with normal control subjects, the dementia patients were significantly more distracted in the auditory modality, but not in the visual modality. However, as Miller (1977, p. 72) points out, because the two conditions (visual and auditory) were not matched in terms of their potency as distractors, no conclusions can be drawn about any modality difference in the effects of distraction.

Selective attention within the visual modality has often been studied with digit (Lewis and Kupke, 1977) or letter (Talland and Schwab, 1964) cancellation tasks. In these tasks, the subject must cross out a particular printed digit or letter with a pencil every time it occurs within a string of other digits or letters. Using the digit cancellation task, Allender and Kaszniak (1985) found moderately demented AD patients to be impaired relative to age and education-matched healthy control subjects. The set of tasks within the "attention" subscale of the Mattis Dementia Rating Scale (MDRS) (Mattis, 1976) includes a similar letter cancellation task. In one study, impairment was not seen on the MDRS attention subscale for mild AD patients relative to normal control subjects (Vitaliano, Russo, Breen, Vitiello, and Prinz, 1986). However, impairment was found on this subscale as the patients' dementia progressed over time and as their ability to function in their home environment decreased. Thus, impairment of selective attention sufficient to interfere with digit or letter cancellation performance does not seem to occur until the AD patient is moderately demented.

Another study that can be considered to assess an aspect of selective attention was reported by Hutton, Johnston, Shapiro, and Pirozzolo (1979). Examining eye movements with a photoelectric infrared technique, Hutton and colleagues documented what they termed "oculomotor programming disturbances" in three AD patients of unspecified dementia severity. That is, the pattern of the AD patients' visual scanning of simple and complex visual stimuli, in response to the examiner's questions, was poorly regulated and planned, in comparison with that of control subjects. Thus, the AD patients were impaired in their ability to systematically search their visual environment. A clinical implication of this deficit is that AD patients do not "take in" important information present in the visual environment. Some of the disorientation of AD patients, as well as some instances of inappropriate behavior, likely reflect a failure to selectively focus the gaze upon salient visual cues.

Attentional Capacity in AD

While available research documents a deficit in the selective attention of AD patients, the status of their *attentional capacity*, as it has been studied in normal aging, is unclear. To the authors' knowledge, no research on attentional capacity in dementia, comparable with that found in the normal aging literature (e.g., employing dual-task methodologies) has been reported. However, the present authors' clinical experience suggests that attentional capacity is impaired in AD, relative to healthy persons of comparable age.

Summary

The striate cortex and prestriate visual information processing in AD patients is comparable with that of healthy older persons. However, the central processes that contribute to iconic memory are more slowed in AD. This slowing likely contributes to those severe visual-perceptual and visual-constructive deficits frequently noted by clinical observers.

Further research on attention in dementia is needed. Available research does argue for deficit in selective aspects of attention in AD, but insufficient data are presently available on attentional capacity.

Problems in attention and perception can significantly contaminate the measurement of other constructs, particularly memory. A better understanding of the nature of attentional and perceptual problems in AD and other dementing illnesses would assist the clinician and investigator in developing procedures to minimize the influence of these deficits in the assessment of other cognitive domains.

CLINICAL IMPLICATIONS

1. Age-associated changes in sensory processes necessitate that modifications in illumination, size of visual stimuli, and complexity of visual presentations be considered when working with the older adult.
2. Reduction in attentional capacity with aging implies that task complexity be carefully considered in clinical interactions with older individuals. Multiple task processing demands, particularly when each component task is relatively complex, and therefore demanding of greater effortful processing resources, will place the older person at a disadvantage.
3. Directing the older person's selective attention (e.g., spatial or temporal cuing) can be expected to improve performance to the same degree as that of younger adults.
4. AD patient deficits in both perception and attention must be taken into account in any attempt to assess other aspects of cognition and communication.
5. Reduction in stimulus complexity, and procedures designed to increase the degree to which stimuli are attended to (e.g., through increasing stimulus size, novelty, or color) will be necessary to insure that information "enters" the patient's processing system.
6. The selective attention deficits of AD patients likely contribute to their spatial disorientation and the occurrence of behavior inappropriate to a particular context. Emphasizing those visual cues important to orientation (e.g., the sink, stove, and refrigerator indicate that we are in the kitchen), through pointing and verbal description, may improve the orientation of mildly demented patients. However, moderately to severely demented patients may lack the ability to utilize these cues in guiding their visual attention.

REFERENCES

Albert, M., and Moss, M. (1984). The assessment of memory disorders in patients with Alzheimer's disease. In L.R. Squire and N. Butters (Eds.), *Neuropsychology of memory* (pp. 236-246). New York: Guilford.

Allender, J., and Kaszniak, A.W. (1985, February). *Processing of emotional cues and personality change in dementia of the Alzheimer's type.* Paper presented at the 13th annual meeting of the International Neuropsychological Society, San Diego, CA.

Benton, A.L., and Van Allen, M.W. (1968). Impairment in facial recognition in patients with cerebral disease. *Cortex*, *4*, 344-358.

Benton, A.L., Varney, N.R., and Hamsher, K. (1978). Visuospatial judgment: A clinical test. *Archives of Neurology*, *35*, 364-367.

Berg, L., Danziger, W.L., Storandt, M., Coben, L.A., Gado, H., Hughes, C.P., Knesevich, J.W., and Botwinick, J. (1984). Predictive features in mild senile dementia of the Alzheimer type. *Neurology (Cleveland)*, *34*, 563-569.

Brouwers, P., Cox, C., Martin, A., Chase, T., and Fedio, P. (1984). Differential perceptual-spatial impairment in Huntington's and Alzheimer's diseases. *Archives of Neurology*, *41*, 1073-1076.

Cerella, J., Poon, L.W., and Fozard, J.L. (1982). Age and iconic read-out. *Journal of Gerontology*, *37*, 197-202.

Changeux, J.P. (1985). *Neuronal man: The biology of mind.* New York: Pantheon.

Cotman, C.W., and Holets, V.R. (1985). Structural changes at synapses with age: Plasticity and regeneration. In C.E. Finch and E.L. Schneider (Eds.), *Handbook of the biology of aging* (pp. 617-644). New York: Van Nostrand Reinhold.

Crowder, R.G. (1980). Echoic memory and the study of aging memory systems. In L.W. Poon, J.L. Fozard, L.S. Cermak, D. Arenberg, and L.W. Thompson (Eds.), *New directions in memory and aging* (pp. 181-204). Hillsdale, NJ: Lawrence Erlbaum.

Crystal, H.A., Horoupian, D.S., Katzman, R., and Jotkowitz, S. (1982). Biopsy-proved Alzheimer disease presenting as a right parietal lobe syndrome. *Annals of Neurology*, *12*, 186-188.

Devaney, K.O., and Johnson, H.A. (1980). Neuron loss in the aging visual cortex of man. *Journal of Gerontology*, *35*, 836-841.

Ernst, B., Dalby, A., and Dalby, M.A. (1970). Gnostic-praxic disturbances in presenile dementia. *Acta Neurologica Scandinavica, Supplement*, *43*, 101-102.

Eslinger, P.J., and Benton, A.L. (1983). Visuoperceptual performances in aging and dementia: Clinical and theoretical implications. *Journal of Clinical Neuropsychology*, *5*, 213-220.

Farkas, M.S., and Hoyer, W.J. (1980). Processing consequences of perceptual grouping in selective attention. *Journal of Gerontology*, *35*, 207-216.

Fodor, J.A. (1983). *The modularity of the mind.* Cambridge, MA: MIT Press.

Fozard, J.L., Wolf, E., Bell, B., McFarland, R.A., and Podolsky, S. (1977). Visual perception and communication. In J.E. Birren and K.W. Schaie (Eds.), *Handbook of the psychology of aging* (pp. 497-534). New York: Van Nostrand Reinhold.

Geldard, F.A. (1972). *The human senses.* New York: John Wiley.

Gilmore, G.C., Allan, T.M., and Royer, F.L. (1986). Iconic memory and aging. *Journal of Gerontology*, *41*, 183-190.

Gilmore, G.C., Tobias, T.R., and Royer, F.L. (1985). Aging and similarity grouping in visual search. *Journal of Gerontology*, *40*, 586-592.

Hasher, L., and Zacks, R.T. (1979). Automatic and effortful processes in memory. *Journal of Experimental Psychology: General*, *108*, 356-388.

Hoyer, W.J., and Plude, D.J. (1980). Attentional and perceptual processes in the study of cognitive aging. In L.W. Poon (Ed.), *Aging in the 1980's: Psychological issues* (pp. 227-238). Washington, DC: American Psychological Association.

Hubel, D.H., and Wiesel, T.N. (1968). Receptive fields and functional architecture of the monkey striate cortex. *Journal of Physiology*, *195*, 215-243.

Hubel, D.H., Wiesel, T.N., and Stryker, M.P. (1978). Anatomical demonstration of orientation columns in the macaque monkey. *Journal of Comparative Neurology*, *177*, 361-379.

Hutton, J.T., Johnston, C.W., Shapiro, I., and Pirozzolo, F.J. (1979). Oculomotor programming disturbance in the dementia syndrome. *Perceptual and Motor Skills*, *49*, 312-314.

James, W. (1890). *The principles of psychology.* New York: Holt.

Kahneman, D. (1973). *Attention and effort.* Englewood Cliffs, NJ: Prentice-Hall.

Kline, D.W., and Schieber, F. (1985). Vision and aging. In J.E. Birren and K.W. Schaie (Eds.), *Handbook of the psychology of aging* (2nd ed.) (pp. 296-331). New York: Van Nostrand Reinhold.

Lawson, J.S., McGhie, A., and Chapman, J. (1967). Distractability in schizophrenics and organic cerebral disease. *British Journal of Psychiatry, 113*, 527-535.

Layton, B. (1975). Perceptual noise and aging. *Psychological Bulletin, 82*, 875-883.

Lewis, R. and Kupke, T. (1977). *The Lafayette Clinic repeatable neuropsychological test battery: Its development and research applications*. Paper presented at the annual meeting of the Southeastern Psychological Association, Hollywood, Florida.

Mattis, S. (1976). Mental status examination for organic mental syndrome in the elderly patient. In R. Bellack and B. Karasu (Eds.), *Geriatric psychiatry* (pp. 77-121). New York: Grune and Stratton.

Miller, E. (1977). *Abnormal aging: The psychology of senile and presenile dementia*. New York: John Wiley

Mountcastle, V.B. (1976). An organizing principle for cerebral function: The unit module and the distributed system. In G.M. Edelman and V.B. Mountcastle (Eds.), *The mindful brain* (pp. 7-50). Cambridge, MA: MIT Press.

Nebes, R.D., and Madden, D.J. (1983). The use of focused attention in visual search by young and old adults. *Experimental Aging Research, 9*, 139-143.

Neisser, U. (1967). *Cognitive psychology*. New York: Appleton-Century-Crofts.

Nissen, M.J., and Corkin, S. (1985). Effectiveness of attentional cueing in older and younger adults. *Journal of Gerontology, 40*, 185-191.

Posner, M., and Snyder C.R.R. (1975). Attention and cognitive control. In R.L. Solso (Ed.), *Information processing and cognition: The Loyola Symposium*. Potomac, MD: Lawrence Erlbaum.

Prinzmetal, W., and Banks, W.P. (1977). Good continuation affects visual detection. *Perception and Psychophysics, 21*, 389-395.

Rabbitt, P.M.A. (1965). An age decrement in the ability to ignore irrelevant information. *Journal of Gerontology, 20*, 233-238.

Reed, S.K. (1982). *Cognition: Theory and applications*. Monterey, CA: Brooks/Cole.

Rogers, J., and Bloom, F.E. (1985). Neurotransmitter metabolism and function in the aging central nervous system. In C.E. Finch and E.L. Schneider (Eds.), *Handbook of the biology of aging* (pp. 645-691). New York: Van Nostrand Reinhold.

Rumelhart, D.E. (1977). *Introduction to human information processing*. New York: John Wiley.

Salthouse, T.A. (1982). *Adult cognition: An experimental psychology of human aging*. New York: Springer-Verlag.

Salthouse, T.A., Rogan, J.D., and Prill, K.A. (1984). Division of attention: Age differences on a visually presented memory task. *Memory and Cognition, 12*, 613-620.

Scheibel, M.E., Lindsay, R.D., Tomiyasu, U., and Scheibel, A.B. (1975). Progressive dendritic changes in aging human cortex. *Experimental Neurology, 47*, 392-403.

Schlotterer, G., Moscovitch, M., and Crapper-McLachlon, D. (1983). Visual processing deficits as assessed by spatial frequency contrast sensitivity and backward masking in normal aging and Alzheimer's disease. *Brain, 107*, 309-325.

Schneider, W., and Schiffrin, R.M. (1977). Controlled and automatic information processing: I. Detection, search and attention. *Psychological Review, 84*, 1-66.

Schonfield, D. (1974). Translations in gerontology—from lab to life: Utilizing information. *American Psychologist, 29*, 796-801.

Somberg, B.L., and Salthouse, T.A. (1982). Divided attention abilities in young and old adults. *Journal of Experimental Psychology: Human Perception and Performance, 8*, 651-663.

Sperling, G. (1960). The information available in brief visual presentations. *Psychological Monographs, 74*, 1-29.

Storandt, M., Botwinick, J., Danziger, W.L., Berg, L., and Hughes, C.P. (1984). Psychometric differentiation of mild senile dementia of the Alzheimer type. *Archives of Neurology, 41*, 497-499.

Talland, G.A., and Schwab, R.S. (1964). Performance with multiple sets in Parkinson's disease. *Neuropsychologia, 2*, 45-53.

Terry, R., and Katzman, R. (1983). Senile dementia of the Alzheimer's type: Defining a disease. In R. Katzman and R. Terry (Eds.), *The neurology of aging* (pp. 51-84). Philadelphia: F.A. Davis.

Vitaliano, P.P., Russo, J., Breen, A.R., Vitiello, M.V., and Prinz, P.N. (1986). Functional decline in the early stages of Alzheimer's disease. *Psychology and Aging, 1*, 41-46.

Walsh, D.A., Till, R.E., and Williams, M.V. (1978). Age differences in peripheral perceptual processing: a monoptic backward masking investigation. *Journal of Experimental Psychology: Human Perception and Performance, 4*, 232-243.

Weale, R.A. (1963). *The aging eye*. London: H.K. Lewis.

Wickelgren, W.A. (1979). *Cognitive psychology*. Englewood Cliffs, NJ: Prentice-Hall.

Wilson, R.S., Kaszniak, A.W., Bacon, L.D., Fox, J.H., and Kelly, M.P. (1982). Facial recognition memory in dementia. *Cortex*, *18*, 329-336.

Wright, L.L., and Elias, J.W. (1979). Age differences in the effects of perceptual noise. *Journal of Gerontology*, *34*, 704-708.

Wright, R.E. (1981). Aging, divided attention, and processing capacity. *Journal of Gerontology*, *36*, 605-614.

Chapter 12

Memory in Normal Aging

"Each man's memory is his private literature."

Aldous Huxley

Mr. R is a 72-year-old widower who lives with his son and daughter-in-law. His favorite pastime is reading novels. He has been an active participant in a book club for the past 12 years, and enjoys exchanging descriptions of recent books he has read with fellow club members. Over the past 6 or 7 years, he has become concerned that something is wrong with his memory. Remembering the detail of recently read novels now seems to require much more effort. He also experiences difficulty in remembering the names of new club members, something that was always very easy for him. Although no one else seems to notice anything wrong with him, he fears that his difficulties may be the beginning of a progressive deterioration.

Are Mr. R's fears justified, or is he experiencing the memory changes of normal aging? In order to address this question, it is helpful to first explore how healthy older persons experience their memory functioning.

COMPLAINTS OF MEMORY CHANGE IN NORMAL AGING

Older persons complain more than younger adults of memory difficulty (Zelinski, Gilewski, and Thompson, 1980). In general, older individuals appear to be accurate judges of their memory functioning. Older subjects' "feeling of knowing" (Lachman and Lachman, 1980) or evaluation of everyday memory functioning (Zelinski et al., 1980) is significantly correlated with laboratory memory task performance. Many elderly complain of decreased ability to remember recent and remote events, names, dates, phone numbers, and appointments. Complaints also often include trouble in remembering what has been read, the thread of thought in conversation, where something has been put, and what one had gone to the store to buy. Older persons may report more frequent use of mnemonics, such as keeping appointment books and making reminder notes.

Memory complaints appear quite common among healthy older individuals. In one study, based upon a survey of 111 normal older men participating in the Baltimore Longitudinal Study of Aging, 80 percent made complaints about memory difficulty (Sluss, Rabins, Gruenberg, and Reedman, 1980). Kral (1962) was the first to use the term "benign senescent forgetfulness" to describe these memory complaints. Kral observed that most older persons with complaints of forgetfulness, but without severe memory deficit, have a benign prognosis. Similarly, Reisberg and Ferris (1982) reported a study of 17 independently living older persons (mean age = 68.5) who complained of forgetting names and the location of objects. At follow-up examination, an average of 27 months later, none showed worsened health or cognitive functioning.

CURRENT THEORIES OF NORMAL MEMORY FUNCTIONING

In Chapter 2, the reader was introduced to current models employed to conceptualize how human memory processes operate. In order to understand the present status of research in memory, aging, and dementia, it is helpful to briefly review the history of information processing approaches to the study of memory. This review is limited to a description of approaches that have been most widely applied in research on dementia, amnesia, and aging. For a more complete overview of the history of the development of various memory theories, the reader is referred to Schacter (1982).

Information Processing Approaches to Memory

While memory research conducted during the 1940s and 1950s focused primarily upon stimulus–response theories of learning, by the 1970s emphasis had shifted to an information processing approach. This "paradigm shift" occurred primarily because of the inability of then popular behaviorist models to adequately explain emerging empirical data. In particular, it became clear that stimulus–response chain accounts could not adequately explain either the learning or the execution of complex, serially ordered behavior, such as speaking or playing a musical instrument (c.f. Lashley, 1951).

The information processing model of memory is based upon three basic assumptions: (1) that humans actively participate in learning and information retrieval, (2) that responses can be analyzed quantitatively and qualitatively, and (3) that information flow can be traced through a number of hypothetic memory processes (Kaszniak, Poon, and Riege, 1986; Poon, 1985).

Until fairly recently, a "linear" model of information processing has dominated memory research. This model assumes that information flows from input to output through a series of sequential stages, or memory "stores. At the very early stage of information registration is sensory memory, a preattentive and highly unstable system characterized by rapid decay of information representation. Perceptual (pattern recognition) and attentional processes serve to transfer information out of sensory stores and into the next stage. Sensory memory, and perceptual and attentional processes, were discussed in the previous chapter. The next stage involves the division of primary (short-term) and secondary (long-term) memory (Waugh and Norman, 1965), which is responsible for the acquisition and retention of new information. Primary memory is thought of as a limited-capacity store in which information is still "in consciousness" as it is being used. The process of rehearsal is postulated to transfer information from primary to secondary memory (see Murdock, 1967). If the information is not rehearsed instantly, so that it can be stored in secondary memory, it will be lost. The reader will recall the example, in Chapter 2, looking up and rehearsing a telephone number.

Within the linear information processing model, memory failures are attributed to a variety of factors, which include (1) reduced capacity of the hypothetic stores, particularly the short-term store, (2) a decay, or "forgetting," of information from one or more stores, (3) a failure of the transfer processes (i.e., pattern recognition, attention, rehearsal) in which information is moved from one store to the next, and (4) a combination of these factors. If there is difficulty at any stage of the sequence, an information "bottleneck" is hypothesized to occur, and memory performance suffers (c.f. Atkinson and Shiffrin, 1971; Kaszniak et al., 1986). In addition to these stages or stores, several other interacting dimensions are hypothesized. One such dimension consists of dynamic processes related to the encoding, storage, and retrieval of information. Another dimension defines the modality-specific (e.g., auditory, visual, olfactory) or other properties (e.g., verbal, spatial) of the incoming information. The functioning of any or all of these multiple dimensions of memory is affected by differences in intelligence, education, and socioeconomic status, as well as neurologic, hormonal, and physiologic states. Thus, given the many factors that can influence memory, it is clear that the level of functional memory is fluid and subject to both intra- and interpersonal variability (Kaszniak et al., 1986). This explains why memory performance fluctuates somewhat, from one examination to the next, in both healthy and ill individuals.

As described later in this chapter, research results indicate that secondary memory encoding and retrieval processes decline with normal aging. However, in dementia (the focus of the next chapter), all hypothetic stages and processes appear to be affected with disease progression. Thus, the healthy older person will appear able to briefly retain new information with accuracy, but may complain of difficulty retrieving the information at some later time.

Modifications of the Linear Model of Information Processing in Memory

The linear information processing model of memory has many attractions. It allows for testable hypotheses to be derived and has permitted investigators to draw conclusions concerning the apparent loci of age- and dementia-related memory change. However, this model also has significant drawbacks and requires modification. Within the following discussion, these modifications, and examples of the research motivating such changes, are presented. These more recent information processing models also help in explaining differences between the memory changes of normal aging and those more severe memory deficits of dementia. Research employing these models has made it clear, for example, that much of the AD patient's deficit in memory for events (episodic memory) is attributable to problems in the access to, and possibly the structure of, semantic memory. Normal older persons do not carry out effective encoding and retrieval operations, although semantic memory processes and structure are generally intact and can be accessed under appropriate conditions.

Levels of Processing: An Alternative to the Memory Stores Model

The recent shift away from the linear information processing model of memory has been prompted by the accumulating evidence indicating that characteristics of the hypothetic memory stores vary considerably with changes in tasks, materials, and strategies. As Craik (1984) states, "Whereas it is plausible that mental *processes* might be context-dependent, it is surely less reasonable for mechanisms to vary in this respect" (p. 3). Within a process-oriented model of memory, as first proposed by Craik and Lockhart (1972), short-term, or primary, memory is seen as the continued processing (or activation) of a part of the memory system. What the linear information processing model saw as evidence of information "stored" in primary memory was now seen as continued activation or "attention paid to" an event (Craik, 1984, p. 4). Primary memory thus is viewed as the reflection of a process, rather than as a store. Similarly, the previous distinctions between primary and secondary memory are viewed in terms of encoding processes, retrieval processes, and their interaction. In other words, instead of a series of discrete stages through which a mental representation is sequentially moved, event or episodic memory is conceived as a continuous process of elaboration of new information. The extensiveness and distinctiveness of elaboration determines how well events will later be retrieved.

Encoding Processes. Craik (1984) provides the following description of the process of encoding:

> Encoding processes are seen as interpretations of the stimulus pattern in terms of qualitatively different types of past experience (or in terms of innate analyzing procedures, in the case of basic pattern-recognition operations). Thus, an event can be analyzed in terms of its sensory qualities, or (in addition) in terms of its meaning and significance in various different dimensions. . . . an event will be remembered, provided, first, that some well-organized body of past experience (schema or expertise) is brought to bear on the event, and, second, that the resulting analysis is somewhat different from highly practiced routine proce-

> dures performed by the schemas in question. . . . Such distinctive encodings naturally require more attention and processing resources. . . . (Craik, 1984, p. 5).

Thus, within this view, an event will be well remembered only if it is both meaningful, in terms of past experience, and also distinct from routine past applications of analytic procedures employed in its encoding. Such distinctive encoding necessarily involves greater processing resources or effort than more routinely or automatically encoded events. A corollary of these assumptions is that if available processing resources are insufficient, for whatever reason, then the system must revert to relatively automatic procedures. Automatic or routine encoding leads to analysis "that is very similar to many previous analyses, and thus to a nondistinctive encoding and poor subsequent recollection of the event" (Craik, 1984, p. 5). As should be obvious from this description, the encoding of events is heavily dependent upon the access to, and integrity of, semantic memory. It is within semantic memory that concepts and schema necessary for understanding and encoding events are stored.

Retrieval Processes

Retrieval processes, within this view, are seen as being very similar to (perhaps even identical with) encoding processes. Remembering or retrieval can be thought of as a process by which the cognitive system returns to the same configuration or state it was in at the time the event was originally encoded. In the performance of some types of tasks, such as those involving recognition memory paradigms, stimulus conditions at the time of retrieval are very similar to those at the time of encoding. Within a typical recognition memory paradigm, a series of words or other stimuli is presented for memorization. Either immediately afterward or at a later time, a recognition list is presented, containing the original stimuli ("targets") mixed among new stimuli ("distractors"). The subject's task is to indicate those stimuli that were originally presented for memorization. The similarity between the material within the recognition targets and the originally presented material is so high that the recognition stimuli can be thought to "drive" the system back into the original configuration.

In free recall memory paradigms, words or other stimuli are similarly presented for memorization. However, the subject's task is then to immediately, or at a later time, recall the original stimuli without the aid of any cues. For these types of tasks, the retrieval environment does not itself induce the original encoding configuration, and retrieval processes must hence be initiated by the rememberer. Such self-initiated (as contrasted with retrieval-environment–driven) processing consumes greater attentional resources and is hence more "effortful" (Hasher and Zacks, 1979). As demonstrated by research discussed in the present chapter, normal older individuals generally show episodic memory problems only for those tasks requiring greater processing resources. In contrast, dementia patients show deficit in both effortful, as well as automatic, memory tasks. This contrast, as well as episodic memory processing differences between persons with dementia, various amnesic syndromes, and depression, will be shown to have important implications for clinical assessment.

Given the foregoing discussion, it should by now be obvious to the reader that it is not possible to understand the nature of episodic memory functioning in aging or dementia without also understanding other cognitive process contributing to it. The critical relationship between episodic and semantic memory was already described. Age- or disease-related slowing of information processing, perceptual impairment, and limitations in the focusing or capacity of attention can all have a marked impact upon episodic memory. For this reason, concepts and research results presented in the previous several chapters remain critical for understanding memory impairment.

MEMORY AND AGING FROM A LINEAR INFORMATION PROCESSING PERSPECTIVE

In order to comprehend recent developments in memory and aging, it is necessary to first briefly review the conclusions of research employing the linear information processing model. Two broad conclusions are drawn from the results of this body of research: (1) that there is an age-related decline in memory retrieval speed from the various memory store, and (2) that the largest age group differences are seen in secondary memory.

Evidence for the Sparing of Primary Memory Processes in Normal Aging

Overall, minimal or no adult age group differences have been found in primary (short-term) memory. A commonly used task in evaluation of primary memory is that involving forward memory span. Typically, the subject is presented with an auditory or visual sequence of stimuli, and required to repeat the sequence back to the examiner (see Botwinick and Storandt, 1974). Stimuli may be digits, letters, words, or spatially arranged blocks that are tapped by the examiner in a particular order. When the number of items is approximately seven or less, the presumed capacity of primary memory, minimal age group differences have been found, in either capacity or speed of retrieval (see review by Poon, 1985).

Significant differences between younger and older adults have been found in backward memory span tasks, in which the participant must immediately reproduce the stimuli in the reverse order from which they were presented. However, it has been hypothesized that the cognitive operations necessary to perform the backward memory span task may exceed the capacity of primary memory (Botwinick and Storandt, 1974).

Another example of a task employed to examine retrieval speed and capacity in primary memory is that of the continuous recognition memory task employed by Poon and Fozard (1978). The participant in this task is presented a sequence of words and told that some of the words will be repeated a second time. The individual is then required to say whether each word is being shown for the first or second time, and the speed of this decision is measured. The intervals between the first and second presentations of a word are varied so that they are within either primary memory capacity (seven items or less) or secondary memory (more than seven items). Thus, both speed and accuracy of retrieval from primary and secondary memory can be determined. Older age groups were not significantly slower, and were no less accurate in retrieval of items in the primary memory range. They were significantly slower and less accurate in retrieval from secondary memory (Poon and Fozard, 1978). Thus, neither primary memory retrieval speed nor recall accuracy changes greatly with older age, provided that the assumed capacity of this hypothetic store is not exceeded.

Evidence for Secondary Memory Changes in Normal Aging

In contrast to the minimal age differences in primary memory, relatively large age effects are reported whenever the items to be remembered exceed primary memory capacity (see Poon, 1985). Adult age group differences have been reported with meaningful and meaningless verbal material, spatial displays, and recognition of pictures and geometric drawings (see Salthouse, 1982, pp. 127–128, for brief review of relevant studies). Age-related changes in secondary memory are thus seen across different stimulus types and modalities of stimulus presentation. Given the consistency of results, considerable effort has gone into examining whether encoding, storage, or retrieval processes are responsible for the secondary memory deficit of older persons. Reviewers of this body of investigation (e.g., Fozard, 1980; Poon, 1985) are in general agreement that age differences are most evident in the encoding and retrieval processes, and least evident in storage.

Lack of Age Differences in Secondary Memory Storage

Estimations of the integrity of storage are typically based upon an evaluation of forgetting rate after information has been adequately encoded. Forgetting rates, measured by the accuracy of recall at different intervals following initial encoding, have been found to be comparable in younger and older adults. Various tasks have failed to demonstrate age differences in rate of forgetting. These include (1) paired-associate learning, requiring the participant to learn a list of word pairs over repeated presentations (Thomas and Ruben, 1973), (2) recognition memory, requiring the participant to select, from a list of words or other stimuli, those which were presented before (Poon and Fozard, 1978), and (3) recall of common events that happened long ago (Warrington and Silberstein, 1970).

Age-Related Encoding Deficits

Age-related encoding deficits have been identified employing tasks that manipulate verbal or visual elaboration and stimulus organization. Verbal elaboration is defined by amount of verbal association that occurs when an event is encoded. Visual elaboration is defined by the amount of visual imagery involved in encoding an event. Organization is defined by the degree of relatedness among stimuli. A comprehensive review of research concerned with secondary memory encoding deficits in older age has been provided by Smith (1980). Similar to the presentation provided by Kaszniak and colleagues (1986), the following discussion serves merely to highlight some of this work.

A typical approach to the study of verbal elaboration deficit in older adults is provided by Eysenck (1974). Young adult and elderly subject groups were required to count letters of words, to generate rhymes, or to generate appropriate adjectives to words presented in a list-learning paradigm. Age-matched control groups received no elaboration instructions. In a later free recall test, the participants were asked to recall as many of the words as possible, in any order. In comparison with younger adults, older participants demonstrated increasing decrements, from letter to rhyme to adjective conditions. Thus, the more elaboration required in processing words, the larger the age difference found in later recall performance.

Evidence in support of age-related deficits in visual elaboration has been obtained from studies contrasting younger and older groups in verbal learning tasks. These studies manipulate the presence or absence of instructions to mentally "picture" what the words in the list refer to (e.g., Hulicka and Grossman, 1967; Poon, Walsh-Sweeney and Fozard, 1980). Imagery instructions improve the recall of older persons and reduce the size of age-group differences. This has been interpreted as evidence that older adults do not make as much spontaneous use of visual elaboration encoding processes as younger adults.

Evidence for age-associated deficits in the use of organization at encoding comes from studies in which the amount of inherent stimulus organization is manipulated. Few or no age differences are found in recall of difficult-to-organize material, such as color names or random letters. Older adults are significantly worse in recall of material that can be easily organized, such as text sentences or letters grouped into words (Taub, 1974).

Age-Related Retrieval Deficits

Conclusions regarding the presence of retrieval deficits in older persons typically come from studies in which recall and recognition memory performances are compared (e.g., Shonfield and Robertson, 1966). Small age group differences are repeatedly found for recognition memory, compared with large differences for recall. These observations were taken as support for the idea that age-related changes were greatest in retrieval, rather than storage. This is based upon the assumption that the information must have been effectively encoded and stored in secondary memory in order to have been correctly identified in the recognition task. Free recall was assumed to differ from recognition memory in placing greater demands upon retrieval mechanisms. Results of other types of studies were also interpreted as consistent with age differences in retrieval rather than storage. These included comparisons of performance in free versus cued recall (e.g., Hultsch, 1975) and comparisons of the presence versus absence of organization cues at input and output (e.g., Smith, 1977). As described later in this chapter, investigators working within the levels of processing framework (e.g., Craik and Lockhart, 1972; Craik, 1984) have reinterpreted these results.

Summary

The linear information processing approach to the study of memory and aging has produced a large body of research, leading to the following general conclusions: (1) speed and accuracy of recall from primary memory show little, if any, age group differences, provided that information load does not exceed the capacity of this store, (2) there is an age-related slowing of retrieval from secondary memory, (3) secondary memory accuracy shows relatively large age group differences, and (4) older adults are deficient in secondary memory encoding and retrieval processes, but not in storage. The following sections of this chapter will explore contributions of recent research and theory that have elaborated upon and modified these conclusions.

AGE-RELATED MEMORY CHANGES FROM THE LEVELS-OF-PROCESSING PERSPECTIVE

The levels-of-processing model hypothesizes memory to be a continuous process, rather than a series of discrete stages or stores. Within this framework, event encoding and retrieval are highly similar processes requiring the effortful activation of schemas and concepts that make the mental representation of an event more distinctive. It will also be recalled from the previous chapter that older adults are characterized by more limited attentional capacity resources than younger adults. The levels-of-processing and capacity limitation hypotheses have been used to reinterpret much of the evidence previously considered as relevant to secondary memory encoding, storage, and retrieval.

For example, these hypotheses predict that age group differences will be largest in free recall tasks, for which considerable attentional resources are necessary for effective encoding and retrieval. Somewhat smaller age group differences are predicted to occur in cued recall tasks. In these tasks, the "cue," such as a phonemic or semantic associate of the word to be remembered, is thought to reinstate a portion of the initial encoding configuration. Even smaller age group differences are predicted for recognition memory tasks. In recognition memory tasks, reinstatement of most of the encoding configuration is assumed to be automatically "driven" by the recognition choices. Finally, age group differences should often be nonexistent in priming tasks, where activation of the mental representation is assumed to be entirely automatic.

The results of recent studies have generally supported these predictions. Rabinowitz (1986) demonstrated a rank-ordering of age group differences across experimental tasks, as follows: the greatest age differences were found for a cued-recall task, followed by a recognition memory task. No age difference was obtained for a task in which reaction time to a word was primed by a related or unrelated word with which it had been paired in a previous learning trial. Lexical priming paradigms, wherein previous presentation of a word results in faster response to a semantically associated word, have generally shown an absence of age group differences (e.g., Byrd, 1984). These results are consistent with the hypothesis of an age-related impairment in effortful retrieval processes.

Episodic and Semantic Memory

As described earlier in the book, Tulving (1972, 1983, 1984, 1985) has proposed an influential distinction between *episodic* and *semantic* memory systems. Tulving conceptualizes episodic memory as a system that receives and stores information about "temporally dated episodes or events, and temporal-spatial relations among them" (Tulving, 1984, p. 223). Semantic memory is distinguished as

> "the memory necessary for the use of language. It is a mental thesaurus, organized knowledge a person possesses about words and other verbal symbols, their meaning and referents, about relations among them, and about rules, formulas, and algorithms for the manipulation of the symbols, concepts, and relations." (Tulving, 1972, p. 386)

Within the older linear information processing "stores" model of memory, episodic and semantic memory would generally be considered as subdivisions of secondary memory. However, Tulving (1985) conceives of these as hierarchically related, with episodic memory "embedded within" semantic memory. Each system is characterized by a distinct information source (episodic = events or episodes; semantic = facts, ideas, concepts), organization (episodic = temporal; semantic = symbolic), and processing characteristics. A full detailing of the differences between episodic and semantic memory is clearly beyond the scope of the present chapter. Of importance for the present purposes is that various investigators have interpreted available data as suggesting that age decrements occur in episodic but not in semantic memory (e.g., Perlmutter, 1978).

While much available data argues for a differential age vulnerability of episodic versus semantic memory, Craik (1984) has noted some exceptions. Craik argues that these exceptions indicate age differences to be more "a function of the degree of active, novel manipulation required by the task, not simply as a function of the "system" involved" (Craik, 1984, p. 9).

Age differences have not been obtained within studies employing lexical decision–semantic priming paradigms (Byrd, 1984; Howard, McAndrews, and Lasaga, 1981). However, the recent report of Howard, Shaw, and Heisey (1986) does suggest some slowing in the time course of semantic activation for older, as compared with younger, adults. Thus, "automatic" (Hasher and Zacks, 1979) aspects of semantic memory activation do not appear affected by aging, except for small age differences in activation time course. Other semantic memory tasks, such as generating as many words as possible beginning with a particular letter, do show age group differences. Craik (1984) argues that word fluency tasks involve more effortful semantic memory retrieval processes than do priming paradigms. The reader will recall that results from episodic memory tasks are given similar interpretation by Craik. Older adults perform episodic memory tasks inefficiently, "unless the operations are induced and guided by the task, by specific instructions, or by other supportive aspects of the current environment" (Craik, 1984, p. 10). This conclusion is of practical importance, in its suggestion that there should be specific instructional and environmental manipulations capable of minimizing age-related deficits in memory for events. The following sections discuss recent research indicating potential causes of, and possible modes of compensation for, age-related deficits in effortful memory processing.

Possible Causes of Age-Related Changes in Effortful Encoding/Retrieval

What might account for the failure of older persons to carry out effective effortful encoding/retrieval operations? A particularly interesting recent report by Riege, Metter, Kuhl, and Phelps (1985) sheds some light on this question. Positron emission tomography (PET) scan measures of regional brain glucose metabolism were correlated with 18 multivariate memory tests in 23 healthy adults, ranging in age from 27 to 78 years. Among other relationships, Riege and colleagues found that glucose metabolism in the left frontal cerebrum decreased with age. Further, this age-related left frontal hypometabolism correlated highly with performance on those memory tasks requiring greater verbal mediation and elaboration. This observation is consistent with the hypothesis (Albert and Kaplan, 1980) that arousal and attention systems, critically dependent upon structures within the frontal lobes of the cerebrum, may become impaired in older age. Age-related impairment in arousal and attention systems would result in a decrease in spontaneous utilization of elaborative encoding/retrieval strategies, unless such strategies are "driven" by particular task design or task instructions.

Compensating for Age-Related Changes in Effortful Encoding/Retrieval

Thus, considerable evidence argues that older adults do not spontaneously process items in memory to the same "depth" or degree of elaboration as do young adults (e.g., Rankin and Collins, 1985; Simon, 1979). However, much of the episodic memory deficit of older adults can be overcome if instructions are given in the use of various elaboration (e.g., visual imagery) and mediation strategies (Perlmutter, 1979; Poon and Walsh-Sweeney, 1981; Rissenberg and Glanzer, 1986; Treat and Reese, 1976; Yesavage, Rose, and Bower, 1983). Because of the age-related reduction in processing resources, older persons often fail to carry out effective encoding and retrieval operations. Yet, the consequences of reduced attentional capacity can often be overcome if the task, the environment, or both are structured so as to induce effective encoding and retrieval processes. Once events have been effectively encoded, there is little evidence for any greater rate of forgetting in older than in younger persons (e.g., Poon and Fozard, 1980).

These findings give cause for some optimism. Experimental manipulations, such as instruction in the use of elaboration and encoding strategies, could be developed into standard intervention procedures. These procedures could then be tested in large samples of normal elderly persons with memory complaints. If they are proved effective, with improvements maintained over time, the clinician would then have an approach to offer the large number of persons with "benign senescent forgetfulness." One important question that future clinical research must address is how to get persons to continue using the encoding techniques in their daily lives. Studies examining the prolonged use of mnemonic strategies find that older persons do not use the techniques unless they are reminded to do so (e.g., Schaffer and Poon, 1982).

Summary

The theoretic approach that views memory as a continuous process, and the research motivated by this theory, suggest that age-related change in episodic memory is due to decreased spontaneous use of elaborative encoding/retrieval strategies. Those semantic memory processes involving automatic activation of concepts, schema, and other contents are not greatly affected by aging. The decreased use of effortful encoding/retrieval strategies is likely secondary to the age-related reduction in attentional capacity. Recent research employing neuroradiologic measures of regional brain metabolism suggests that this may be due to a hypometabolism, with aging, of frontal cerebral structures subserving attentional functions. A cause for clinical optimism is provided by observations of episodic memory improvement when older persons are supplied with instructions to facilitate encoding elaboration.

CLINICAL IMPLICATIONS

1. **Normal age-related changes in memory are "benign," in that there is not rapid progression to more severe impairment. It is important to reassure healthy older individuals that some increased difficulty in remembering events and retrieving information is to be expected with aging. This difficulty does not indicate impending deterioration.**
2. **Digit- or word-span tests will not be useful in attempting to clinically document age-related memory changes, since primary memory tasks are little affected by normal aging.**
3. **Because normal age-related changes do occur, clinical memory assessment instruments *must* have available normative data for older age groups if they are to be useful in differential diagnosis.**
4. **Current theory and data concerning memory and aging stress the importance of assisting the older individual in more elaborate and distinctive encoding of events and information to be remembered. One way in which this can be accomplished is through emphasis on the relationship of new information not only to what the person already knows or understands, but also to what is unique and distinctive. Another way is through encouraging the visual imaging of new events and information.**

5. **Similarly, instruction concerning the reinstatement of visual images, semantic associations, or other elaborative processing, at the time of attempted retrieval, may assist the older person in more effective recall.**

6. **Empiric evaluations of the effectiveness of mnemonic strategies will need to address the problem of how to facilitate the continued daily use of techniques.**

REFERENCES

Albert, M.S., and Kaplan, E. (1980). Organic implications of neuropsychological deficits in the elderly. In L.W.Poon, J.L.Fozard, L.S.Cermak, D.Arenberg, and L.W.Thompson (Eds.), *New directions in memory and aging* (pp.403-432). Hillsdale, NJ: Lawrence Erlbaum.

Atkinson, R.C., and Shiffrin, R.M. (1971). The control of short-term memory. *Scientific American*, *225*, 82-90.

Botwinick, J., and Storandt, M. (1974). *Memory and related functions and age*. Springfield, IL: Charles C Thomas.

Byrd, M.(1984). Age differences in the retrieval of information from semantic memory. *Experimental Aging Research*, *10*, 29-33.

Craik, F.I.M. (1984). Age differences in remembering. In L.R. Squire and N. Butters (Eds.), *Neuropsychology of memory* (pp. 3-12). New York: Guilford.

Craik, F.I.M., and Lockhart, R.S. (1972). Levels of processing: A framework for memory research. *Journal of Verbal Learning and Verbal Behavior*, *11*, 671-684.

Eysenck, M.W. (1974). Age differences in incidental learning. *Developmental Psychology*, *10*, 936-941.

Fozard, J.L. (1980). The time for remembering. In L.W. Poon (Ed.), *Aging in the 1980's: Psychological issues* (pp. 273-290). Washington, DC: American Psychological Association.

Hasher, L., and Zacks, R.T. (1979). Automatic and effortful processes in memory. *Journal of Experimental Psychology: General*, *108*, 356-388.

Howard, D.V., McAndrews, M.P., and Lasaga, M.I. (1981). Semantic priming of lexical decisions in young and old adults. *Journal of Gerontology*, *36*, 707-714.

Howard, D.V., Shaw, R.J., and Heisey, J.G. (1986). Aging and the time course of semantic activation. *Journal of Gerontology*, *41*, 195-203.

Hulicka, I.M., and Grossman, J.L. (1967). Age-group comparisons for the use of mediators in paired-associate learning. *Journal of Gerontology*, *22*, 46-51.

Hultsch, D. (1975). Adult age differences in retrieval: Trace-dependent and cue-dependent forgetting. *Developmental Psychology*, *11*, 197-201.

Kaszniak, A.W., Poon, L.W., and Riege, W.R. (1986). Assessing memory deficits: An information processing approach. In L.W. Poon, B.J. Gurland, C. Eisdorfer, T. Crook, L.W. Thompson, A.W. Kaszniak, and K. Davis, (Eds.), *Handbook of clinical memory assessment of the older adult*. Washington, DC: American Psychological Association.

Kral, V.A. (1962). Senescent forgetfulness, benign and malignant. *Canadian Medical Association Journal*, *86*, 257-260.

Lachman, J.L., and Lachman, R. (1980). Age and the actualization of world knowledge. In L.W. Poon, J.L. Fozard, L.S. Cermak, D. Arenberg, and L.W. Thompson (Eds.), *New directions in memory and aging* (pp. 285-311). Hillsdale, NJ: Lawrence Erlbaum.

Lashley, K. (1951). The problem of serial order in behavior. In L.A. Jeffress (Ed.), *Cerebral mechanisms in behavior* (pp.112-136). New York: John Wiley.

Murdock, B.B. (1967). Recent developments in short-term memory. *British Journal of Psychology*, *58*, 421-433.

Perlmutter, M. (1978). What is memory aging the aging of? *Developmental Psychology*, *14*, 330-345.

Perlmutter, M. (1979). Age differences in adults' free recall, cued recall, and recognition. *Journal of Gerontology*, *34*, 533-539.

Poon, L.W. (1985). Differences in human memory with aging: Nature, causes, and clinical implications. In J.E. Birren and K.W. Schaie (Eds.), *Handbook of the psychology of aging* (pp. 427-462). New York: Van Nostrand Reinhold.

Poon, L.W., and Fozard, J.L. (1978). Speed of retrieval from long-term memory in relation to age, familiarity and datedness of information. *Journal of Gerontology*, *5*, 711-717.

Poon, L.W., and Fozard, J.L. (1980). Age and word frequency effects in continuous recognition memory. *Journal of Gerontology*, *35*, 77-86.

Poon, L.W., and Walsh-Sweeney, L. (1981). Effects of bizzare and interacting imagery on learning and retrieval of the aged. *Experimental Aging Research*, *7*, 65-70.

Poon, L.W., Walsh-Sweeney, L., and Fozard, J.L. (1980). Memory skill training for the elderly: Salient issues on the use of imagery mnemonics. In L.W. Poon, J.L. Fozard, L.S. Cermak, D. Arenberg, and

L.W. Thompson (Eds.), *New directions in memory and aging* (pp. 461-484). Hillsdale, NJ: Lawrence Erlbaum.

Rabinowitz, J.C. (1986). Priming in episodic memory. *Journal of Gerontology, 41*, 204-213.

Rankin, J.L., and Collins, M. (1985). Adult age differences in memory elaboration. *Journal of Gerontology, 40*, 451-458.

Riege, W.H., Metter, E.J., Kuhl, D.E., and Phelps, M.E. (1985). Brain glucose metabolism and memory functions: Age decrease in factor scores. *Journal of Gerontology, 40*, 459-467.

Reisberg, B. and Ferris, S.H. (1982). Diagnosis and assessment of the older patient. *Hospital and Community Psychiatry, 33*, 104-110.

Rissenberg, M., and Glanzer, M. (1986). Picture superiority in free recall: The effects of normal aging and primary degenerative dementia. *Journal of Gerontology, 41*, 64-71.

Salthouse, T.A. (1982). *Adult cognition: An experimental psychology of human aging*. New York: Springer-Verlag.

Schacter, D.L. (1982). *Stranger behind the engram: Theories of memory and the psychology of science*. Hillsdale, NJ: Lawrence Erlbaum.

Schaffer, G., and Poon, L.W. (1982). Individual variability in memory training with the elderly. *Educational Gerontology, 8*, 217-229.

Shonfield, D., and Robertson, B.A. (1966). Memory storage and aging. *Canadian Journal of Psychology, 20*, 228-236.

Simon, E. (1979). Depth and elaboration of processing in relation to age. *Journal of Experimental Psychology: Human Learning and Memory, 5*, 115-124.

Sluss, T.K., Rabins, P., Gruenberg, E.M., and Reedman, G. (1980). Memory complaints in community residing men. *The Gerontologist, 20*, 201.

Smith, A.D. (1977). Adult age differences in cued recall. *Developmental Psychology, 13*, 326-331.

Smith, A.D. (1980). Age differences in encoding, storage, and retrieval. In L.W. Poon, T.L. Fozard, L.S. Cermak, D. Arenberg, and L.W. Thompson (Eds.), *New directions in memory and aging* (pp. 23-46). Hillsdale, NJ: Lawrence Erlbaum.

Taub, H.A. (1974). Coding for short-term memory as a function of age. *Journal of Genetic Psychology, 125*, 309-314.

Thomas, J.C., and Ruben, H. (1973). *Age and mnemonic techniques in paired-associate learning*. Paper presented at the Annual Meeting of the Gerontological Society, Miami, FL.

Treat, N., and Reese, H.W. (1976). Age, pacing and imagery in paired-associate learning. *Developmental Psychology, 12*, 119-124.

Tulving, E. (1972). Episodic and semantic memory. In E. Tulving and W. Donaldson (Eds.), *Organization of memory*. New York: Academic Press.

Tulving, E. (1983). *Elements of episodic memory*. New York: Oxford University Press.

Tulving, E. (1984). Precis of elements of episodic memory. *The Behavioral and Brain Sciences, 7*, 223-268.

Tulving, E. (1985). How many memory systems are there? *American Psychologist, 40*, 385-398.

Warrington, E.K., and Silberstein, M. (1970). A questionnaire technique for investigating very long term memory. *Quarterly Journal of Experimental Psychology, 22*, 508-512.

Waugh, N.C., and Norman, D.A. (1965). Primary memory. *Psychological Review, 72*, 89-104.

Yesavage, J.A., Rose, T.L., and Bower, G.H. (1983). Interactive imagery and affective judgments improve face-name learning in the elderly. *Journal of Gerontology, 38*, 197-203.

Zelinski, E.M., Gilewski, M.J., and Thompson, L.W. (1980). Do laboratory tests relate to self-assessment of memory ability in the young and old? In L.W. Poon, J.L. Fozard, L.S. Cermak, D. Arenberg, and L.W. Thompson (Eds.), *New directions in memory and aging* (pp. 519-544). Hillsdale, NJ: Lawrence Erlbaum.

Chapter 13

Memory in Dementia

"It would be unbearable if memory didn't exist . . . I hear your laughter. I see you writing in your office, the smoke from your cigarette forcing you to blink. At will, I can spend hours with you."

Jeanne Moreau
(on the death of her best friend, Francois Truffaut)

Mrs. M is a 68-year-old retired high-school principal who continues to be very active in local civic affairs. She has always taken pride in her ability to remember names and faces of new people she meets. In her community activities, others have relied upon her for accurate recall of the details of events and conversations. However, over the last 2 years, she has experienced a marked and progressive change in her memory. She began experiencing difficulty in recalling the names of new acquaintances. Now, she is often unable to recall names of people with whom she has frequent contact. When a close friend expressed concern, Mrs. M dismissed her forgetfulness as being due to her being "too busy." Over the past several weeks she has been avoiding social situations in which her memory difficulties might become apparent. Yesterday, her friend called and tried to persuade her to see a physician, after Mrs. M was unable to remember ever having been at a full-day meeting they attended just last week.

Mrs. M illustrates the marked impairment of memory for events that is the hallmark of the early stage of AD. It is the failure to remember events or episodes that most often brings the patient in the early stage of AD to professional attention. As the disease progresses, memory becomes ever more severely impaired, until all ability to recall recent and most remote events is lost. As noted in the previous chapter, there are also changes in event memory that occur with normal aging. This contributes to difficulty in the clinical differentiation of normal aging memory changes from those of the early stage of dementia. Further complicating clinical diagnosis is the fact that memory deficit can also occur with certain focal cerebral lesions in other neurologic disorders. Recent research indicates that the memory changes of normal aging, dementia, and these various neurologic disorders can be differentiated on the basis of the specific aspects of memory processing that are impaired. It is the purpose of this chapter to review research concerned with the *nature* of memory change in dementia and in select amnesic disorders. Before beginning this review, it is useful to first examine the progression of memory impairment in dementia. In order to enable the reader to appreciate the clinical impact of progressive memory deficit, it is described in relation to other cognitive and emotional features characterizing the stages of dementia.

PROGRESSIVE DETERIORATION OF MEMORY AND OTHER CLINICAL FEATURES OF AD

While longitudinal studies of the course of memory deterioration in AD have begun to appear (e.g., Berg et al., 1984; Kaszniak, Wilson, Fox, and Stebbins, in press; Storandt, Botwinick, and Danziger, 1986; Wilson and Kaszniak, 1986), there remains a lack of empirical data on the characteristics of the earliest features of dementia. Even when extensive efforts are made to recruit mild AD patients into prospective longitudinal studies (e.g., Berg et al., 1982), it is still likely that patients are already several years into the course of their illness (see Roth, 1980). Consequently, the researcher must rely upon information gained from clinical anecdotal and family member reports. Both anecdotal reports and prospective longitudinal data (e.g., Wilson and Kaszniak, 1986) indicate that for most cases of AD, cognitive deterioration is gradual, rather than occurring in discrete stages. However, it is useful to reconstruct a series of "snapshots," or "phases," of the clinical course. This reconstruction will focus upon the typical course of dementia in Alzheimer's disease (AD).

Clinical Phases of AD

First Phase

Investigators at the New York University Geriatric Study and Treatment Program (Reisberg, 1983; Reisberg, and Ferris, 1982; Schneck, Reisberg and Ferris, 1982) have suggested three phases in the progression of AD. In the earliest, or "forgetfulness," phase, the patient, and occasionally other close family members, notice increasing forgetfulness, often accompanied by anxiety. Common symptoms include reading a newspaper article and forgetting the beginning before reaching the end, or seeing a movie and, a week later, not remembering having seen it at all (Reisberg and Ferris, 1982). In this phase, differentiation from the memory changes of normal aging is difficult or impossible. Katzman (1981) has cautioned that with increasing public and professional awareness of AD, there may be a growing tendency to confuse "benign senescent forgetfulness" (Kral, 1962) with senile dementia. Important distinctions include the progressive nature of the memory impairment in AD, as well as severity sufficient to interfere with work, social functioning, or both.

Schneck and colleagues (1982) focus their discussion of this stage upon memory difficulty. Certainly, most clinical observers agree that memory deficit is the most obvious early symptom of AD (e.g., Katzman, 1986; Miller, 1977; Rosen and Mohs, 1982; Sim and Sussman, 1962). The present authors, on the basis of clinical experience and discussion with families of AD patients, would add that conceptual and communicative functioning also show subtle impairment very early, but may be less obvious than memory deficit.

Second Phase

The next stage, termed the "confusional phase" by Schneck and colleagues (1982), is characterized by particularly severe deficit in memory for recent events. In addition, there is difficulty in orientation and concentration, and more obvious communication deficits, despite generally intact vocabulary and syntax. The person may begin to miss appointments and forget the names of familiar people. Significant events may be entirely forgotten soon after they occur. Simple arithmetic calculations may become extremely difficult. At this phase, the patient more clearly fits the diagnostic criteria for dementia set forth in the DSM-III. The importance of obtaining information from a spouse, or other informant close to the patient, is emphasized by the apparent denial that patients can manifest at this stage. As Reisberg and Ferris state:

> patients . . . devise strategies for avoiding conscious recognition of their intellectual decline. Although they watch the news on television every night, they may excuse their lack of knowledge for major current events by saying, "I'm not interested in those things." A retired accountant explains his inability to do simple arithmetic by saying, "I'm bad at numbers." Thus even the most astute clinician will find the presence of a spouse essential for an adequate evaluation of the patient. (Reisberg and Ferris, 1982, p. 106)

Third Phase

The third, or "dementia," phase is characterized by severe disorientation and memory deficit. It is also marked by more severe abnormalities of communication, perception, and praxis. Behavioral problems, including motor restlessness, wandering, and psychotic symptoms (e.g., paranoid ideation, delusions, hallucinations) occur in some patients. It is at this phase that somatic and neurologic abnormalities (e.g., incontinence, abnormal reflexes) are most likely to appear. Typically, the patient at this phase will show little knowledge of recent events, often having difficulty describing any recent activities. As dementia progresses within this phase, all memory for recent events is lost, and memory for remote personal history also deteriorates. Eventually, even the name of one's spouse, or one's own name, is forgotten. Familiar activities, such as handling utensils when eating, or the routines of proper toileting, become impaired.

Personality and Emotional Changes

In addition to the cognitive deficits of AD, personality and emotional changes occur with disease progression. As Roth (1980, p. 211) describes, personality may become "a caricature of its worst features, and undesirable traits such as meanness, tactlessness, impulsiveness, hypochondriasis, (and) disinhibition of sexually deviant conduct formerly held in check" may appear. Such behavior is often the most distressing aspect of a patient's dementia for other family members (Rabins, Mace, and Lucas, 1982). Social judgment may become progressively impaired, with decreasing concern for others and narrowing of interest. This impairment of social judgment is likely due, in part, to the deficits in perception, attention, memory, and conceptual reasoning, which limit appreciation of social context and expectations. It has also been demonstrated that AD patients are impaired in recognizing emotion communicated in facial expression or voice characteristics (Allender and Kaszniak, 1985). However, the specific relationship between the deficit in processing emotional cues and the behavior exhibiting poor social judgment remains to be determined.

Early in the course of AD, withdrawal and a flattening of emotional expression may be noted (Reisberg and Ferris, 1982). When required to perform a task that exceeds their abilities, patients will often become anxious. Increased anxiety can frequently be seen when patients forget where familiar cooking utensils are placed, or have difficulty comprehending a conversation. Signs of anxiety, such as motor restlessness and autonomic arousal, can be observed by the clinician, even when the AD patient may deny experiencing excessive anxiety (Kaszniak, 1985). Withdrawal from anxiety-provoking activities and social interactions is a frequent response.

Depression may also accompany AD, either early or later in the course of illness. Kaszniak (1985) compared 40 mild to moderate AD patients and 43 healthy older individuals, matched for age, occupation, and previous occupation, on a series of self-report and clinician-observer measures of depression. The AD patient group was found to be significantly more depressed on all measures. Differentiating primary depression from depression in dementia can be quite difficult. Detailed discussion of this issue is contained in the subsequent chapter.

Particularly distressing for family members are the increased suspiciousness and hostility typically seen in the middle to later phases of AD. Often, the suspiciousness appears related to memory impairment, as when the patient who forgets where he or she has placed something accuses a family member of stealing it. Hostility frequently is triggered by the frustration encountered by a patient who is unable to remember an event or perform a previously easy task.

Clinical Course in Other Dementias

The clinical course of other dementias may be quite different from that seen in AD. In multi-infarct dementia (MID), clinical features are believed to be secondary to the accumulation of abrupt vascular episodes ("strokes"). Consequently, the onset of dementia in MID is typically abrupt, with a stepwise course of deterioration, focal neurologic signs and symptoms, a history consistent with cerebrovascular accident (CVA), and a history or presence of hypertension (Brust, 1983; Hachinski, Lassen, and Marshall, 1974). Initially, memory deficit may be greatest for particular types of material. For example, the MID patient with more abundant infarctions in the left than in the right temporal lobe would be expected to have more difficulty in memory for linguistic than nonlinguistic material. The differences between MID and AD, in clinical presentation and course, were described in Chapter 1, as were the major characteristics of HD and PD.

While the foregoing clinical descriptions are of value in gaining a general overview of the presentation and course of dementia, they do not provide sufficiently detailed accounts to understand what specifically is changing in the memory functioning of dementia patients. In the remainder of this chapter, research providing this detail is discussed, and clinical implications are derived.

THE NATURE OF MEMORY DEFICIT IN DEMENTIA

If changes in memory with normal aging are due to decreased spontaneous use of elaborate and distinctive encoding/retrieval strategies, can the more severe memory deficit of AD be considered an exaggeration of this problem? Research on memory in AD suggests not. Rather, memory deficit in AD has been shown to differ from memory change in normal aging along two major dimensions.

The Authors' Claims About the Memory Disorder of AD

First, AD patients show abnormally rapid forgetting of information stored in episodic memory. In this respect, AD patients are similar to amnesic patients with medial temporal lobe cerebral damage. Second, much of the severity of episodic memory deficit in AD appears to be due to deterioration in the access to, and possibly the structure of, semantic memory. In this respect, AD patients are different from most patients with amnesia due to focal cerebral damage. The remainder of this chapter will review the evidence in support of these claims. Their clinical importance is primarily in implications for assessment. The abnormally rapid forgetting of events in AD suggests that clinical assessment of episodic memory should include instruments that allow the measurement of information loss over time. Further, the differentiation of AD from normal aging, as well as various amnesic disorders, will be heavily dependent upon the inclusion of instruments to assess aspects of semantic memory.

Much of the research on memory in dementia was designed to address issues motivated by a linear information processing model of memory. Consequently, the present discussion will initially describe results of this research, under the headings of primary and secondary memory. However, since much recent research has addressed more current models, such as the levels-of-processing approach, data relevant to these alternative models will follow. Finally, a major emphasis will be placed upon studies designed to address issues concerning the status of episodic, semantic, and procedural memory in dementia.

Linear Information Processing Approaches to Memory in Dementia

Primary Memory

Memory Span Paradigms. The most frequently applied procedure for the study of primary memory is Forward Digit Span. While reflecting mostly primary memory, Digit Span may also contain a small secondary memory component (Craik, 1977). Most investigators (e.g., Corkin, 1982; Crook, Ferris, McCarthy, and Rae, 1980; Kaszniak, Garron, and Fox, 1979; Larner, 1977) find Digit Span impaired in AD patients. However, this impairment may not be seen in mildly demented patients (Storandt, Botwinick, Danziger, Berg, and Hughes, 1984). Digit Span performance does deteriorate over time in AD, as dementia severity increases (Berg, et al., 1984). Digit Span performance has been found to be negatively correlated with severity of EEG slowing in AD (Kaszniak, Garron, Fox, Bergen, and Huckman, 1979), as well as with degree of impairment in activities of daily living (ADL) (Corkin, 1982). Word Span (employing words rather than Digits) and Block Span (requiring the subject to tap spatially arranged blocks in the sequence indicated by the examiner) tasks demonstrate similar impairment in AD (Corkin, 1982; Miller, 1973).

The Brown-Peterson Paradigm. Another task traditionally employed to examine primary memory is the Brown (1958) or Peterson and Peterson (1959) technique, in which either three words or a consonant trigram is presented. Recall is then tested either immediately, or following various delay intervals (typically 1 to 18 seconds) filled with distracting cognitive activity, such as counting backwards by twos. Since the distracting activity is presumed to prevent rehearsal, any decrease in recall, with increasing distraction interval, is taken to reflect a loss of information from primary memory.

Employing this procedure, Corkin (1982) found no difference between AD patients and control subjects in immediate recall. The performance of AD patients was, however, impaired with increasing distraction intervals. Corkin also found the Brown-Peterson performance of AD patients to be negatively correlated with ADL impairment. While interpretation of the Brown-Peterson technique as reflecting primary memory processes has been questioned (Baddeley, 1976), AD patient deficits in performing this task are similar to those obtained with span tasks.

Free Recall Paradigms. Still another task that has been used to examine primary memory in dementia is based upon the free recall paradigm. In this procedure, the subject is presented a sequence of, typically, 12 or more words and instructed to recall as many words as possible immediately following the last presented word. When probability of recall is plotted against the serial position in which the word was presented, normal individuals demonstrate a U-shaped curve, in which the first few words and the last few words are recalled better than those presented in the middle of the list. Following Glanzer and Cunitz (1966), the relatively good recall of words from the end of the list has been interpreted as reflecting short-term or primary memory. Words recalled from the beginning of the list are presumed to reflect material that has passed into secondary or long-term storage.

Miller (1971) was the first to report free recall serial position data comparing presenile AD patients and matched control subjects. Control subjects demonstrated the expected U-shaped curve. Words from the end of the list (primary memory component) were recalled more poorly by the presenile AD patients, although the group difference was even more marked for words from the beginning of the list (secondary memory component). These results are consistent with a reduced primary memory capacity or efficiency, or both, in presenile AD. Discussion of the markedly reduced secondary memory component of the serial position curve will shortly be reviewed. Using a similar verbal free recall procedure, Kaszniak, Wilson, and Fox (1981) obtained the same evidence of reduced primary memory in AD patients, compared with age-matched control subjects.

The interpretation of recency and primacy effects, in free recall serial position data, as reflecting primary and secondary memory, respectively, has been subject to criticism. Baddeley (1976) has questioned whether the recency effect results from a retrieval strategy that uses serial position as a cue, rather than reflecting primary memory. Further, recency effects in verbal recall have been obtained under conditions in which their origin in primary memory can be ruled out (e.g., Bjork and Whitten, 1974; Tzeng, 1973).

Tulving and Colotla (1970) described a procedure for defining primary and secondary memory components in free recall data, which takes into account both serial list position of word presention and serial order of word recall. In this procedure, each word that is recalled within six or fewer intervening word presentations and recall productions is assigned to primary memory. All other recalled words are assigned to secondary memory. The Tulving and Colotla procedure has found considerable empirical support, both in experimental investigations of normal memory functioning (Watkins, 1974) and in neuropsychologic studies of amnesia (Moscovitch, 1982). Employing this scoring procedure, Wilson, Bacon, Fox, and Kaszniak (1983) found primary memory to be impaired in AD patients, relative to matched healthy control subjects (Figure 13-1), and further showed that the size of the patients' primary memory deficit increased linearly with an increasing number of items between presentation and recall. Longitudinal study demonstrated the primary memory score to deteriorate over time for the AD patients, but not for the control subjects (Wilson and Kaszniak, 1986).

Summary. In summary, while no single experimental procedure for defining primary memory has escaped theoretic debate, all have shown impairment in AD. Collectively, the available research suggests that impairment of primary memory is

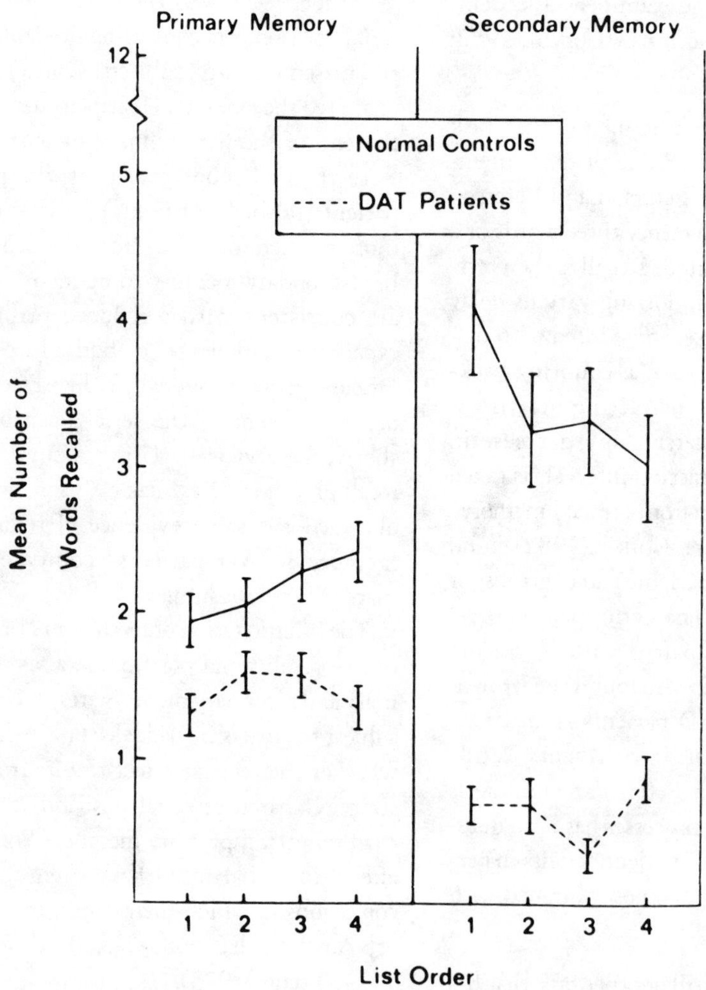

Figure 13-1. *Primary and secondary memory scores, across consecutive free recall lists, for normal control and dementia of the Alzheimer type (DAT) patients. (From Wilson, R S., Bacon, L. D., Fox, J. H., and Kaszniak, A. W. (1983). Primary memory and secondary memory in dementia of the Alzheimer type.* Journal of Clinical Neuropsychology, *5, 337–344, by permission. Copyright 1983 by Swets and Zeitlinger, B.V., Lisse.)*

mild early in the course of AD and increases over time with greater severity of dementia. Primary memory for both linguistic and nonlinguistic material is impaired in AD, and the degree of impairment corresponds to the severity of EEG slowing. The impairment of primary memory in AD contrasts with the lack of normal aging effects upon primary memory. This also contrasts with the relative preservation of primary memory in amnesic patients with cerebral damage limited to medial temporal areas (Corkin, 1982; Drachman and Arbit, 1965; Miller, 1973; Warrington, 1982).

Secondary Memory

Verbal Learning Paradigm. Recall of material presented in verbal learning tasks has been considered to reflect at least some secondary memory, since word lists employed have been longer than presumed primary memory capacity. In a typical verbal learning task, a list of ten or more words is repeatedly presented, and the number of trials necessary for accurate recall is recorded. AD patients require a much greater number of trials than age-matched control subjects (McCarthy, Ferris, Clark, and Crook, 1981). Studies employing verbal learning tasks, which assess recall accuracy for lists of progressively longer length, also reveal impairment in AD (Miller, 1973).

Paired-Associate Paradigm. Paired-associate learning tasks repeatedly present lists of word pairs, or other stimulus pairs, and record the number of trials necessary for correct recall of the second word of the pair when the first is provided. Studies employing a verbal paired-associate learning paradigm consistently document deficit in AD (Barbizet and Cany, 1969; Caird, Sanderson and Inglis, 1962; Corkin, 1982; Danziger and Storandt, 1982; Inglis, 1959; Inglis and Caird, 1963; Kaszniak, Garron, and Fox, 1979; Rosen and Mohs, 1982; Wilson, Bacon, Kaszniak, and Fox, 1982). Paired-associate learning for geometric forms shows impairment similar to that seen with verbal paired-associate learning tasks (Corkin, 1982). For AD patients, the level of performance in verbal paired-associate learning has been shown to be negatively correlated with the degree of cerebral atrophy seen on CT scan (DeLeon, Ferris, George, Reisberg, Kricheff, and Gershon, 1980; Kaszniak, Garron, Fox, Bergen, and Huckman, 1979), and with the severity of EEG slowing (Johannesson, Hagberg, Gustafson, and Ingvar, 1979; Kaszniak, Garron, Fox, Bergen, and Huckman, 1979).

Studies of regional cerebral blood flow distribution in presenile dementia patients have found verbal paired-associate learning impairment to be most closely associated with left temporal lobe blood flow reductions (Hagberg, 1978; Hagberg and Ingvar, 1976). This suggests that paired-associate learning deficit in dementia is particularly related to abnormal functioning of those same brain regions (i.e., medial temporal lobes, particularly the hippocampal bodies) known to be affected in certain amnesic disorders (Milner, 1971).

Text Recall Paradigms. Recall of verbal textual material, such as short stories, is another task considered to involve predominantly secondary memory. AD patients demonstrate impairment, relative to matched control subjects, in immediate recall of spoken short stories (Brinkman, Largen, Gerganoff, and Pomara, 1983; Danziger and Storandt, 1982; Logue and Wyrick, 1979; Osborne, Brown and Randt, 1982). The level of performance in story recall shows the same negative correlations with degree of cerebral atrophy and EEG slowing, as was described for paired-associate learning (DeLeon et al., 1980; Kaszniak, Garron, Fox, Bergen, and Huckman, 1979). When recall of short stories is tested immediately after presentation as well as after a delay interval, AD patients show a lower percentage of retention than matched control subjects (Brinkman et al., 1983; Logue and Wyrick, 1979). These results indicate that secondary memory in AD is characterized by an abnormally rapid rate of forgetting.

Rapid Forgetting from Secondary Memory in AD

Additional evidence for abnormally rapid rate of forgetting in AD has been presented by Moss, Albert, Butters, and Payne (1986). Moss and colleagues compared AD, HD, and alcoholic Korsakoff's (an amnesic syndrome typically associated with chronic alcoholism) patients with normal control subjects on a task involving delayed recall of 16 nouns and verbs. Following several trials, in which the subjects read the words, recall was tested at 15 seconds and at 2 minutes later. The interval between presentation and recall testing was filled by unrelated conversation with the examiner, to prevent rehearsal. Because the list of words was longer than the presumed capacity of primary memory, and rehearsal was prevented, it can be assumed that recall was from secondary memory. All three patient groups were equally impaired, relative to normal control subjects, at the shorter delay interval. However, the Korsakoff's and HD groups had significantly better recall scores than the AD group at the longer delay interval. Thus, the pattern of recall performance argues that patients with AD experience a more rapid rate of forgetting than healthy control subjects, HD patients, or Korsakoff's patients.

Several other investigators have also reported that Korsakoff's amnesia patients (with greatest locus of cerebral damage within the dorsomedial thalamus of the diencephalon) exhibit a relatively normal rate of forgetting. However, patients with amnesic syndromes secondary to hippocampal damage exhibit abnormally rapid forgetting (see Squire and Cohen, 1984, for a review of this literature). Monkeys with hippocampal ablations demonstrate similar rapid forgetting, while those with dorsomedial thalamic lesions show normal forgetting rates (Zola-Morgan, 1984). The marked accumulation of neuritic plaques and neurofibrillary tangles, within the hippocampi of AD patients, has been described in Chapter 1. As Moss and colleagues (1986) have hypothesized, the rapid decay of stored information in AD might be attributable to the severity of hippocampal damage.

Basal forebrain cell loss (i.e., in the nucleus basalis of Meynert) is also marked in AD. Recently, basal forebrain cell loss has been demonstrated to be present in Korsakoff's patients (see Moss et al., 1986). It was hypothesized by Moss and associates (1986) that this locus of cell loss in both Korsakoff's and AD patients might play a common role in a neuronal processing system that underlies registration and immediate-retention mechanisms. This would account for Moss and colleagues' observation of equivalent impairment of immediate recall in these two groups. In the sections to follow, deficits shown by AD patients in registration (encoding) of new information will be further discussed.

Summary of Evidence from the Linear Information Processing Perspective

Available data on the memory disorder of AD, conceptualized with a linear information processing model, argue for impairment in both primary and secondary memory. As will be recalled from evidence reviewed in the previous chapter, the memory changes of normal aging are limited to secondary memory. The primary and secondary memory deficits of AD patients are manifest across stimulus types, including both linguistic and nonlinguistic material. AD patients show rapid forgetting of information from secondary memory, likely associated with the severity of plaque and tangle accumulation within the hippocampal bodies. The rate of forgetting is not altered in normal aging, or in amnesic syndromes due to dorsomedial thalamic damage.

THE MEMORY DEFICIT OF AD FROM A LEVELS-OF-PROCESSING PERSPECTIVE

As was discussed in the previous chapter, recent theory has moved away from a memory "stores" model to a conceptualization in which memory is seen as involving a continous processing of mental representation. Thus, secondary memory is seen not as a "store" into which information is placed and from which it is retrieved, but rather as a *process*. The efficiency and accuracy of this process is dependent upon the degree of elaboration and distinctiveness of encoding, as well as reinstatement of the same effortful processing at the time of retrieval.

Encoding/Retrieval Deficit in AD

Research concerned with encoding/retrieval processes has documented a pervasive encoding deficit in AD. Further, unlike the memory changes of normal aging, AD patients' memory is not facilitated by various task or environment manipulations (e.g., cuing, instruction in verbal elaboration of stimuli). Normal older persons often fail to adequately encode new information because of limitations in effortful processing capacity. AD patients have an impairment in access to, and possibly the structure of, previously acquired facts, concepts, and schema, which are necessary for adequate encoding of new information. This impairment is observed even when the effort required for such access is reduced. The nature of these deficits, and their relationship to the encoding of new information, will be discussed under the heading of *episodic and semantic memory*.

Free Recall Paradigms

The application of scoring procedures for separating primary and secondary memory components in free recall reveals progressive impairment of secondary memory in AD (Wilson, Bacon, Fox, and Kaszniak, 1983; Wilson and Kaszniak, 1986). It is of particular interest to note that primary and secondary memory scores are independent in healthy elderly control subjects, but significantly correlated in AD patients (Wilson, Bacon, Fox, and Kaszniak, 1983). Further, the size of AD patients' primary memory deficit increases linearly with the number of items between presentation and attempted recall. These observations led Wilson and colleagues to argue that the secondary memory deficit in AD is at least partially due to impaired primary memory. Other investigators (Miller, 1971; Diesfeldt, 1978) employing the free recall paradigm with AD patients have come to the same conclusion. Within a continuous process view of memory, these observations can be interpreted as suggesting that new information rapidly dissipates in AD because of deficits in initial encoding.

Corroboration from the Study of Proactive Interference

Consistent with this view are data concerning proactive interference. Proactive interference occurs when previously learned information interferes with recall of more recent material. Wilson, Bacon, Fox, and Kaszniak (1983) examined proactive interference in AD in two ways. The first measured the decline in free recall across four consecutive list presentations. The second measured the number of words from a previous list produced during attempt at recall of a subsequent list, termed "prior item intrusions." While the control group showed the expected linear decline in recall over lists, the AD patients did not. This can be seen in Figure 13-1, presented earlier in this chapter. Further, the patients showed fewer prior list intrusions than the controls. This lack of proactive interference effects for the AD patients suggests that the initially presented information was never sufficiently encoded and therefore failed to interfere with recall of later presented information.

This contrasts with the pattern observed in alcoholic Korsakoff's amnesia, in which there is increased susceptibility to proactive interference (Cermak and Butters, 1972; Kinsbourne and Winocur, 1980; Warrington and Weiskrantz, 1974). Korsakoff's patients have clear encoding deficits (see Butters and Cermak, 1980, for a review of evidence for this conclusion). It has been suggested by Jacoby (1982) that despite these encoding deficits, Korsakoff's patients retain "automatic" memory activation processes, as reflected in priming phenomena (Jacoby and Witherspoon, 1982). Jacoby argues that the susceptibility of Korsakoff's amnesia patients to proactive interference reflects the effects of priming by prior presentation. The lack of susceptibility of AD patients to proactive interference suggests that they are impaired in even automatic aspects of the encoding of recent events. Both the lack of proactive interference and the marked impairment of secondary memory in AD may thus reflect initial effortful and automatic processing failure.

Evidence from Recognition Memory Paradigms

Recognition memory paradigms have provided additional insight into the mechanisms of memory impairment in AD. Such paradigms involve the forced choice recognition, following target stimulus presentation, of mixed target and distractor stimuli. An advantage of recognition memory tasks is that they allow for examination of variables (e.g., response bias) not easily evaluated in free recall tasks.

Recognition memory has been shown to be impaired in AD, employing both verbal and nonverbal (faces) stimuli (Martin, Brouwers, Cox, and Fedio, 1985; Miller, 1975, 1978; Wilson, Kaszniak, Bacon, Fox, and Kelly, 1982). Signal detection analysis (Marcer, 1979; Swets, 1973) indicates this deficit to be due to a problem in the memory discrimination of target versus distractor stimuli, rather than to any response bias (Miller and Lewis, 1977; Wilson, Kaszniak, Bacon, Fox, and Kelly, 1982).

Miller (1975, 1978) had proposed that this recognition memory deficit is predominantly one of retrieval, since it worsens as the number of recognition alternatives increases, and improves when testing employs a partial information rather than uncued recognition procedure. However, it has been shown that both of these findings can be reproduced in normal individuals if the length of time between target presentation and retention testing is increased, so that normal performance is in a range similar to that seen in immediate recognition testing of dementia patients (Mayes and Meudell, 1981; Meudell and Mayes, 1981). Thus, it is possible that poor initial encoding of information accounts for the recognition memory deficit in AD.

Several recent observations support this interpretation. First, Wilson, Kaszniak, Bacon, Fox, and Kelly (1982) found verbal, but not facial, recognition memory performance in AD to be negatively correlated with the severity of language impairment, as measured by a summary index of performance on the Boston Diagnostic Aphasia Examination. This suggests that linguistic processing deficits limit verbal episodic encoding in AD and make a specific contribution to verbal recognition memory impairment. Conversely, Martin, Cox, Brouwers, and Fedio (1985) found that AD patients' recognition memory for nonverbal (complex random shapes) stimuli was related to a nonverbal reasoning task (WAIS Block Design performance) but not to object naming ability. Thus, material-specific (i.e., linguistic and nonlinguistic) conceptual processing deficits in AD predictably relate to material-specific recognition memory performance. As will be discussed later in the chapter, a breakdown in the processes, and likely also the content of semantic memory, contribute to insufficient encoding of information in episodic memory.

Experimental Manipulation of Encoding Variables in Recognition Memory Paradigms. Manipulation of depth of processing of verbal stimuli can be accomplished by asking orienting questions, prior to the presentation of each stimulus word, which focus the subject upon either phonemic or semantic aspects (Craik and Tulving, 1975). This manipulation has less effect upon the verbal recognition memory performance of AD patients than on that of matched control subjects (Corkin, 1982; Wilson, Kaszniak, Bacon, Fox, and Kelly, 1982). Similarly, AD patients are less responsive to verbal imagery manipulations in free recall tasks than are matched controls (Kaszniak, Wilson, and Fox, 1981). As was noted in the previous chapter, instructing normal older subjects in the use of either imagery or verbal elaboration can greatly reduce the magnitude of age differences in episodic memory. Rissenberg and Glanzer (1986) found that whereas instruction in verbal elaboration improved free recall for the names of pictures presented to normal older persons, it did not have this effect in a group of AD patients.

These observations support the hypothesis of defective encoding of information contributing to the episodic memory deficit of AD. Unlike the case with normal older individuals, this encoding deficit is not improved by task or instructional manipulations of encoding strategies. Thus, while normal older persons may fail to activate sufficiently distinctive encoding operations, because of attentional capacity limitations, AD patients have a deficit in the access to, and likely the structural integrity of, semantic memory, which is necessary for adequate encoding.

Word Frequency Effect in Recognition Memory Paradigms. Another examination of the hypothesis that encoding deficits contribute to the impaired recognition memory performance of AD patients was provided by Wilson, Bacon, Kramer, Fox, and Kaszniak (1983). In normal younger and older individuals, recognition memory for rare words is superior to that for common words (Kinsbourne and George, 1974; Poon and Fozard, 1980; Shepard, 1967). This "rare word advantage" is thought to be dependent upon more active attention to, and semantic analysis of, the rare words as they are initially presented. Wilson, Bacon, Kramer, Fox, and Kaszniak (1983) reasoned, therefore, that analysis of the word frequency effect would provide another way of examining the efficiency of encoding operations in AD. Consistent with their hypothesis, the AD patients failed to show the normal rare word advantage in their hit rate, despite the fact that they showed a normal tendency to give false-alarm responses to common words (Figure 13-2).

In a second experiment (Wilson, Bacon, Kramer, Fox, and Kaszniak, 1983), normal subjects were examined both immediately after word list presen-

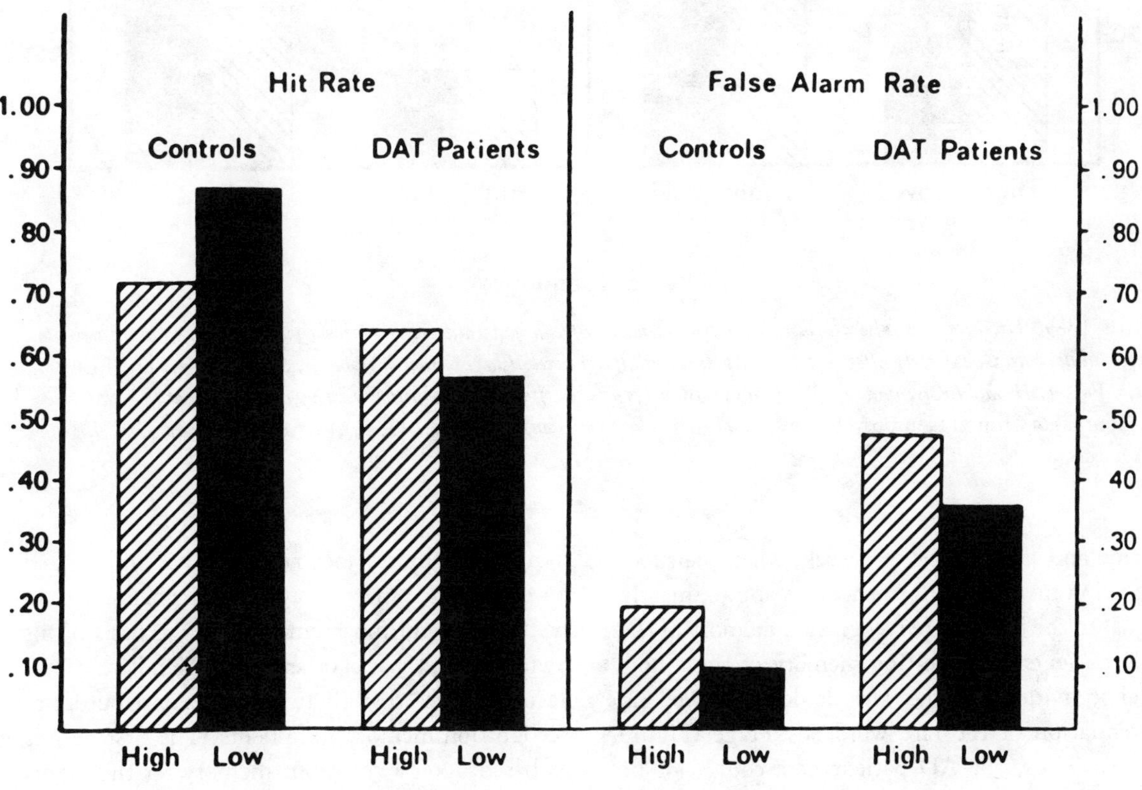

Figure 13-2. *Hit rate and false alarm rate for high-and low-rate frequency words in recognition memory task. (From Wilson, R. S., Bacon, L. D., Kramer, R. L., Fox, J. H., and Kaszniak, A. W. (1983). Word frequency effect and recognition memory in dementia of the Alzheimer type.* Journal of Clinical Neuropsychology, 5, *97–104, by permission. Copyright 1983 by Swets and Zeitlinger, B.V., Lisse.)*

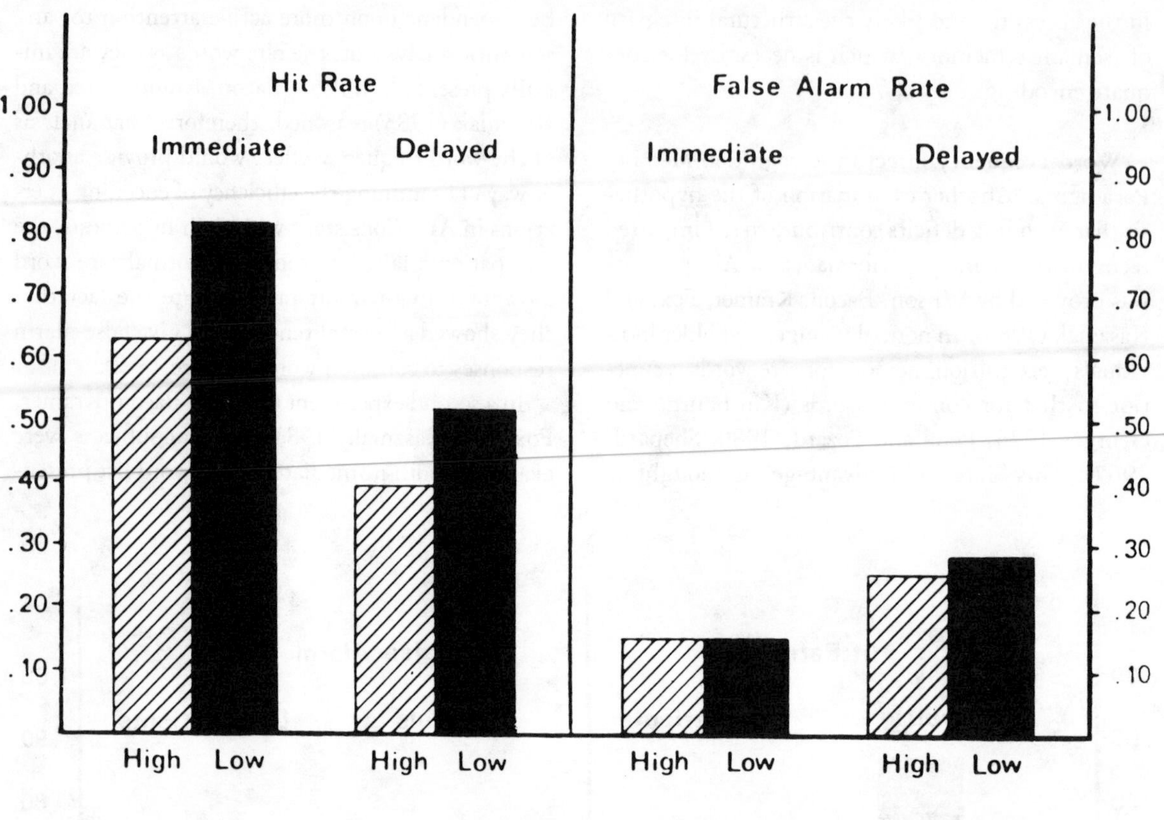

Figure 13-3. *Hit rate and false alarm rate for high- and low-frequency words in recognition memory task, administered to normal adults both immediately after target list exposure and at a 1-week delay. (From Wilson, R. S., Bacon, L. D., Kramer, R. L., Fox, J. H., and Kaszniak, A. W. {1983}. Word frequency effect and recognition memory in dementia of the Alzheimer type.* Journal of Clinical Neuropsychology, 5, *97–104, by permission. Copyright 1983 by Swets and Zeitlinger, B.V. Lisse.)*

tation and after a delay of 1 week, when their recognition memory performance was approximately equal to the immediate recognition memory of the AD patients. Recognition memory of these normal individuals at the 1-week delay showed no attenuation of the rare word advantage (Figure 13-3). Thus, the AD patient data could not be explained simply as the result of poor retention (i.e., rapid forgetting) or as an artifact of the difficulty of the memory test.

Effortful and Automatic Processes in Recognition Memory. There has been considerable speculation concerning the memory processes reflected in recognition memory. Jacoby (1982) has emphasized an important aspect of associative phenomena in tests of recognition memory. On the basis of his own work and that of others (e.g., Mandler, 1979), Jacoby argues that there are two contributors to recognition memory judgments. The first he sees as based upon a conscious memory for the events of the previous presentation of the items. The second he sees as based on assessment of the "trace strength." This is similar to the account of recognition memory suggested by Huppert and Piercy (1976), who argued that recognition memory could depend either on a judgment of "list membership," a conscious or effortful process, or on familiarity determined by "trace strength," an automatic priming process. At present, the degree to which automatic aspects (e.g., priming) of episodic or semantic memory activation are intact in AD remains controversial.

Semantic Context and Cuing Fail to Facilitate Pictorial Recognition Memory in AD Patients

Butters et al., (1983) compared patients with AD, HD, Korsakoff's syndrome and right cerebral hemisphere damage with normal control subjects on a picture recognition task. In this task, subjects were to associate specific human and animal figures with particular scenic backgrounds. Two conditions were employed: one in which no specific verbal cues were provided, and one in which stories linking the figures to the background scenes were read to subjects. Although all four patient groups were impaired in the no-story condition, the groups significantly differed in ability to use the stories to improve their pictorial memory. The AD and Korsakoff's syndrome groups failed to benefit from the verbal context material. In contrast, the HD and right-hemisphere lesion groups showed significant improvement when stories were provided.

Further, illustrating the heterogeneity of the dementias, Moss and colleagues (1986) have shown AD, HD, and Korsakoff's syndrome patients to be impaired on a recognition memory task when spatial, color, pattern, or facial stimuli were used. However, when verbal stimuli were used, AD and Korsakoff's patients were impaired, but HD patients were not. Moss and colleagues suggest that this difference between their patient groups may reflect a greater preservation of verbal encoding and storage processes in HD, as compared with AD and Korsakoff's syndrome. The comparable recognition memory deficit for nonlinguistic stimuli might reflect the visuospatial deficits that occur in HD.

Other investigators, employing various cuing techniques, have also come to the conclusion that AD is characterized by a deficit in episodic memory encoding processes that likely reflects problems in the accessing of semantic memory, its structure, or both. Davis and Mumford (1984), for example, examined AD patients and age-matched healthy control subjects on recall for lists of words, using a cued recall technique. Word list memory was tested either with no cues given at the time of recall, or alternatively by cuing the subjects either with the target word's first letter or with a word representing its semantic category. Semantic category cuing significantly increased the recall accuracy of the control subjects, but not of the AD patients. Davis and Mumford interpret this observation as being consistent with a deficit in initial semantic encoding. Martin and colleagues (1985) have similarly reported failure of AD patients to benefit from a selective cuing procedure, and argue for an explanation in terms of insufficient encoding into episodic memory of the semantic dimensions of stimuli.

Episodic and Semantic Memory in Dementia

The available research provides ample evidence of deficit in the episodic memory of AD patients. Regardless of whether the "episodes" or "events" involve linguistic or nonlinguistic information, AD patients are impaired. From the studies just reviewed, there are two distinguishable components to this episodic memory deficit. The first is an increased rate of forgetting, assumed to reflect impairment within the storage or consolidation processes of episodic memory. The second reflects inadequate encoding, caused by problems in the access to semantic memory, its structure, or both. Within the present section, more specific examination of both forgetting and semantic encoding in the episodic memory of AD will be presented.

Memory for Remote Episodes

Memory for remote episodes involves recall of events that occurred in the distant past. Forgetting over time is a characteristic of normal episodic memory. Bahrick, Bahrick, and Wittlinger (1975) illustrated this in their study of episodic memory for names of high-school classmates. Using a cross-sectional approach, they tested 392 high-school graduates and found that free recall of names declined, with negative acceleration, by 60 percent, over an interval ranging from 2 weeks to 57 years.

Albert, Butters, and Levin (1979) tested recognition of faces and events that became famous during the 1920s through the 1970s. As would be anticipated from the results of Bahrick and colleagues (1975), normal individuals were more accurate at identifying famous people and events from more recent decades. However, Korsakoff's amnesia patients were considerably better at identification of faces and events from the more distant, than from more recent, decades.

Recently, Cermak (1984) has suggested an interpretation of such "retrograde gradients" in terms of the operations of both episodic and semantic memory. Cermak argues, as do other theorists, that normal individuals remember fewer episodes from their youth and childhood than they do from more recent years. Further, he states:

> Even those distant episodes that do appear vivid may actually be more familial folklore than truly retained

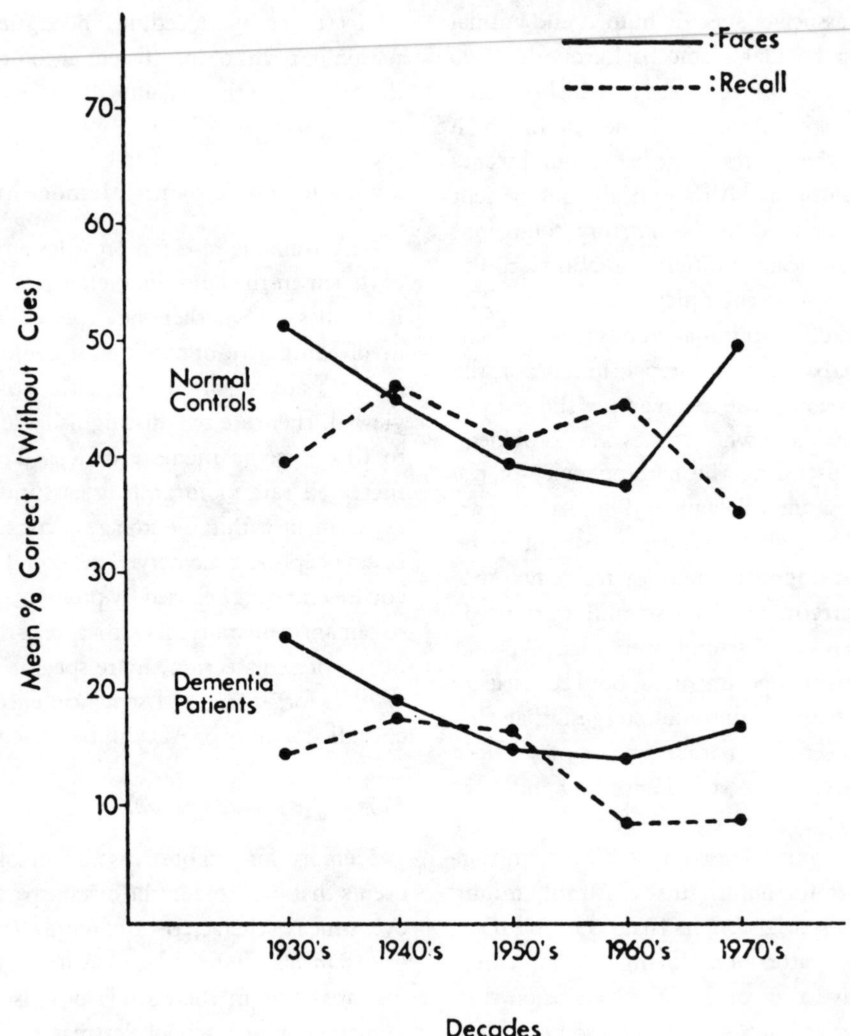

Figure 13-4. *Performance of Alzheimer's disease patients and normal control subjects on famous faces ("faces") and famous events ("recall") remote memory test. (From Wilson, R. S., Kaszniak, A. W., and Fox, J. H., {1981}. Remote memory in senile dementia.* Cortex *17, 41–48. With permission of Masson Italia Periodici S.r.l.)*

> episodes. . . . As a consequence, normal subjects may tend to answer more of the queries about distant decades on a retrograde-memory test from their semantic memory and more of the recent items from their episodic memory. An event from the 1950s might be remembered more as a matter of general knowledge, while an event from the 1970s might still retain a personal episodic component. An individual might recall where he or she was when Nixon resigned, but not know where he or she was when Eisenhower had a heart attack. (Cermak, 1984, p. 59)

Hence, normal retrograde retrieval may change from being primarily from semantic memory to primarily from episodic memory, as the events in question become nearer to the present. There is ample evidence that Korsakoff's patients have more intact semantic than episodic memory (see review by Cermak, 1984). The shifting bias, from semantic to episodic memory retrieval, could explain the apparent "shrinking" retrograde amnesia of Korsakoff's patients.

Clinical observation of dementia patients suggests that remote memory for distant episodes might be relatively spared. Mild and moderately demented patients often seem able to recall childhood or other remote events, despite a severe deficit in recall of recent events. Interpretation of such clinical observations, however, is problematic. The remote events recalled not only occurred in the more distant past, but also are typically of greater emotional significance, than recent events, or have been more frequently rehearsed.

Wilson, Kaszniak, and Fox (1981) attempted to systematically investigate memory for remote events in AD. Remote memory was assessed with the procedure constructed by Albert, Butters, and Levin (1979) to examine the temporal gradient of remote memory in alcoholic Korsakoff's amnesia. Wilson, Kaszniak, and Fox (1981) found AD patients to be significantly impaired, relative to age-matched control subjects, on these tests. As shown in Figure 13-4, the AD patients showed a relatively consistent recall deficit over the time period examined (i.e., persons and events that became famous between 1930 and 1975). This contrasts with the retrograde gradient that characterizes the remote memory deficit of Korsakoff's patients.

Albert, Butters, and Brandt (1981) have observed a similar remote memory deficit, without retrograde gradient, in HD patients. Further, Cermak and O'Connor (1983), reporting on a case study of a postencephalitic dementia patient, found a flatter retrograde gradient of remote recall than seen in Korsakoff's syndrome. They interpret this observation as consistent with the possibility that the postencephalitic dementia patient's semantic memory is not as normal as that of Korsakoff's patients. This semantic memory deficit is presumed to be due to the greater cortical cerebral damage in encephalitis than in Korsakoff's amnesia. Thus, AD, HD, and some amnesic syndromes with significant cortical involvement appear to include impairment in retrieval from both episodic and semantic memory components of remote memory tests.

Relations between Episodic and Semantic Memory Deficit in AD

Weingartner and colleagues (1982) compared 14 very mildly demented AD patients with a group of matched control subjects, on a word learning task. Subjects were presented with two different sets of common words, presented in randomized sequences. One list had 20 random words, and the other had words drawn from two superordinate categories (10 words each) of semantically related words. All subjects were tested for free recall. The word lists were then presented five additional times, always in a different random order, with a test of free recall after each presentation. Delayed recall was also examined, at 10 minutes for AD patients and at 1 day for normal subjects. These different recall testing intervals were used to equate the groups for overall rate of forgetting. The AD patients were unable to effectively use the semantic organizational or relational properties of word lists, on free recall, list learning, or delayed recall. The control subjects remembered more related than random words, and this was increasingly evident as list learning continued. The normal subjects' recall of related words was also better than that for random words, when they were tested 1 day later. Weingartner and associates concluded that AD patients do not make use of semantic features.

In a separate study reported in the same paper, Weingartner and colleagues (1982) examined 20 moderately depressed patients who had similar psychometric intelligence and clinical memory test scores to those of the AD patients. The depressed patients were able to make use of semantic category clusters in facilitating their free verbal recall. This illustrates one type of difference between the dementia of AD and the cognitive/memory impairment associated with depression. This result also suggests that the episodic verbal memory deficit of AD cannot be sufficiently accounted for by a lack of effortful encoding operations, which are characteristic of depression. It appears that a deficit in the access to semantic memory, or its structure, or both must be invoked.

Weingartner, Grafman, Boutelle, Kaye, and Martin (1983) have further reported on a study designed to specifically contrast and relate aspects of episodic and semantic memory. They predicted that AD patients, unlike Korsakoff's patients, would show impaired semantic memory functions, the extent of which would be directly related to the severity of their episodic memory failure. The patient groups (N = 8 each) were matched on age, Wechsler Memory Scale (Wechsler, 1945) Memory Quotient, and a premorbid IQ estimate (Wilson, Rosenbaum, and Brown, 1979), and were compared with a group of eight age-matched control subjects. Three episodic memory tasks were employed: (1) a 20-word delayed free verbal recall task, (2) a 12-word selective reminding list-learning task (on each learning trial only those words not previously recalled are presented), and (3) a 20-picture delayed free recall task. Three semantic memory tasks were also used: (1) tests of phonemic and semantic generative naming, (2) a sentence completion task, and (3) a task requiring judgment about correct sequences in common themes and activities.

Weingartner and colleagues (1983) found that relative to control subjects, both the Korsakoff's and AD patients were impaired on the selective reminding and on the free recall tasks. The AD patients were impaired on generative naming and the other semantic memory tasks, but Korsakoff's patients were not. Episodic memory impairment was unrelated to semantic memory performance in the Korsakoff's patients, but the two were significantly intercorrelated in the AD patients. Weingartner and colleagues concluded that episodic memory failures are associated with a loss of access to semantic knowledge in AD. Korsakoff's patients, who show equally profound episodic memory impairment, have intact semantic memory.

Declarative versus Procedural Knowledge

Another distinction, which has assisted in the interpretation of studies of amnesic disorders, is that between declarative and procedural knowledge (e.g., Squire, 1982). Declarative knowledge involves information based on specific items or data, whereas procedural knowledge involves information based on rules or procedures (Squire, 1982, p. 259). Tulving (1985) has theorized that procedural memory is a primitive associative memory system, within which are hierarchically embedded semantic and episodic memory.

Mirror Reading and Rotary Pursuit Tasks

One type of task that has been used to examine procedural memory is that of mirror reading. When amnesic patients are asked to read sets of words that are reversed by a mirror, they improve their skill at a normal rate, over 3 days of practice. Further, amnesic patients retain the skill at a normal level when tested 3 months later. However, they continue to show a profound amnesia for the specific words they have read, as well as for other aspects of the testing situation (Cohen and Squire, 1980).

Another type of task used to examine procedural memory is that of motor skill learning, such as that reflected in rotary pursuit tasks. Patients with amnesia secondary to bilateral temporal lobe damage, as well as Korsakoff's syndrome patients, show normal motor learning on this type of task (Brooks and Baddeley, 1976; Cermak, Lewis, Butters, and

Goodglass, 1973; Corkin, 1968; Starr and Phillips, 1970).

Priming

Still another phenomenon that some theorists (e.g., Tulving, 1984) have included within the domain of procedural memory is that of priming effects, the influence of recently perceived material upon subsequent performance. Priming in tasks requiring the completion of three letter stems into full words (Diamond and Rozin, 1984; Graf, Squire, and Mandler, 1984), and in tasks requiring subjects to list members of a semantic category (Graf, Shimamura, and Squire, 1985) appears intact in amnesic syndromes.

Procedural Memory in Dementia

Data concerning procedural memory in dementia are just becoming available, and have thus far generated more mixed results, than those reported for amnesic patients. One preliminary paper has reported motor skill learning to be relatively intact in AD (Eslinger and Damasio, 1985). Other research relevant to the concept of procedural memory has also recently been reported. In a study by Moscovitch (1984), elderly memory-impaired subjects required less time to read transformed text over repeated sessions, despite an impaired ability to recognize which sentences they had previously read. Grober (1986), reporting on preliminary data, found repetition priming effects to occur in a group of mixed AD and MID patients. Not only were the dementia patients faster to read an item the second time they saw it, but they displayed priming effects that were as large as those in a group of matched normal elderly control subjects. In contrast, Gordon (1984) provided some preliminary evidence of impaired repetition priming in a single AD patient. Although patients with right or left temporal lobectomies demonstrated preserved repetition priming effects in word reading, Gordon's AD patient did not. Martone, Butters, Payne, Becker, and Sax (1984) report finding evidence of repetition priming for mirror image words, in HD patients who were unable to recognize the stimuli they read.

Thus, while replication of these studies with larger series of AD and other dementia patients is necessary, these recent reports suggest that procedural memory may be relatively preserved in some dementia patients. It remains unclear whether the different phenomena considered to reflect procedural memory (e.g., mirror reading, motor skill learning, priming) all really involve the same process. In addition, it is not clear whether procedural memory remains intact across the range of dementia severity. Further experiments along this line would be of considerable interest, since it has been hypothesized that neural systems subserving procedural learning may be different, and phylogenetically more primitive, than those subserving declarative learning (e.g., Squire, 1982, p. 260).

Summary

A fairly large body of literature has accumulated concerning the nature of memory impairment in dementia, particularly in AD. Those studies employing a linear information processing model of memory lead to the conclusion that both primary and secondary memory are impaired in AD. Further, deficit in primary memory appears to limit the adequacy of encoding of information into secondary memory.

Recent research, viewing memory as a continuous process, has provided evidence of AD patient deficits in encoding events, along contextual, imagery, and verbal elaboration dimensions. Several studies have indicated this episodic memory encoding deficit to be largely due to impairment in access to, and possibly in the structure of, semantic memory. Unlike normally aging individuals, who can overcome inadequate episodic memory encoding when appropriate environmental or instructional conditions exist, AD patients cannot. AD, as well as HD, patients show impaired memory for remote events. Recent research and theory suggest that deficits in both episodic and semantic memory contribute to this remote memory impairment. AD patients also show rapid forgetting of events, similar to that of certain amnesic patients, likely due to their particularly abundant hippocampal lesions.

Research employing various approaches to the assessment of procedural memory in dementia has, thus far, produced mixed results. However, some studies exist that indicate preservation of some aspects of procedural learning in AD and HD. Further research in this area is necessary to clarify whether different measures of procedural memory really reflect a single domain, or are dissociable in dementia. Additional research concerning procedural memory in dementia would be of importance, given the theoretic differences in the ontogeny and underlying brain processes between procedural, semantic, and episodic memory. The study of dementia provides a unique "experiment of nature" for exploring the complexities of human memory. Relationships between, and dissociations among, hypothetic memory domains in dementia differ from those seen in either normal aging or amnesic syndromes. The study of memory in dementia is therefore of both clinical and theoretic importance.

CLINICAL IMPLICATIONS

1. Memory for events is impaired early in the course of AD, and this impairment becomes increasingly severe with dementia progression. Tests of episodic memory therefore should be included within any dementia assessment battery.

2. Semantic memory is also impaired in AD, contributing significantly to episodic memory deficit. Evidence of semantic memory impairment helps to differentiate dementia from amnesia patients, the latter generally showing intact semantic memory. Tests of semantic memory are therefore also a critical component in assessment.

3. Unlike normally aging individuals, AD patients show rapid forgetting of events. Clinical memory assessment should therefore include measures of both immediate and delayed recall.

4. Various procedures designed to increase the distinctiveness of encoding of events, useful in healthy older individuals, produce little memory improvement in the AD patient. Clinical interventions with AD patients, employing such mnemonic techniques, are therefore not likely to be successful.

5. As yet, it is unclear whether procedural learning is preserved in AD or the other dementias, across levels of dementia severity. The possibility of relatively intact procedural learning ability, at least in early dementia, suggests that patients may be able to learn certain skills, with sufficient practice, provided that conscious recollection of the specific events or context of the skill is not required.

REFERENCES

Albert, M.S., Butters, N., and Brandt, J. (1981). Patterns of remote memory in amnesic and demented patients. *Archives of Neurology*, *38*, 495-500.

Albert, M.S., Butters, N., and Levin, J. (1979). Temporal gradients in the retrograde amnesia of patients with alcoholic Korsakoff's disease. *Archives of Neurology*, *36*, 211-216.

Allender, J., and Kaszniak, A.W. (1985, February). *Processing of emotional cues and personality change in dementia of the Alzheimer's type.* Paper presented at the 13th annual meeting of the International Neuropsychological Society, San Diego, CA.

Baddeley, A.D. (1976). *The psychology of memory*. New York: Basic Books.

Bahrick, H.P., Bahrick, P.S., and Wittlinger, R.P. (1975). Fifty years of memory for names and faces: A cross-sectional approach. *Journal of Experimental Psychology: General*, *104*, 54-75.

Barbizet, J., and Cany, E. (1969). A psychometric study of various memory deficits associated with cerebral lesions. In G.A. Talland and N.C. Waugh (Eds.), *The pathology of memory* (pp. 49-64). New York: Academic Press.

Berg, L., Hughes, C.P., Coben, L.A., Danziger, W.L., Martin, R.L., and Knesevich, J. (1982). Mild senile dementia of the Alzheimer type: Research diagnostic criteria, recruitment and description of a study population. *Journal of Neurology, Neurosurgery and Psychiatry, 45*, 962-968.

Berg, L., Danziger, W.L., Storandt, M., Cohen, L.A., Gado, H., Hughes, C.P., Knesevich, J.W., and Botwinick, J. (1984). Predictive features in mild senile dementia of the Alzheimer type. *Neurology (Cleveland), 34*, 563-569.

Bjork, R.A., and Whitten, W.B. (1974). Recency-sensitive retrieval processes in long-term free recall. *Cognitive Psychology*, 6, 173-189.

Brinkman, S.D., Largen, J.W., Gerganoff, S., and Pomara, N. (1983). Russell's revised memory scale in the evaluation of dementia. *Journal of Clinical Psychology, 39*, 989-993.

Brooks, D.N., and Baddeley, A. (1976). What can amnesic patients learn? *Neuropsychologia, 14*, 111-122.

Brown, J. (1958). Some tests of the decay theory of immediate memory. *Quarterly Journal of Experimental Psychology, 10*, 12-21.

Brust, J.C.M. (1983). Dementia and cerebrovascular disease. In R. Mayeux and W.G. Rosen (Eds.), *The dementias* (pp. 131-147). New York: Raven Press.

Butters, N., Albert, M.A., Sax, D.S., Miliotis, P., Nagode, J., and Sterste, A. (1983). The effect of verbal mediation on the pictorial memory of brain-damaged patients. *Neuropsychologia, 21*, 307-323.

Butters, N., and Cermak, L.S. (1980). *Alcoholic Korsakoff's syndrome: An information processing approach to amnesia*. New York: Academic Press.

Caird, W.K., Sanderson, R.E., and Inglis, J. (1962). Cross validation of a learning test for use with elderly psychiatric patients. *Journal of Mental Science, 108*, 368-370.

Cermak, L.S., (1984). The episodic-semantic distinction in amnesia. In L.R. Squire and N. Butter (Eds.), *Neuropsychology of memory* (pp. 55-62). New York: Guilford.

Cermak, L.S., and Butters, N. (1972). The role of interference and encoding in the short-term memory deficits of Korsakoff patients. *Neuropsychologia, 10* 89-96.

Cermak, L.S., Lewis, R., Butters, N., and Goodglass, H. (1973). Role of verbal mediation in performance of motor tasks by Korsakoff's patients. *Perceptual and Motor Skills, 37*, 259-262.

Cermak, L.S., and O'Connor, M. (1983). The retrieval capacity of a patient with amnesia due to encephalitis. *Neuropsychologia, 21*, 213-234.

Cohen, N.J., and Squire, L.R. (1980). Preserved learning and retention of pattern analyzing skill in amnesia: Dissociation of knowing how and knowing that. *Science, 210*, 207-209.

Corkin, S. (1968). Acquisition of motor skill after bilateral medial temporal lobe excision. *Neuropsychologia*, 6, 225-265.

Corkin, S. (1982). Some relationships between global amnesias and the memory impairments in Alzheimer's disease. In S. Corkin, K.L. Davis, J.H. Growdon, E. Usdin, and R.L. Wurtman (Eds.), *Aging: Vol. 19. Alzheimer's disease: A report of progress* (pp. 149-164). New York: Raven Press.

Craik, F.I.M. (1977). Age differences in human memory. In J.E. Birren and K.W. Schaie (Eds.), *Handbook of the psychology of aging* (pp. 384-420). New York: Van Nostrand Reinhold.

Craik, F.I.M. and Tulving, E. (1975). Depth of processing and the retention of words in episodic memory. *Journal of Experimental Psychology: General, 104*, 268-294.

Crook, T., Ferris, S., McCarthy, M., and Rae, D. (1980). Utility of digit recall tasks for assessing memory in the aged. *Journal of Consulting and Clinical Psychology, 48*, 228-233.

Danziger, W.L. and Storandt, M. (1982, November). *Psychometric performance of healthy and demented older adults: A one-year follow-up.* Paper presented at the Annual Meeting of the Gerontological Society of America, Boston, MA.

Davis, P.E., and Mumford, S.J. (1984). Cued recall and the nature of memory disorder in dementia. *British Journal of Psychiatry, 144*, 383-386.

DeLeon, M.J., Ferris, S.H., George, A.E., Reisberg, B., Kricheff, I.I., and Gershon, S. (1980). Computerized tomography evaluations of brain-behavior relationships in senile dementia of the Alzheimer's type. *Neurobiology of Aging, 1*, 69-79.

Diamond, R., and Rozin, P. (1984). Activation of existing memories in the amnesic syndrome. *Journal of Abnormal Psychology, 93*, 98-105.

Diesfeldt, H.F.A. (1978). The distinction between long-term and short-term memory in senile dementia: An analysis of free recall and delayed recognition. *Neuropsychologia, 16*, 115-119.

Drachman, D.A. and Arbit, J. (1965). Memory and the hippocampal complex. *Archives of Neurology*, *15*, 52-61.

Eslinger, P.J., and Damasio, A.R. (1985). Alzheimer's disease spares motor learning. *Society for Neurosciences Abstracts*, *11*, 459.

Glanzer, M., and Cunitz, A.R. (1966). Two storage mechanisms in free recall. *Journal of Verbal Learning and Verbal Behavior*, *5*, 351-360.

Gordon, B. (1984, February). *Perceptual repetition memory spared by medial temporal lesions but not by Alzheimer's disease.* Paper presented at the Annual Meeting of the International Neuropsychological Society, Houston, TX.

Graf, P., Squire, L.R., and Mandler, G. (1984). The information that amnesic patients do not forget. *Journal of Experimental Psychology: Learning, Memory and Cognition*, *10*, 164-168.

Graf, P., Shimamura, A.P., and Squire, L.R. (1985). Priming across modalities and priming across category levels: Extending the domain of preserved function in amnesia. *Journal of Experimental Psychology: Learning, Memory and Cognition*, *11*, 386-396.

Grober, E. (1986, February). *Encoding of item-specific information in Alzheimer's disease.* Paper presented at the Annual Meeting of the International Neuropsychological Society, Denver, CO.

Hachinski, V.C., Lassen, N.A., and Marshall, J. (1974). Multi-infarct dementia, a cause of mental deterioration in the elderly. *Lancet*, *2*, 207-210.

Hagberg, B. (1978). Defects of immediate memory related to the cerebral blood flow distribution. *Brain and Language*, *5*, 366-377.

Hagberg, B., and Ingvar, D.H. (1976). Cognitive reduction in presenile dementia related to regional abnormalities of the cerebral blood flow. *British Journal of Psychiatry*, *128*, 209-222.

Huppert, F.A., and Piercy, M. (1976). Recognition memory in amnesia patients: Effect of temporal context and familiarity of material. *Cortex*, *12*, 3-20.

Inglis, J. (1959). A paired associate learning test for use with elderly psychiatric patients. *Journal of Mental Science*, *105*, 440-448.

Inglis, J., and Caird, W.K. (1963). Modified-digit spans and memory disorder. *Diseases of the Nervous System*, *24*, 46-50.

Jacoby, L.L. (1982). Knowing and remembering: Some parallels in the behavior of Korsakoff patients and normals. In L.S. Cermak (Ed.), *Human memory and amnesia* (pp. 97-122). Hillsdale, NJ: Lawrence Erlbaum.

Jacoby, L.L., and Witherspoon, D. (1982). Remembering without awareness. *Canadian Journal of Psychology*, *36*, 300-324.

Johannesson, G., Hagberg, B, Gustafson, L., and Ingvar, D.H. (1979). EEG and cognitive impairment in presenile dementia. *Acta Neurological Scandinavica*, *59*, 225-240.

Kaszniak, A.W. (1985). Personality and emotional change in dementia of the Alzheimer's type: Issues in the investigation of individual differences. *Journal of Clinical and Experimental Neuropsychology*, *7*, 611.

Kaszniak, A.W., Garron, D.C., and Fox, J.H. (1979). Differential effects of age and cerebral atrophy upon span of immediate recall and paired-associate learning in older patients suspected of dementia. *Cortex*, *15*, 285-295.

Kaszniak, A. W., Garron, D.C., Fox, J.H., Bergen, D., and Huckman, M. (1979). Cerebral atrophy, EEG slowing, age, education, and cognitive functioning in suspected dementia. *Neurology*, *29*, 1273-1279.

Kaszniak, A.W., Wilson, R.S., and Fox, J.H. (1981). Effects of imagery and meaningfulness on free recall and recognition memory in presenile and senile dementia. *International Journal of Neuroscience*, *12*, 264.

Kaszniak, A.W., Wilson, R.S., Fox, J.H., and Stebbins, G.T. (in press). Cognitive assessment in Alzheimer's disease: Cross-sectional and longitudinal perspectives. *Canadian Journal of Neurological Sciences*.

Katzman, R. (1981). Early detection of senile dementia. *Hospital Practice*, *16*, 61-76.

Katzman, R. (1986). Alzheimer's disease. *New England Journal of Medicine*, *314*, 964-973.

Kinsbourne, M., and George, J. (1974). The mechanism of the word frequency effect on recognition memory. *Journal of Verbal Learning and Verbal Behavior*, *13*, 63-69.

Kinsbourne, M., and Winocur, G. (1980). Response competition and interference effects in paired-associate learning by Korsakoff amnesics. *Neuropsychologia*, *18*, 541-548.

Kral, V.A. (1962). Senescent forgetfulness, benign and malignant. *Canadian Medical Association Journal*, *86*, 257-260.

Larner, S. (1977). Encoding in senile dementia and elderly depressives: A preliminary study. *British Journal of Social and Clinical Psychology*, *16*, 379-390.

Logue, P., and Wyrick, L. (1979). Initial validation of Russell's revised Wechsler Memory Scale: A comparison of normal aging versus dementia. *Journal of Consulting and Clinical Psychology*, *47*, 176-178.

Mandler, G. (1979). Organization and repetition: Organizational principles with special reference to rote learning. In L. Nillson (Ed.), *Perspectives on memory research* (pp. 293-327). Hillsdale, NJ: Lawrence Erlbaum.

Marcer, D. (1979). Measuring memory change in Alzheimer's disease. In A.I.M. Glen and L.J. Whalley (Eds.), *Alzheimer's disease: Early recognition of potentially reversible deficits* (pp. 117-121). London: Churchill Livingstone.

Martin, A., Brouwers, P., Cox, C., and Fedio, P. (1985). On the nature of verbal memory deficit in Alzhiemer's disease. *Brain and Language*, *25*, 323-341.

Martin, A., Cox, C., Brouwers, P., and Fedio, P. (1985). A note on different patterns of impaired and preserved cognitive abilities and their relation to episodic memory deficits in Alzhiemer's patients. *Brain and Language*, *26*, 181-185.

Martone, M., Butters, N., Payne, M., Becker, J., and Sax, D.S. (1984). Dissociations between skill learning and verbal recognition in amnesia and dementia. *Archives of Neurology*, *41*, 965-970.

Mayes, A., and Meudell, P. (1981). How similar is the effect of cueing in amnesics and in normal subjects following forgetting? *Cortex*, *17*, 113-124.

McCarthy, M., Ferris, S.H., Clark, E., and Crook, T. (1981). Acquisition and retention of categorized material in normal aging and senile dementia. *Experimental Aging Research*, 7, 127-135.

Meudell, P., and Mayes, A. (1981). A similarity between weak normal memory and amnesia with two and eight choice word recognition: A signal detection analysis. *Cortex*, *17*, 19-29.

Miller, E. (1971). On the nature of memory disorder in presenile dementia. *Neuropsychologia*, *9*, 75-78.

Miller, E. (1973). Short- and long-term memory in presenile dementia (Alzheimer's disease). *Psychological Medicine*, *3*, 221-224.

Miller, E. (1975). Impaired recall and memory disturbance in presenile dementia. *British Journal of Social and Clinical Psychology*, *14*, 73-79.

Miller, E. (1977). *Abnormal aging: The psychology of senile and presenile dementia*. New York: John Wiley.

Miller, E. (1978). Retrieval from long-term memory in presenile dementia: Two tests of an hypothesis. *British Journal of Social and Clinical Psychology*, *17*, 143-148.

Miller, E., and Lewis, P. (1977). Recognition memory in elderly patients with depression and dementia: A signal detection analysis. *Journal of Abnormal Psychology*, *86*, 84-86.

Milner, B. (1971). Interhemispheric differences in the localization of psychological processes in man. *British Medical Bulletin*, *27*, 272-277.

Moskovitch, M. (1982). Multiple dissociations of function in amnesia. In L.S. Cermak (Ed.), *Human memory and amnesia* (pp. 337-370). Hillsdale, NJ: Lawrence Erlbaum.

Moskovitch, M. (1984). The sufficient conditions for demonstrating preserved memory in amnesia: A task analysis. In L.R. Squire and N. Butters (Eds.), *Neuropsychology of memory* (pp. 104-114). New York: Guilford.

Moss, M.B., Albert, M.S., Butters, N., and Payne, M. (1986). Differential patterns of memory loss among patients with Alzheimer's disease, Huntington's disease, and alcoholic Korsakoff's syndrome. *Archives of Neurology*, *43*, 239-246.

Osborne, D.P., Brown, E.R., and Randt, C.T. (1982). Qualitative changes in memory functioning: Aging and dementia. In S. Corkin, K.L. Davis, J.H. Growdon, E. Usdin, and R.L. Wurtman (Eds.), *Alzheimer's disease: Aging: Vol. 19. A report of progress* (pp. 165-169). New York: Raven Press.

Peterson, L.R., and Peterson, M.J. (1959). Short-term retention of individual items. *Journal of Experimental Psychology*, *58*, 193-198.

Poon, L.W., and Fozard, J.L. (1980). Age and word frequency effects in continuous recognition memory. *Journal of Gerontology*, *35*, 77-86.

Rabins, P.V., Mace, N.L., and Lucas, M.J. (1982). The impact of dementia on the family. *Journal of the American Medical Association*, *248*, 333-335.

Reisberg, B. (1983). Clinical presentation, diagnosis and symptomatology of age-associated cognitive decline in Alzheimer's disease. In B. Reisberg (Ed.), *Alzheimer's disease: The standard reference* (pp. 173-187). New York: Free Press.

Reisberg, B, and Ferris, S.H. (1982). Diagnosis and assessment of the older patient. *Hospital and Community Psychiatry*, *33*, 104-110.

Rissenberg, M., and Glanzer, M. (1986). Picture superiority in free recall: The effects of normal aging and primary degenerative dementia. *Journal of Gerontology*, *41*, 64-71.

Rosen, W.G., and Mohs, R.C. (1982). Evolution of cognitive decline in dementia. In S. Corkin, K.L. Davis, J.H. Growdon, E. Usdin, and R.L. Wurtman (Eds.), *Aging: Vol. 19. Alzheimer's disease: A report of progress* (pp. 183-188). New York: Raven Press.

Roth, M. (1980). Senile dementia and its borderlands. In J.O. Cole and J.E. Barrett (Eds.), *Psychopathology in the aged* (pp. 205-232). New York: Raven Press.

Schneck, M.K., Reisberg, B., and Ferris, S.H. (1982). An overview of current concepts of Alzheimer's disease. *American Journal of Psychiatry*, *139*, 165-173.

Shepard, R.N. (1967). Recognition memory for words, sentences and pictures. *Journal of Verbal Learning and Verbal Behavior*, 6, 156-163.

Sim, A., and Sussman, I. (1962). Alzheimer's disease: Its natural history and differential diagnosis. *Journal of Nervous and Mental Disorders*, *135*, 489-499.

Squire, L. R. (1982). The neuropsychology of human memory. *Annual Review of Neurosciences*, *5*, 241-273.

Squire, L.R., and Cohen, N.J. (1984). Human memory and amnesia. In G. Lynch, J.L. McGaugh, and N.M. Weinberger (Eds.), *Neurobiology of learning and memory* (pp. 3-61). New York: Guilford.

Starr, A., and Phillips, L. (1970). Verbal and motor memory in the amnesic syndrome. *Neuropsychologia*, *8*, 75-88.

Storandt, M., Botwinick, J., and Danziger, W.L. (1986). Longitudinal changes: Mild SDAT and matched healthy controls. In L.W. Poon, B.J. Gurland, C. Eisdorfer, T. Crook, L.W. Thompson, A.W. Kaszniak, and K. Davis (Eds.), *The handbook of clinical memory assessment of older adults*. Washington, DC: American Psychological Association.

Storandt, M., Botwinick, J., Danziger, W.L., Berg, L., and Hughes, C.P. (1984). Psychometric differentiation of mild senile dementia of the Alzheimer type. *Archives of Neurology*, *41*, 497-499.

Swets, J.A. (1973). The relative operating characteristic in psychology. *Science*, *182*, 990-1000.

Tulving, E. (1984). Precis of elements of episodic memory. *The Behavioral and Brain Sciences*, *7*, 223-268.

Tulving, E. (1985). How many memory systems are there? *American Psychologist*, *40*, 385-398.

Tulving, E., and Colotla, V.A. (1970). Free recall of trilingual lists. *Cognitive Psychology*, *1*, 86-98.

Tzeng, O.J.L. (1973). Positive recency effects in delayed free recall. *Journal of Verbal Learning and Verbal Behavior*, *12*, 436-439.

Warrington, E.K. (1982). The double dissociation of short- and long-term memory deficits. In L.S. Cermak (Ed.), *Human memory and amnesia* (pp. 61-76). Hillsdale, NJ: Lawrence Erlbaum.

Warrington, E.K., and Weiskrantz, L. (1974). The effect of prior learning on subsequent retention in amnesic patients. *Neuropsychologia*, *12*, 419-428.

Watkins, M.J. (1974). Concept and measurement of primary memory. *Psychological Bulletin*, *81*, 695-711.

Weingartner, H., Grafman, J., Boutelle, W., Kaye, W., and Martin, P.R. (1983). Forms of memory failure. *Science*, *221*, 380-383.

Weingartner, H., Kaye, W., Smalling, S., Cohen, R., Ebert, M.H., Gillin, J.C., and Gold, P. (1982) Determinants of memory failure in dementia. In S. Corkin, K.L. Davis, J.H. Growdon, E. Usdin, and R.J. Wurtman (Eds.), *Aging: Vol. 19. Alzheimer's disease: A report of progress in research* (pp. 171-176). New York: Raven Press.

Wilson, R.S., Bacon, L.D., Fox, J.H., and Kaszniak, A.W. (1983). Primary memory and secondary memory in dementia of the Alzheimer type. *Journal of Clinical Neuropsychology*, *5*, 337-344.

Wilson, R.S., Bacon, L.D., Kaszniak, A.W., and Fox, J.H. (1982). The episodic-semantic memory distinction and paired-associate learning. *Journal of Consulting and Clinical Psychology*, *50*, 154-155.

Wilson, R.S., Bacon, L.D., Kramer, R.L., Fox, J.H., and Kaszniak, A.W. (1983). Word frequency effect and recognition memory in dementia of the Alzheimer type. *Journal of Clinical Neuropsychology*, *5*, 97-104.

Wilson, R.S., and Kaszniak, A.W. (1986). Longitudinal changes: Progressive idiopathic dementia. In L.W. Poon, B.J. Gurland, C. Eisdorfer, T. Crook, L.W. Thompson, A.W. Kaszniak, and K. Davis (Eds.), *The handbook of clinical memory assessment of older adults*. Washington, DC: American Psychological Association.

Wilson, R.S., Kaszniak, A.W., Bacon, L.D., Fox, J.H., and Kelly, M.P. (1982). Facial recognition memory in dementia. *Cortex*, *18*, 329-336.

Wilson, R.S., Kaszniak, A.W., and Fox, J.H. (1981). Remote memory in senile dementia. *Cortex*, *17*, 41-48.

Wilson, R.S., Rosenbaum, G., and Brown, G. (1979). The problem of premorbid intelligence in neuropsychological assessment. *Journal of Clinical Neuropsychology*, *1*, 49–53.

Zola-Morgan, S. (1984). Toward an animal model of human amnesia: Some critical issues. In L.R. Squire and N. Butters (Eds.), *Neuropsychology of Memory* (pp. 316-329). New York: Guilford.

Chapter 14

Neuropsychologic Assessment of the Dementia Patient

Neuropsychologic assessment can play an important part in the clinical diagnosis of dementia and can add important information to the planning of intervention and patient management. A work group organized by the National Institute of Neurological, Communicative Disorders and Stroke (NINCDS) and the Alzheimer's Disease and Related Disorders Association (ADRDA) reviewed clinical experience and available research concerning the diagnosis of Alzheimer's disease and other dementias. They recommended that neuropsychologic evaluation be included as a necessary part of the clinical diagnostic protocol in assessing suspected dementia (McKhann et al., 1984).

NEUROPSYCHOLOGIC ASSESSMENT IN DIAGNOSIS

In present clinical practice, the diagnosis of dementia relies heavily upon clinical examination, neuropsychologic testing, CT scanning, and certain laboratory procedures (Roth, 1980). Results of a number of previous studies (e.g., Fleiss, Gurland, and Des Roche, 1976; Kendrick and Post, 1967; Roth and Hopkins, 1953; Trier, 1966) have indicated that various psychologic assessment instruments are reasonably successful in differentiating the moderately demented patient from healthy members of his or her age cohort. However, difficulty in diagnosis does occur when dementia is relatively early in its course, or when dementia must be differentiated from cognitive deficits associated with other disorders, such as depression.

Accuracy and Sources of Error in Diagnosis

Research concerning accuracy in the diagnosis of dementia has indicated a range of 10 to 30 percent of inaccurate diagnoses in the general medical population (National Institute on Aging Task Force, 1980). A substantial portion of such diagnostic errors appear to be false negative diagnoses, that is, failing to diagnose a dementia when present. One recent review (McCartney, 1986) has attributed the high rate of false negative diagnoses to inadequate assessment of intellectual functioning in older medical patients by physicians. However, particular concern has also been raised over false-positive diagnoses, which Heston and Mastri (1982), evaluating clinical diagnoses against autopsy criteria, found to be approximately 30 percent.

The results of a study reported by Garcia, Reding, and Blass (1981) suggest that differentiation of dementia from cognitive deficits accompanying depression may make the most significant contribution to this high false-positive rate. These investigators studied 100 older patients, initially diagnosed as showing evidence of dementia, who were referred to a specialized outpatient dementia clinic. Upon very careful evaluation within the clinic, 26 were found not to be demented. Of these, 15 were diagnosed as depressed, 7 as having other miscellaneous neuropsychiatric disorders, and 4 as being normal. Ron, Toone, Garralda, and Lishman (1979) report similar data from a study of 51 patients discharged from the Bethlehem Royal and Maudlsey Hospitals with a firm diagnosis of presenile dementia. All were below the age of 65 at the time of diagnosis, and none showed evidence of cerebrovascular disease, severe head injury, space-occupying lesion, intracranial infection, metabolic or endocrine disorder, alcoholism, or drug addiction. All patients were hospitalized between 1963 and 1972. At follow-up study in 1977, 33 patients had died, and 18 were still alive. Neurologic, psychiatric, and psychologic test examinations were conducted on survivors at the time of follow-up, and clinical records were carefully reviewed on those patients who had died. From these data, the original diagnosis of presenile dementia was confirmed in 35 cases (69 percent) and rejected in 16 (31 percent). Twelve of this later group were alive and four had died. Of the 16 cases in which the diagnosis was rejected, retrospective diagnoses of affective illness were made in eight patients, paranoid psychosis in one, schizophrenic illness in one, and a range of other diagnoses in the remainder.

Why should the differentiation of dementia from depression in older age be so difficult? As will be reviewed here, there appear to be several reasons, that can be summarized as follows: First, there are changes in cognitive functioning that accompany normal aging, somewhat blurring the distinction between normal age changes and early indicators of dementia. Second, cognitive difficulty frequently accompanies depression in the elderly, and it can be of sufficient severity to be confused with dementia. Third, the signs and symptoms of neurologic disorders in which dementia can occur (e.g., Alzheimer's disease, Huntington's disease, Parkinson's disease) do have some overlap with those of depression. Finally, dementia can be accompanied by depression in some patients. Within the following section, evidence for these contributors to difficulty in differentiating dementia from depression will be briefly reviewed, with implications drawn for approaches to clinical assessment. A fuller discussion of this literature can be found in Kaszniak, Sadeh, and Stern (1985).

Problems in Differentiating Dementia from Depression

Cognitive Change in Normal Aging

As reviewed in previous chapters, research has documented the presence of some changes in cognitive functioning with normal aging. The major implication of these changes, for clinical assessment, is that age-appropriate normative expectations must be employed in the interpretation of cognitive tests. Certainly, the application of normative data based upon younger adults would be inappropriate for judging the intelligence test performance of elderly individuals. Fortunately, the most frequently employed measure of adult intelligence, the Wechsler Adult Intelligence Scale (WAIS) (Wechsler, 1958), is a reliable test instrument with age-stratified norms. The revised WAIS (WAIS-R) (Wechsler, 1981) improved upon the sampling procedures employed for obtaining older individuals in the normative standardization data. It provides, therefore, adequate age norms for seven groups from 20 through 74 years of age.

Similarly, age-related changes in memory functioning require that age-appropriate normative expectations be employed in evaluating performance on standardized clinical memory assessment instruments. One such instrument is the Wechsler Memory Scale (WMS) (Wechsler, 1945) and its revised version (Russell, 1975). Both cross-sectional and longitudinal data show age-related decline in WMS performance (McCarty, Siegler, and Logue, 1982). The original WMS norms (Wechsler, 1945) did not extend beyond 65 years of age. Haaland, Linn, Hunt, and Goodwin (1983) have provided revised WMS norms for ages 65 to over 80. However, the volunteer subjects in the normative sample of Haaland and colleagues were better educated than is typical for the general population of this age range. The number of years of formal education has been shown to have a significant relationship with WMS performance among older patients suspected of having dementia (Kaszniak, Garron, Fox, Bergen, and Huckman, 1979). Consequently, caution must be employed in using the WMS norms provided by Haaland and colleagues, unless the patient being examined has had nearly the same number of years of education as the normative sample.

Similar considerations can be outlined for a range of other frequently employed neuropsychologic assessment instruments. Comprehensive discussion of age effects upon various neuropsychologic tests, as well as normative data for different adult age groups, can be found in Schear (1984) and in Heaton, Grant, and Matthews (1986). Additional discussion of age-appropriate normative expectations will appear here, when specific neuropsychologic assessment instruments are described.

Depression and Cognitive Deficit

A second factor contributing to difficulties in differential diagnosis is the presence of memory complaint and memory deficit in depression. Research and clinical experience have suggested that older depressed patients frequently complain of memory difficulty, even when objective assessment of memory fails to document a deficit (Kahn, Zarit, Hilbert, and Niederehe, 1975). Kahn and colleagues speculated that this discrepancy between memory complaint and memory performance in older depressed patients may reflect a general tendency toward pessimistic self-assessment.

In addition to increased memory complaint, research documents the presence of memory deficit, as well as other cognitive difficulties, among many depressed patients (see reviews by Caine, 1986; McAllister, 1981; Miller, 1975). Further, it appears that such cognitive deficits are more likely to manifest in older, as compared with younger, depressed patients (Donnelly, Waldman, Murphy, Wyatt, and Goodwin (1980). These deficits have been shown to be reversible following successful treatment of the depression, with the degree of memory improvement being correlated with the degree of resolution of depression (Sternberg and Jarvik, 1976; Stromgren, 1977). Although memory is not the only cognitive function impaired in depression, it has been one of the most frequently documented areas of deficit (McAllister, 1981).

Pseudodementia. The appearance of marked cognitive deficit in the absence of evidence of neurologic or other medical origin has often been labeled "pseudodementia," a term first introduced by Kiloh (1961). Kiloh's original description was of ten patients with functional psychiatric disorders who manifested features such as impairment of orientation, memory, intellect, and judgement. Kiloh emphasized depressive illness in the etiology of pseudodementia, and others have employed the term almost exclusively in reference to depressed patients (e.g., Post, 1975). However, pseudodementia can also occur in various other disorders, including hysterical syndromes and schizophrenia (Kiloh, 1961; Wells, 1979; Bienenfeld and Hartford, 1982; Maletta, Pirozzolo, Thompson, and Mortimer, 1982).

The patient with the syndrome of pseudodementia is difficult to differentiate from the demented patient. Recent research suggests that even experienced clinicians tend to misdiagnose depression as dementia, when the syndrome of pseudodementia is present in older patients. This bias was illustrated in an interesting study published by Perlick and Atkins (1984). A sample of 36 experienced clinical psychologists were presented a tape recording of the psychiatric interview of a 64-year-old depressed man with pseudodementia. The diagnosis of pseudodementia had previously been confirmed through the negative results of neurologic workup and remission of depressive symptoms and cognitive deficits following treatment. The clinician/subjects were randomly assigned to one of three experimental conditions: 12 of them were told that the patient was 75 years old, 12 were told that he was 55 years old, and 12 were not supplied with any age information. Ratings of the patient by these clinicians, on a structured diagnostic questionnaire, revealed a bias, with a greater attribution of dementia and fewer judgments of depression when the patient was described as elderly.

Clinical Features Differentiating Dementia from Pseudodementia. The problem of differentiating dementia from pseudodementia has attracted considerable recent attention from the psychiatric community. Several case studies, observations on small series of patients, and some systematic prospective studies have been published. From available reviews of this literature (Post, 1975; Wells, 1979; Roth, 1980; Janowsky, 1982; McAllister, 1983; Caine, 1986), several useful clinical features, which assist in differentiating depressive pseudodementia from dementia, can be abstracted. Most authors emphasize the importance of careful history-taking in this differential diagnostic process. Typically, except for multi-infarct dementia, dementing illness begins insidiously, with a history extending back for several years. In contrast, the patient with depressive pseudodementia has often experienced symptoms of short duration (no more than a few weeks to a month) before seeking medical help, and there is apparent rapid progression of symptoms after onset. A history of previous psychiatric dysfunction is also much more common in pseudodementia than in true dementia.

Careful interview concerning presenting symptoms is also helpful. Whereas the dementia patient, at least in the middle to later stages of the disorder, may complain very little of memory or other cognitive deficit, the depressive pseudodementia patient will complain considerably of these difficulties. These complaints often include elaborate detail and examples, emphasizing disability and highlighting failures. The dementia patient's complaints, when they occur, are typically more vague, with efforts to conceal disability, and evidence of pride in even trivial accomplishments. The dementia patient may hence appear relatively unconcerned about his or her illness, whereas the depressive pseudodementia patient usually communicates a strong sense of distress. The dementia patient's behavior is typically consistent with the clinically observed severity of cognitive dysfunction. For example, the dementia patient with psychometrically documented memory deficit will be observed to forget a variety of day-to-day events. The depressive pseudodementia patient will often demonstrate incongruities between behavior and apparent severity of cognitive deficit.

The above observations underscore the necessity for careful history-taking, behavior observation, and comprehensive evaluation of affective and cognitive features. Characteristics of cognitive test performance that can help in differentiating dementia from pseudodementia will be discussed within the context of the individual neuropsychologic assessment instruments reviewed here.

Depression and Depression-Like Symptoms in Dementing Illness

The final contributors to difficulty in differentiating dementia from depression are (1) the occurrence of depression coexisting with a dementing illness and (2) the resemblance of certain features of dementing illnesses to those of depression.

Depression in Alzheimer's Disease. Several authors (e.g., Demuth and Rand, 1980; Miller, 1980; McAllister and Price, 1982; Reifler, Larson, and Hanley, 1982; Kaszniak, 1986) have recently drawn attention to the occurrence of coexisting depression and cognitive deficit in AD. Older references to this coexistence (e.g., English, 1942) can also be found. The importance of diagnosing coexisting depression in AD is emphasized by the occurrence of suicide and suicide attempt in these patients (Post, 1962), as well as indirect self-destructive behavior, which may serve as an alternative form of suicide (Nelson and Faberow, 1980). Efforts at differential diagnosis are further encouraged by case reports of depression in AD patients responding to treatment, such as electroconvulsive therapy (Demuth and Rand, 1980).

Although some authors (Busse, 1975; Pfeiffer, 1977) have suggested that depressive symptoms are most common in the early stages of dementia, others (e.g., Demuth and Rand, 1980) have observed depression in patients with severe dementia. Similarly, within studies of larger series of patients, some (Reifler et al., 1982) have found the prevalence of coexisting depression to decrease significantly with greater severity of cognitive impairment. Others (Kaszniak, Wilson, Lazarus, Lessor, and Fox, 1981; Kaszniak, 1985) fail to find any significant relationship between severity of depressive symptoms and severity of cognitive impairment. At present, it would appear most prudent to conclude that depressive symptoms can occur at any point in the course of dementia.

To date, relatively little systematic research has focused upon the nature of depression in AD. Available research does suggest that different approaches to the assessment of depression may yield quite different results (Miller, 1980; Kaszniak, 1985). Most apparent from this research is that self-report measures give different estimates of the presence and severity of depression in dementia than do examiner-administered or observation-based instruments. Such discrepancies should not be surprising, given the difficulties in insight and self-report frequently manifested by dementia patients.

A final difficulty in attempting to diagnose coexistent depression in Alzheimer's disease is generated by the similarity of certain features of dementia and depression. For example, the dementia patient may be careless in personal grooming, suggesting the possibility of depression-related apathy. Decreased variability of facial expression in dementia may be interpreted as the loss of interest or pleasure seen in depression. For at least some clinicians, a tendency toward such interpretation may be increased by the desire to find a treatable disorder, such as depression, in the dementia patient (Mortsyn, Hachanadel, Kaplan, and Gutheil, 1982).

Depression in Parkinson's Disease. The symptoms of depression have long been known to be associated with PD. Mayeux, Williams, Stern, and Cote (1984), in their review of relevant literature, found estimates of significant depression in PD patients to range from 37 to 90 percent, in comparison with age-matched control subjects without neurologic disease. Such estimates likely vary not only because of differences in the composition of the research samples, but also because of difficulties in the assessment of depression in PD.

Bradykinesia contributes to difficulties in diagnosis of depression. Patients with PD have delayed initiation of movements, general poverty of motor activity, and reduced facial gestures, which are difficult to differentiate from the psychomotor slowing and constricted emotional expression of depression. In addition to bradykinesia, there may be bradyphrenia, with both this feature and movement slowing possibly being more common in older PD patients (Wilson, Kaszniak, Klawans, and Garron, 1980). Thus, the relatively immobile, slowly responsive patient with a mask-like expression may easily be thought to be apathetic or depressed, although the patient's subjective mood may not be markedly altered. This emphasizes the necessity of evaluating psychologic symptoms as well as physical signs in the diagnosis of PD.

The etiology of depression in PD is not well understood. Whether this depression is reactive to the disabling nature of PD or rather reflects some neurochemical aspect of the disease itself remains in debate.

The diagnosis of depression in PD is further complicated in those patients with dementia accompanying their disease. All of the difficulties just described in the assessment of depression in AD would equally apply to the demented PD patient.

Depression in Huntington's Disease. In addition to the neurologic features and progressive dementia of HD, personality and emotional changes are pervasive. Psychiatric manifestations of the disease include personality changes, schizophrenia-like syndromes, paranoid delusions, and affective disorders, with some authors (e.g., McHugh and Folstein, 1975; Folstein, Folstein, and McHugh, 1979) believing depression to be the most prominent manifestation. In a study of 30 HD patients, carefully employing DSM-III diagnostic criteria, Caine and Shoulson (1983) found 24 of the patients to demonstrate substantial behavioral abnormality, including affective and schizophrenic syndromes, personality disorders, and syndromes that could not be classified adequately. However, Caine and Shoulson found no correlation between the severity of dementia and the type or severity of psychopathologic features in their group of HD patients. They also found antidepressant pharmacotherapy to benefit the somatic signs of their patients' affective disorders without altering their dysphoric mood. As with depression in PD, the etiology of depression in HD is unclear. The possibility of the depression being reactive, perhaps to the knowledge of the hereditary nature and prognosis of the disease, has been raised (see Pearson, 1973). However, depression, and attempted suicide, may occur many years prior to the onset of the involuntary movement disorder of HD.

ASSESSMENT OF COGNITIVE FUNCTION IN DEMENTIA

The purpose of the following review is to critically evaluate the available research literature, as well as provide some guidance in selection of appropriate assessment instruments. This review progresses from general assessment instruments (i.e., mental status examination protocols) through more specific neuropsychologic tests designed to evaluate particular aspects of cognition.

Mental Status Examination

Clinical mental status examination, and a thorough history, preferably from a reliable family member who is close to the patient, will typically enable recognition of the syndrome of dementia, once the patient is several years into the course of illness (Folstein and McHugh, 1978). However, the clinician must be cautious not to apply inappropriate expectations for cognitive functioning in the elderly. As discussed in previous chapters, sensory, perceptual, attentional, processing speed, memory, and intellectual functioning all show age-related changes in adulthood. Consequently, the use of mental status examination protocols with age-appropriate normative data is of importance. The present discussion will focus only on those most frequently employed instruments for which adequate information concerning reliability and validity is available.

The Geriatric Mental Status Interview

The Geriatric Mental Status Interview (GMS), developed by Gurland, Copeland, Sharpe, and Kelleher (1976), is one of the more comprehensive mental status examinations available. The GMS is a semistructured interview technique, which can be administered by a trained interviewer in typically less than 1 hour. Between 100 and 200 questions, concerning dimensions such as cognitive functioning, affective state, behavioral symptoms, result in ratings on 500 items. On the basis of data from both the United States and the United Kingdom (Gurland, Fleiss, Goldberg, Sharpe, Copeland, Kelleher, and Kellet 1976), 21 factors have been found to characterize these 500 ratings. Normative data are available for each of these factors. Interrater reliability is acceptable (Gurland, Copeland, Sharpe, and Kelleher, 1976), although items based on patient self-report and specific tests of memory and orientation yield higher agreement than observation of the patient's expression, speech pattern, and spontaneous behavior. Valid discrimination of dementia from functional psychiatric disorders, including depression, has been demonstrated for the GMS (Fleiss, Gurland, and DesRoche, 1976; Gurland and Toner, 1983).

The Comprehensive Assessment and Referral Evaluation

The GMS has been expanded and incorporated into the Comprehensive Assessment and Referral Evaluation (CARE), which covers the psychiatric, medical, nutritional, economic and social problems of which older persons are at risk. Those items of the CARE most relevant to the assessment of dementia demonstrate high interrater reliability (Gurland et al., 1977–78). Two relatively short CARE scales, for assessment of cognitive impairment and depression, respectively, together misclassified only 2 percent of a sample of 10 depressed and 31 demented older persons (Gurland, Golden, and Challop, 1982).

Brief Mental Status Examination Protocols

While these and other (Pfeiffer, 1976; Fillenbaum, and Smyer, 1981; Lawton, Moss, Fulcomer, and Kleban, 1982) comprehensive interview protocols for assessment of mental status provide reliable and valid diagnostic information, they are relatively lengthy to administer and require specific training. Brief, specific mental status examination protocols are available for the examination of patients with known or suspected dementia.

The Blessed Orientation and Memory Examination. One example is the orientation and memory examination of Blessed, Tomlinson, and Roth (1968), which the authors have shown to correlate well with the average number of neuritic plaques observed at postmortem microscopic examination of cerebral grey matter. Fuld (1978) has created a 33-item modification of this instrument, appropriate for examination of patients within the United States. High test–retest reliability (Spearman rank order correlation coefficient = 0.96) was found for this modified test, reexamining 17 demented and nondemented patients after 3 weeks (Fuld, 1978). Scores of eight or more errors on this test differentiated community dwelling (N = 54) from nursing home resident (N = 500) elderly (Fuld, 1978). Follow-up evaluation of the nursing home sample revealed error scores to correlate well (r = .59) with neuritic plaque count in the cortex. One-year follow-up of the community sample showed that five to eight errors at first examination were predictive of deterioration into the dementia range of scores (Fuld, 1982a).

The Mini Mental State Examination. Another of the more popular brief mental status screening protocols is the Mini-Mental State (MMS) examination of Folstein, Folstein, and McHugh (1975). The MMS consists of 11 items, which have been divided into two different sets of tests. The first set consists of items evaluating orientation and memory. These test items require vocal responses from the patient and yield a maximum score of 21. The second set consists of items examining ability to follow verbal and written commands, name objects, write a spontaneous sentence, and copy a geometric figure. This latter set of items requires the ability to read and write and yields a maximum score of 9. Thus, the total MMS has a maximum score of 30. Adequate test-retest reliability, and valid discrimination of demented from depressed patients and from normal older persons, has been demonstrated. Significant correlations with Wechsler Adult Intelligence Scale (WAIS) (Wechsler, 1958) IQ scores have also been shown (Folstein et al., 1975; Folstein and McHugh, 1978). Recent research has found specific MMS items to correlate with age and education, and false-positive errors in diagnosing dementia are more frequent for older, less educated patients (Anthony, LeResche, Niaz, von Korff, and Folstein, 1982). These observations underscore the need for caution in comparing any particular patient to normative standards. This same caution, of course, should be exercised with the use of similar mental status screening instruments, such as the Mental Status Questionnaire (MSQ) (Kahn, Goldfarb, Pollak, and Peck, 1960), the Short Portable Mental Status Questionnaire (SPMSQ) (Brink, Capri, DeNeeve, Janakes, and Oliveira, 1978; Fillenbaum, 1980; Haglund and Schuckit, 1976; Pfeiffer, 1975), or those contained within the GMS and CARE.

The Need for a Representative Normative Data Base to Interpret Mental Status Examination Results

The availability of a larger base of normative data for any of these instruments, truly representative of the entire population of elderly persons, would likely lessen such diagnostic errors. The mental status examination score of a given patient could, if such data were available, be compared with normative expectation based upon individuals of similar age, sex, education, and possibly other demographic variables. Such national population norms may soon be available for the MMS, through data being collected through the National Institute of Mental Health catchment area program (Regier, et al., 1984).

The Advantage of Combining Mental Status Examination Protocols with Other Assessment Instruments

Instruments such as the Blessed et al. (1968) protocol, as well as the MMS, MSQ, and SPMSQ have the advantage of brevity and ease of administration. Further, brief mental status screening instruments can be administered to those more severely demented patients who may not be examinable with more complex psychometric instruments, thus allowing repeat examination over several years of the patient's illness (Wilson and Kaszniak, 1986). However, these advantages also result in unacceptably high false negative errors for patients early in the course of dementia (Pfeffer et al., 1981; Wilson and Kaszniak, 1986). Some (e.g., Pfeffer, et al., 1981; Whelihan, Lesher, Kleban, and Granick, 1984) have addressed this problem by combining brief mental status screening measures with performance-based psychometric instruments, resulting in markedly improved sensitivity, at the cost of some decrease in specificity (Pfeffer et. al., 1981). Thus, although various available mental status examination protocols are able to reliably and validly demonstrate relatively marked cognitive impairment, when employed alone they are inadequate for assessment of mild dementia. Further, as Cohen, Eisdorfer, and Holm (1984) state, in their review of mental status examinations in aging, "existing mental status examinations of cognitive status do not provide more than a gross estimate of generalized deficit in an individual" (p. 221). These authors recommend that mental status examination protocols be followed by a evaluation of a wide range of intellectual abilities, such as that represented by comprehensive neuropsychologic assessment batteries. Components of such batteries are critically reviewed here.

Dementia Rating Scales

The Mattis Dementia Rating Scale

Another approach to this problem involves the construction of an examination protocol that maintains some of the brevity of brief mental status screening instruments, yet samples a more comprehensive range of cognitive functioning. One of the more widely used examples of such an instrument is the Mattis Dementia Rating Scale (MDRS) (Coblentz et al., 1973; Mattis, 1976). Items of the MDRS are grouped into five areas, respectively designed to assess attention, initiation and perseveration, construction, conceptualization, and memory. Scores from all five areas are also summed to provide a general index of dementia severity (maximum total score = 142). High (.97) test–retest reliability has been reported for a group of 30 presenile AD patients (Coblentz et al., 1973), and impressive split-half reliability (.90) was found for a sample of 25 older (65 to 94 years of age) institutionalized dementia patients (Gardner, Oliver-Munoz, Fisher, and Empting, 1981). Correlation between the MDRS and WAIS full scale IQ was reported as .75 for a group of 20 patients with presenile dementia of mixed etiology (Coblentz et al., 1973). Relatively high correlation between the MDRS and other psychometric instruments (e.g., WAIS vocabulary subtest, Benton Visual Retention Test) has also been reported for a sample of 85 normal elderly (Montgomery and Costa, 1983). Normal elderly have generally been found to score at or near the ceiling score of the MDRS (Coblentz et al., 1973; Montgomery and Costa, 1983), while our own experience, and that of others (e.g., Gardner et al., 1981) indicates institutionalized demented patients to almost always score below 100. Various clinicians (e.g., Albert, 1981) anecdotally report the MDRS to be useful in evaluating the mild to moderately demented AD patient. A recent study (Vitaliano, Breen, Albert, Russo, and Prinz, 1984) found MDRS scores (particularly those concerned with memory recall) to significantly differ between healthy elderly and mildly demented AD patients living in the community. This study also found that MDRS item scores were predictive of independent measures of functional competence in their AD patients. The same team of investigators (Vitaliano et al., 1986), reporting on a 2-year follow-up of 15 mild AD patients who had participated in their previous study, found MDRS total scores, as well as certain MDRS subscale scores, to predict amount of decline in functional competence over the 2 years.

Hersch (1979) has expanded and modified the scoring of the MDRS, employing weighting of items based on their empirically determined relative difficulty. Based on data from 90 psychogeriatric inpatients, Hersch found high internal consistency for the scale as a whole, and valid discrimination of demented from nondemented inpatients. Hersch also showed the scale to correlate with an independent rating scale completed by ward staff, and a significant decline in the scores of dementia patients retested after 6- and 12-month intervals was found.

The Global Deterioration Scale

Since dementias are progressively deteriorative conditions, there is a need for assessment instruments capable of repeated administration throughout the disease course. As was noted, some of the briefer mental status examination protocols, and possibly the MDRS, are able to fill this need. Observation-based rating scales are a useful addition to such instruments, as they often do not necessitate patient cooperation and provide ratings of behavioral features observed later in the course of dementia. An example of a rating scale, developed specifically for the evaluation of various "stages" throughout the course of dementia, is the Global Deterioration Scale of Primary Degenerative Dementia (GDS) (Reisberg, Ferris, and Crook, 1982). This instrument defines seven stages in the course of dementia, with well specified observational criteria. Levin and Peters (1982) report preliminary support for interrater reliability. GDS ratings correlate well with various independent psychometric measures of cognitive impairment, as well as with CT and PET measures in AD patients (Reisberg et al., 1982). While further characterization of the psychometric properties of the GDS is needed (e.g., more information on reliability and on age, sex, educational, and cultural influences), it provides a promising approach to the difficult task of classifying dementia severity. Such classification is necessary in order to compare research based on different AD or other dementia patient samples.

Rating Scales for Application in the Patient's Residential Environment

In addition to the type of rating scale represented by the GDS, there is need for observation-based rating scales that can be completed by persons familiar with the patient's behavior in his or her residential environment, whether community, hospital, or nursing home. Reviews of such instruments, appropriate for use with impaired older patients, are available (Kaszniak and Allender, 1985; Robinson, 1979; Salzman, Shader, Kochansky, and Cronin, 1972), and only a brief review of selected measures will be presented here.

The Geriatric Rating Scale. One of the earliest rating scales developed specifically for geriatric inpatients is the Stockton Geriatric Rating Scale (SGRS) (Meer and Baker, 1966), and its revised version, usually referred to as the Geriatric Rating Scale (GRS) (Plutchik et al., 1970). Good interrater reliability has been found when the GRS has been applied to both organically and functionally impaired elderly, and reliabilities do not appear to significantly differ across rater types, such as nurse aides, RNs, and psychologic assistants (Taylor and Bloom, 1974). The 24-item GRS has been found to be characterized by three factors: (1) withdrawal/apathy, (2) antisocial and disruptive behavior, and (3) deficits in activities of daily living (Smith, Bright, and McCloskey, 1977). Validity studies of the SGRS and GRS have shown differentiation of elderly patients with functional versus organic disorders, agreement between the scale scores and independent clinical evaluation, prediction of hospital discharge, and prediction of patient participation in hospital activities (Meer and Baker, 1966; Plutchik et al., 1970; Plutchik and Conte, 1972; Taylor and Bloom, 1974).

The London Psychogeriatric Rating Scale. The London Psychogeriatric Rating Scale (LPRS) (Hersch, Krall, and Palmer, 1978) is basically an extension of the SGRS, with additional items designed to improve observer ratings of patient cognitive functioning. Predictive validity has been established against criteria of diagnosis, outcome (continued hospitalization, discharge, or death), ward placement, and ability of the patient to benefit from particular treatment programs (Hersch et al., 1978; Hersch, Merskey, and Palmer, 1980).

Other Observation-Based Rating Scales. More recently, rating scales have been developed specifically for evaluation of behavior reflecting cognitive deficits in older patients. Lawson, Rodenburg, and Dykes (1977) have reported on the development of a dementia rating scale, with evidence of acceptable internal consistency, interrater and test–retest reliability, and criterion-related validity. While this instrument has been carefully developed from a psychometric perspective, the available data are based upon a relatively small number of patients, and independent replication has not been reported.

Another instrument, the Inventory of Psychic and Somatic Complaints in the Elderly (IPSC-E) (Reisberg et al., 1981), contains a subset of 19 (out of a total of 80) items rating aspects of cognitive functioning. Significant correlations between IPSC-E items and independent psychometric measures of cognitive functioning (Reisberg et al., 1981) encourage the further development of this instrument.

Functional Competence Rating Scales. Finally, the existence of rating scales for the evaluation of the functional competence in activities of daily living of dementia patients should be noted. Lawton and Brody (1969) describe their Independent Activities of Daily Living (IADL) instrument, and Pfeffer, Kurosaki, Harrah, Chance, and Filos (1982) have demonstrated reliability and validity against clinical diagnosis of the IADL in rating normal and mildly demented elderly who are living in the community. Further, they supply supporting data on a new instrument, the Functional Activities Questionnaire (FAQ), for assessing social function.

Comprehensive Neuropsychologic Assessment

Although mental status examination protocols and dementia rating scales play an important role in diagnostic assessment and patient follow-up, such procedures are often alone inadequate. Typically, they are relatively insensitive to very mild dementia (e.g., Whelihan et al., 1984) and lack sufficient specificity in the separation of the various disorders presenting as dementia. Consequently, neuropsychologists experienced in the assessment of older patients suspected of having dementia (e.g., Albert, 1981; Fuld, 1978; Kaszniak et al., 1979; Klisz, 1978; Miller, 1977, 1981; Pirozzolo and Lawson-Kerr, 1980; Rosen, 1983) recommend the use of more extensive neuropsychologic assessment batteries. While there is some variability in the specific tests included by each author in a recommended battery, most agree on the need to sample a range of cognitive functions, including general intelligence, memory, attention, language, perception, and praxis. Within the following subsections, the status of knowledge concerning the diagnostic utility of representative instruments for such assessment will be reviewed. The use of neuropsychologic assessment instruments in the examination of older patients requires the consideration of special issues in test administration and interpretation. While space does not allow a comprehensive discussion of these issues, a brief review of the major considerations follows. The reader is directed to other available reviews (e.g., Albert, 1981; Heaton, Grant, and Matthews, 1986; Kaszniak and Allender, 1985; Klisz, 1978) for more detailed information.

Psychometric Issues in the Neuropsychological Assessment of Dementia

There are several risks to the reliability and validity of psychologic assessment instruments when employed in the evaluation of older persons. One important threat to reliability and validity concerns differences between adult age groups in motor, sensory, and cognitive functioning, as were reviewed in previous chapters.

Age-Related changes in Sensory Functioning. Changes in visual acuity with aging can affect ability in a range of tasks in which questions or other stimuli are visually presented. One implication of this is that higher levels of illumination should be employed in assessment of the older patient. In addition, enlargement of type for printed material and increased size of other visual stimuli may prove helpful. Similarly, changes in auditory acuity (e.g., presbycusis) with aging may particularly affect perception of speech and other high-frequency sounds. Since much of cognitive, as well as communicative, evaluation depends upon spoken instructions and the presentation of auditory stimuli, age-related auditory changes can have a marked impact upon assessment results. Practical implications of auditory problems in the elderly, as well as special considerations in evaluating auditory functioning in the older person, are reviewed by Orchik (1981).

Age-Related Slowing. Behavioral slowing with aging is a pervasive phenomenon. Application of performance-based measures, in which total time to task completion or response initiation forms part of the dependent variable, must be approached with caution. Adequate age-appropriate normative data are a necessity for interpretation of such measures when used with the elderly.

Fatigue. Clinical lore suggests that older individuals tire more rapidly than younger persons, and it is therefore often recommended that testing sessions be kept as short as possible (e.g., Piper, 1979). Empirical studies that have either manipulated or controlled fatigue effects have either failed to demonstrate significant differences (Cunningham, Sepkoski, and Opel, 1978; Rust, Barnard, and Oster, 1979) or have found only slight effects (Furry and Baltes, 1973) upon cognitive test performance of healthy elderly versus younger adults. Thus, it appears that fatigue has relatively little specific effect upon cognitive task performance of healthy older persons. However, acute or chronic illness and depression all are generally associated with the symptom of increased fatigability. Therefore, it indeed seems advisable for the clinician to keep testing sessions as brief as possible, and to preferentially select shorter instruments in the psychologic assessment of older persons in clinical settings.

Test-Taking Attitudes and Response Biases. Test-taking attitudes and response biases, such as the tendency to choose socially desirable responses, are particular threats to the reliability and validity of self-report psychologic inventories (Anastasi, 1982). Klassen, Homstra, and Anderson (1975) have reported the degree of social desirability response bias to increase with adult age. Older persons may also differ from younger adults in other attitudes relevant to test performance. Various studies (e.g., Botwinick, 1966) have suggested a relationship between adult age and increasing cautiousness. This increased cautiousness among the aged is observed in responses to questions concerning life situations with high relevance for the older person (Wallach and Kogan, 1961). When provided with a list of risky alternatives, older individuals tend to choose one that involves little risk, unless risk cannot be avoided (Botwinick, 1969). In addition to this apparent cautiousness, or reluctance to act, when faced with questions concerning relevant life situations, older persons have also been shown to be more cautious in their response to a range of other kinds of tasks. For example, in the assessment of auditory threshold, older adults tend to report a sound only when certain about it (Rees and Botwinick, 1971). One practical consequence of this cautiousness is that traditional hearing tests may overestimate the magnitude of auditory deficit in later life (Botwinick, 1973, p. 115). Such response biases have also been shown to be of importance in the interpretation of data from various perceptual and memory tasks employed with older persons (see Danziger, 1980).

The Need for Age-Appropriate Reliability and Validity Data. The foregoing discussion merely highlights some of the difficulties in the use of all psychologic assessment instruments with the elderly. In general, it cannot be assumed that those assessment instruments known to be reliable and valid in application to younger adults will have the same reliability and validity when applied to older individuals. Schaie (1978) finds that the external validity of intellectual assessment in adulthood is not constant either across situations or across different adult age groups. Similarly, self-report instruments that are externally valid when used with younger adults cannot be assumed to have the same validity for older persons. Further limiting measurement validity is the fact that several psychologic assessment instruments contain content that is either irrelevant or inappropriate to older persons (Oberleder, 1967).

Several authors (e.g., McNair, 1979) have questioned whether there is presently sufficient information on the reliability of psychologic test responses of elderly adults to allow informed evaluation of them. Further, it has been pointed out (Kochansky, 1979; McNair, 1979) that there is a relative lack of empirical comparison of the validity of various assessment procedures, thus making it difficult to make educated choices among them.

In part, this paucity of comparative validity data reflects the magnitude of both conceptual and methodologic problems facing the investigator interested in determining the external validity of assessment procedures appropriate for the elderly. Kaszniak and Davis (1986) have reviewed those problems in determining the external validity of memory assessment instruments for older adults, and most of the same considerations apply equally to other measures of cognitive function. Several of these issues, of particular relevance for the interpreting results of cognitive research in normal aging and dementia, were discussed in Chapter 9. In the review that follows, efforts will be made to alert the reader to these problems as they specifically manifest in attempting to determine the reliability or validity, or both, of a given assessment instrument. Despite these problems, the clinician or investigator faced with making diagnostic or management decisions needs some guidance in selecting assessment approaches that suit his or her particular needs. It is in the service of such guidance that the following review is provided.

Assessment of Intelligence

Since impairment in intellectual functioning is one of the defining features of dementia, most neuropsychologists include formal intelligence testing in their assessment battery. The most frequently used instrument is the Wechsler Adult Intelligence Scale (WAIS) (Wechsler, 1958), or its revised version (WAIS-R) (Wechsler, 1981). Miller (1977, pp. 33–42) reviews the results of several investigations in which the WAIS (or the older Wechsler-Bellevue Scale) was applied to dementia patients. Of ten studies reviewed, only one failed to find average IQs below the expected population mean of 100, and those testing control groups always found the dementia group to show lower scores. While the WAIS thus validly reflects the intellectual impairment of dementia, there is greater variability in the subtest scores of demented persons compared with healthy elderly individuals, and overlap of respective score distributions (see Miller, 1977, pp. 35-36).

Estimating Premorbid Intelligence. One attempt to improve the accuracy of the WAIS in the diagnosis of dementia involves procedures to estimate intellectual decline. Wechsler's (1958) deterioration index, along with many suggested alternatives, use several of the WAIS subtests showing the least decline with age as indicators of premorbid levels. Other subtests, more sensitive to the effects of age, are used as measures of present levels. Such approaches are problematic in that they assume the manifestations of dementia to be similar to those of normal aging. Further, the results of validation studies employing such deterioration indices have generally not been encouraging (see Miller, 1981, pp. 126–127).

An alternative approach is to estimate premorbid intelligence through application of an equation differentially weighting age, sex, race, years of formal education, and occupation. The application of such a formula, based upon a regression equation derived from analysis of the original WAIS standardization data, has been supported in a validation study (Wilson, Rosenbaum, and Brown, 1979). This approach to the estimation of premorbid intelligence has recently been cross-validated and extended by an independent group of investigators (Karzmark, Heaton, Grant, and Matthews, 1985). However, given the variation in IQ among people with comparable educational and occupational backgrounds (see Matarazzo, 1972), caution needs to be exercised in the clinical application of this estimation equation.

WAIS Scores Are Not Helpful in Differentiating Dementia from Pseudodementia. In addition to the investigations concerned with the sensitivity of the WAIS to dementia, other studies have been concerned with the possibility of WAIS subtest pattern specificity in the differentiation of various causes of dementia. One of the more frequent, and more difficult, of diagnostic questions asked of the clinical neuropsychologist concerns the differentiation of dementia from pseudodementia. Pseudodementia can occur in various syndromes, including hysterical disorders and schizophrenia, although depressive illness appears to be the most frequent cause (Bienenfeld and Hartford, 1982; Kiloh, 1961; Maletta et al., 1982; Wells, 1982). Various investigations have documented the presence of cognitive deficit in depression (see reviews by McAllister, 1981; Miller, 1975), and older depressed patients may be more likely to show such deficits (Donnelly et al., 1980).

Crookes (1974) found the WAIS to be useful in differentiating between dementia and depression, with diagnosis based upon 1-year follow-up clinical examination. However, little other convincing data on the validity of the WAIS for such differential diagnosis exists. Whitehead (1973), comparing elderly patients with depression versus those with diffuse brain damage, found the brain-damaged patients to score at generally lower levels on the WAIS. However, there was no evidence that the patterns of scores were related to diagnosis. Similar WAIS subtests were impaired for both groups. Thus, interpretation of WAIS performance, in attempting to differentiate depression from dementia, requires the exercise of considerable caution. In the present authors' experience, differentiation of dementia from depressive pseudodementia is not greatly assisted by the examination of WAIS score patterns or levels alone. However, the observation of qualitative features in intelligence test performance may be helpful. For example, the pseudodementia patient will frequently give "don't know" answers in response to intelligence test items, whereas the dementia patient shows fewer such responses and often makes several "near miss" errors or shows obvious guessing (Wells, 1979).

Application of the WAIS in Differentiating AD from MID. Several attempts have also been made to determine the utility of the WAIS in differentiating AD from MID. Perez, Rivera, Meyer, Gay, Taylor, and Mathew (1975) reported a 74 percent accuracy of classification of AD, MID, and demented vertebrobasilar insufficiency (VBI) patients, via a discriminant analysis of WAIS subtests. While successful cross-validation has been reported (Perez, Stump, Gay, and Hart, 1976), clinical application of the resultant regression formula is not warranted. In both studies reported by Perez and colleagues, the AD patients were more educated than the MID patients. Further, the AD patients were, overall, more severely impaired than the MID group. Such confounding of diagnostic group with education and dementia severity invalidates the discriminant analysis results. Brinkman (1983) analyzed WAIS IQ and subtest scores of 20 MID and 16 AD patients, matched for age, education, and dementia severity, and failed to find any significant differences.

Fuld (1982b) has suggested that although WAIS IQ or individual subtests do not effectively differentiate AD from other dementia patients, the relationship between WAIS subtests might. Fuld presents a formula based upon the WAIS profile shown by young subjects treated with scopolamine (an anticholinergic) (Drachman and Leavitt, 1974). Of 31 consecutive patients with dementia, 10 of 17 patients with a diagnosis of AD and 1 of 14 patients with other diagnoses showed this profile. Brinkman and Braun (1984), comparing 39 MID and 23 AD patients, found 13 of the AD and only 2 of the MID patients to show Fuld's WAIS profile. This profile was unrelated to age, sex, or overall impairment severity.

Brust (1983), however, cautions against reliance upon WAIS or other psychologic testing in attempts to differentiate AD from MID, given the range of possible anatomic locations of infarcts and consequent possible deficits in MID. Further, it should be remembered that cases of AD initially resembling focal aphasic (Wechsler, 1977) or right parietal lobe (Crystal, Horoupian, Katzman, and Jotkowitz, 1982) syndromes have been reported. Such cases would be easily confused with MID cases, in which relatively focal cognitive deficits are often observed.

Memory Assessment

In addition to loss of intellectual ability, memory impairment is another necessary feature for the diagnosis of dementia. Neither most mental status examination protocols nor the WAIS provide sufficiently sensitive or comprehensive memory evaluation.

Wechsler Memory Scale. The most frequently employed instrument for clinical memory assessment is the Wechsler Memory Scale (WMS) (Wechsler, 1945). The WMS has been frequently criticized (e.g., Erickson, 1978; Erickson and Scott, 1977). Prigatano (1978) has summarized the weaknesses of the WMS as follows: (1) absence of scaled or standard scores for individual subtests; (2) problems in scoring the Logical Memory subtest, a task involving immediate recall of short spoken stories; (3) lack of adequate norms for the sexes and for various age groups, based on large, representative samples; (4) lack of sufficient information on test-retest reliability of Memory Quotient (MQ) scores for normal individuals; (5) lack of data concerning the distribution of WAIS Full Scale IQ minus WMS MQ scores, particularly for persons with superior IQ scores; and (6) the need for restandardization of the MQ scores with WAIS, or preferably WAIS-R, Full Scale IQ. Albert (1981) adds to these criticisms the confounding of perceptual and constructional skills with nonverbal memory in the Visual Reproduction subtest, and the omission of delayed recall assessment.

Despite these difficulties, the WMS continues to be widely employed, and several of the criticisms have been addressed by recent improvements. Russell (1975) has provided a revision of the WMS in which both immediate and delayed recall of both verbal (i.e., the Logical Memory subtest) and nonverbal (i.e., the Visual Reproduction subtest) material is assessed. When specific scoring conventions are adopted, this revised WMS demonstrates good interrater reliability (Power, Logue, McCarty, Rosenstiel, and Ziesat, 1979). Alternate form reliability for the revised WMS has been found to be adequate for immediate recall on both subtests, but less adequate for delayed recall and inadequate for percentage retained scores (McCarty, Logue, Power, Ziesat, and Rosenstiel, 1980).

The revised WMS has been shown to validly differentiate dementia patients from appropriately matched normal groups (Logue and Wyrick, 1979). WMS subtests are also helpful in differentiating elderly psychiatric patients with functional disorders from those with a variety of organic brain syndromes (Gilleard, 1980). Recently (Brinkman, Largen, Gerganoff, and Pomara, 1983), the revised WMS was shown to validly differentiate carefully diagnosed AD patients from age- and education-matched healthy elderly persons. However, a bimodal distribution of percent retained (delayed recall/immediate recall) scores was noted in the patient group, but not in the control group, suggesting the possibility of subgroups of AD patients. Perez, Gay, Taylor, and Rivera (1975) reported the subtests of the original WMS to accurately discriminate between AD, MID, and demented vertebrobasilar insufficiency patients. However, the same problems concerning group differences in education and dementia severity, as was discussed regarding WAIS scores, also applies to this study and confounds interpretation of the results.

Clinical interpretation of WMS and revised WMS scores depends upon the application of age-appropriate norms. Both cross-sectional and longitudinal data show age-related decline in WMS performance (McCarty, Siegler, and Logue, 1982). Recently, Haaland et al., (1983) provided revised WMS norms for ages 65 through over 80 years. While such normative data have been badly needed, some caution should be exercised in the application of these norms. The volunteer subjects composing the normative sample were better educated than is typical for the general population of these ages. The number of years of formal education has a significant correlation with WMS performance of older individuals (Bak and Green, 1981). Further, the magnitude of this correlation may independently account for as much of the variance in WMS subtest scores as do relationships with age, degree of cerebral atrophy, and EEG slowing in older patients suspected of having dementia (Kaszniak, Garron, Fox, Bergen, and Huckman, 1979).

One further caution is required in any attempt at clinical interpretation of any observed differences between verbal ("semantic") and nonverbal ("figural") initial or delayed recall scores on the revised WMS. One approach to interpretation would associate such differences with asymmetric status of particular hemispheric structures. That is, semantic scores are expected to be more affected by left hemispheric damage, and figural scores by right hemispheric damage. Although there is some support for the validity of this interpretation, when the revised WMS is used with younger adult patients (Russell, 1975), several factors argue against similar interpretation for older patients. First, there are differences in factor structure of the WMS for older versus younger adults (Dye, 1982). Such alteration in factor structure suggests that those processes contributing to WMS performance differ with aging. Second, there are data to indicate that adult age effects are stronger for the figural than for the semantic subtests (Bak and Green, 1981). Finally, as Albert (1981) and Rosen (1983) remind us, perceptual, constructional, and nonverbal memory skills are confounded in the figural subtest of the revised WMS. Both suggest including conditions of copying and matching of visual reproductions, although normative data for such procedures do not yet exist.

Other Memory Assessment Instruments. While the WMS is the most widely used of memory assessment instruments, there are others that hold promise for the evaluation of dementia. The Benton Revised Visual Retention Test (BVRT-R) (Benton, 1974) is a figural retention task often employed in neuropsychologic assessment. As with the figural subtests of the revised WMS, aging appears to markedly affect performance on this instrument (Arenberg, 1978), and age-appropriate normative data (Benton, Eslinger, and Damasio, 1981) should be employed. The BVRT-R has been shown to effectively differentiate normal and demented elderly persons (Eslinger, Damasio, Benton, and Van Allen, 1985; LaRue, D'Elia, Clark, Spar, and Jarvik, 1986). However, depressed older persons may show a large number of errors on this test, resulting in great difficulty in differentiating them from demented patients (Crookes and McDonald, 1972; LaRue et.al., 1986).

The Guild Memory Test. The Guild Memory Test (GMT) (Crook, Gilbert, and Ferris, 1980) is another instrument employing immediate and delayed recall of paragraphs and paired-word associates and recall of visuospatial designs. Normative data for older individuals are available, and GMT performance is significantly correlated with WMS subtest performance (Crook et al., 1980).

The Misplaced Objects Test. Another task developed by this group of investigators, the Misplaced Objects Task (Crook, Ferris, and McCarthy, 1979), employs a board upon which a cross-section of a seven-room furnished house is depicted. Ten magnetized vinyl shapes of frequently misplaced objects (e.g., keys) are identified and placed on the board, representing where in the home they would likely be kept. Following removal of the board for an interval, the patient is asked to replace the objects in their original position. With this task, Crook and colleagues (1979) have demonstrated valid differentiation of older individuals with intact versus impaired memory functioning. Its high face validity, and the possibility that it therefore would elicit greater patient cooperation, encourages the further development of this task, particularly for application with moderately to severely demented patients.

The Fuld Object Memory Evaluation. Another recently developed instrument with promise for utility with more demented patients is the Fuld Object Memory Evaluation (Fuld, 1980; 1981). This test employs a modification of the Buschke and Fuld (1974) procedure of selective reminding, allowing for differential evaluation of storage and retrieval processes from within a single testing session. In addition, the test also evaluates ability to retrieve words rapidly from familiar semantic categories. The test "guarantees" stimulus processing by presenting ten common objects in a bag and having the subject identify and describe each object by touch, and afterward by visual identification, with correction by the examiner of any identification errors. This procedure circumvents the visual and auditory impairments common in the elderly, as well as the perceptual and naming difficulties frequently observed in dementia patients. Following a 60-second distraction, during which the semantic category naming task is administered, recall is assessed over five consecutive recall trials. Selective reminding is employed for the items omitted. Scoring allows separate estimates of storage and retrieval processes.

Fuld (1980) has reported good internal reliability (coefficient alpha = .84) for this instrument. Storage scores were found to be correlated (r = .72) with retention after 3 weeks, for a sample of nursing home residents. Further, Fuld demonstrated significant differences on the test, comparing moderately impaired and unimpaired elderly nursing home residents, grouped on the basis of an independent mental status examination (Blessed et al., 1968).

Finally, intrusion errors on this test have been shown to be correlated with choline acetyltransferase levels and neuritic plaque counts in the brain tissue of nursing home residents at autopsy (Fuld, Katzman, Davies, and Terry, 1982). Norms for the Fuld Object Memory Evaluation are available for community active, as well as nursing home residing, 70- and 80-year-olds (Fuld, 1980).

The New York University Memory Test. Finally, note should be taken of the recently developed New York University Memory Test (Osborne, Brown, and Randt, 1982; Randt, Brown, and Osborne, 1980). This test allows for immediate and delayed recall (at 10 seconds, 3 minutes, and 24 hours) assessment for objects, words, short stories and pictures, and provides selective reminding and incidental learning procedures. Five equivalent alternate forms are available, facilitating longitudinal study and application to treatment evaluation. Normative data are available on 300 subjects, grouped by decade from 20 to 80 years. The instrument has been shown to differentiate normal from memory impaired elderly subjects (Osborne et al., 1982). If future research continues to support the reliability and validity of this test battery, it may prove an excellent instrument for the detailed evaluation of various memory processes in persons with mild to moderate memory loss, including patients early in the progression of dementia.

Assessment of Other Cognitive Processes

Although intellectual and memory assessment typically occupy the largest portion of the neuropsychologic assessment of patients suspected of having dementia, assessment of other areas should also be included in any comprehensive evaluation.

Selective Attention

The most frequently employed procedures for evaluating selective attention are the visual letter (Talland and Schwab, 1964) and digit (Lewis and Kupke, 1977) cancellation tasks. In these tasks, the person crosses out a particular digit or letter every time it appears on a printed page. Although mild AD patients may not show deficits on this type of task (Vitaliano, Russo, Breen, Vitiello, and Prinz, 1986), moderately demented AD patients typically do (Allender and Kaszniak, 1985).

Abstraction

Abstract thinking ability is most frequently evaluated by examining WAIS Similarities and Comprehension ("proverbs" items) subtests. Other procedures for evaluating abstraction ability and cognitive flexibility, such as the Wisconsin Card Sorting Test (Berg, 1948), are available, but adequate norms for older age groups are typically not available, and specific validity in assessment of dementia remains to be empirically demonstrated. The Picture Absurdities subtest of the Stanford-Binet Intelligence Scale (Terman and Merril, 1973) provides a useful index of the patient's ability to make judgments concerning the appropriateness of actions pictured within a setting. Performance on this measure has been shown to be negatively correlated with degree of EEG slowing, within a sample of older patients suspected of having dementia (Kaszniak, Garron, Fox, Bergen, and Huckman, 1979). Within a small sample of AD patients, Picture Absurdities performance was found to be significantly poorer for those patients deceased, versus those still alive, at 1 year after examination (Kaszniak, Fox, Gandell, Garron, Huckman, and Ramsey, 1978).

Constructional Praxis

Constructional ability is most frequently examined by the Block Design subtest of the WAIS or by various drawing tasks. Studies comparing WAIS performance of demented and nondemented elderly have consistently demonstrated Block Design impairment in moderate to severe dementia (see review by Miller, 1977, pp. 33–42). WAIS Block Design performance has also recently been shown to be impaired in mildly demented AD patients (Storandt, Botwinick, Danziger, Berg, and Hughes, 1984). Longitudinal deterioration of WAIS Block Design performance by AD patients has been documented (Berg et al., 1984). Similarly, the ability to copy two-dimensional geometric forms has been shown to be impaired in dementia, with the degree of impairment generally proportional to the overall severity of dementia (Ajuriaguerra and Tissot, 1968). Mildly demented AD patients show significantly more errors than age-matched control subjects in drawing the Bender-Gestalt (Bender, 1938) geometric figures (Storandt et al., 1984). Longitudinal deterioration of AD patient performance in the Bender-Gestalt test has been demonstrated (Berg et al., 1984).

Visual-Perceptive Ability

As noted in Chapter 11, clinical observers have noted visual-perceptual deficits in AD and other dementia patients, increasing as dementia progresses. Eslinger and Benton (1983) compared a group of 40 patients with dementia of mixed etiology and 40 appropriately matched normal volunteers, employing the Benton Facial Recognition Test (Benton and Van Allen, 1968) and the Benton Line Orientation Test (Benton, Varney, and Hamsher, 1978). The Facial Recognition Test requires the identification of one or more black-and-white photographs of unfamiliar faces in a matching-to-sample multiple choice display. In this test, the choice foils vary in lighting conditions and angle of photograph. The Line Orientation Test requires identification of pairs of lines differing in slope on a matching-to-sample multiple choice display. Conversion of raw scores to T scores, on the basis of a larger referent sample of 178 normal subjects, showed that the normal control subjects had almost identical performances on the two tests and progressive decline with advancing age. However, large and significant differences emerged on both tests in the comparison of the dementia and matched normal groups, supporting the validity of these instruments in the assessment of dementia. Further, dissociations in performance on the two tests were common for the dementia patients but rare for the normal subjects, suggesting that dementia may manifest in differential perceptual deterioration. Normative data are available on these tests for subjects aged 65 to 84 years, grouped by 5-year intervals (Benton et al., 1981).

Generative and Confrontation Naming Ability

Evaluation of naming ability forms another important component of the comprehensive neuropsychologic assessment of dementia. Approaches to the comprehensive evaluation of communication deficit in dementia were provided in Chapters 6 and 7. For the purposes of this chapter, it is sufficient to note that generative naming tasks, in combination with episodic memory tasks, are among the most sensitive measures for differentiating mild AD patients from normal older persons (e.g., Storandt et al., 1984).

SUMMARY

This chapter has reviewed critical issues in the neuropsychologic assessment of dementia patients. One of the most difficult problems in neuropsychologic diagnostic assessment is the differentiation of dementia from pseudodementia. Pseudodementia most frequently occurs in the context of depression. However, depression and depression-like features often occur in dementing illnesses. Although quantitative aspects of intelligence, and other psychometric, test performance are not helpful in differentiating dementia from depressive pseudodementia, particular qualitative features are.

Neuropsychologic assessment of older persons faces several threats to validity. Consideration of these threats underscores the need for age-appropriate normative data for the interpretation of test scores. Further, tests with known reliability and validity in application to assessment of younger adults cannot be assumed to have comparable psychometric properties when applied to older persons. In order to assist the clinician in selecting appropriate assessment instruments, this chapter reviewed those tests and protocols with known reliability and validity for older individuals. Mental status examination instruments, dementia rating scales, and behavior-observation protocols were described.

Although necessary and helpful in the evaluation of dementia, these instruments do not provide sufficiently detailed assessment of cognition. Tests appropriate for the evaluation of memory, selective attention, visual-constructive skill, visual-perceptual ability, and naming were therefore reviewed. The careful application of these assessment instruments can contribute substantially to the diagnosis and clinical management of dementia.

REFERENCES

Ajuriaguerra, J. de, and Tissot, R. (1968). Some aspects of psycho-neurologic disintegration in senile dementia. In C. Muller and I. Ciompi (Eds.), *Senile dementia* (pp. 69-79). Switzerland: Huber.

Albert, M.S. (1981). Geriatric neuropsychology. *Journal of Consulting and Clinical Psychology*, *49*, 835-850.

Allender, J., and Kaszniak, A.W. (1985, February). *Processing of emotional cues and personality change in dementia of the Alzheimer type.* Paper presented at the Annual meeting of the International Neuropsychological Society, San Diego, CA.

Anastasi, A. (1982). *Psychological Testing (5th ed.).* New York: Macmillan.

Anthony, J.D., LeResche, L., Niaz, V., von Korff, M.R., and Folstein, M.F. (1982). Limits of the 'Mini-Mental State' as a screening test for dementia and delirium among hospital patients. *Psychological Medicine, 12*, 397-408.

Arenberg, D. (1978). Differences and changes with age in the Benton Visual Retention Test. *Journal of Gerontology*, *33*, 534-540.

Bak, J.S., and Greene, R.L. (1981). A review of the performance of aged adults on various Wechsler Memory Scale subtests. *Journal of Clinical Psychology*, *37*, 186-188.

Bender, L.A. (1938). *A visual-motor gestalt test and its clinical use.* New York: American Orthopsychiatric Association.

Benton, A.L. (1974). *Revised visual retention test: Clinical and experimental application*, (4th ed.). New York: The Psychological Corporation.

Benton, A.L., Eslinger, P.J., and Damasio, A.R. (1981). Normative observations on neuropsychological test performances in old age. *Journal of Clinical Neuropsychology*, *3*, 33-42.

Benton, A.L., and Van Allen, M.W. (1968). Impairment in facial recognition in patients with cerebral disease. *Cortex*, *4*, 344-358.

Benton, A.L., Varney, N.R., and Hamsher, K. (1978). Visuospatial judgement: A clinical test. *Archives of Neurology*, *35*, 364-367.

Berg, E.A. (1948). A simple objective test for measuring flexibility in thinking. *Journal of General Psychology*, *39*, 15-22.

Berg, L., Danziger, W.L., Storandt, M., Coben, L.A., Gado, M., Hughes, C.P., Knesevich, J.W., and Botwinick, J. (1984). Predictive features in mild senile dementia of the Alzheimer type. *Neurology (Cleveland)*, *34*, 563-569.

Bienenfeld, D., and Hartford, J.T. (1982). Pseudodementia in an elderly woman with schizophrenia. *American Journal of Psychiatry*, *139*, 114-115.

Blessed, G., Tomlinson, B.E., and Roth, M. (1968). The association between quantitative measures of dementia and of senile change in the cerebral grey matter of elderly subjects. *Journal of Psychiatry*, *114*, 797-811.

Botwinick, J. (1966). Cautiousness in advanced age. *Journal of Gerontology*, *21*, 347-353.

Botwinick, J. (1969). Disinclination to venture response versus cautiousness in responding: Age differences. *Journal of Genetic Psychology*, *115*, 55-62.

Botwinick, J. (1973). *Aging and Behavior.* New York: Springer.

Brink, T.L., Capri, D., DeNeeve, V., Janakes, C., and Oliveira, C. (1978). Senile confusion: Limitations of assessment by the face-hand test, mental status questionnaire, and staff ratings. *Journal of the American Geriatrics Society*, *26*, 380-382.

Brinkman, S.D., (1983). Neuropsychological differences between Alzheimer's disease and multi-infarct dementia. Paper presented at the Talland Memorial Conference on Clinical Memory Assessment of Older Adults, Wakefield, Mass, October.

Brinkman, S.D., and Braun, P. (1984). Classification of dementia patients by a WAIS profile related to central cholinergic deficiencies. *Journal of Clinical Neuropsychology*, *6*, 393-400.

Brinkman, S.D., Largen, J.W., Gerganoff, S., and Pomara, M. (1983). Russell's revised Memory Scale in the evaluation of dementia. *Journal of Clinical Psychology*, *39*, 989-993.

Brust, J.C.M. (1983). Dementia and cerebrovascular disease. In R. Mayeux and W.G. Rosen (Eds.), *The dementias* (pp. 131-147). New York: Raven Press.

Buschke, H., and Fuld, P.A. (1974). Evaluating storage, retention and retrieval in disordered memory and learning. *Neurology*, *24*, 1019-1025.

Busse, E.W. (1975). Aging and psychiatric diseases of late life. In S. Arieti (Ed.), *American handbook of psychiatry (2nd ed.): Vol. IV. Organic disorders and psychosomatic medicine* (pp. 67-89). New York: Basic Books.

Caine, E.D. (1986). The neuropsychology of depression: The pseudodementia syndrome. In I. Grant and K.M. Adams (Eds.), *Neuropsychological assessment of neuropsychiatric disorders* (pp. 221-243). New York: Oxford University Press.

Caine, E.D., and Shoulson, I. (1983). Psychiatric syndromes in Huntington's Disease. *American Journal of Psychiatry*, *140*, 728-733.

Christensen, A.L. (1979). *Luria's neuropsychological investigation: Text (2nd ed.).* Copenhagen: Munksgaard.

Coblentz, J.M., Mattis, S., Zingesser, L.H., Kassoff, S.S., Wisniewski, H.M., and Katzman, R. (1973). Presenile dementia: Clinical evaluation of cerebrospinal fluid dynamics. *Archives of Neurology*, *29*, 299-308.

Cohen, D., Eisdorfer, C., and Holm, C.L. (1984). Mental status examinations in aging. In M.L. Albert (Ed.), *Clinical neurology of aging* (pp. 219-230). New York: Oxford University Press.

Corso, J.F. (1981). *Aging sensory systems and perception.* New York: Praeger.

Crook, T., Ferris, S., and McCarthy, M. (1979). The misplaced-objects task: A brief test for memory dysfunction in the aged. *Journal of the American Geriatrics Society*, *27*, 284-287.

Crook, T., Gilbert, J.G., and Ferris, S. (1980). Operationalizing memory impairment for elderly persons: The Guild Memory Test. *Psychological Reports 47*, 1315-1318.

Crookes, T.G. (1974). Indices of early dementia on WAIS. *Psychological Reports*, *34*, 734.

Crookes, T.G., and McDonald, K.G. (1972). Bentons Visual Retention Test in the differentiation of depression and early dementia. *British Journal of Social and Clinical Psychology*, *11*, 66-69.

Crystal, H.A., Horoupian, D.S., Katzman, R., and Jotkowitz, S. (1982). Biopsy-proved Alzheimer disease presenting as a right parietal lobe syndrome. *Annals of Neurology*, *12*, 186-188.

Cunningham, W.R., Sepkoski, C.M., and Opel, M.R. (1978). Fatigue effects on intelligence test performance in the elderly. *Journal of Gerontology*, *33*, 541-545.

Danziger, W.L.(1980). Measurement of response bias in aging research. In L.W. Poon (Ed.), *Aging in the 1980s: Psychological issues* (pp. 552-557). Washington, DC: American Psychological Association.

Demuth, G.W., and Rand, B.S. (1980). Atypical major depression in a patient with severe primary degenerative dementia. *American Journal of Psychiatry*, *137*, 1609-1610.

Donnelly, E.F., Waldman, I.N., Murphy, D.L., Wyatt, R.J., and Goodwin, F.K. (1980). Primary affective disorder: Thought disorder in depression. *Journal of Abnormal Psychology*, *89*, 315-319.

Drachman,D.A., and Leavitt, J. (1974). Human memory and the cholinergic system: A relationship to aging? *Archives of Neurology*, *30*, 113-121.

Dye, C.J. (1982). Factor structure of the Wechsler Memory Scale in an older adult population. *Journal of Clinical Psychology*, *38*, 163-166.

English, W.H. (1942). Alzheimer's disease: Its incidence and recognition. *Psychiatric Quarterly*, *16*, 91-94.

Erickson, R.C. (1978). Problems in the clinical assessment of memory. *Experimental Aging Research*, *4*, 255-272.

Erickson, R.C., and Scott, M.L. (1977). Clinical memory testing: A review. *Psychological Bulletin*, *84*, 130-1149.

Eslinger, P.J., and Benton, A.L. (1983). Visuoperceptual performances in aging and dementia: Clinical and theoretical implications. *Journal of Clinical Neuropsychology*, *5*, 213-220.

Eslinger, P.J., Damasio, A.R., Benton, A.L., and Van Allen, M. (1985). Neuropsychologic detection of abnormal mental decline in older persons. *Journal of the American Medical Association*, *253*, 670-674.

Fillenbaum, G.G. (1980). Comparison of two brief tests of organic brain impairment, the MSQ and the Short Portable MSQ. *Journal of the American Geriatrics Society*, *8*, 381-384.

Fillenbaum, G.G., and Smyer, M. (1981). The development, validity and reliability of the OARS multidimensional functional assessment questionnaire. *Journal of Gerontology*, *36*, 428-434.

Fleiss, J., Gurland, B., and Des Roche, P. (1976). Distinctions between organic brain syndrome and functional psychiatric disorders based on the Geriatric Mental State interview. *International Journal of Aging and Human Deveopment*, 7, 323-330.

Folstein, M.F., Folstein, S.E., and McHugh, P.R. (1975). Mini-mental state: A practical method for grading the cognitive state of patients for the clinician. *Journal of Psychiatric Research*, *12*, 189-198.

Folstein, M.F., and McHugh, P.R. (1978). Dementia syndrome of depression. In R. Katzman, R.D. Terry, and K.L. Bick (Eds.), *Alzheimer's disease: Senile dementia and related disorders* (pp. 87-93). New York: Raven Press.

Fuld, P.A. (1978). Psychological testing in the differential diagnosis of the dementias. In R. Katzman, R.D. Terry, and K.L. Bick (Eds.), *Alzheimer's disease: Senile dementia and related disorders* (pp. 185-193). New York: Raven Press.

Fuld, P.A. (1980). Guaranteed stimulus-processing in the evaluation of memory and learning. *Cortex*, *16*, 255-271.

Fuld, P.A. (1981). *The Fuld object memory evaluation*. Chicago, IL: Stoelting Instrument Co.

Fuld, P.A. (1982a). *Mental status examination of 80 year olds—what is normal?* Paper presented at the Annual Scientific Meeting of the Gerontological Society of America, Boston, MA.

Fuld, P.A. (1982b). Behavioral signs of cholinergic deficiency in Alzheimer dementia. In S. Corkin, K.L. Davis, H.H. Growdon, E. Usdin, and R.L. Wurtman (Eds.), *Aging: Vol. 19. Alzheimer's disease: A report of Progress*, (pp. 193-196). New York: Raven Press.

Fuld, P.A., Katzman, R., Davies, P., and Terry, R.D. (1982). Intrusions as a sign of Alzheimer dementia. Chemical and pathological verification. *Annals of Neurology*, *11*, 155-159.

Furry, C.A., and Baltes, P.B. (1973). The effect of age differences in ability-extraneous performance variables on the assessment of intelligence in children, adults, and the elderly. *Journal of Gerontology*, *28*, 73-79.

Garcia, C.A., Reding, M.J., and Blass, J.P. (1981). Overdiagnosis of dementia. *Journal of the American Geriatrics Society*, *29*, 407-410.

Gardner, R., Oliver-Munoz, S., Fisher, L., and Empting, L. (1981). Mattis Dementia Rating Scale: Internal reliability study using a diffusely impaired population. *Journal of Clinical Neuropsychology*, *3*, 271-275.

Gilleard, C.J. (1980). Wechsler memory scale performance of elderly psychiatric patients. *Journal of Clinical Psychology*, *36*, 958-960.

Gurland, B.J., Copeland, J., Sharpe, L., and Kelleher, M. (1976). The Geriatric Mental Status Interview (GMS). *International Journal of Aging and Human Development*, 7, 303-311.

Gurland, B.J., Fleiss, J.L., Goldberg, K., Sharpe, L., Copeland, J.R.M., Kelleher, M.J., and Kellet, J.M. (1976). A semi-structured clinical interview for the assessment of diagnosis and mental state in the elderly: The Geriatric Mental State Schedule II, A factor analysis. *Psychological Medicine*, *6*, 451-459.

Gurland, B., Golden, K., and Challop, J. (1982). Unidimensional and multidimensional approaches to the differentiation of depression and dementia in the elderly. In S. Corkin, K.L. Davis, J.H. Growdon, E Usdin, and R.L. Wurtman, (Eds.), *Aging: Vol. 19. Alzheimer's disease: A report of progress* (pp. 119-125). New York: Raven Press.

Gurland, B., Kuriansky, T., Sharpe, L., Simon, R.,

Stiller, P., and Birkett, P. (1977-78). The Comprehensive Assessment and Referral Evaluation (CARE): Rationale, development and reliability. *International Journal of Aging and Human Development, 8*, 9-42.

Gurland, B., and Toner, J. (1983). Differentiating dementia from nondementing conditions. In R. Mayeux and W.G. Fosen (Eds.), *The dementias* (pp. 1-17). New York: Raven Press.

Haaland, K.Y., Linn, R. T., Hunt, W.C., and Goodwin, J.S. (1983). A normative study of Russell's variant of the Wechsler Memory Scale in a healthy elderly population. *Journal of Consulting and Clinical Psychology, 51*, 878-881.

Haglund, R.M.J., and Schuckit, M.A. (1976). A clinical comparison of tests of organicity in elderly patients. *Journal of Gerontology, 31*, 654-659.

Heaton, R.K., Grant, I., and Matthews, C.G. (1986). Differences in neuropsychological test performance associated with age, education and sex. In I. Grant and K.M. Adams (Eds.), *Neuropsychological assessment of neuropsychiatric disorders* (pp. 100-120). New York: Oxford University Press.

Hersch, E.L. (1979). Development and application of the extended scale for dementia. *Journal of the American Geriatrics Society, 27*, 348-354.

Hersch, E.L., Krall, V.A., and Palmer, R.B. (1978). Clinical value of the London Psychogeriatric Rating Scale. *Journal of the American Geriatrics Society, 26*, 348-354.

Hersch, E.L., Merskey, H., and Palmer, R.B. (1980). Prediction of discharge from a psychogeriatric unit: Development and evaluation of the LPRS prognosis index. *Canadian Journal of Psychiatry, 25*, 234-241.

Heston, L.L., and Mastri, A.R. (1982). Age at onset of Pick's and Alzheimer's dementia: Implications for diagnosis and research. *Journal of Gerontology, 37*, 422-424.

Janowsky, D.S. (1982). Pseudodementia in the elderly: Differential diagnosis and treatment. *Journal of Clinical Psychiatry, 43*, 19-26.

Kahn, R., Goldfarb, A., Pollack, M., and Peck, A. (1960). Brief objective measures for the determination of mental status in the aged. *American Journal of Psychiatry, 117*, 326-328.

Kahn, R.L., Zarit, S.H., Hilbert, N.M., and Niederehe, G. (1975). Memory complaint and impairment in the aged. *Archives of General Psychiatry, 32*, 1569-1573.

Karzmark, P., Heaton, R.K., Grant, I., and Matthews, C.G. (1985). Use of demographic variables to predict full scale IQ: A replication and extension. *Journal of Clinical and Experimental Neuropsychology, 7*, 412-420.

Kaszniak, A.W. (1985). Personality and emotional change in dementia of the Alzheimer's type: Issues in the investigation of individual differences. *Journal of Clinical and Experimental Neuropsychology, 7*, 611.

Kaszniak, A.W. (1986). The neuropsychology of dementia. In I. Grant, and K.M. Adams (Eds.), *Neuropsychological assessment of neuropsychiatric disorders* (pp. 172-220). New York: Oxford University Press.

Kaszniak, A.W., and Allender, J.A. (1985). Psychological assessment of depression in older adults. In G.M. Chaisson-Stewart (Ed.), *Depression in the elderly: An interdisciplinary approach* (pp. 107-160). New York: John Wiley.

Kaszniak, A.W., and Davis, K. (1986). Instrument and data review: The quest for external validators. In L.W. Poon, B.J. Gurland, C. Eisdorfer, T. Crook, L.W. Thompson, A.W. Kaszniak, and K. Davis (Eds.), *The handbook of clinical memory assessment of older adults.* Washington, DC: American Psychological Association.

Kaszniak, A.W., Fox, J., Gandell, D.L, Garron, D., Huckman, M.S., and Ramsey, R.G. (1978). Predictors of mortality in presenile and senile dementia. *Annals of Neurology, 3*, 246-252.

Kaszniak, A.W., Garron, D.C., Fox, J.H., Bergen, D., and Huckman, M. (1979). Cerebral atrophy, EEG slowing, age, education, and cognitive functioning in suspected dementia. *Neurology, 29*, 1273-1279.

Kaszniak, A.W., Sadeh, M., and Stern, L.Z. (1985). Differentiating depression from organic brain syndromes in older age. In G.M. Chaisson-Stewart (Ed.), *Depression in the elderly: An interdisciplinary approach* (pp. 161-189). New York: John Wiley.

Kaszniak, A.W., Wilson, R.S., Lazarus, L., Lessor, J., and Fox, J.H. (1981, February). *Memory and depression in dementia.* Paper presented at the Ninth Annual Meeting of the International Neuropsychological Society, Atlanta, GA.

Kendrick, D.C., and Post, F. (1967). Differences in cognitive status between healthy, psychiatrically ill, and diffusely brain-damaged elderly subjects. *British Journal of Psychiatry, 113*, 75-81.

Kiloh, L.G. (1961). Pseudo-dementia. *Acta Psychiatrica Scandinavica, 37*, 336-351.

Klassen,D., Homstra, R.K., and Anderson, P.B. (1975). Influence of social desirability on symptom and mood reporting in a community survey. *Journal of Consulting and Clinical Psychology*, *43*, 448-452.

Klisz, D. (1978). Neuropsychological evaluation in older persons. In M. Storandt, I. Siegler, and M. Elias (Eds.), *The clinical psychology of aging* (pp. 71-96). New York: Plenum.

Kochansky, G.E. (1979). Psychiatric rating scales for assessing psychopathology in the elderly: A critical review. In A. Raskin, and L.F. Jarvik (Eds.), *Psychiatric symptoms and cognitive loss in the elderly* (pp. 125-156). Washington, DC: Hemisphere.

LaRue, A., D'Elia, L.F., Clark, E.O., Spar, J.E., and Jarvik, L.F. (1986). Clinical tests of memory in dementia, depression, and healthy aging. *Journal of Psychology and Aging*, *1*, 69-77.

Lawson, J.S., Rodenburg, M., and Dykes, J.A. (1977). A dementia rating scale for use with psychogeriatric patients. *Journal of Gerontology*, *32*, 153-159.

Lawton, M.P., and Brody, E.M. (1969). Assessment of older people. Self-maintaining and instrumental activities of daily living. *Gerontologist*, *37*, 179-186.

Lawton, M.P., Moss, M., Fulcomer, M., and Kleban, M.H. (1982). A research and service oriented multilevel assessment instrument. *Journal of Gerontology*, *37*, 91-99.

Levin, H.S., and Peters, B.H. (1982). Appendix: Report of the ad hoc committee for the classification of the severity of Alzheimer's disease. In S. Corkin, K.L. Davis, J.H. Growdon, E. Usdin, and R.L. Wurtman (Eds.), *Aging: Vol. 19. Alzheimer's disease: A report of progress*. (pp. 501-506). New York: Raven Press.

Lewis, R., and Kupke, T. (1977). *The Lafayette Clinic repeatable neuropsychological test battery: Its development and research applications*. Paper presented at the annual meeting of the Southeastern Psychological Association, Hollywood, FL.

Logue, P., and Wyrick, L. (1979). Initial validation of Russell's revised Wechsler Memory Scale: A comparison of normal aging versus dementia. *Journal of Consulting and Clinical Psychology*, *47*, 176-178.

Maletta, G.J., Pirozzolo, F.J., Thompson, G., and Mortimer, J.A. (1982). Organic mental disorders in a geriatric outpatient population. *American Journal of Psychiatry*, *139*, 521-523.

Matarazzo, J. D. (1972). *Wechsler's measurement and appraisal of adult intelligence*. Baltimore: Williams and Wilkins.

Mattis, S. (1976). Mental Status examination for organic mental syndrome in the elderly patient. In R. Bellack and B. Karasu (Eds.), *Geriatric psychiatry* (pp. 77-121). New York: Grune and Stratton.

Mayeux, R., Williams, J.B.W., Stern, Y, and Cote, L. (1984). Depression and Parkinson's disease. In R.G. Hassler, and J.F. Christ (Eds.), *Advances in Neurology, Vol. 40*. New York: Raven Press.

McAllister, T.W. (1981). Cognitive functioning in the affective disorders. *Comprehensive Psychiatry*, *22*, 572-586.

McAllister, T.W. (1983). Overview: Pseudodementia. *American Journal of Psychiatry*, *140*, 528-533.

McAllister, T.W., and Price, T.R.P. (1982). Severe depressive pseudodementia with and without dementia. *American Journal of Psychiatry*, *139*, 626-629.

McCartney, J.R. (1986). Physician's assessment of cognitive capacity: Failure to meet the needs of the elderly. *Archives of Internal Medicine*, *146*, 177-178.

McCarty, S.M., Logue, P.E., Power, D.G., Ziesat, H.A., and Rosenstiel, A.K. (1980). Alternate-form reliability and age-related scores for Russell's revised Wechsler Memory Scale. *Journal of Consulting and Clinical Psychology*, *48*, 296-298.

McCarty, S.M., Siegler, I.C., and Logue, P.E. (1982). Cross-sectional and longitudinal patterns of three Wechsler Memory Scale subtests. *Journal of Gerontology*, *37*, 169-175.

McHugh, P.R., and Folstein, M.F. (1975). Psychiatric syndromes of Huntington's chorea: A clinical and phenomenologic study. In D.F. Benson and D. Blumer (Eds.), *Psychiatric aspects of neurological diseases* (pp. 267-286). New York: Grune and Stratton.

McKahnn,G., Drachman,D., Folstein, M., Katzman, R., Price, D., Stadlin, E.M. (1984). Clinical diagnosis of Alzheimer's disease: Report of the NINCDS-ADRDA work group under the auspices of the Department of Health and Human Services Task Force on Alzheimer's disease. *Neurology*, *34*, 939-944.

McNair, D.M. (1979). Self-rating scales for assessing psychopathology in the elderly. In A. Raskin and L.F. Jarvik (Eds.), *Psychiatric symptoms and cognitive loss in the elderly* (pp. 157-168). Washington, DC: Hemisphere.

Meer, B., and Baker, J.A. (1966). The Stockton Geriatric Scale. *Journal of Gerontology*, *21*, 392-403.

Miller, E. (1977). *Abnormal ageing: The psychology of senile and presenile dementia*. New York: John Wiley.

Miller, E. (1981). The differential psychological evaluation. In N.E. Miller and G.D. Cohen (Eds.), *Aging: Vol. 15. Clinical aspects of Alzheimer's disease and senile dementia* (pp. 121-138). New York: John Wiley.

Miller, N.E. (1980). The measurement of mood in senile

brain disease: Examiner ratings and self-reports. In J.O. Cole and J.E. Barrett (Eds.), *Psychopathology in the aged* (pp. 97-122). New York: Raven Press.

Miller, W.R. (1975). Psychological deficit in depression. *Psychological Bulletin, 82*, 238-260.

Montgomery, K., and Costa, L. (1983, February). *Neuropsychological test performance of a normal elderly sample*. Paper presented at the annual meeting of the International Neuropsychological Society, Mexico City, Mexico.

Mortsyn, R., Hachanadel, G., Kaplan, E., and Gutheil, T.G. (1982). Depression versus pseudodepression in dementia. *Journal of Clinical Psychiatry, 43*, 197-101.

National Institute on Aging Task Force (1980). Senility reconsidered: Treatment possibilities for mental impairment in the elderly. *Journal of the American Medical Association, 244*, 259-263.

Nelson, F.L., and Faberow, N.L. (1980). Indirect self-destructive behavior in the elderly nursing home patient. *Journal of Gerontology, 35*, 949-957.

Oberleder, M. (1967). Adapting current psychological techniques for use in testing the aging. *Gerontologist*, 7, 188-191.

Orchik, D.J. (1981). Peripheral auditory problems and the aging process. In D.S. Beasley, and G.A. Davis (Eds.), *Aging: Communication process and disorders* (pp. 243-255). New York: Grune and Stratton.

Osborne, D.P., Brown, E.R., and Randt, C.T. (1982). Qualitative changes in memory function: Aging and dementia. In S. Corkin, K.L. Davis, J.H. Growdon, E. Usdin, and R.L. Wurtman (Eds.), *Aging: Vol. 19. Alzheimers disease: A report of progress*. (pp. 165-169). New York: Raven Press.

Pearson, J.S. (1973). Behavioral aspects of Huntington's chorea. In A. Barbeau, T.M. Chase, and G.W. Paulson (Eds.), *Advances in neurology, Volume 1: Huntington's chorea* (pp. 701-712). New York: Raven Press.

Perez, F.I., Gay, J.R.A., Taylor, R.L., and Rivera, V.M. (1975). Patterns of memory performance in the neurologically impaired aged. *Canadian Journal of Neurological Sciences, 2*, 347-355.

Perez, F.I., Rivera, V.M., Meyer, J.S., Gay, J.R.A., Taylor, R.L., and Mathew, N.T. (1975). Analysis of intellectual and cognitive performance in patients with multi-infarct dementia, vertebrobasilar insufficiency with dementia, and Alzheimer's disease. *Journal of Neurology, Neurosurgery, and Psychiatry, 38*, 533-540.

Perez, F.I., Stump, D.A., Gay, J.R., and Hart, B.R. (1976). Intellectual performance in multi-infarct dementia and Alzheimer's disease: A replication study. *Canadian Journal of Neurological Science, 3*, 181-187.

Perlick, D., and Atkins, A. (1984). Variation in the reported age of a patient: A source of bias in the diagnosis of depression and dementia. *Journal of Consulting and Clinical Psychology, 52*, 812-820.

Pfeffer, R.I., Kurosaki, T.T., Harrah, C.H., Chance, J.M., Bates, D., Detels, R., Filos, S., and Butzke, C. (1981). A survey diagnostic tool for senile dementia. *American Journal of Epidemiology, 114*, 515-527.

Pfeffer, R.I., Kurosaki, T.T., Harrah, C.H., Chance, J.M., and Filos, S. (1982). Measurement of functional activities in older adults in the community. *Journal of Gerontology, 37*, 323-329.

Pfeiffer, E. (1975). A short portable mental status questionnaire for the assessment of organic brain deficit in elderly patients. *Journal of the American Geriatrics Society, 23*, 433-441.

Pfeiffer, E. (1976). *Multidimensional functional assessment: The OARS methodology*. Durham, NC: Duke University Center for the Study of Aging and Human Development.

Pfeiffer, E. (1977). Psychopathology and social pathology. In J.E. Birren and K.W. Schaie (Eds.), *Handbook of the psychology of aging* (pp. 650-671). New York: Van Nostrand Reinhold.

Piper, M. (1979). Practical aspects of psychometric testing in the elderly. *Age and Ageing, 8*, 299-303.

Pirozzolo, F.J., and Lawson-Kerr, K. (1980). Neuropsychological assessment of dementia. In F.J. Pirozzolo and G.J. Maletta (Eds.), *Advances in neurogerontology; Vol. 1. The aging nervous system* (pp. 175-186). New York: Praeger.

Plutchik, R., and Conte, H. (1972). Change in social and physical functioning of geriatric patients over a one-year period. *Gerontologist, 12*, 181–184.

Plutchik, R., Conte, H., Lieberman, M., Bakur, M., Grossman, J., and Lehrman, N. (1970). Reliability and validity of a scale for assessing the function of geriatric patients. *Journal of the American Geriatrics Society, 18*, 491-500.

Power, D.E., Logue, P.E., McCarty, S.M., Rosenstiel, A.K., and Ziesat, H.A. (1979). Inter-rater reliability of the Russell revision of the Wechsler Memory Scale: An attempt to clarify some ambiguities in scoring. *Journal of Clinical Neuropsychology, 1*, 343-345.

Post, F. (1975). Dementia, depression, and pseudodementia. In D.F. Benson, and D. Blumer (Eds.), *Psychiatric aspects of neurologic disease* (pp. 99-120). New York: Grune and Stratton.

Prigatano, G.P. (1978). Wechsler Memory Scale: A selective review of the literature. *Journal of Clinical Psychology*, *34*, 816-832.

Randt, C.T., Brown, E.R., and Osborne, D.P. (1980). A memory test for longitudinal measurement of mild to moderate deficits. *Clinical Neuropsychology*, *2*, 184-194.

Rees, J., and Botwinick, J. (1971). Detection and decision factors in auditory behavior of the elderly. *Journal of Gerontology*, *26*, 133-141.

Regier, D.A., Myers, J.K., Kramer, M., Rabins, L.N., Blazer, D.G., Hough, R.L., Eaton, W.W., and Locke, B.Z. (1984). The NIMH epidemiologic catchment area program. *Archives of General Psychiatry*, *41*, 934-942.

Reifler, B.V., Larson, E., and Hanley, R. (1982). Coexistence of cognitive impairment and depression in geriatric outpatients. *American Journal of Psychiatry*, *139*, 623-626.

Reisberg, B., Ferris, S.H., and Crook, T. (1982). Signs, symptoms, and course of age-associated cognitive decline. In S. Corkin, K.L. Davis, J.H. Growdon, E. Usdin, and R.L. Wurtman (Eds.), *Aging: Vol. 19. Alzheimer's disease: A report of progress* (pp. 177-181). New York: Raven Press.

Reisberg, B., Ferris, S.H., De Leon, M.J., and Crook, T. (1982). The global deterioration scale for assessment of primary degenerative dementia. *American Journal of Psychiatry*, *139*, 1136-1139.

Reisberg, B., Ferris, S.H., Schneck, M.K., deLeon, M.J., Crook, T.H., and Gershon, S. (1981). The relationship between psychiatric assessments and cognitive test measures in mild to moderately cognitively impaired elderly. *Psychopharmacology Bulletin*, *17*, 99-101.

Robinson, R.A. (1979). Some applications of rating scales in dementia. In A.I.M. Glen and L.J. Whalley (Eds.), *Alzheimer's disease: Early recognition of potentially reversible deficits* (pp. 108-114). New York: Churchill Livingstone.

Ron, M.A., Toone, B.K., Garralda, M.E., and Lishman, W.A. (1979). Diagnostic accuracy in presenile dementia. *British Journal of Psychiatry*, *134*, 161-168.

Rosen, W.G. (1983). Clinical and neuropsychological assessment of Alzheimer's disease. In R. Mayeux and W.G. Rosen (Eds.), *The dementias* (pp. 51-63). New York: Raven Press.

Roth, M. (1980). Senile dementia and its borderlands. In J.O. Cole and J.E. Barrett (Eds.), *Psychopathology in the aged* (pp. 205-232). New York: Raven Press.

Roth, M., and Hopkins, B. (1953). Psychological test performance in patients over 60: I. Senile psychosis and the affective disorders of old age. *Journal of Mental Science*, *99*, 439-450.

Russell, E.W. (1975). A multiple scoring method for the assessment of complex memory functions. *Journal of Consulting and Clinical Psychology*, *43*, 800-809.

Rust, J.O., Barnard, D., and Oster, G.D. (1979). WAIS verbal-performance differences among the elderly when controlling for fatigue. *Psychological Reports*, *44*, 489-496.

Salzman, C., Shader, R.I., Kochansky, G.E., and Cronin, D.M. (1972). Rating scales for psychotropic drug research with geriatric patients: I. Behavior ratings. *Journal of the American Geriatrics Society*, *20*, 209-214.

Schaie, K.W. (1978). External validity in the assessment of intellectual development in adulthood. *Journal of Gerontology*, *33*, 695-701.

Schear, I.M., (1984). Neuropsychological assessment of the elderly in clinical practice. In P.E. Logue and I.M. Schear (Eds.), *Clinical neuropsychology: A multidisciplinary approach* (pp. 199-236). Springfield, IL: Charles C Thomas.

Smith, J.M., Bright, B., and McCloskey, J. (1977). Factor analytic composition of the Geriatric Rating Scale (GRS). *Journal of Gerontology*, *32*, 58-62.

Sternberg, D.E., and Jarvik, M.E. (1976). Memory function in depression. *Archives of General Psychiatry*, *33*, 219-228.

Storandt, M., Botwinick, J., Danziger, W.L., Berg, L., and Hughes, C.P.(1984). Psychometric differentiation of mild senile dementia of the Alzheimer type. *Archives of Neurology*, *41*, 497-499.

Stromgren, L.S. (1977). The influence of depression on memory. *Acta Psychiatrica Scandinavica*, *56*, 109-121.

Talland, G.A., and Schwab, R.S. (1964). Performance with multiple sets in Parkinson's disease. *Neuropsychologia*, *2*, 45-53.

Taylor, H.G., and Bloom, L.M. (1974). Cross-validation and methodological extension of the Stockton Geriatric Rating Scale. *Journal of Gerontology*, *29*, 190-193.

Terman, L.M., and Merrill, M.A. (1973). *Stanford-Binet intelligence scale. Manual for the third revision, form L-M*. Boston: Houghton Mifflin.

Trier, T.R. (1966). Characteristics of mentally ill aged: A comparison of patients with psychogenic disorders and patients with organic brain syndromes. *Journal of Gerontology*, *21*, 354-364.

Vitaliano, P.P., Breen, A.R., Albert, M.S., Russo, J., and Prinz, P.N. (1984). Memory, attention, and functional status in community-residing Alzheimer type dementia patients and optimally healthy aged individuals. *Journal of Gerontology*, *39*, 58-64.

Vitaliano, P.P., Russo, J., Breen, A.R., Vitiello, M.V., and Prinz, P.N. (1986). Functional decline in the early stages of Alzheimer's disease. *Journal of Psychology and Aging*, *1*, 41-46.

Wallach, M.A., and Kogan, N. (1961). Aspects of judgments and decision making: Interrelationships and changes with age. *Behavioral Sciences*, 6, 23-28.

Wechsler, A.F. (1977). Presenile dementia presenting as aphasia. *Journal of Neurology, Neurosurgery, and Psychiatry*, *40*, 303-305.

Wechsler, D. (1945). A standardized memory scale for clinical use. *Journal of Psychology*, *19*, 87-95.

Wechsler, D. (1958). *The measurement and appraisal of adult intelligence*, (4th ed.). Baltimore: Williams and Wilkins.

Wechsler, D. (1981). *Wechsler Adult Intelligence Scale-Revised Manual*. New York: The Psychological Corporation.

Wells, C.E. (1979). Pseudodementia. *American Journal of Psychiatry*, 136, 895–900.

Wells, C.E. (1982). Pseudodementia and the recognition of organicity. In D.F. Benson and D. Blumer (Eds.), *Psychiatric aspects of neurologic disease* (Vol. II) (pp. 167-178). New York: Grune and Stratton.

Whelihan, W.M., Lesher, E.L., Kleban, M.H., Granick, S. (1984). Mental status and memory assessment as predictors of dementia. *Journal of Gerontology*, *39*, 572-576.

Whitehead, A. (1973). The pattern of WAIS performance in elderly psychiatric patients. *British Journal of Social and Clinical Psychology*, *12*, 435-436.

Wilson, R.S., and Kaszniak, A.W. (1986). Longitudinal changes: Progressive idiopathic dementia. In L.W. Poon, B.J. Gurland, C. Eisdorfer, T. Crook, L.W. Thompson, A.W. Kaszniak, and K. Davis (Eds.), *The handbook of clinical memory assessment of older adults*. Washington, DC: American Psychological Association.

Wilson, R.S., Kaszniak, A.W., Klawans, H.L., and Garron, D.C. (1980). High speed memory scanning in Parkinsonism. *Cortex*, *16*, 67-72.

Wilson, R., Rosenbaum, G., and Brown, G. (1979). The problem of premorbid intelligence in neuropsychological assessment. *Journal of Clinical Neuropsychology*, *1*, 49-53.

Chapter 15

Management of Dementia

There is a destiny that makes us brothers;
 None goes his way alone:
All that we send into the lives of others
 Comes back into our own.

Edwin Markham

The psychologic and communicative capacities of dementia patients continuously change, a consideration fundamental to effective patient management. Continuous behavioral change demands a dynamic management approach because diagnostic tests appropriate for the assessment of cognitive and communicative disorders early in the course of dementing illness may later be inappropriate. Techniques for maximizing the ability of demented individuals to function in their environments will differ as dementing disease progresses; and behavioral management strategies will vary across the different stages of the syndrome.

The second fact that is fundamental to planning effective patient management is that the progressive decline of the patient imposes progressively greater responsibility on the caregiver. Clinicians must understand the course of dementing illnesses and the behaviors associated with the different stages for productive patient interaction and caregiver counseling.

The third fundamental consideration when planning a management program for demented patients and their caregivers is that both the patient and the caregiver are likely to be older individuals. Knowledge of the process of normal aging and the educational, economic, social, and emotional characteristics of the elderly is beneficial to the professional responsible for making patient care recommendations. In the first section of this chapter, the characteristics of the normal elderly individual will be reviewed to help clinicians who are inexperienced with the elderly build an appreciation for the uniqueness of the geriatric population.

PROFILE OF THE NORMAL ELDERLY

Education, Income, Living Arrangements, Family Support

Individuals over the age of 65 are likely to have 12 years of education, and an annual income of less than $17,000, and live independently, though close to their children. Between 1970 and 1983 there was a rise in the average number of years of education among the over 65 population, increasing from

8.7 to 11.0 years of education (American Association of Retired Persons [AARP], 1984). Not surprisingly, as the number of years of education increased, average income rose.

According to the 1982 census, the annual income of most elders was between $5,000 and $17,499 (mean = $9,366). Only ll percent made more than $17,500, and 32 percent realized less than $5,000 (Table 15-1).

Most elders do not work. Of those between the ages of 65 and 69, 72 percent do not work even part time; of those 70 to 72 years, 83 percent do not work, and among those above the age of 73, 93 percent are unemployed. When asked if they would rather be working (AARP, 1983), the majority (63 percent) were glad to be retired, but 33 percent expressed a desire to work, and 4 percent were undecided. When attitudes toward working were related to income, a not surprising 46 percent of those whose income was less than $6,999 wanted to be employed. The reason most individuals gave for not working was a lack of desire or need. In 25.8 percent, health was reported as the reason for not working (Table 15-2).

According to the American Association of Retired Persons (1984) the major source of income for elders in 1982 was Social Security. It accounted for 37 percent, followed by earnings at 24 percent, asset income 23 percent, public and private pensions 13 percent, and "transfer" payments 2 percent. Transfer payments include supplemental security, unemployment, and veterans' payments.

In terms of living arrangements, since 1970 a notable decline has occurred in the number of men and women who live with someone other than a spouse, especially among those over 75 (U.S. Office of Technology Assessment [OTA], 1985). In 1981, 79 percent of men between the ages of 65 and 74 years lived with a spouse, and approximately 9 percent lived with someone else. Of women in the same age range, 47 percent lived with a spouse, and less than 20 percent lived with someone else. More than four times as many elderly women as men live alone, approximately 6.2 million women and 1.6 million men (OTA, 1985). In the next few years women will constitute about 84 percent of the single nonfamily households in the over 75 population.

Institutionalization rates for the young old (persons aged 65 to 74) have fallen, especially for elderly men, but among the old old (persons aged 75 to 84), these rates have increased, particularly for women. Those elderly women most likely to be institutionalized are poor, widowed, living alone, and very old.

The elderly are generally well integrated into an informal social network of family, friends, and neighbors (Silverstone, 1985). Most elders have regular contact with their children. A surprising 75 percent live within a 30-minute drive of a child (Shanas, 1979), and 80 percent report seeing their children at least once a week. In a study by Bengston and Treas (1980), the elderly viewed their children as confidants, and Troll (1979) reports a mutual exchange of goods and services between the elderly and their offspring.

Within the extended families of the elderly, the adult daughter is the most important and reliable source of family help (Brody, 1979). In the Brody study, daughters (with a mean age of 49 years) provided help to their mothers an average of 8.6 hours per week, an amount that increased to 28.5 hours per week if the mother resided in the home. Daughters older than 50 averaged more than 15 hours per week.

Health Status

Four out of five seniors report the presence of one or more chronic health conditions (Siegler et al., 1980), but nonetheless, most function adequately. Among all age segments from 65 to 93 years, arthritis is the most commonly reported disease (Siegler, et al., 1980). Other common diseases are hypertension, heart disease, diabetes, stroke, emphysema, peptic ulcer, and cancer. After the turn of the century, infectious diseases were no longer the most common cause of death but were replaced by cardiovascular disease and cancer (OTA, 1985). The three most common causes of death, in both the general population and elderly, are heart disease, cancer, and stroke, in that order. To-

Table 15-1. Total Income for Families and Unrelated Individuals, by Age, 1982

	Under 65		65 and Over	
Income Class	Percent	Number	Percent	Number
Families				
<$7,499	11	5,697,560	14	1,343,580
$7,500–12,499	10	5,179,600	22	2,111,340
$12,500–17,499	11	5,697,560	18	1,727,460
$17,500–24,499	18	9,323,280	19	1,823,430
$25,000+	50	25,898,000	26	2,501,000
Mean income		$28,585		$20,990
Total number		51,796,000		9,597,000
Unrelated individuals				
<$5,000	21	4,095,420	32	2,689,920
$5,000–5,999	6	1,170,120	14	1,176,840
$6,000–6,999	3	585,060	9	797,000
$7,000–9,999	11	2,145,220	17	1,400,000
$10,000–17,499	28	5,460,560	17	1,408,000
$17,500+	31	6,045,620	11	936,000
Mean income		$14,602		$9,366
Total number		19,502,000		8,406,000

Adapted from U.S. Bureau of the Census (1982). *Current Population Reports*, Series P-60, No. 140, Money Income and Poverty Status of Families and Persons in the United States: 1982 (Table 6, p. 12).

gether they account for three of every four deaths.

The likelihood of disease increases with age, and 85 percent of the elderly have at least one chronic health problem. Indeed, "multiple pathology" and "illness clustering" are terms frequently used to describe the health status of our seniors. In a random sample of community dwelling adults over age 65, 3.5 significant disabilities per person were found.

According to a Department of Health, Education and Welfare survey (1978), only nine percent of elders rate their health as poor, whereas 22.3 percent rate it as fair, 39 percent as good, and 29 percent as excellent. In general, self-report mea-

Table 15-2. Reported Reason* for Not Working, 1980–83 (Percent)

	Average 1980–83	1980	1981	1982	1983
Don't want or need to	31.3	32	27	34	32
Too old	21.8	17	19	24	27
Health	25.8	24	33	23	23
No work available	4.0	2	4	5	5
Rules (retirement test)	2.3	2	3	2	2
Don't know/other	13.8	23	14	12	6

Adapted from AARP (July, 1983). *AARP Annual Survey of Opinions of Older Americans* AARP: Washington, D.C.
*Note: Response is to question: "Is there any particular reason why you are not currently working?"

sures have been found to correlate well with the results of physical examination (LaRue, Bank, Jarvik, and Hetland, 1979; Maddox and Douglass, 1973).

Interestingly, the health of married elders may be influenced by the health of their spouses. Satariano, Minkler, and Langhauser (1984) surveyed 678 elderly residents of Alameda County, California, and found that respondents who reported their spouses as being ill in the last 6 months were more likely to report their own health as poor. Health of spouse was a better predictor of the respondent's health than number of social contacts, socioeconomic status, years of education, financial need, average length of sleep, and whether they had primary responsibility for making the decisions that affect them.

One of the most important health problems, from the perspective of the clinician, is hearing loss. Although this problem was discussed earlier, its prevalence is worth emphasizing. Hearing impairment is the third most prevalent chronic condition among the noninstitutionalized elderly (OTA, 1985). As the elderly population grows, the number of hearing impaired persons will dramatically increase. The term "hearing impaired" includes individuals who are deaf, as well as those who have

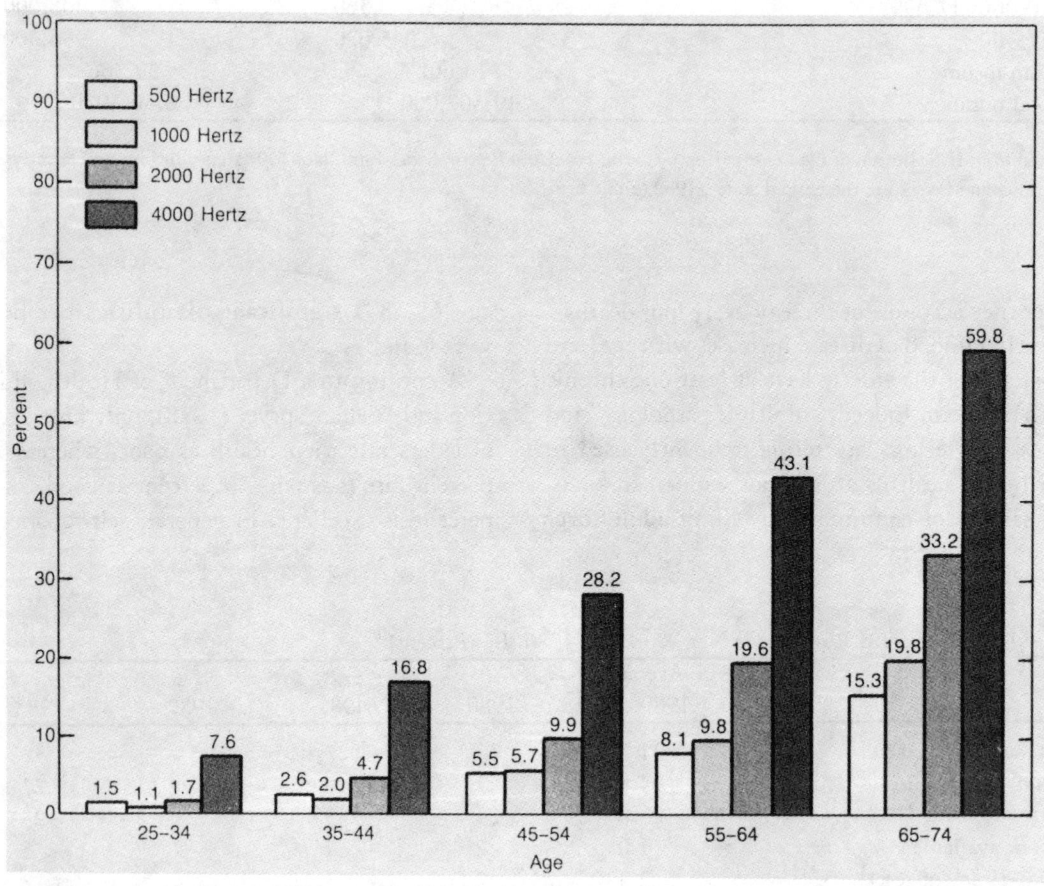

Figure 15-1. *Percent of adults aged 25 to 74 with hearing impairment, by frequency of tone in the United States, 1971–1975. (Source: National Center for Health Statistics, Basic Data on Hearing Level of Adults 25-74, Office of Health Research Statistics and Technology, 1980).*

diminished sensitivity and acuity. The clinician must consider changes in both hearing sensitivity and acuity. Not only can the ability to perceive sound be diminished (a sensitivity change), but age effects are common in the ability to discriminate speech sounds, even when they are sufficiently audible (an acuity change). Patients and caregivers with acuity changes may complain of not understanding what they hear. This condition is sometimes referred to as a central processing disorder. It results from disorders in the ascending auditory pathways.

The most common type of hearing loss among the aged is *presbycusis*, a term that literally means "old hearing." It results from changes in the inner ear and is therefore called a *sensorineural loss*. In sensorineural loss, individuals suffer damage to the inner ear, the cochlea, the fibers of the eighth cranial nerve, or two or more of those structures. The other major type of hearing loss is *conductive*, which results from damage or blockage in the outer ear, middle ear, or both. Some individuals have both sensorineural and conductive losses, or a *mixed* hearing loss.

Ringing or buzzing in the ears is a frequent complaint of the elderly, a condition known as *tinnitus*. Tinnitus is more common in women, and its prevalence increases with age (Leske, 1981). Yet another prevalent disorder in the hearing impaired elderly is *recruitment*, an inability to tolerate loud sounds. This condition may affect the ability of an individual to use a hearing aid.

In Figure 15-1, the percentage of adults with hearing impairment has been specified in relation to sound frequency. As can be seen, the elderly have considerably greater hearing loss for high-frequency sounds. In English therefore, the most imperceptible sounds are s, t, k, and p. Because hearing loss is invisible, it is often denied. Clinicians must consider the hearing status of both the dementia patient and the caregiver.

Drugs and the Elderly

Related to health status is drug consumption. Although the elderly constitute 11 percent of the population, they consume 25 to 30 percent of all medications (Besdine, 1980; Ouslander, 1981; Thompson, Moran, and Nies, 1983). Drug purchases constitute the elderly's largest out-of-pocket health care expense. Ninety percent of the prescriptions taken by elders are for long-term use to treat chronic medical conditions (OTA, 1985).

The average elder takes 6.1 drugs at a time and an average of 14 to 18 different drugs during the course of a year. Ouslander (1981) discovered that ten drugs are typically prescribed for an elderly patient during a hospital stay. The most frequently prescribed drugs are cardiovascular (cardiac stimulants, diuretics, antihypertensives), psychotropics (sedatives, hypnotics, antipsychotics), analgesics, and laxatives (Lamy, 1980; Williamson and Chopin, 1980).

The use of many medications during the same time period is known as polypharmacy. Bressler and Conrad (1983) warn that the consumption of two or more drugs simultaneously can result in drug potency alterations and possibly adverse drug reactions. When 6 to 10 drugs are taken simultaneously, there is a 7 percent chance of the patient experiencing an adverse drug reaction. When 16 to 20 drugs are taken, the adverse reaction rate rises to 40 percent (Hurwitz, 1969; Smith, Seidel, and Cluff, 1966).

Several studies have shown that adverse drug reactions are more common in the aged. In a survey of 700 hospitalized individuals, drug-induced illness was detected in 25 percent of those patients older than 80 years as compared with 12 percent among individuals between 41 and 50 years (Seidel, Thornton, Smith, and Cluff, 1966). In a 3-year study of drug-induced illness in a teaching hospital, 40 percent of the patients with drug-induced illness were older than 60, a rate 15 times greater than that of younger patients (Caranasos, Stewart, and Cluff, 1974).

The pharmacologic action of drugs differs in the elderly because of age-related physiologic changes related to absorption, distribution, metabolism, excretion, and receptor sensitivity. Recent studies of pharmacokinetics (how drugs are distributed and metabolized in the body) and pharmacodynamics (how drugs act) show marked differences between older and younger users (OTA, 1985). Older adults have significantly altered drug reaction time and metabolism (Greenblatt, Divoll, Abernathy, and Shader, 1982; Lamy, 1982; McGlone, 1982). As one example, older persons have a higher percentage of fatty tissue, causing them to have increased concentrations of water-soluble drugs and prolonged retention of fat-soluble drugs.

Personality and Emotional Status

The characteristics of long-lived individuals are flexibility, resourcefulness, and optimism (Butler and Lewis, 1982). The elderly, by virtue of their survival, have demonstrated adaptability. The most obvious and important age-related changes they experience are slowing in the ability to respond (Birren, Woods, and Williams, 1980) and decrements in the ability to process complex information. The sensitive clinician will slow the pace of information presentation and make explicit those points of importance to maximize the ability of the elder to comprehend.

A frequently noted characteristic of the aged is cautiousness (Botwinick, 1973; Schaie and Marquette, 1972). Unresponsive elders may be mistaken as ignorant when in fact they are cautious and introverted.

Depression is more common among the elderly segment. In the over 65 age group, 2 to 3 percent suffer severe depression and 3 to 4 percent suffer mild depression. The prevalence of depression increases with each decade of life after the age of 60, and is more common among females (Myers et al., 1982). Clinicians should screen both patients and their caregivers for depression. Depressed individuals should be referred for treatment.

Related to depression is the incidence of suicide. Whereas the elderly account for approximately ll percent of the United States population, they are responsible for 25 percent of the suicides (Pfeiffer and Busse, 1975). With age, suicide rates rise among men; the highest rate occurs in those over the age of 80. Among men 65 to 69 years of age, suicides number 31.9 per 100,000, compared with 9.0 per 100,000 in women. The rate increases to 45.8 per 100,000 for men in the over 85 age group, while in women, the rate drops to 4.2 per 100,000 (U.S. National Center for Health Statistics, 1981a).

Summary

In summary, the typical elder has 12 years of education, is self-sufficient, unemployed, living on a modest income, likely to have a hearing loss, and coping with at least one chronic disease. Throughout adulthood, the elder has experienced gradual slowing in the ability to process information and respond and has become increasingly cautious. An appreciation of these characteristics provides the clinician with a foundation for developing a deeper understanding of the effects of the imposition of a dementing illness and the challenge of caregiving.

WHAT DOES IT MEAN TO BE THE PERSONAL CAREGIVER OF A DEMENTIA PATIENT?

The challenge of caregiving is so immense that caregivers have been described as having "36-hour" days (Mace and Rabins, 1981). Caregivers cope with increased physical demands, financial burdens, changes in social status and family relationships, and what Rabins (1984) calls "chronic grief."

Throughout the course of dementing illness, the caregiver must consider the patient's safety, for demented individuals are often restless and wander aimlessly. If left unattended, they may become lost. In the later stages of the syndrome, patients are incontinent, and diapering and personal hygiene routines become the responsibility of the caregiver. The execution of these responsibilities requires increased physical energy at a time when the elderly are slowing.

Caregivers fortunate enough to have access to a day care facility may be unable to afford it. The average cost of one day of care is $52.00, but some facilities cost as much as $88.00. Though caregivers may receive advice and help through home health care services, the per-visit charge typically ranges between $27.00 and $33.00. When patients are in the advanced stages of dementing illness, skilled nursing care is frequently necessary, an option so frighteningly expensive that many families wait as long as possible to seek help. The average cost for skilled nursing care ranges between $38 and $41.80 per day. Yearly per-patient nursing home costs range between $17,000 and $30,000 (Richards, Zuckerman, and West, 1985). National nursing home costs exceed 16 billion dollars per year for the estimated 2.5 million persons currently affected with Alzheimer's disease in the United States (Brody, Lawton, and Liebowitz, 1984).

Caregivers of dementia patients are at risk of becoming social isolates. As the dementia progresses, their reluctance to entertain at home or attend social events with the patient increases because such events may confuse the patient. Then too, the patient's behavior embarrasses the caregiver. Feeling embarrassed by the behavior of a dementia patient is commonly reported by caregivers (Mace and Rabins, 1981). The continuous supervision required by the patient ties the caregiver to the home, and as the years pass, visits with old friends become rare. Hirschfeld (1983) reported that the most frequently reported feeling of caregivers was that of being "tied down."

For many caregivers the advent of dementing disease causes a change in both their responsibilities and their role in the family. Whatever responsibilities were assumed by the patient must be taken over by the caregiver. For some individuals this means learning, for the first time, about businesses, taxes, automobile maintenance, and insurance. For others, cooking, gardening, sewing, and shopping must be mastered. More difficult to accept than new responsibilities are role changes (Rabins, 1984), particularly when the caregiver is the patient's child. Accepting one's parents as dependents is psychologically and emotionally difficult. Rabins recommends that clinicians identify for caregivers "role conflict" as a source of psychologic distress, and provide counseling.

Caregivers ride an emotional roller-coaster as they helplessly witness the gradual intellectual deterioration of someone they love. Because they can do nothing to stop the disease, a disease that has made their lives so difficult, they feel angry. On the heels of anger is guilt—guilt because they are spared, or want to be free of the worry and responsibility. Sanford (1975) and Zarit, Reever, and Bach-Peterson (1980) emphasize that caregivers report a lack of time for themselves as especially frustrating. Finally, occasional resentment becomes virtually unavoidable as the caregiver fatigues, endures financial hardship, and becomes socially isolated. The following experiences of the Adams family are a moving introduction to the emotional upheaval experienced by caregivers.

Mrs. Adams was diagnosed as having Alzheimer's disease three years ago. Within the past 6 months, she has experienced substantial decline in the ability to complete the activities of daily living. Her husband has observed her gradual decline, noticing the loss of her sense of humor and interest in gardening and art. Mrs. Adams, who had been a vivacious, enthusiastic woman, is now unable to discuss their children or travels. Mr. Adams misses his wife's companionship and agonizes over her inability to remember their children. Mrs. Adams still attempts to prepare meals and bake her favorite pastries, but the recipes are too complex for her limited attention span and memory. She is incapable of organizing the ingredients or following the prescribed mixing sequence and leaves the kitchen strewn with dirty dishes. The kitchen messes occasionally anger Mr. Adams, but after he becomes angry, he feels guilty because he reminds himself that his wife's behaviors are unintentional. Yet, in the last 6 months, he acknowledges a feeling of persistent resentment, not towards his wife as she once was, but towards the person who is making life so miserable now. He has extra duties, among them cooking, a skill he never acquired. He has had to leave his bowling league and can no longer attend church. Bridge was a pastime he and his wife enjoyed but no longer share. The primary activity left to them is watching television, but because of his hearing loss, watching television is not particularly enjoyable.

Most Difficult Problems of Caregiving

The problems confronting caregivers primarily come from three sources: (l) the patient's behavior pattern, (2) the caregiver's own limitations related to the dependent patient, and (3) environmental and social conditions (Sanford, 1975).

The Patient's Behavior. Rabins, Mace, and Lucas (1982) interviewed family caregivers of dementia patients to identify the type of behavior problems encountered and their frequency. The problems most commonly encountered are listed in Table 15-3, as well as the percentage of families acknowledging the problem (Rabins et al., 1982). Caregivers have to cope with the majority of these problems but find some more burdensome than others. In Sanford's caregiver survey, sleep disturbance was the most commonly mentioned intolerable problem related to the patients' behavior. In a study by Sainsbury and Grad de Alarcon (1970), being troublesome at night, restlessness, behaving oddly, and being potentially harmful to self and others were the most frequently mentioned behavioral problems.

Kaszniak and Schechner (1981) studied the relationship of patient symptoms to caregiver distress. According to the responses of 75 caregivers, those patient characteristics that were most distressing were mental confusion, anxiety, and depression. Caregivers found these problems more wearing than sensorimotor impairment, ambulatory dependence, and self-care dependence, a finding that corroborated the earlier similar reports of Grad de Alarcon

Table 15-3. Behavior Problems of Patients Cited by Families

Behavior	No. of Families Responding*	Families Reporting Occurrence		Families Reporting Behavior to be a Problem	
		Number	(percent)	Number	(percent)
Memory disturbance	55	55	(100)	51	(93)
Catastrophic reactions	52	45	(87)	40	(89)
Demanding/critical behavior	52	37	(71)	27	(73)
Night waking	54	37	(69)	22	(59)
Hiding things	51	35	(69)	25	(71)
Communication difficulties	50	34	(68)	25	(74)
Suspiciousness	52	33	(63)	26	(79)
Making accusations	53	32	(60)	26	(82)
Meals	55	33	(60	18	(55)
Daytime wandering	51	30	(59)	21	(70)
Bathing	51	27	(53)	20	(74)
Hallucinations	49	24	(49)	16	(42)
Delusions	49	23	(47)	19	(83)
Physical violence	51	24	(47)	22	(94)
Incontinence	53	21	(40)	18	(86)
Cooking	54	18	(33)	8	(44)
Hitting	50	16	(32)	13	(81)
Driving	55	11	(20)	8	(73)
Smoking	53	6	(11)	4	(67)
Inappropriate sexual behavior	51	1	(2)	0	(0)

*"Don't know" answers excluded.

(Source: Rabins, P.V., Mace, N.L., and Lucas, M.J. (1982). The impact of dementia on the family. *Journal of the American Medical Association, 248,* 333–335. Copyright 1982, American Medical Association.)

and Sainsbury, (1963, 1965) and Isaacs, Livingstone and Neville, (1972).

Caregiver Limitations Related to the Dependent Patient. The lion's share of the caregiver's time is consumed by helping the patient with the activities of daily living, according to Zarit et al. (1980). In their study, the problems contributing most to the caregiver's perception of burden was lack of time for oneself, excessive dependency of the patient on the caregiver, and the caregiver's fears about further deterioration in the patient's behavior.

Fitting, Rabins, Lucas, and Eastham (1986) interviewed 54 spouse caregivers and compared them on psychologic adjustment and feelings of burden. Female caregivers were found to be more distressed than male caregivers, and younger caregivers were lonelier and more resentful of their role than those older.

George and Gwyther (1986) also studied the well-being of family caregivers in terms of physical health, mental health, financial resources, and social participation. Among this sample of 510 family caregivers, burden was experienced primarily in the areas of mental health and social participation. Spouse caregivers exhibited lower levels of well-being in all four dimensions studied than adult child caregivers or other relatives. Across the entire sample, caregivers averaged nearly three times as many stress symptoms as the comparison sample. Then too, caregivers had considerably lower life satisfaction. A substantially higher percentage (28 percent) reported using psychotropic drugs as compared with the comparison sample (19 percent). Finally, 59 percent of the caregiver sample expressed a need for more assistance.

Environmental and Social Conditions. The results of a study of family experiences in relation to obtaining a diagnosis (Chenoweth and Spencer, 1986) reveal that most families are under-informed about the nature of dementing disease by their physicians. Then too, they report being ill-prepared for the behavioral changes that occurred. Fifty-four percent, of the 289 caregivers surveyed, perceived the explanation by health care professionals (primarily physicians) as focusing almost entirely on the hopeless nature of the dementing disease. Only 28 percent of the families reported that a factual and adequate explanation was given without undue focus on the hopelessness of the condition. Twenty-two percent could recall no explanation at the time of diagnosis! In only three cases did the physician arrange a family conference to educate the family members and provide a forum for questions.

According to Chenoweth and Spencer, the information received by the majority of the families did not enable them to predict the difficulty with day-to-day activities the patients experienced. These authors write,

> Families had difficulty understanding that a person eventually would not be able to read or write, or that wandering, lack of manners, or constant pacing could be part of the disease. . . . Until families received thorough explanations of the progression of the disease, they tended to believe that their relatives had more control over their behaviors than was likely, and expected that reasoning and past means of communication would still work. With few exceptions, families were astonished when they recognized the extent of impairment in thought, judgment, and reasoning. (p. 269)

The environmental and social conditions in which caregivers cope with dementia patients vary markedly. Adequacy and environmental comfort are closely related to the economic well-being of the family. A safe environment, in which the dementia patient is free to move about unrestrained, is best for both the patient and caregiver. Also of importance is proximity to a commercial center and community services. Caregivers with accessible shopping, medical facilities, and recreation cope better.

Formal and Informal Social Support. Several investigators suggest that formal and informal social support acts to moderate the psychologic impact of stressful life events (Brown and Harris, 1978; Caplan, 1974; Cassel, 1976; Cobb, 1976; Dean and Lin, 1977; Eaton, 1978; Henderson, 1977; and Myers, Lindenthal, and Pepper, 1975). Cantor (1980) has defined a social support system as "a pattern of continuous or intermittent ties and interchanges of mutual assistance that plays a significant role in maintaining the psychological, social and physical integrity of the individual over time" (p. 133). Cantor further identified two major subsystems: formal and informal support. Formal support consists of governmental, community, and voluntary service agencies, and health and other service programs that provide long-term care services to elderly living in the community. Informal support is generally provided by an elder's family, friends, and neighbors, individuals with whom the elder has the most frequent interaction.

Cobb (1976) defines social support as "information leading the caregiver to believe that he or she is cared for and loved, esteemed and a member of a network of mutual obligations" (p. 300). He observed that when people were classified by high and low life change and high and low social supports, the group most susceptible to a variety of illness was the group with high life change and low social supports. Social support appears to provide some protection from the physiologic and psychologic consequences of the stresses of caregiving (Cassel, 1976; Henderson, 1977; Rabkin and Streuning, 1976). This mediating effect has been termed the "social support hypothesis" and is defined as the phenomenon in which individuals with a strong social support system are believed to be better able to cope with stressful events, and those individuals with little or no social support are believed to be more vulnerable to the effects of life changes, particularly undesirable ones (Thoits, 1982).

For caregivers of dementia patients, relief from stress may be difficult to obtain. Brocklehurst (1977) reported that in his study of 57 community dwelling dementia patients, 29 percent of the caregivers found taking vacations impossible. Only thirty-seven caregivers left the patient to go shopping.

Gilhooly (1984) investigated the factors affecting the psychologic wellbeing of persons caring for dementing old persons in the community. None of the 37 caregivers had psychiatric problems or intellectual impairment. Factors found to affect the morale of caregivers were (a) sex of the patient (morale was higher when the patient was female), (b) sex of the caregiver (male caregivers were found to have higher morale, possibly in relation to the greater tendency for males to leave the patient unattended for social outings), (c) satisfaction with help received (more important than amount of help was whether it was perceived as good), (d) home help services (caregivers with more home help had higher morale), and (e) duration of caregiving (the longer the caregiver had been giving care, the higher the morale). This last finding suggests that with time, some caregivers adapt to caring for a mentally diminished individual.

Gilhooly did not find a positive correlation between the number of social visits received by caregivers and their morale. The opposite was true in the study of Zarit et al. (1980). Frequency of visits from family members was the best predictor of burden for caregivers of dementia patients; the more visits, the less the burden.

Institutionalization is likely to occur when there are no family members to provide care (Bergmann, Foster, and Matthews, 1978) or the caregiver's health fails (Isaacs et al., 1972). Lowenthal (1964) reported that family caregivers were most likely to institutionalize dementia patients if they were unduly restless, behaved oddly, and were troublesome at night. Zarit (1982) reported that tolerance of memory and behavior problems were the strongest predicting variables related to the likelihood of institutionalization.

SUPPORT SERVICES AVAILABLE TO CAREGIVERS

Support services are of three basic types: those related to household management, caregiver counseling, and patient care (Table 15-4). Household management services can take the form of home helpers, cleaning services, kitchen aides, cooks, gardeners, and business managers. Clinicians designing a management plan should systematically evaluate whether the routines of household management are within the capability of the caregiver, remembering that the responsibilities of the caregiver will gradually increase as the dementia worsens.

Table 15-4. Important Support Services

Type of Service	Definition or Function
SERVICES FOR CAREGIVER	
Household management	
Homemakers	Manage the household (shopping, laundry, repairs)
Cleaning services	Provide individuals who perform housekeeping chores
Home caterers	Prepare and deliver food to the home
Gardeners	Maintain grounds
Business managers	Oversee and conduct business
Home maintenance managers	Maintain and repair the physical structure of the home
Counseling	
Private counselers	Provide counseling and therapeutic intervention to relieve psychologic stress
Support groups	Community organizations that provide education and assistance
SERVICES FOR THE PATIENT	
Day care and rehabilitation	Patient supervision and activity sponsor for adults in a protective setting; therapeutic services offered
Day maintenance care	Patient supervision and meal service in a protective setting
Respite care	Temporary care to provide relief for caregiver
Hospice	Support program for terminally ill
Home health care	Variety of nursing and rehabilitation services provided in patient's home
Skilled nursing care	Nursing service provided by licensed individual
Foster care	Private homes providing meals and personal care
Board and care	Provision of 24-hour protective supervision and meals
Nursing home	Provision of long-term medical and personal care
Transportation	Provision of travel to and from community resources
Escort	Companionship to patient and/or caregiver
Mental health	Diagnostic, therapeutic, and educational services
Physical therapy	Rehabilitative care to restore or maintain physical function
Speech–language therapy	Diagnostic, therapeutic, and counseling services related to the disorders of human communication

Caregiver Counseling

The caregivers of dementia patients need emotional support and guidance to cope with the multiplicity of stresses they will endure throughout the disease course. Once the diagnosis is known, access to a knowledgeable person, from whom information about the disease and the dementia syndrome can be obtained, is valuable to caregivers for several reasons. First, caregivers can be guided to other forms of support; second, caregivers can learn to manage their stress before its effects are too deleterious; and third, caregivers can learn strategies for solving the problems they will encounter.

Patient Care

Adult Day Care Programs

An important service for caregivers, although not available in all communities, is day care or respite care. This type of service is relatively new, having expanded from 20 service centers in the United States in 1970 to 800 in 1983 (Aaronson, 1983).

Adult day care programs are designed for two purposes: first, to provide rehabilitation-oriented programs, and second, to provide multipurpose programs in which participants receive social stimulation and families receive respite (Weissert, 1976). Day care programs offer a stable, calm, predictable environment conducive to creating feelings of security among participants while at the same time affording them opportunities for social interaction. Activities are selected that enable patients to use their retained functions, thereby building their feelings of self-esteem. Activities typically include dance, music, art therapy, and reality orientation. Current events are reviewed, and patients may participate in the preparation of the noon meal. Such programs operate between 6 and 8 hours per day.

The availability of transportation to and from day care programs varies. If transport services are provided, it is best if the driver–patient relationship is maintained over time. Having the same driver each day gives the patient and family security and enhances the opportunity for social interaction before and after the daily program (Rosin, Abramowitz, Diamond, and Jesselson, 1985).

Day care programs vary considerably in the composition of their staff. The following personnel may be included: registered nurse; geriatric nurse specialist; social worker; psychologist; geropsychiatrist; social gerontologist; recreation, dance, and art therapists; volunteers; students; and activity aides. Physicians generally are not involved on a regular basis, although they may monitor patient health status. The staff-to-patient ratio is an important determinant of the adequacy of the day care program. A common ratio is one to five (Sands and Suzuki, 1983).

The typical participant in adult day care programs is 74 years old, mildly to moderately impaired in the activities of daily living, ambulatory, and capable of some social interaction. Day care participants are not typically incontinent of bladder or bowel. Most participants live with their spouses or grown children and attend the day care program an average of 70 days per year (OTA, 1985).

The cost per day of adult day care services ranges from $18.00 to $88.00 (average cost = $52.00). The higher cost of some programs results from the provision of transportation and rehabilitation services. Participants and their families often pay for some, if not all, of the cost of day care. Medicare does not pay for adult day care programs, although some rehabilitative services provided through day care are covered.

In 1980, the Subcommittee on Health and Long-Term Care of the House Select Committee on Aging recommended the establishment of a national policy on day care. In 1981, the Omnibus Budget Reconciliation Act, under Title XXI, Section 2176, was enacted; it permits states to request a waiver to allow Medicaid coverage for day care services. In 1982, the Economic Recovery Act was passed; it offers tax credit to families with elderly dependents in day care programs. The largest tax breaks are available to families earning $10,000 or less per year.

Board and Care Facilities

Board-and-care facilities are designed to provide residents with 24-hour protective supervision, personal care assistance, cooking, cleaning, and laundry services. They are not, however, medical care programs. Currently, 30,000 board-and-care facilities exist in the United States, though some care exclusively for the mentally retarded. Between one-third to one-half of the residents, or between 150,000 and 200,000, are elderly (Reichstein and Bergofsky, 1980).

A dearth of information is available about the characteristics of the typical resident of a board-and-care facility. However, results of a recent seven-state study indicate that a large percentage of residents need assistance with home management activities such as laundry (64 percent), cleaning (55 percent), managing money (46 percent), shopping (43 percent), and taking medications (43 percent) (Bennett, Gruen, and Tepper, 1983). The surprising finding of this survey was that approximately 40 percent of the residents had mental disorders; in fact, about 28 percent had previously been institutionalized for mental illness.

The average daily cost of board-and-care facilities is $10. Approximately one-third of the expense is covered through private payment (OTA, 1985), and the other two-thirds is supplied by Federal Supplemental Security Income (SSI) payments and state supplements to SSI benefits.

Home Health Agencies

A variety of organizations sponsor home health services, which have developed with increased Medicare and Medicaid support for these services. The organizations providing these services are enumerated in Table 15-5. The government is the largest provider, followed by private nonprofit organizations. The services given to home-bound patients are as varied as the organizations providing them. Services range from nursing and rehabilitation, to medical education, to assistance with activities of daily living.

Nursing Homes

In the United States at present are approximately 20,000 nursing homes, which accomodate about one and a half million individuals, 85 percent of whom are elderly (OTA, 1985). This represents 5 percent of the over 65 population. Nursing homes may be owned and operated by private individuals or nonprofit organizations and government. They may or may not be certified. Approximately 19 percent of all nursing homes are certified as skilled nursing facilities, 24 percent as skilled nursing and intermediate care facilities, and 32 percent as intermediate care facilities; 25 percent are uncertified (U.S. National Center for Health Statistics, 1977, 1979). Skilled nursing facilities are those which provide 24-hour skilled nursing care under the supervision of a physician. Intermediate care facilities are not required to provide the level of service provided by a skilled nursing facility and are designed for patients requiring less intensive care.

The staff-to-patient ratio varies considerably among nursing homes and is influenced by the type of care the facility is certified to provide. The highest ratios are associated with skilled nursing facilities, which in 1977 averaged 52.7 staff per 100 beds. Intermediate care facilities had an average staff to bed ratio of 40.7 (staff per 100 beds), and uncertified homes 29.2 (U.S. Office of the Inspector General, 1981). On an encouraging note, the overall average is rising, though staff recruitment and maintenance remain major problems for the nursing home industry.

Nursing homes offer an around-the-clock protective environment in which some level of medical care and meals, housekeeping, and recreation are provided. Residents are heterogeneous and include the terminally ill, convalescents, and medically stable but functionally impaired patients. Most services are provided under the supervision of a registered nurse. Patients who are acutely ill are generally sent to the hospital (Bruer, 1982), although there is a trend toward treating more acute illness in nursing home facilities.

One-fourth of the individuals receiving long-term nursing home care have a primary diagnosis of mental disorder or dementia, compared with only 3 percent of those who have short stays (Keeler, Kane, and Solomon, 1981). Between one-third and one-half of all nursing home residents are discharged within 3 months (Keeler et al., 1981; Liu and Palesch, 1981). Short-stay residents typically are convalescents or terminally ill individuals who are

Table 15-5. Home Health Agencies, Percentage Distribution by Type of Agency, 1977 and 1981

Type of Agency	1977	1981
Visiting nurse association	19	17
Government	47	40
Hospital-based	11	14
Proprietary	5	8
Private nonprofit	14	18
Other	4	3
Total	100	100

Source: Staff. (1982, February 26). VNA's will "hold" their own, proprietary to "gain force," PNP's to "lose force," hospital-based HHA's to "gain ground," hospital discharge planning rules should be updated — says FDA expert. *Home Health Line, 6,* p.2. Data from Health Care Financing Administration.

admitted from a hospital. Long-term residents are typically admitted from home.

Nursing home care is the most expensive of the available patient care services. The average daily cost is $75, or $27,000 per year (Piktialis, 1986). The cost of nursing care would impoverish 63 percent of all individuals over age 65 within 13 weeks. Families and patients pay directly for about half the costs. More than half the cost is funded by government programs, particularly Medicaid. Private insurance pays less than 2 percent (U.S. General Accounting Office 1983; OTA, 1985).

The typical nursing home patient is in the old old segment of the population. The median age at admission is 80, and the median age of residents is 83. More than half the patients in nursing homes require assistance with mobility, bathing, dressing, and toileting. Forty-five percent require assistance with bowel and bladder control and 32 percent with eating (U.S. National Center for Health Statistics, 1981b).

The factors most predictive of whether an individual (demented or nondemented) will be placed in a nursing home are (1) dependency in toileting and eating, (2) dependency in bathing and dressing, and (3) mental disorders (Weissert and Scanlon, 1982). Other important factors are the ability of the family to bear the financial burden of nursing home costs (Kaszniak and Schechner, 1981) and availability of a living spouse or relative to provide care (Brody, Poulshock, and Masciocchi, 1978).

Clinicians may have to counsel families in the selection of a nursing home. The factors to be considered in nursing home selection include those listed in Table 15-6. An indispensable step in choosing a nursing home is a visit to any candidate facility. Providing families with a list of factors to consider in choosing a nursing home will make them more observant when they visit.

Two reasons for the marked variation in the quality of nursing home care are differences in regulations and reimbursement policies (Rango, 1982). Rango writes that the worst instances of poor quality are in proprietary facilities. When undesirable patient outcomes occur, they typically result from two types of errors: "unnecessary clinical interventions and failure to intervene with appropriate diagnostic and therapeutic measures" (p. 886). In a quality-of-care survey conducted in seven Salt Lake City nursing homes, high rates of infection were found, as well as decubitus ulcers, conjunctivitis, urinary tract infections, and lower respiratory tract infections (Garibaldi, Brodine, and Matsumiya, 1981). The most common patient management error is overmedication of patients (Ray, Federspiel, and Schaffner, 1980).

Table 15-6. Factors to Consider in Choosing a Nursing Home

- Type of medical care provided
- Staff-to-patient ratio
- Training of staff
- Experience of staff
- Rate of attrition of staff
- Psychologic support services offered residents
- Physical support services offered residents
- Safety features
- Security
- Attractiveness
- Cleanliness
- Design features enhancing patient ability to hear/see
- Quality of design for accommodating wheelchair users
- Cost
- Use of medications

A final consideration in the nursing home placement of dementia patients is whether the facility has a special unit for their care. Many nursing homes do not. Although a trend has developed to create special units, most nursing care facilities are designed to treat the physically ill (Sands and Suzuki, 1983). In such facilities the dementia patient, who is prone to aimless wandering, must be restrained, a less desirable management approach (Cornbleth, 1977; Pajk, 1984). Cornbleth studied the relative effects of freedom to wander and restriction on the physical status of wandering and nonwandering patients. Nonwanderers decreased in physical function on the locked ward and improved in the less protected environment, and wanderers improved in the protected ward only.

Creation of special units for AD and other dementia patients allows the recruitment of interested professional staff, specialized care, and staff efficiency (Rabins, 1986). For those conducting research with AD and other dementia patients, the specialized dementia patient units make it easier to obtain important data about the behavioral consequences of the disease. The special units are a place where the behavior of many dementia patients can be observed as they engage in a variety of tasks.

Paying for Long-Term Care

Public funds pay for approximately 61 percent of long-term care costs, 19 percent of which are covered by the state (Gibson and Waldo, 1981). Private insurance contributes a small percentage of nursing home expenses, only 0.2 percent in 1981 (Gibson and Waldo, 1981).

Medicare is designed to cover the costs of short-term acute care. In the area of home health services, however, Medicare is somewhat responsive, although there are limitations on the amount of time that can be given to a particular individual in any week. Medicaid is the principal source of public funds for reimbursement of long-term care services. Title XX of the Social Security Act of 1974 makes available federal block grants to the states for a variety of services, one of which is social service to the elderly (Schram, 1982). The Older Americans Act of 1965 and its amendments created a service program for those older than 60 years that includes funding of visiting nurses, homemaker aides, health education, screening and immunization, nutrition support, and home maintenance work. The last important source of long-term care monies is the Veterans Administration (VA) Program. The VA is the nation's largest medical service provider and has an extensive geriatric program, which includes long-term care.

LEGAL INFORMATION CLINICIANS SHOULD KNOW

Because patients with irreversible dementia suffer progressive deterioration of intellect, they ultimately become incompetent to manage their own affairs. Under the law, several different arrangements can be made for the protection of their interests. The following information about the guardian/conservatorship roles were obtained through E. Pollock, Esq. (personal communication, April 4, 1986). The information in this section is not intended as legal advice nor as a substitute for it. Caregivers needing legal advice are referred to their local support groups or national chapters. For example, the Tucson chapter of the Alzheimer's Disease and Related Disorders Association, and the ADRDA national office, both can help families obtain qualified legal counsel.

Guardianship

All guardians must be court appointed. The court, before appointing a guardian, must decide that the proposed ward is an "incapacitated" person. Incapacitated persons are those unable to make or communicate responsible decisions concerning their person because of mental or physical disability. Once the court has determined the proposed ward to be incapacitated, a guardian can be appointed.

Guardians make decisions regarding their wards' medical care, place of residence, and therapy. A guardian is not, however, personally financially liable for the ward's debts or actions. If no conservator (conservatorship is discussed in next section) has been appointed, the guardian may receive funds on behalf of the ward that can be applied to the ward's needs. Guardians may not, however, use the ward's funds to pay themselves for room and board furnished to the ward, or room and board furnished by another member of the guardian's family, without prior court approval.

Guardianship is generally appropriate for elderly persons with serious mental or physical disability, but it can make inpatient hospital treatment for the ward more difficult to obtain. Difficulty arises when the guardian is unavailable or opposes the recommendations of the medical professionals. Guardians cannot commit their wards to an institution.

The guardianship status is initiated by filing a petition for appointment, and filing typically is done by the proposed guardian. After the petition is filed, a hearing date is set. The filing fee and costs of serving and publishing the notice are paid through an attorney by the proposed guardian, or the estate if there is a conservator. If the ward has no funds, the proposed guardian is responsible for the payment of legal fees incurred in the guardianship proceedings. Other court fees commonly incurred are for a court attorney who has been appointed to represent the wishes of the proposed ward. The attorney will interview the proposed ward, and sometimes the proposed guardian, prior to the hearing. In most cases, the petitioner—that is, the proposed guardian—pays these costs.

To declare an individual incapacitated and in need of a guardian, a report from a physician must be submitted to the court. Usually the attending physician of the proposed ward is the one appointed to prepare the report. The physician is responsible for outlining the conditions that make the proposed ward unable to make decisions, and for including an opinion as to whether a guardian should be appointed.

Before the court makes a decision regarding the appointment of a guardian, the proposed guardian is asked to attest to the statements contained in the petition. If proper documentation is presented, the court will sign an order appointing the guardian. The clerk's office will then issue "Letters of Guardianship." This document is the official one evidencing the guardian's appointment.

The guardian is not required to report back to the court following the appointment proceedings, though the appointment is permanent. The appointment terminates only on the death of the ward or when terminated by court order. If the ward dies, the guardian should notify the attorney, who can determine what needs to be done to close the guardianship. If the guardian dies or is no longer willing or able to serve, a petition must be filed with the court to appoint a successor guardian.

Conservatorship

Conservatorship is a legal proceeding designed to protect persons with property or income who are unable to manage their financial affairs because of a mental or physical impairment. A person under conservatorship is referred to as a "protected person." The property of a protected person is referred to as the "conservatorship estate."

It is common to have both a guardian and a conservator appointed for a disabled person. Although the guardian and conservator are usually the same person, they may be different.

A conservatorship carries with it requirements for bonding the conservator, filing an inventory of the assets, and making an annual accounting to the court of the receipts and expenditures from the conservatorship funds. Because of the time and expense involved, possible alternatives to conservatorship should be discussed by the family with the attorney before making the decision to proceed.

If the proposed conservator is the spouse of the protected person, a conservatorship may not be necessary if all the assets are in both names. In community property states, such as Arizona, either spouse has the authority to manage the community assets. However, if real estate is involved, or if there are assets in the protected person's name only, conservatorship may then be necessary to effectively manage the assets. If the only assets of the proposed protected person are Veterans Administration or Social Security benefits, a responsible person may apply to the Veterans Administration or Social Security to be named a "representative payee" without court proceedings.

All conservators must post a bond with the court. The bonding company agrees that in return for the payment of a yearly premium, it will repay to the estate any funds wrongfully spent by the conservator. The bond protects the protected person, not the conservator.

Annual bond premiums generally range from $50 to $500, depending upon the size of the estate. The bond premium is payable from the estate funds, not by the conservator personally. Legal fees connected with the conservatorship are also payable from estate funds.

A conservator manages the financial affairs of the protected person. The conservator must first collect all the assets of the protected person and submit an inventory of the estate to the court. The inventory is due 90 days after the date of the conservator's appointment.

Estate funds must be used by the conservator only for the support, care, and benefit of the protected person and those legally dependent on the protected person. The conservator pays the bills of the protected person from estate funds. Comingling of estate funds with the personal funds of the conservator are not permitted, nor can conservators lend to themselves money from the estate. The conservator is required to keep accurate records of all receipts to and expenditures from the estate. The conservator must file an accounting with the court at least once a year. Yearly filing does involve a court proceeding and legal fees, expenses to be considered along with the yearly bond premium.

The prospective conservator initiates the appointment procedure by filing a petition, after which a hearing date is established. The petitioner is generally asked to advance to the attorney the legal fees and costs incurred during the conservatorship proceedings, but is reimbursed from the conservatorship estate upon appointment. If the petition is in order, and the signed order and approved bond presented to the court, the clerk will issue the "Letters of Conservatorship."

Following the appointment as a conservator, the appointee must supply the court with a yearly accounting of the conservatorship estate. The conservator is responsible to the court for the financial transactions related to the funds of the protected person.

ROLE OF THE NEUROPSYCHOLOGIST IN THE MANAGEMENT OF THE DEMENTIA PATIENT

Diagnosis

The responsibilities of the neuropsychologist in the management of dementia patients include diagnosis, monitoring, therapy, and counseling. In terms of diagnosis, it is the neuropsychologist who is best prepared to determine whether a patient suspected of having a dementing disease is experiencing progressive deterioration in memory, personality, and intellect—those characteristic features, according to DSM-III (American Psychiatric Association, 1980) criteria, of the dementia syndrome. As explained in Chapter 14, the neuropsychologist should evaluate mental status, affective state, memory, associative reasoning, attention, and visuospatial ability. The performance of the patient should be evaluated in relation to age- appropriate norms and estimated premorbid intelligence, and a judgment made about to whether deterioration has occurred.

When dementia is present, the neuropsychologist judges its severity, specifying in operational terms the limitations of the patient. Caregivers will want practical information about what it means to have mild or moderate dementia. Another piece of information appreciated by caregivers is the patient's understanding of basic concepts, such as same/different, hot/cold, yes/no, open/close, and on/off.

Monitoring

The second responsibility of the neuropsychologist is monitoring intellectual and behavioral change during the course of the disease. Some readers may wonder why it is necessary to reevaluate the patient with dementia. Can't they just be expected to get worse? Several reasons justify periodic reevaluation, not the least of which is that the patient may have a reversible dementia, or pseudodementia. When progressive deterioration is not observed in individuals diagnosed as having irreversible dementing disease, particularly after a year has elapsed, the diagnosis should be reevaluated. Another motivation for monitoring the patient is to educate the family members about the patient's capacities and help them to develop appropriate and effective behavioral management strategies. Finally, when a reliable assessment has been made of the patient's abilities, performance on behavioral measures can be used to assess the efficacy of pharmacologic and other therapies. To quantify the degree to which a drug may be having deleterious effects on mental status, repeated testing during drug therapy and in its absence are required.

Therapy

The term "therapy" is not used with the dementia patient to suggest that the clinician will be able to eliminate the patient's cognitive problems, but to suggest that the clinician can help the patient cope with cognitive loss. As was emphasized in Chapter 1, dementia patients with the same disease vary markedly in the degree to which particular cognitive functions are affected. Some individuals may have greater visuospatial than language problems, or suffer more from depression, or behavioral slowing. Knowledge of the intellectual and affective strengths and weaknesses of the patient enables the clinician to recommend the best way of imparting information to the patient. During the therapy session, the clinician can systematically identify what techniques improve the patient's performance.

Counseling

Counseling dementia patient caregivers, both professional and personal, is one of the most important responsibilities of the neuropsychologist. Caregivers need to be informed of the capabilities of their patients, what can reasonably be expected of them, and how to modify the environment and their behavior to maximize the patient's ability to function. To accomplish these goals, practitioners must analyze each case individually, being careful not to make assumptions about caregiver needs (Zarit, Orr, and Zarit, 1985). Zarit and colleagues (1985) suggest that for each case clinicians "assess relevant clinical dimensions, including the problem behaviors currently present, the caregiver's reactions to them, social support available to the caregiver, current stress or burden on the caregiver, and the family's values and preferences" (p. 86).

It will be the caregiver's understanding of the dementing disease, the environmental variables they can control to help the patient, and motivation that will make the greatest difference in the patient's performance. It is as important for the neuropsychologist to know the caregiver as the patient.

Getting to Know the Caregiver

Information about the emotional, physical, cognitive, social, and financial status of the caregivers is requisite for the development of recommendations about patient management and caregiver support. However, before discussing the ways in which clinicians can help caregivers, it is important to mention that at present, insurance companies and federal health care programs do not pay for caregiver evaluation, counseling, case management, guardianship services, or day care (Piktialis, 1986). Costs incurred by a service delivery unit for supportive counseling of caregivers will, in most cases, be the responsibility of caregivers. Professionals concerned with dementia victims and their families should advocate for third-party payment for caregiver support services. Indeed, to the degree that the caregiver can be sustained, the patient is likely to remain noninstitutionalized, and caregiver support costs are vastly lower than the cost of institutional care.

Even though third party payment is lacking, the authors believe the services that clinicians can offer caregivers are so important that caregivers should be made aware of their existence. Clinicians should interview caregivers about their physical health, use of drugs, and feelings about the disease effects on the patient and themselves. Additionally, caregivers should be screened for depression and mental status impairment and ability to manage the dementia patient. Mental status and depression screening instruments, with adequate normative data for older adults, were reviewed in Chapter 14. In relation to social status, the neuropsychologist should ascertain the type and amount of support being given the caregiver. Before making a judgment as to the adequacy of social support, the clinician will need to know which of the patient problems, of those listed in Table 15-3, or others, the caregiver is encountering.

Numerous well-developed, interview-based rating scales exist that can help the neuropsychologist and other clinicians in assessing the status and needs of a caregiver. Since many caregivers are themselves older adults, such assessment instruments need to have a content and structure appropriate for older persons. The three instruments reviewed below have been specifically developed to assess older adults across a number of dimensions, including psychologic, medical, nutritional, economic, and social.

The CARE. One such instrument is the Comprehensive Assessment and Referral Evaluation (CARE)(Gurland et al., 1977–78). The CARE has been shown to reliably record and classify information on the health and social problems of older individuals. It consists of a semistructured interview guide with an inventory of defined ratings. Because it covers psychiatric, nutritional, medical, economic, and social problems, it is quite well suited to assist in determining whether a caregiver is experiencing difficulties that require professional intervention. One particular advantage of this instrument is that because of its multidimensional content, sections of it can be administered by various members of a multidisciplinary team.

The OARS. The Older Americans Resources and Services Questionnaire (OARS) (Pfeiffer, 1976) is a multidimensional evaluation technique developed for the Duke University Longitudinal Study of Aging. It is based on a semistructured interview with ratings of physical and mental health, as well as social and economic resources.

Fillenbaum and Smyer (1981) have demonstrated adequate interrater reliability for the OARS. This feature is important because the various parts of the OARS were specifically designed to be completed by different multidisciplinary team members working independently. Fillenbaum and Smyer (1981) also demonstrated acceptable criterion validity, employing such criteria as an objective economic scale, ratings based on personal interviews by geropsychiatrists, and ratings by physician's associates and physical therapists. As with the CARE, the OARS thus appears to be very useful in selecting among various referral and service alternatives for the older adult.

The Philadelphia Geriatric Center Multilevel Assessment Instrument. The final instrument to be reviewed here is the Philadelphia Geriatric Center Multilevel Assessment Instrument (MAI) (Lawton, Moss, Fulcomer and Kleban, 1982), designed to assess the well-being of older persons in a range of particular areas. Behavioral competence in the domains of activities of daily living, cognition, health, time use, and social interaction is assessed, as well as subjective psychologic well-being and perceived environmental quality.

Lawton and colleagues (1982) evaluated the psychometric qualities of these measures by administration of the instrument to 590 older persons from various groups (independent community residents, in-home services clients, and people awaiting admission to an institution). The summary rating scales of the instrument demonstrated agreement between an interviewer and an independent rater, with either a zero or a one-point discrepancy in 95 percent of all instances. Intraclass correlations (another reliability index) ranged from a high of .88 for the rating of activities of daily living competence to a low of .58, for the rating of social interaction. Other measures of reliability (internal consistency and retest reliability), although not impressively high, were found to be acceptable. Validity, assessed by contrasting the different criterion groups (e.g., independently living people versus those awaiting admission to an institution), as well as by comparison to clinician and administrator ratings, also generally supported the validity of the MAI.

The present authors have routinely administered combined portions of the OARS and MAI in the assessment of caregivers seen during evaluation of dementia patients in the University of Arizona Memory Disorders Clinic, and have found this approach quite useful in helping to determine what combination of services, referrals, or both best meets the caregiver's needs.

Helping the Caregiver Manage the Patient

An important early step in the counseling process is to educate the caregiver as to the type and availablility of support services. Have a handout prepared with the name and type of service, eligibility criteria and cost. Also, provide addresses and phone numbers of local and national support groups. A brief list of national organizations is presented at the end of this chapter.

Caregivers should be encouraged to define the skills retained by the patient and provide an opportunity for the patient to use these skills. Such opportunities may give the patient satisfaction and be useful to the caregiver. For example, patients may be able to fold clothes, stir food, or water the lawn. The oral reading ability of dementia patients typically remains intact, and one creative caregiver had the patient read aloud to her every night while she did the dishes. This enabled the caregiver to read books for which she would otherwise have had no time.

Because clinicians can not anticipate every challenge the caregiver will encounter, it is valuable to provide caregivers with a problem-solving approach that will enable them to cope with problems as they arise, a procedure recommended by Zarit and colleagues (1985). Teaching an approach to problem-solving will strengthen the independence of the caregiver. The components of problem-solving are as follows:

1. Problem identification
2. Generation and recording of all possible solutions
3. Consideration of the pros and cons of possible solutions
4. Selection of the most promising
5. Evaluation of the effectiveness of the approach used
6. If the approach was unsuccessful, selection of another approach

Of course, when the clinician can offer a concrete suggestion for solving a problem, it should be given. Coming away from a counseling session knowing a specific strategy makes caregivers feel that something has been acomplished. When offering specific suggestions, demonstrate how these solutions could have been arrived at by using the problem-solving technique just described.

Some commonly reported problems and suggested strategies follow:

Affective/Behavioral Problems

Paranoia. Do not become defensive or argumentative; distract the patient if possible. Suspiciousness reflects memory failure (e.g., Who stole my jacket? Why do you never call me anymore?), and accusations are transient.

Irritability. Do not take the comments and actions personally; watch for antecedent conditions that exacerbate problems (e.g., frustration with a task that cannot be performed by the patient).

Mood Changes. Make sure medications are not responsible. If uncertain, have the physician evaluate all the drugs being taken by the patient.

Physical Problems

Night Wandering. Place a sensor under a mat by the patient's bed, which will sound an alarm near the caregiver. Install a complex lock on the inside of the door.

Wandering and Getting Lost. Make sure the patient has identification, preferably a Med-alert bracelet. Install a photoelectric cell to alert a monitor when the front or back door opens.

Incontinence. Establish a regular fluid intake and elimination pattern so that at regular intervals the patient can be assisted or reminded. If the problem is due to the patient forgetting how to get to the bathroom, a marker system may help.

Sleeping Difficulty. Have the patient exercise more during the day.

Dressing. The patient may be unable to dress because of an inability to choose what to wear. If this is the case, make the selection for the patient. If the problem is manipulation of buttons, bows, and clasps, use simpler closures such as Velcro squares.

Eating. Patients may appear overly selective in the food they will eat. It may be that there are too many foods for the patient to choose among. Try limiting the number of food items offered.

Cognitive Problems

Forgetfulness. Use memory aids; try different kinds: small notebooks, calendars, calendar watches, blackboard with the day's schedule. Place family pictures around the home to maintain orientation to family. In social situations, provide information indirectly: "You remember Mr. and Mrs. Doe from our bridge club."

Learning New Skills. As a function of dementing disease, patients will have difficulty learning new skills. Expect difficulty. Minimize the necessity for learning new skills and routines. Capitalize on the familiar.

To cope with the problems of an individual caregiver, have the caregiver make a record of problems that arise, the presumed cause of the problem, approaches considered, approaches tried, and outcomes. Such a record may reveal a pattern of events that triggers a problem. Emphasize that this need not be a formal report, just notes that can be reviewed in subsequent counseling sessions. A beneficial by-product of having the caregiver keep such a record is that the act of recording the information may serve as an outlet for frustration.

For a caregiver to cope with the "36-hour day" of caring for a dementing individual, it is of utmost importance that the caregiver remain in adequate psychologic and physical health. If the neuropsychologist or other clinician finds the caregiver to be depressed, appropriate professional treatment should be recommended. If the neuropsychologist is trained in psychotherapy, he or she may be the individual to initiate such treatment. If not, referral should be made to a professional experienced in the psychotherapeutic treatment of depressed older individuals. In some cases, consultation with a psychiatrist experienced in the diagnosis and treatment of depression in older persons may be necessary. Useful guidance in determining indicators for appropriate referral, as well as assistance in planning treatment approaches, can be found in Chaisson-Stewart (1985).

For many depressed caregivers, participation in a group treatment setting, where the person can have contact with others in similar situations, and hence learn from their coping successes and failures, is very helpful. In their experience at the University of Arizona, the present authors have found cognitive/behavioral approaches to group treatment of depressed elders to be particularly useful in the management of caregiver depression. Guidance in the application of cognitive/behavioral techniques in group settings can be found in Yost, Beutler, Corbishley, and Allender (1986).

Whereas caregivers showing signs or symptoms of stress-related physical disorders (e.g., cardiovascular, gastrointestinal, repetitive infectious) are obviously in need of medical attention, they may benefit from psychologic interventions designed to reduce the risk of future stress-related physical symptoms. Stressful responsibilities like caring for a dementia patient can lead to physical symptoms, including increased susceptibility to infectious illness (see Gunderson and Rahe, 1974). Psychologic interventions designed to enable the caregiver to better cope with stress may reduce the risk of such symptoms. In a carefully controlled study, Kiecolt-Glaser and colleagues (1985) demonstrated the effectiveness of relaxation training (a structured training program designed to increase the ability to relax and reduce stress) in enhancement of immunocompetence in older adults. In a sample of 45 community-living elderly persons, relaxation training (compared with equivalent social-contact and no-contact control groups) was associated with improved immunocompetence. The procedure involved 45-minute relaxation sessions, three times per week for 1 month. This training was associated with an increase in natural killer cell activity (associated with antiviral and antitumor functions) as well as other indicators of improved virus control. Subjects also reported improvement in the quality of their sleep. Although the no-contact and social-contact control groups did not show comparable results, the authors suggest that social-contact interventions may have some effect with those elderly who have greater environmental restrictions (such as dementia patient caregivers).

The availability of social contact and support has received much attention of late as a variable mediating stress and "burnout" in caregiving (e.g., Etzion, 1984; Morycz, 1985). While the clinician may be able to do little to facilitate increased contact with the caregiver's endogenous informal social support system, a range of formal social support options exists that can be of assistance. Perhaps the most relevant of these is the variety of services and information available through the local chapters of the Alzheimer's Disease and Related Disorders Association (ADRDA). The local chapters of this national organization typically sponsor support groups, provide referrals to services within the community, and offer considerable information on dementing illnesses. Referring the caregiver to the local ADRDA chapter can be one of the most helpful of interventions available to the clinician.

At the close of a caregiver counseling session, be certain the caregiver knows what has transpired. Forecast expected changes in the patient's behavior. Do not, however, overwhelm the caregiver by enumerating all possible future changes, but rather those likely to arise in the near future. Knowing what to expect will enable caregivers to prepare themselves and anticipate solutions to problems. End counseling sessions by providing recognition to the caregivers for their efforts.

In follow-up sessions, plan to assess change in the patient since the last visit; an informal assessment may be all that is necessary. Consider the possibility of change in the caregiver as well. If mental or physical deterioration is observed in the caregiver, make appropriate referrals. Review the effectiveness of behavioral management strategies suggested during the previous visit. If they were unsuccessful, determine why and modify your recommendations. Review the caregiver's daily records about the behavior of the patient and make recommendations when possible. Finally, discuss the caregiver's support system with attention to those which are unused but potentially beneficial.

Personal caregivers will benefit inestimably from counseling with the neuropsychologist. The counseling agenda can help them cope with the patient's behavioral problems, their personal sacrifices in caring for the patient, the anger and grief they feel, and their plans for their own and the patient's future.

THE ROLE OF THE SPEECH–LANGUAGE PATHOLOGIST IN THE MANAGEMENT OF THE DEMENTIA PATIENT

The speech–language pathologist, like the neuropsychologist, has responsibilities in diagnosis, monitoring, therapy, and counseling. In fact, the speech-language pathologist and the neuropsychologist will be interested in much of the same information about the patient and caregiver. In those settings where both types of professionals are on the staff, the labor of obtaining information about the patient and caregiver can be divided, saving the patient and caregiver time. In many geographically remote settings, a single psychologist or speech–language pathologist may be responsible for assessing and managing dementia patients. The authors recognize that some professionals will argue about the boundaries of the domains of neuropsychology and speech–language pathology. Our view is that neuropsychologists must by necessity be concerned with language and communicative ability and speech-language pathologists must, by necessity, be concerned with cognitive functions essential to the ability to meaningfully communicate. Cognition involves language, and communication and language involve cognition. The authors also recognize that not all psychologists and speech–language pathologists have had training or experience with geriatric neurologically impaired individuals. The competency of each professional to care for the dementia patient, regardless of professional title, must be judged individually until professional training programs require, for certification, clinical practicum with the geriatric neurologically impaired.

Diagnosis

The performance data obtained in the communication evaluation of the dementia patient, like the performance data from neuropsychologic tests, are valuable in confirming the diagnosis of dementia. Communicative impairment, as an omnipresent feature of the dementia syndrome, should be considered by clinicians before designating an individual as demented.

Tests and techniques appropriate for assessment of communicative function in dementia patients were discussed in Chapters 6 and 7, and the more practical aspects of evaluation will be discussed in this chapter. At the conclusion of the communication evaluation of the dementia patient, the clinician must translate the patient's performance into practical terms for the benefit of the caregivers. Test scores are meaningless without interpretation as to what they reveal about the patient's communication ability in the real world. Caregivers will be interested in knowing how well the patient understands television, what is read in the newspaper, and what is said by family members at dinner. They will want to know which words confuse the patient. Can the patient follow instructions? At what level of complexity does an instructional command become incomprehensible? Does the patient require a step-by-step reiteration of the components of a task in order to complete it? Caregivers will want to know if there is anything they can do to improve the patient's ability to communicate.

To demonstrate how test performance on a communication battery might be translated into practical information for the caregiver, some practical implications of performance on subtests in the Arizona Battery for Communication Disorders (ABC) (Chapter 7) are suggested:

Subtest 1: Auditory Discrimination: Knowledge of concepts "same" and "different"; ability to remember a one level command (e.g., say if two words are same or different); possibility of hearing loss or speech discrimination deficit.

Subtest 2: Mental Status Examination: Orientation to time, place, and person; comprehension of single sentences.

Subtest 3: Story-Retelling Task: Ability to follow a verbal description of a daily event or anecdote; indication of how fast information is forgotten.

Subtest 4: Delayed Recognition Span Test: Memory for words and locations of things.

Subtest 5: Verbal Description Task: Ability to describe a common object; knowledge of English grammar.

Subtest 6: Reading Comprehension Task: Ability to read and understand words, single sentences, and short paragraphs.

Subtest 7: Sentence Disambiguation Task: Ability to understand sentences; ability to reason.

Subtest 8: Pantomimic Expression Task: Ability to use common objects correctly.

Subtest 9: Drawing Task: Ability to conceptualize simple spatial relationships.

Subtest 10: Generative Naming Task: Ability to think up answers or solutions to a problem.

Subtest 11: Contrast Test of Oral and Written Discourse: Ability to write a meaningful paragraph, ability to describe a picture or event.

Subtest 12: Peabody Picture Vocabulary Test: Ability to understand words.

Monitoring

As discussed in earlier chapters, the pattern of decline in communicative function reflects the progression of dementing disease. Thus, changes in performance on measures of communicative function signal changes in disease state. This is just one justification for periodic reevaluation of the dementia patient. Additionally, because clinicians now have tools with which to reliably evaluate the communicative ability of dementia patients, communicative performance can be used to assess the efficacy of drug and other therapies. A measure of communicative function can be given to a dementia patient as a baseline performance measure, after which a drug can be administered and the communicative test readministered to ascertain whether it was efficacious in improving cognitive and communicative functioning. This is yet another reason for periodically evaluating the communicative competence of the dementia patient but these are not the only reasons for patient monitoring. An even more basic reason is to obtain information about how the patient comprehends, processes, and produces linguistic information in the different stages of the disease. One of the questions most frequently asked by personal caregivers is whether patients understand as much as they did earlier in the disease course.

Therapy

Speech–language pathologists may be able to improve the ability of dementia patients, particularly those in the early mild stages, to communicate. They may accomplish this *not* by teaching the patient a new technique, but by systematically defining the effect(s) of manipulation of environmental and linguistic variables on communicative performance. Clinicians should schedule a period of therapy for the purpose of systematically exploring the effect(s) of linguistic and environmental variables on the the patient's communicative ability. As Golper and Rau (1983) have eloquently stated,

> Any therapeutic approach that requires the learning of new behavior or purports to "stimulate" or reestablish previously learned abilities will, in large measure, be undermined by diffuse disease. Treatment, therefore, is better directed toward therapies that require little cognitive flexibility or learning. The therapies most likely to be recommended are highly pragmatic, that is, they are directed toward adjustments in the environment that can enhance functional and interpersonal communication, and ameliorate some of the concerns of the family or custodial personnel. (p. 123)

Environmental variables likely to affect performance are the number of individuals in the communicative interaction, the number of distractions, existence of cues as to topic, and the patient's familiarity with the environment. The greater the number of individuals participating in a communicative interaction, the more information the patient must track, because every additional conversant adds another set of facial expressions, reactions, and comments to be interpreted. Dementia patients communicate best face-to-face with a single individual. Not surprisingly, they also do better in quiet, ordered environments. Finally, they are benefited by having visual and tactile access to the object of discussion.

Linguistic variables manipulable by the clinician include level of syntactic complexity, use of reference, verbal cue strength, directness, literality, input modality, abstractness of topic, propositionality, word frequency, rate of speech, word class, and imageability of word. To date, empirical data about the effect of these variables on dementia patients of varying severity are virtually nonexistant. The single exception may be the data from a study by Obler, Obermann, Samuels, and Albert (1985), in which the effect of input modality (written, verbal, combined) on comprehension was studied in dementia patients and a facilitation effect was reported in the combined condition.

Our clinical experience has led us to believe that all of these variables are important in the processing of linguistic information. By using single-subject experimental designs (Kazdin, 1982; McReynolds and Kearns, 1982), clinicians can systematically and reliably determine the effect of variable manipulation on the capacity of the dementia patient to comprehend information.

One possible confounding variable that must be mentioned is the effect of memory. In a study by Bayles, Slauson, Tomoeda, and Boone (1986) dementia patients were asked to recall and recognize words from a list of 12 presented in three conditions: orally, visually, orally and visually. In the pilot study, the research question about the effect of input modality on word recall and recognition was unanswerable because the stimulus word lists were too long. When the word lists were composed so that the number of stimulus words exceeded the patients' immediate sensory memory by approximately 50 percent, rather than 100 percent, the effect of modality could be determined (note: a significant effect was not obtained for input modality on either word recall or recognition).

Counseling

The first item on the speech–language pathologist's caregiver counseling agenda should be a caregiver interview to obtain information about the caregiver's perception of disease effects on the patient's communication. Variability in the knowledge of caregivers is so pronounced that a structured interview, or paper-and-pencil test, is recommended to provide the clinician with an understanding of the caregivers' educational needs. The interview or test should include questions about the nature of the dementing disease; behavioral consequences associated with disease progression; linguistic communication; the capacities necessary to meaningfully communicate; those aspects of speech, language, and communication most vulnerable to the effects of dementing disease; types of language to avoid with the dementia patient; and behavioral management of communication disorders. Some portion of the interview should be devoted to asking the caregiver about the premorbid communicative style of the dementia patient: was the patient gregarious, quiet, verbally humorous, in a job that required considerable talking, a reader, addicted to cross-word puzzles, and so forth. The purpose is to develop in the clinician an appreciation for what the loss of communicative function means in terms of that patient and caregiver.

Once the clinician has assessed the level of knowledge of the caregiver, an educational program can be developed to correct misconceptions, develop appropriate expectations, and learn techniques to maximize the patient's abilities. The clinician should emphasize the relation between the type of brain damage the patient is experiencing and its effect on cognition and communication. For many caregivers, it is comforting to be reassured that the bizarre utterances of the patient are not motivated by negative feelings about the caregivers, or any limitation in their caregiving, but result from brain injury.

While every clinician will be challenged to develop behavioral management techniques suitable for the unique problems of their client caregivers, the following techniques will be useful for most:

Modifying Question Asking. Avoid open-ended questions: "What would you like to do this afternoon?" "Where should we go on our drive?" As dementia worsens, affected individuals are increasingly unable to think of possibilities, and the ability to generate ideas deteriorates. Therefore, ask either yes/no or either/or questions: "Do you want to go to the store?" "Do you want to drive to the lake?" "Do you want fish or chicken for supper?"

Help Minimize the Effects of Poor Memory on Communication. The suggestions for modifying question asking apply here as well. Short, simple questions enhance comprehension (Pajk, 1984). Do not leave the patient guessing about what or whom you are talking about. Avoid frequent use of pronouns; it is better to repeat the name of the person or thing to which you are referring.

Be Redundant. Assume that previously given information is gradually being forgotten, so restate critical facts during the recitation of an anecdote or explanation. The following two explanations are responses to the same question, but they differ in the amount of redundancy used by the speaker.

Example of nonredundant explanation: Mr. Ferguson is here to repair the air-conditioner. Maybe he can fix the dishwasher too.

Example of redundant explanation: Mr. Ferguson is here to fix the air-conditioner. If Mr. Ferguson can fix the air-conditioner, maybe Mr. Ferguson can fix the dishwasher. Both the air-conditioner and dishwasher are broken. Let's see if Mr. Ferguson will repair the broken air-conditioner and dishwasher.

Remind dementia patients of what is expected of them throughout a task. Performance errors may occur simply because the patient does not remember the purpose of the task or your instructions, not because of an incapacity to do the task.

Use right-branching sentences rather than left-branching. As Kynette and Kemper (1986) have demonstrated, left-branching sentences, place a greater load on memory. Left-branching sentences such as "Because Tom left (the house without his keys), Bob was upset" are more difficult to process than right-branching, such as "Bob was upset because Tom left (the house without his keys)." Simple short sentences are easiest to comprehend (Tomoeda, Bayles, and Slauson, 1986).

Modify Topic. Because of their diminished ability to reason and generate ideas, dementia patients will not be able to participate in philosophically oriented dicussions, follow complex argumentation, or consider hypothetic situations. Talk with the patient about that which is directly observable and familiar. Urge families to refrain from logical arguments when these are no longer meaningful (Reifler and Wu, 1982).

Be direct. Requiring dementia patients to process implied information will handicap them. Say what you mean; be explicit about what you want them to understand. For example, if you are busy and have no time to talk, don't say something like "Do I look like I have nothing to do?" Rather, say "I am too busy to talk."

Avoid Using Analogies. An analogy is a logical inference based on the assumption that if two things are alike in some respects, then they must be alike in other respects: Participating in a team sport is like being a member of the corporation board; being a good friend is like being a good gardener. Difficulty seeing the relation between objects and events is precisely the kind of processing problem that defines dementia.

Restate and Paraphrase That Which the Patient Has Not Understood. Although dementia patients suffer deterioration in conceptual knowledge, it is lost gradually, and not all members in a category are necessarily lost simultaneously. Therefore, when the patient fails to understand an idea stated in one form, it may be comprehensible in another.

Be Literal. Much of what people say is expressed in nonliteral terms: "This mousse is heaven" and "That writer is dynamite." A dessert is not really heaven, whatever heaven is, and no writer is a cylindrical container filled with explosive material. The use of nonliterality is a way of expressing degree of feeling, being humorous, and being polite. Dementia patients have progressive difficulty inferring the sense of nonliteral utterances.

Provide Illustrations of What You Are Talking About. Photographs and illustrations will make it easier for dementia patients to grasp word meaning.

Establish Eye Contact Before Addressing the Patient. Securing eye contact will help the patient attend to what you are saying. Being able to see your face and expressions makes it easier to derive the intended message.

Enhance What You Say with Frequent Gestures. Dementia patients seem to retain some appreciation for body language (Bartol, 1979; Hoffman, Platt, Barry, and Hamill, 1985). Being physically expressive may make it easier to derive the sense of your words.

Much has been said in this book about linguistic communication, the use of words to share information. Little has been said about nonverbal communication. Nonverbal communication is the message humans impart by virture of the tone of voice, facial expressions, body posturing, the distances maintained from other conversants, and the use of gestures and touch. The authors are convinced that when the dementia patient's knowledge of words is lost and linguistic comprehension is minimal, the patient may still respond, at some elemental level, to the nonverbal body language of the caregiver. Some support for this belief comes from the work of Hoffman and colleagues (1985). These investigators used live actors to convey affective cues to ten normal subjects and 44 demented residents of a nursing home. The study participants were evaluated for their recognition, liking, and nonverbal reactions to pleasant and unpleasant affective messages presented by means of voice tone, touch, and facial expression. The subjects' responses were videotaped and later analyzed. Results indicated that responsivity to nonverbal affective stimuli are well maintained in even the extremely demented. When given negatively biased unpleasant stimuli, the demented patients withdrew and appeared uncomfortable, but pleasant stimuli elicited positive verbal and nonverbal responses.

Many times we have calmed an agitated patient with a smile, embrace, and soothing voice. Many times the laughter in our voices and the happiness in our faces have brought a smile to the face of an individual who could not understand our words. We caution the clinician against believing that all channels of communication are closed even with severely demented patients.

THE ROLE OF OTHER PROFESSIONALS IN PATIENT MANAGEMENT

Because this book is authored by a speech–language pathologist and a neuropsychologist, the roles of these professionals have received special attention. It is important to acknowledge, however, that certain of the responsibilities attributed to the neuropsychologist and speech–language pathologist often are assumed by other professionals, such as the social worker, the nurse, and the geriatrician. Indeed, the responsibilities of health professionals frequently overlap. It is the opinion of these authors that management of persons with dementia and their families is best when it is a multidisciplinary team effort. The geriatric assessment/management team is greater than the sum of its parts. Certainly, mention must be made of those professionals who are most likely to be team participants and who individually represent an important resource for the patient and caregiver.

The geriatrician is a physician with specialized training in the medical care of the elderly. Not only do geriatricians play an important role in the diagnosis of dementing disease, they are primarily responsible for managing the patient's physical health and treating intercurrent disease. In many geographic areas, when specially trained geriatricians are unavailable, internists and family practioners perform these duties.

The neurologist is a physician specialized in the diagnosis and treatment of nervous system disorders. These specialists are routinely consulted to make or help in the differential diagnosis of primary degenerative dementing disorders.

The psychiatrist is a physician trained in the diagnosis and treatment of mental disorders. Psychiatrists are frequently involved in the differential diagnosis of dementing diseases, particularly in their differentiation from depression. Pharmacologic intervention may be supervised by the psychiatrist, especially for depression. In terms of counseling and psychotherapy, the role of the psychiatrist overlaps with that of the clinical psychologist.

Clinical psychologists are educated through the doctoral degree and have specialized training in the assessment and psychotherapeutic treatment of mental disorders. They are an excellent referral source for those caregivers having difficulty with the mental stresses of caregiving.

The primary caregiver of the dementia patient is often the nurse. Nurses with specialized training in the care of the elderly are geriatric nurses, whereas psychiatric nurses are specialized in the care of individuals with mental disorders. In addition to being indispensable in the day-to-day care in institutional settings, they are an excellent resource for advising families in the management of health problems.

Another key professional serving the dementia patient is the gerontologic social worker. Members of this profession have been educated at the master's and doctoral level in the social behaviors and social resources relevant to aging individuals. They are often the facilitators who guide caregivers to community resources.

Many other professionals may participate in the geriatric management team. Physical therapists, specialized in accomodating and rehabilitating physical disabilities, provide therapy to those dementia patients with physical problems, such as HD and PD patients, and in some cases the MID patient. In particular situations, other specialists are needed, such as the nutritionist and occupational therapist. Finally, the clergy are represented on many geriatric assessment/management teams and provide spiritual guidance to families.

An Educational Training Program for Caregivers

Merely providing caregivers with descriptions of the aforementioned techniques is, in itself, insufficient if they are to learn to incorporate the techniques into routine communicative interchanges with the patient. The procedures will be better assimilated if practiced under the supervision of the clinician.

In the authors' clinical experience, the most effective way of teaching caregivers communication modification techniques has been to follow these steps: (1) provide an oral and written description of the technique, (2) show a demonstration videotape of the technique being used, (3) demonstrate the technique with the patient while the caregiver observes, (4) have the caregiver try using the technique with the clinician, (5) when the technique is understood, have the caregiver practice the technique with the patient, (6) videotape the caregiver during the patient practice session, and (7) review the practice session with the caregiver offering encouragement. Reviewing the tape with the caregivers will enable the them to evaluate their proficiency as well as the technique's usefulness.

Recommend to caregivers that they keep a home record of their questions about the use of the techniques they have learned or about any communication behavior the patient exhibits. Such records should be brought to subsequent counseling sessions and discussed. The use of a notebook by the caregiver is advantageous because it insures that the therapist can address questions that are genuinely important to the caregiver. Finally, any new information the therapist provides about management of the patient to the caregiver should be in writing so that the caregiver can keep it in the notebook. In the counseling session, caregivers may not be able to absorb all the important points made by the speech–language pathologist. By having the information in writing, they can review it at home at their own pace.

High-Tech Help

The incredible technologic advances of this century can help patients and caregivers cope with the challenges of dementia and aging. Clinicians are encouraged to become informed about the technologic advances that can improve the coping strategies of patients and caregivers. In 1980, Danowski and Sacks reported results of a study of computer communication and the elderly. They found the elderly highly receptive to computer use and appreciative of the control it offered them. An excellent source of information about the technologic advances that can improve the lives of the chronically ill and disabled is *Technology and Aging in America* (U.S. Office of Technology Assessment, 1985). Within this document, numerous currently available devices for handicapped individuals have been described. Consider the potential of just the following devices for helping caregivers and patients cope with aging and dementia:

Talking computer: Provides speech output of data on computer monitor.

Talking caliper: Audioizes measurement functions from digital readout.

Portable telephone: Allows mobility of individual while talking.

Closed circuit TV magnification system: Magnifies material read from computer terminals, typewriters, and microfilm up to 60 times.

Large print computer: Magnifies print on monitor 2 to 16 times.

Telecommunications device for hearing impaired: Provides printout or digital display of information transmitted over telephone. Allows hearing impaired to type and receive messages over the phone from other TDD users.

Amplified speech headset: Telephone handset with adjustable volume for speech transmission.

Electronic safety system: Allows users to program appliances to turn off.

In-home computer: Provides self-instruction for medication, nutrition, and other self-care assistance.

Closed circuit television: Allows individual to monitor other areas of the home.

Talking clock: Time of day is spoken audibly.

Silent communications alarm network: Ultrasonic pen-size transmitter that sounds an alarm in a central office and indicates the user's location.

Lifeline: A personal security system that links users electronically to 24-hour assistance.

The devices mentioned here represent a small sample of those currently available with potential for aiding the ill or handicapped. Imagine the comfort a frail elderly caregiver would receive from having a home alarm system through which a medical emergency could be signaled, a closed circuit television system that permitted the viewing of the dementia patient in other areas of the home, and a home computer that enabled the caregiver to keep track of medications, conduct banking transactions, and select groceries for home delivery.

SUMMARY

To adequately plan the care of dementia patients, three facts must be acknowledged: first, their behavior continuously and insidiously changes; second, as the dementia worsens, the burdens of caregiving increase; and third, both the caregiver and dementia patient are likely to be elderly. The responsibilities of clinicians to dementia victims are long-term, and periodic reevaluation of both the caregiver and patient should be pro forma. In addition to ascertaining dementia-related changes in psychologic and communicative status, sufficient time in therapy should be allowed for identifying the best method of presenting information to the patient. Knowing how to manipulate environmental, situational, and linguistic variables to improve the patient's comprehension can serve as the basis of a caregiver training program.

In the initial meetings with the caregiver, information should be obtained about medical, emotional, financial, and social status. Such information is essential for guiding the caregiver in decision-making. At first, caregivers require emotional support to cope with the shock of the diagnosis. Counseling will help them bear their grief, understand their anger, and accept the future. Sessions with a knowledgeable professional of whom they can ask questions is particularly comforting.

Education of caregivers in the early stages enables them to prepare for the consequences of dementing illness, but clinicians must be careful not to inundate caregivers with excessive information about disease sequelae. Forecast only the most probable short-term behavioral changes. Because it is impossible for clinicians to anticipate all the problems each caregiver will experience, teaching stress-reducing strategies and problem-solving methods is valuable.

Both the neuropsychologist and the speech–language pathologist have critical roles on the dementia patient management team: roles in diagnosis, monitoring, therapy, and counseling. The information these professionals obtain about the psychologic and communicative functioning of patients benefits other professionals, especially when it is interpreted for them in relation to their patient care responsibilities. Because the population of dementia victims is growing, and the cost of institutional care is rising, interest in learning behavioral management techniques, helpful for maintaining patients at home, is also rising. Now is the time for professionals to prepare for the challenges of dementia.

NATIONAL ORGANIZATIONS

Community support groups provide caregivers with a long-term support system. The services they sponsor vary, depending upon the size and enthusiasm of the group, but at the very least they provide education, socialization, and a forum for questions. Many sponsor respite programs for caregivers, and most have a hotline for the caregiver faced with an emergency. As this book closes, it is appropriate to identify and give credit to the following national organizations, which offer support to dementia patients and their caregivers.

National Institute on Aging
Building 31, Room 5C35
9000 Rockville Pike
Bethesda, MD 20205
(for literature on AD)

Alzheimer's Disease and Related Disorders Association, Inc.
(ADRDA)
70 E. Lake St., Suite 600
Chicago, IL 60601
(312) 853-3060

Huntington's Disease Society of America
140 West 22nd Street, 6th Floor
New York, NY 10011
(212) 242-1968

Parkinson's Disease Foundation
William Black Medical Research Building
Columbia Presbyterian Medical Center
640 West 168th Street
New York, NY 10032
(212) 923-4700

United Parkinson's Foundation
360 W. Superior St.
Chicago, IL 60610
(312) 664-2344

National Parkinson's Foundation
1501 N.W. 9th Avenue
Miami, FL 33136
(305) 547-6666

GENERAL SUMMARY AND CLINICAL IMPLICATIONS

1. Because dementia patients and their caregivers are generally elderly, clinicians need to be familiar with the characteristics of the elderly. The average person older than 65 has 12 years of education, suffers from at least one chronic disease, is not working, and receives an annual income of less than $17,000.
2. Most elders are well integrated into an informal social network and have weekly contact with their children, who in most cases live within driving distance.
3. Though the elderly are sometimes more cautious than younger adults, they are generally flexible, resourceful, and optimistic.
4. The most common health problems of the elderly are arthritis and high blood pressure. Ninety percent of the elderly report their health as being fair, good, or excellent.
5. Hearing impairment is the third most prevalent chronic condition of the noninstitutionalized elderly. Because of the prevalence of hearing problems, clinicians should evaluate the hearing of all their elderly patients and caregivers.
6. The average elder takes six drugs at a time, a fact that increases the probability of an adverse drug interaction. Clinicians should review the drug regimens of the patient and their caregivers.
7. Caregivers of dementia patients experience changes in their responsibilities and role within the family. They are at risk for becoming social isolates and financially depleted.
8. Clinicians should review caregiver needs in providing patient care, managing the household, and personally coping with the demands of caregiving. Clinicians can offer caregivers education about the disease and its effects, behavioral management strategies, and stress reductions techniques, as well as refer them to support groups, day care programs, and health care options.
9. Many clinicians may become involved in helping families select a nursing home. Families should be made aware of the certification criteria, staff-to-patient ratio, types of services available, cost, and other factors influencing patient care.
10. Speech–language pathologists and neuropsychologists have an important role in the management of dementia patients, a role that includes diagnosis, monitoring, therapy, and counseling.
11. The speech–language pathologist is uniquely prepared to assess communicative functioning, identify the best ways of communicating with the dementia patient, and train professional and personal caregivers in communication facilitation techniques.

12. The neuropsychologist is uniquely prepared to assess cognitive functioning, identify the best behavior management strategies, counsel the caregiver about the patient's cognitive status, and help the caregiver emotionally cope with the burdens of dementia.
13. The management of dementia is best accomplished by an interdisciplinary effort between health professionals. As part of a team, or individually, the geriatrician, neurologist, psychiatrist, clinical psychologist, geriatric social worker, physical therapist, clergyman, and nurse are important referral sources for the dementia patient and caregiver.

REFERENCES

Aaronson, L. (1983). Adult day care: A developing concept. *The Journal of Gerontological Social Work, 5*, 35-47.

American Association of Retired Persons (1983). *ARP 4th Annual Survey of Opinions of Older Americans*, Washington, DC: author.

American Association of Retired Persons (1984). *A profile of older Americans: 1984*. Washington, DC: author.

American Psychiatric Association (1980). *Diagnostic and statistical manual of mental disorders* (3rd ed.). Washington, DC: author.

Bartol, M.A. (1979). Nonverbal communication in patients with Alzheimer's disease. *Journal of Gerontological Nursing, 5*, 21-31.

Bayles, K.A., Slauson, T.J., Tomoeda, C.K., and Boone, D.R., (1986). [Effect of input modality on word recognition and recall]. Unpublished raw data.

Bengston, V.L., and Treas, J. (1980). The changing family context of mental health and aging. In J.E. Birren, and R.B. Sloane (Eds.), *Handbook of mental health and aging* (pp. 400-428). Englewood Cliffs, NJ: Prentice-Hall.

Bennett, R., Gruen, G., and Tepper, L. (1983, September). *Interactions among citizens, providers and technologies in various settings.* Paper prepared for the Conference on the Impact of Technology on Long-Term Care.

Bergmann, E.M., Foster, A.W., and Matthews, V. (1978). Management of the demented elderly patient in the community. *British Journal of Psychiatry, 132*, 441-449.

Besdine, R.W. (1980). The data base of geriatric medicine. In J.M. Rowe and R.W. Besdine (Eds.), *Health and disease in old age* (pp. 1-24). Boston: Little, Brown.

Birren, J.E., Woods, A.M., and Williams, M.V. (1980). Behavioral slowing with age: Causes, organization, and consequences. In L.W. Poon (Ed.), *Aging in the 1980's: Psychological issues* (pp. 293-308). Washington, DC: American Psychological Association.

Botwinick, J. (1973). *Aging and behavior*. New York: Springer.

Bressler, R., and Conrad, K.A. (1983). Clinical pharmacology. In F.U. Steinberg (Ed.), *Care of the geriatric patient* (pp. 256-274). St. Louis, MO: C.V. Mosby.

Brocklehurst, J.C. (1977). Brain failure in old age—social implications. *Age and Aging, 6*, (Suppl.), 30-41.

Brody, E.M. (1979). Women's changing roles, and care of the aging family. In *Aging: Agenda for the eighties—A national journal issues book*. Washington, DC: Government Research Corporation.

Brody, E.M., Lawton, M.P., and Liebowitz, B. (1984). Senile dementia: Public policy and adequate institutional care. *American Journal of Public Health, 74*, 1381-1383.

Brody, E.M., Poulshock, S.W., and Masciocchi, C.F. (1978). The family caregiving unit: A major consideration in the long-term support system. *Gerontologist, 18*, 556-561.

Brown, G.W., and Harris, T. (1978). *Social origins of depression: A study of psychiatric disorders in women*. New York: Free Press.

Bruer, J.M. (1982). *A handbook of assistive devices for the handicapped elderly*. New York: Academic Press.

Butler, R.N., and Lewis, M.I. (1982). *Aging and mental health*. St. Louis, MO: C.V. Mosby.

Cantor, M. (1980). The informal support system: Its relevance in the lives of elderly. In E. Borgotta and N. McCluskey (Eds.), *Aging and society* (pp. 131-144). Beverly Hills, CA: Sage Publications.

Caplan, G. (1974). *Support systems and community mental health*. New York: Behavioral Publishing.

Caranasos, G.J., Stewart, R.B., and Cluff, L.E. (1974). Drug-induced illness leading to hospitalization. *Journal of the American Medical Association, 288*, 713-717.

Cassel, J. (1976). The contribution of the social environment to host resistance: The Fourth Wade Hampton Frost Lecture. *American Journal of Epidemiology, 104*, 107-123.

Chaisson-Stewart, G.M. (Ed.). (1985). *Depression in the elderly: An interdisciplinary approach*. New York: John Wiley.

Chenoweth, B., and Spencer, B. (1976). Dementia: The experience of family caregivers. *The Gerontologist*, 26, 267-272.

Cobb, S., (1976). Social support as a moderator of life stress. *Psychosomatic Medicine, 38*, 300-314.

Cornbleth, T. (1977). Effects of protected hospital ward area on wandering and nonwandering geriatric patients. *Journal of Gerontology, 32*, 573-577.

Danowski, J.A., and Sacks, W. (1980). Computer communication and the elderly. *Experimental Aging Research*, 6, 125-135.

Dean, A., and Lin, N. (1977). The stress buffering role of social support. *Journal of Nervous and Mental Disorders, 169*, 403-417.

Eaton, J. (1978). Life events, social supports, and psychiatric symptoms: A re-analysis of the New Haven data. *Journal of Health and Social Behavior, 16*, 421-427.

Etzion, D. (1984). Moderating effect of social support on the stress-burnout relationship. *Journal of Applied Psychology, 69*, 615-622.

Fillenbaum, G., and Smyer, M. (1981). The development, validity, and reliablity of the OARS multidimensional functional assessment questionnaire. *Journal of Gerontology, 36*, 428- 434.

Fitting, M., Rabins, P., Lucas, M.J., and Eastham, J. (1986). Caregivers for dementia patients: A comparison of husbands and wives. *The Gerontologist, 26*, 248-252.

Garibaldi, R.A., Brodine, S., and Matsumiya, S. (1981). Infections among patients in nursing homes: Policies, prevalence and problems. *The New England Journal of Medicine, 305*, 731-735.

Gibson, R.M., and Waldo, D.R. (1981). National health expenditures, 1980. *Health Care Financing Review, 3*, 1-54.

Gilhooly, M.L.M. (1984). The impact of care-giving on care-givers: Factors associated with the psychological well-being of people supporting a dementing relative in the community. *British Journal of Medical Psychology, 57*, 35-44.

George, L.K., and Gwyther, L.P. (1986). Caregiver well-being: A multidimensional examination of family caregivers of demented adults. *The Gerontologist, 26*, 253-259.

Golper, L.C., and Rau, M.T. (1983). Treatment of communication disorders associated with generalized intellectual deficits in adults. In W.H. Perkins (Ed.), *Current therapy of communication disorders: Language handicaps in adults* (pp. 119-129). New York: Thieme-Stratton.

Grad de Alarcon, J., and Sainsbury, P. (1963). Mental illness and the family. *Lancet, 1*, 544-547.

Grad de Alarcon, J., and Sainsbury, P. (1965). An evaluation of the effects of caring for the aged at home. In World Psychiatric Association Symposium, *Psychiatric disorders in the aged*. Manchester: Geigy.

Greenblatt, D.J., Divoll, M., Abernathy, D.R., and Shader, R.I. (1982). Physiologic changes in old age: Relation to altered drug disposition. *Journal of the American Geriatrics Society, 30* (Suppl.), s6-s10.

Gunderson, E.K., and Rahe, R.H. (1974). *Life stress and illness*. Springfield, IL: Charles C Thomas.

Gurland, B.J., Kuriansky, J., Sharpe, L., Simon, R., Stiller, P., and Birkett, P. (1977-1978). The Comprehensive Assessment and Referral Evaluation (CARE)—Rationale, development and reliability. *International Journal of Aging and Human Development, 8*, 9-42.

Henderson, S. (1977). The social network, support and neurosis: The function of attachment in adult life. *British Journal of Psychiatry, 131*, 185-191.

Hirschfeld, M. (1983). Homecare versus institutionalization: Family caregiving and senile brain disease. *International Journal of Nursing Studies, 20*, 23-32.

Hoffman, S.B., Platt, C.A., Barry, K.E., and Hamill, L.A. (1985, July). *When language fails: Nonverbal communication abilities of the demented*. Paper presented to the International Congress of Gerontology, New York.

Hurwitz, N. (1969). Predisposing factors in adverse reactions to drugs. *British Medical Journal, 1*, 536-539.

Isaacs, B, Livingstone, E.M., and Neville, Y. (1972). *Survival of the unfittest: A study of geriatric patients in Glasgow*. London: Routledge and Kegan Paul.

Kaszniak, A.W., and Schechner, E. (1981, August). *Correlates of distress among families of chronically ill elderly*. Paper presented as part of symposium at the 89th Annual Meeting of the American Psychological Association. Los Angeles, CA.

Kazdin, A.E. (1982). *Single-case research designs*. New York: Oxford University Press.

Keeler, E.B., Kane, R. L., and Solomon, D.H. (1981). Short- and long-term residents of nursing homes. *Medical Care, 19*, 363-369.

Kiecolt-Glaser, J.K., Glaser, R., Williger, D., Stout,

J., Messick, G., Sheppard, S., Ricker, D., Romisher, S.C., Briner, W., Bonnell, G., and Donnerberg, R. (1985). Psychosocial enhancement of immunocompetence in a geriatric population. *Health Psychology, 4*, 25-41.

Kynette, D., and Kemper, S. (1986). Aging and the loss of grammatical forms: A cross-sectional study of language performance. *Language and Communication,* 6, 65-72.

Lamy, P.P. (1980). *Prescribing for the elderly*. Littleton, MA: PSG Publishing Company.

Lamy, P.P. (1982). Comparative pharmacokinetic changes and drug therapy in an older population. *Journal of the American Geriatrics Society*, (Suppl. 30), s11- s19.

LaRue, A., Bank, L., Jarvik, L., and Hetland, M. (1979). Health in old age: How do physicians' rating and self-ratings compare? *Journal of Gerontology, 34*, 687-691.

Lawton, M.P., Moss, M., Fulcomer, M., and Kleban, M.H. (1982). A research and service oriented multilevel assessment instrument. *Journal of Gerontology, 37*, 91-99.

Leske, M.C. (1981). Prevalence estimates of communicative disorders in the U.S.: Language, hearing, and vestibular disorders. *American Speech- Language-Hearing Association, 23*, 229-237.

Liu, K., and Palesch, Y. (1981). The nursing home population: Different perspectives and implications for policy. *Health Care Financing Review, 19*, 15- 23.

Lowenthal, M.P. (1964). Social isolation and mental illness in old age. *American Sociological Review, 29*, 54-70.

Mace, N.L., and Rabins, P.V. (1981). *The 36-hour day*. Baltimore: Johns Hopkins University Press.

Maddox, G.L., and Douglass, E.B. (1973). Self-assessment of health. *Journal of Health and Social Behavior, 14*, 87-93.

McGlone, F.B. (1982). Therapeutics and an older population: A physician's perspective. *Journal of the American Geriatrics Society*, (Suppl. 30), s1-s2.

McReynolds, L.V., and Kearns, K.P. (1982). *Single-subject experimental designs in communicative disorders.* Austin, TX: PRO-ED.

Morycz, R.K. (1985). Caregiving strain and the desire to institutionalize family members with Alzheimer's disease: Possible predictors and model development. *Research on Aging,* 7, 329-362.

Myers, J., Lindenthal, J.J., and Pepper, M. (1975). Life events, social integration and psychiatric symptomatology. *Journal of Health and Social Behavior, 16*, 421-427.

Myers, J.K., Weissman, M.W., Tischler, G.L., Leaf, P.J., Holzer, C.E., Orvaschel, H., and Boyd, J. (1982, November). *Depression and perception of health in an urban community*. Paper presented at the meeting of the American Public Health Association, Montreal, Canada.

Obler, L.K., Obermann, L., Samuels, I., and Albert, M.L. (1985, November). *Written input to enhance comprehension in Alzheimer's dementia*. Paper presented to the American Speech-Language-Hearing Association, Washington, DC.

Ouslander, J.G. (1981). Drug therapy in the elderly. *Annals of Internal Medicine, 95*, 711-722.

Pajk, M. (1984). Alzheimer's disease inpatient care. *American Journal of Nursing, 84, 216-222.*

Pfeiffer, E. (1976). *Multidimensional functional assessment: The OARS methodology*. Durham, NC: Center for Study of Aging and Human Development.

Pfeiffer, E., and Busse, E. (1975). Mental disorders in later life, affective disorders, paranoid, neurotic and situational reactions. In E. Busse and E. Pfeiffer (Eds.), *Mental illness in later life* (pp. 107-144). Washington, DC: American Psychiatric Association.

Piktialis, D. (1986). Private long term care insurance: A partial solution?, *The American Journal of Alzheimer's Care and Related Disorders, 1*, 37-43.

Rabins, P.V. (1984). Management of dementia in the family context. *Psychosomatics, 25*, 369-375.

Rabins, P.V. (1986). Establishing Alzheimer's disease units in nursing homes: Pros and cons. *Hospital and Community Psychiatry, 37*, 120-121.

Rabins, P.V., Mace, N.L., and Lucas, M.J. (1982). The impact of dementia on the family. *Journal of the American Medical Association, 248*, 333-335.

Rabkin, J.G., and Streuning, E.L. (1976). Life events, stress and illness. *Science, 194*, 1013-1020.

Rango, N. (1982). Nursing-home care in the United States. *The New England Journal of Medicine, 307*, 883-889.

Ray, W.A., Federspiel, C.F., and Schaffner, W. (1980). A study of antipsychotic drug use in nursing homes: Epidemiologic evidence suggesting misuse. *American Journal of Public Health, 70*, 485-491.

Reichstein, K.J., and Bergofsky, L. (1980). *Summary and report of the National survey of state administered domicilliary care programs in the fifty states and the District of Columbia*. Horizon Institute.

Reifler, B.V., and Wu, S. (1982). Managing families of the demented elderly. *The Journal of Family Practice. 14*, 1051-1056.

Richards, L.D., Zuckerman, D.M., and West, P.R. (1985). Alzheimer's disease: Current congressional response. *American Psychologist. 40*, 1256-1261.

Rosin, A.J., Abramowitz, L., Diamond, J., and Jesselson, P. (1985). Environmental management of senile dementia. *Social Work in Health Care. 11*, 33-43.

Sainsbury, P, and Grad de Alarcon, J. (1970). The psychiatrist and the geriatric patient: The effects of community care on the family of the geriatric patient. *Journal of Geriatric Psychiatry. 1*, 23-41.

Sands, D., and Suzuki, T. (1983). Adult day care for Alzheimer's patients and their families. *The Gerontologist. 23*, 21-23.

Sanford, J.R.A. (1975). Tolerance of debility in elderly dependents by supporters at home: Its significance for hospital practice. *British Medical Journal. 23*, 471-473.

Satariano, W.A., Minkler, M.A., Langhauser, C. (1984). The significance of an ill spouse for assessing health differences in an elderly population. *Journal of the American Geriatrics Society. 32*, 187-190.

Schaie, K.W., and Marquette, B. (1972). Personality in maturity and old age. In R.M. Dreger (Ed.), *Multivariate personality research: Contributions to the understanding of personality in honor of Raymond B. Cattell* (pp. 612-623). Baton Rouge: Claitor's Publishing.

Schram, S.F. (1982). Social services for older people. In B.L. Neugarten (Ed.), *Age or need? Public policies for older people* (pp. 221-246). Beverly Hills, CA: Sage Publications.

Seidel, L.G., Thornton, G.F., Smith, J.W., and Cluff, L.E. (1966). Studies on the epidemiology of adverse drug reactions III. Reactions in patients on a general medical service. *Bulletin Johns Hopkins Hospital, 119*, 299-315.

Shanas, E. (1979). Social myth as hypothesis: The case of the family relations of old people. *The Gerontologist, 19*, 3-9.

Siegler, I.C., Nowlin, J.B., and Blumenthal, J.A. (1980). Health and behavior: Methodological considerations for adult development and aging. In L.W. Poon (Ed.), *Aging in the 1980's: Psychological issues* (pp. 599-612). Washington, DC: American Psychological Association.

Silverstone, B. (1985). Informal social support systems for the frail elderly. In Committee on an Aging Society, *Health in an Older Society* (pp. 153-181). Washington, DC: National Academy of Sciences.

Smith, J.W., Seidel, L.G., and Cluff, L.E. (1966). Studies on the epidemiology of adverse drug reactions. V. Clinical factors influencing susceptibility. *Annals of Internal Medicine. 65*, 629-640.

Staff. (1982, February 26). VNA's will "hold" their own, proprietary to "gain force," PNP's to "lose force," hospital-based HHA's to "gain ground," hospital discharge planning rules should be updated - says FDA expert. *Home Health Line, 6*, p. 2.

Thoits, P. (1982). Conceptual, methodological, and theoretical problems in studying social support as a buffer against stress. *Journal of Health and Social Behavior, 23*, 145-159.

Thompson, T.L., Moran, M.G., and Nies, A.S. (1983). Psychotropic drug use in the elderly (second of two parts). *New England Journal of Medicine, 308*, 194-199.

Tomoeda, C.K., Bayles, K.A., and Slauson, T.J. (1986, February). *Effect of presentation rate and syntactic complexity on sentence comprehension in Alzheimer's patients and the normal elderly*. Poster presented at the 1986 meeting of the International Neuropsychological Society, Denver, CO.

Troll, L.E., Miller, S.J., and Atchley, R.C. (1979). *Families in later life*. Belmont, CA: Wadsworth.

U.S. Current Population Reports, Series P-60, No. 140, "Money Income and Poverty Status of Families and Persons in the United States: 1982," U.S. Bureau of the Census, table 6, p. 12.

U.S. Department of Health, Education, and Welfare (1978). *Health-United States 1978* [DHEW Publication No. (PHS) 78-1232]. Washington, DC: Author.

U.S. General Accounting Office (1983). *Medicaid and nursing home care: Cost increases and the need for services are creating problems for the states and the elderly*. IPE 84-1, Washington, DC: U.S. Congress, U.S. Comptroller General.

U.S. National Center for Health Statistics (1977). *Utilization of nursing homes U.S.: National nursing home survey, August 1973-April 1974*. [DHEW publication no. (HRA) 77-1779]. Washington, DC: Department of Health and Human Services.

U.S. National Center for Health Statistics (1979). *National Nursing Home Survey: 1977 Summary for the U.S.*, [DHEW Publication No. (PHS) 79-1794]. Washington, DC: Department of Health and Human Services.

U.S. National Center for Health Statistics (1980). *Basic data on hearing level of adults 25-74*, Washington, DC: Office of Health Research Statistics and Technology.

U.S. National Center for Health Statistics (1981a). *Vital statistics of the United States: Vol. 2, Mortality*. Washington, DC: Department of Health and Human Services.

U.S. National Center for Health Statistics (1981b). *Characteristics of nursing home residents, health status and care received: National nursing home survey, May-Dec., 1977.* (No. 81-1712). Washington, DC: Department of Health and Human Services.

U.S. Office of the Inspector General (1981). *Long term care: Service delivery assessment.* Report to the Secretary (unpublished). 2 volumes. Department of Health and Human Services.

U.S. Office of Technology Assessment (1985). *Technology and Aging in America* (OTA-BA-264). Washington, DC: U.S. Congress.

Weissert, W.G. (1976). Two models of geriatric day care: Findings of a comparative study. *The Gerontologist, 16*, 420-427.

Weissert, W.B., and Scanlon, W. (1982, November). *Determinants of institutionalization of the aged.* Working paper no. 1466-21. Washington, DC: The Urban Institute.

Williamson, J., and Chopin, J.M. (1980). Adverse reactions to prescribed drugs in the elderly: A multicentre investigation. *Age and Ageing, 9*, 73-80.

Yost, E., Beutler, L., Corbishley, A., and Allender, J. (1986). *Group cognitive therapy with depressed older adults.* New York: Pergamon.

Zarit, J.M. (1982). *Predictors of burden and distress for caregivers of dementia patients.* Unpublished doctoral dissertation, University of Southern California.

Zarit, S.H., Orr, N.K., and Zarit, J.M. (1985). *The hidden victims of Alzheimer's disease: Families under stress.* New York: New York University Press.

Zarit, S.H., Reever, K.E., and Bach-Peterson, J. (1980). Relatives of the impaired elderly: Correlates of feelings of burden. *The Gerontologist, 20*, 649-655.

Glossary

acalculia: an inability to do simple arithmetic calculations as a result of cerebral damage.

acetylcholinesterase (AChE): enzyme catalyzing the hydrolysis of acetycholine to choline and acetic acid; deficient in Alzheimer's disease.

agnosia: loss of the ability to recognize one or more types of sensory stimuli; due to cerebral damage.

agraphia: an inability to write, in the absence of muscular weakness; due to cerebral damage.

alexia: an inability to comprehend written language, due to cerebral damage.

Alzheimer's disease (AD): a degenerative neurologic disorder characterized by behavioral changes (memory, cognition, personality, language, and communication) subsequent to abnormal histopathologic (neurofibrillary tangles, neuritic plaques, granulovacuolar degeneration) and neurochemical changes.

amygdaloid nucleus: corpus amygdaloideum; located within the tip of the temporal cortex; involved in olfaction and emotion.

aneuploidy: state of having an abnormal number of chromosomes.

angular gyrus syndrome: constellation of disorders including fluent aphasia, alexia without agraphia, Gertsmann's syndrome, and constructional apraxia; sometimes confused with Alzheimer's disease.

anomic aphasia: a language impairment characterized by good comprehension and expression, but with pronounced word-finding difficulties, resulting in occasionally fluent but circumlocutory and empty discourse.

anterograde amnesia: condition in which a patient is unable to learn new information from the time of illness onset.

aphasia: loss of language and communicative function (comprehension, processing, and production of linguistic information); due to central nervous system damage.

apraxia: loss of the ability to accurately perform voluntary movements; not due to paresis or paralysis.

atrophy: a reduction in size and function of a cell, tissue, or organ.

autosomal dominance: autosomal refers to any chromosome other than the sex chromosome, and therefore is not sex-linked; dominant means that the defective gene dominates its normal partner gene in its phenotypic expression.

basal ganglia: a collection of nuclei within the cerebral hemispheres and the upper brainstem which are important in the control of motor function; included are the caudate nucleus, putamen, globus pallidus, claustrum, and the substantia nigra.

Binswanger's disease: also subcortical atherosclerotic encephalopathy and encephalitis subcorticalis chronica; loss of subcortical white matter, with sclerotic changes in the supplying blood vessels, resulting in dementia with a typically rapid progression.

board-and-care facilities: an alternative living situation for functionally impaired individuals, providing 24-hour protective care and assistance with daily activities; medical care is not typically provided.

bottom–up activation: activation that proceeds from sensory receptors to higher levels of processing within semantic memory.

bradykinesia: slowness in the ability to initiate and execute movement.

bradyphrenia: slowing of cognition.

Broca's aphasia: initially described by neurologist Paul Broca in 1864; language impairment subsequent to focal lesions in Broca's area (Broadmann's area 44) in the third frontal convolution; may also involve damage to motor regions superior and anterior to area 44; characterized by nonfluent, telegraphic expression with phonemic paraphasias, and omission of function words; frequently accompanied by apraxia of speech.

caudate nucleus: an elongated collection of neurons near the lateral ventricle; forms the corpus striatum with the putamen; part of the basal ganglia, which are important in the control of movement; the primary area of degeneration in Parkinson's disease.

cerebral arteriosclerosis: a thickening and loss of plasticity of the arteries of the brain; assumed to play a causal role in multi-infarct dementia.

cerebral ischemia: disruption of delivery of blood to brain tissue.

cerebrovascular accident (CVA): disruption of the blood supply to, and subsequent necrosis of, brain tissue, following hemorrhagic, thrombolic, or embolic occlusion of the supplying arteries; the primary cause of focal lesion aphasia.

choline acetyltrasferase (ChAT): enzyme motivating the synthesis of acetylcholine; deficient in Alzheimer's disease.

choreiform movements: chorea; complex, jerky, involuntary movements; associated with Huntington's disease.

circumlocution: words and phrases substituted for an intended word; frequently observed during instances of word-finding difficulty.

cogwheel: style of movement resulting from the superimposition of resting tremor on rigidity (increased resting tone); common in Parkinson's disease patients.

coherence: in discourse, the logical ordering of parts, accomplished by a variety of logical and grammatical devices.

cohesive devices: linguistic techniques that function to relate propositions to each other; contribute to discourse or text coherence.

communication: the sharing of information by means of a symbol system; may be linguistic or nonlinguistic.

computerized tomography (CT): radiographic imaging technique wherein relative tissue absorption of the emergent beam is counted and recorded by a computer, and reconstructed on a monitor screen or photographic film to produce an image; useful in determining the presence of intracranial masses and cerebral atrophy, as well as other aspects of intracranial anatomy.

concatenation rules: principles specifying the appropriate ordering and linkage of elements.

concept: the elemental unit of semantic memory; hypothetical mental constructs, a mental representation of a general class or category.

conduction aphasia: language impairment due to focal lesions in the left perisylvian area, involving the primary auditory cortex, a portion of the surrounding association cortex, and portions of the insula, supramarginal gyrus, and arcuate fasciculus; characterized by nonfluent expression with occasional phonemic and semantic paraphasias, good comprehension, and a pronounced inability to repeat or to read aloud.

conductive hearing loss: loss due to interference with sound transmission through the outer or middle ear.

conservator: an individual appointed by the court to manage the property and income of an "incapacitated" person.

constructional apraxia: a perceptual-motor impairment typified by an inability to translate a visual perception into an appropriate action; thus, activities such as assembling, building and drawing are affected.

coreference: two terms referring to the same thing (e.g., **The pastry chef** is French. **He** makes wonderful eclairs.).

cortical dementia: a controversial classification of dementing diseases on the basis of presumed cortical preponderance of pathologic changes; includes Alzheimer's disease, Creutzfeldt-Jakob disease, and Pick's disease.

Creutzfeldt-Jakob spongiform encephalopathy: a viral disease, characterized by partial degeneration of pyramidal and extrapyramidal tracts, with progressive dementia, tremor, athetosis, and spastic dysarthria.

crystallized intelligence: represents the cumulative product of information previously acquired by the activity of fluid intelligence; represents culturally acquired information.

day care services: care programs for cognitively impaired elderly individuals, designed to provide social interaction and stimulation while affording the caregiver temporary respite from the caregiving situation; services may include medical supervision and rehabilitative services.

deixis: linguistic "pointing" terms relating to time, place, and person in a conversation or text (e.g., here/there, today/yesterday).

delirium: typically a short-term syndrome including altered state of consciousness, cognitive change, language impairment, memory disorders, and delusions; typically due to toxic metabolic abnormality.

dementia: a syndrome including decreased intellect, memory, language, and communicative ability and personality change; may result from over 50 reversible and irreversible causes.

dendrites: unipolar, bipolar, or tree-like extensions from the cell body, which receive information from axons of neighboring cells through neurotransmitter activity at specific points of contact (synapses).

disjunction: a type of inferential process of the logical form "p or q" and "not p" therefore "q."

dopamine-β-hydroxylase: a dopamine-converting enzyme located in the basal ganglia; particularly deficient in the brains of Parkinson's disease patients, though concentrations decline with normal aging.

Down syndrome: condition resulting from the presence of a third chromosome 21; includes several skeletal abnormalities and moderate to severe mental retardation.

dysarthria: a variety of motor speech disorders (e.g., spastic, hypokinetic, flaccid); due to central or peripheral neuronal damage.

dyslogia: term suggested by MacDonald Critchley for the language and communication impairment associated with Alzheimer's disease.

dysphagia: difficulty in swallowing.

echoic memory: sensory memory specific to auditory information processing.

ecological validity: degree to which the tested behavior represents or is relevant to the patient's real-life circumstances.

electroencephalogram (EEG): a recording of the electrical activity of brain cells, obtained through electrodes placed on the scalp; useful in the differential diagnosis of neurologic disorders.

ellipsis: omission of a word or phrase whose meaning is implied.

emotional lability: increased variability in emotional states; tendency to the inappropriate expression of emotion; common in patients with brain damage and mental illness.

encephalitis: inflammation of the brain.

episodic memory: that hypothetic system of memory involved in the input, storage, and retrieval of events along with their spatial and temporal relationships; that aspect of human knowledge concerned with autobiographic information.

evoked potentials: discrete electric charges from brain neurons, resulting from the presentation of sensory stimulation.

fluid intelligence: involves processes used in acquiring new information.

formal support: governmental, religous, national, and local support groups; contrasted with informal support.

γ-aminobutyric acid (GABA): the major inhibitory neurotransmitter in the brain; synthesized through the decarboxylation (removal of a carboxyl group) of glutamate, catalyzed by glutamic acid decarboxylase (GAD), a neuroenzyme; deficient in Huntington's disease patients.

generative grammar: also transformational grammar; a set of rules capable of generating an infinite number of sentences in a natural language; a set of rules whereby sentences can be related to each other and transformed.

Gerstmann syndrome: syndrome characterized by acalculia, difficulty with left–right discriminations, finger agnosia. The status of this constellation as a unitary syndrome is controversial.

gist: the moral or implied meaning underlying a segment of discourse, derived through inferential processes.

global aphasia: severe inability to produce, process, and comprehend language; due to brain damage in the language dominant cerebral hemisphere.

glutamic acid decarboxylase (GAD): enzyme responsible for catalyzing the neurotransmitter γ-aminobutyric acid (GABA) through the removal of a carboxyl group (decarboxylation) from glutamates.

granulovacuolar degeneration: an accumulation of fluid-filled vacuoles and granular debris within a cell; occurring primarily in the temporal and frontal regions of Alzheimer's disease patients, and, to a lesser degree, in the normal elderly.

guardian: individual appointed by the court to make decisions regarding medical care, rehabilitative services, and residence for "incapacitated" persons; not liable for the debts or actions of the ward, although the guardian may be responsible for making financial decisions and planning in the absence of a court-appointed conservator.

hallucination: a perceptual experience in the absence of apparent sensory stimulation.

hemianopsia: impaired vision or blindness in half of the visual field.

hereditary dysphasic dementia: deterioration of cognitive and communicative function in older members of successive generations within a single family; combines the characterstic neuropathologic features of both Alzheimer's and Pick's disease.

hippocampus: located in the temporal lobe and considered a component of the limbic system; involved in learning and memory; area that demonstrates particularly severe damage in AD.

histopathologic changes: abnormal changes in the microscopic structure, function, and composition of tissue.

homovanillic acid: the primary metabolite of dopamine; a low level of this chemical in cerebrospinal fluid is a marker of dopamine deficiency.

horizontal activation: spread of activation within a single level of semantic memory (i.e. concept–concept, proposition–proposition, schema–schema).

Huntington's disease (HD): an autosomal dominant, degenerative neurologic condition characterized by low levels of GABA and the development of choreiform movements and dementia.

hyperreflexia: an exaggeration of the reflexes.

hypothalamus: portion of the diencephalon forming the floor and a portion of the wall of the third ventricle; includes the optic chiasm, mammillary bodies, tuber cinereum, infundibulum, and hypophysis; involved in the activation and integration of peripheral autonomic functions, endocrine regulation, and many somatic functions; controls the pituitary gland through secretions of vasopressin and oxytocin.

iconic memory: sensory memory specific to visual information processing.

ideational perseveration: the inappropriate repetition of an idea or concept in the absence of the original elicitor.

idiopathic: without a known cause.

illocutionary: type of utterance that in itself represents the performance of some act; common types are directives, representatives, commissives, expressives, and declarations.

implicature: indication through inference or association, rather than through direct statement.

incontinence: an inability to control excretory functions; incontinence of bladder and bowel are common late stage problems in Alzheimer's disease patients.

infarction: a condition in which death of tissue occurs due to insufficient vascular circulation.

informal support: the support provided by family, friends, neighbors, and other nonprofessional persons with whom the caregiver interacts frequently.

information unit: any new, relevant piece of information; unit used for quantifying the ideational impoverishment of the discourse of dementia patients.

kuru: transmissible spongiform encephalopathy found in cannibalistic native tribes in New Guinea who eat raw brain tissue of recently deceased victims of the disease; characterized by dementia, tremor, ataxia, and dysarthria.

lacunar state: syndrome label applied to patients, typically with a diagnosis of multi-infarct dementia, with large numbers of lacunar infarcts.

lacunes: small cavities of infarcted tissue primarily in the basal ganglia, thalamus, brain stem, and deep cerebral white matter; typically secondary to middle cerebral, posterior cerebral, and basilar artery occlusion; commonly observed in individuals with multi-infarct dementia.

levodopa: 3-hydroxy-L-tyrosine; the levorotatory (left-turning) isomer of dopa; a precursor of dopamine; used in the treatment of Parkinson's disease.

lexical ambiguity: word ambiguity; a word in a phrase or sentence that has more than one meaning (e.g., The boy found the **bat**.).

limbic system: a collection of brain structures, including the amygdala, hippocampus, dentate gyrus, cingulate gyrus, and septal areas and adjacent structures deep within the brain; important in autonomic functions, olfaction, emotion, and memory.

linguistic reference: what the words refer to; may be different from speaker reference.

logical ambiguity: more than one interpretation of subject–verb–object relations (e.g., John wants the presidency more than Martha.).

logoclonia: repetition of the final syllable of a word.

macrostructure: the elements of a text or discourse that constitute the theme.

magnetic resonance imaging (MRI): also nuclear magnetic resonance (NMR); a noninvasive, high-resolution imaging technique in which proton behavior in tissue subjected to a magnetic field is measured; the emitted signals are reconstructed to form an image of the tissue.

Medicaid: a federal health-care reimbursement program, the primary reimbursor for long-term care costs in the United States.

Medicare: a federal health-care reimbursement program, covering short-term, acute care costs.

metaphor: a figure of speech in which a term literally denoting one kind of object or idea is used in place of another to suggest a likeness or analogy between them, as in "the winter of life."

micrographia: tendency for the handwriting to become small; frequently observed in individuals with extrapyramidal damage, particularly Parkinson's disease patients.

modularity: a set of characteristics (see Chapter 2) theorized by Fodor (1983) to define certain cognitive faculties, notably the perceptual input systems.

multi-infarct dementia (MID): a dementia syndrome consequent to repeated cerebral infarctions; characterized by bilateral brain damage.

muscarinic receptors: a type of cholinergic neurotransmitter receptor site.

myoclonus: abrupt contractions of a portion of a muscle, an entire muscle, or a group of muscles; may occur asynchronously or in synchrony.

neglect syndrome: failure to report, respond, or orient to stimuli presented to the side opposite the brain lesion; not attributable to sensory or motor defects.

neuritic plaque: also senile plaque; an aggregation of neuronal debris having an amyloid core surrounded by an outer ring of granular filamentous material; present in small numbers in intellectually intact elderly individuals and to a greater extent in the brains of patients with Alzheimer's disease.

neurofibrillary tangles: twisted intraneuronal fibers or pairs of helically wound filaments within the cytoplasm of the neuronal cell body; characteristic histopathologic sign of Alzheimer's disease.

neuropleptic drugs: drugs that serve to favorably

alter psychotic behaviors; includes phenothiazines, butyrophenones, and thioxanthenes.

neuropeptides: short chains of amino acids found in brain tissue, which act as neurotransmitters and hormones.

nonautomatic language tasks: tasks requiring the creative and intentional use of language.

normal pressure hydrocephalus: condition marked by enlargement of the ventricles and subsequent inadequacy in the subarachnoid space in the presence of normal cerebrospinal fluid pressure; signs include dementia, urinary incontinence, and ataxia.

nuclear magnetic resonance (NMR): also magnetic resonance imaging (MRI).

nucleus basalis of Meynert (nbM): ganglion located directly beneath the globus pallidus; a major component of the substantia innominata; approximately 70 percent of the cholinergic activity in the cortex occurs at terminals with cell bodies located in the nbM.

Older Americans Act of 1965: legislation for the development of service programs designed specifically for the elderly.

on-off phenomenon: rapid unpredictable swings from a hyperkinetic state to one of akinesia and rigidity; commonly observed in Parkinson's disease patients receiving drug therapy.

paralysis agitans: a term for parkinsonism.

paraphasia: linguistic errors, phonemically or semantically related to the intended word.

Parkinson's disease (PD): a neurologic syndrome resulting from disruption of dopaminergic activity in the subcortex; signs include hypokinesia, bradyphrenia, resting tremor, rigidity, and frequently cognitive impairment and dementia.

perseveration: the inappropriate repetition of a response in the absence of the original elicitor.

perlocutionary: a type of speech act; distinguished from an illocutionary act in that it has an observable effect on the listener; for example, the listener is persuaded, cajoled, or comforted.

Pick's disease: a degenerative neurologic disease with particularly marked frontal atrophy resulting in a dementia syndrome characterized by difficulty in reasoning and irrational behaviors.

pharmacodynamics: the study of the effects of medications.

pharmacokinetics: the study of the distribution and metabolism of medications within the body.

phonemic paraphasia: linguistic errors that are phonemically related to the intended word; may include a single phoneme substitution, or may approach neologistic paraphasias, with the production of several incorrect phonemes rendering the intended word nearly unrecognizable.

phonologic knowledge: the rules for ordering the sounds of a language into words, phoneme production, and prosody.

physostigmine: a cholinergic facilitator that inhibits the action of acetylcholinesterase (AChE).

positron emission tomography (PET): an imaging technique during which positron-emitting isotopes are introduced into tissue. The paths of the gamma rays resulting from the collision of positrons and electrons, which are inherent in tissue, are recorded by a computer, generating a tomogram depicting locations of isotope-containing substances. The tomogram may be used as an indicator of metabolic activity.

pragmatic knowledge: knowledge related to the interaction between language structure and language use; includes deixis, conversational implicature, presupposition, speech acts, and discourse construction; entails meaning not apparent through analysis of only language structure and semantics, requires consideration of the context and extralinguistic variables.

praxis: performance of intentional movements.

presupposition: assumptions made by the speaker/writer about the type and extent of the listener's/reader's prior knowledge; the speaker's/writer's concept of the context in which the communicative exchange occurs.

primary memory: short-term memory; stage in information processing model in which new information is acquired and briefly retained; storage is limited.

prions: **pro**tinaceous **in**fectious particles implicated as the infectious agent in slow virus diseases, such as scrapie and Creutzfeldt-Jakob diesease, and hypothesized as being involved in Alzheimer's disease.

proactive interference: occurs when previously learned information interferes with recall of more recent material.

proposition: a structural unit of semantic memory; a relational expression (either linguistic or nonlinguistic) that is grammatically analogous to a clause, composed of a relational term such as a verb, and one or more nouns or noun phrases that function as subjects and objects of the relation.

prosody: the melodic contour, pausal phenomena, and stress of spoken language.

prosopagnosia: impairment in the ability to recognize familiar faces, typically secondary to bilateral brain damage.

pseudodementia: memory loss and cognitive and communicative impairment secondary to mental illness, most frequently depression.

psychomotor agitation: increase in motor activity and restlessness, sometimes present in depression.

psychomotor retardation: marked slowing of movemovement and thought, often present in depression.

putamen: lateral portion of the lentiform nucleus; forms the corpus striatum with the caudate nucleus, within the basal ganglia.

recruitment: increase in loudness sensation at a greater rate than normal.

retrograde amnesia: condition in which a patient is unable to recall events that occurred prior to illness onset.

rigidity: increase in the resting tone of muscle or resistance to passive stretch; present throughout the muscle's range of motion.

schema: a structural unit of semantic memory; formed through the simultaneous activation of a group of concepts and propositions that are related to a specific event, object, or sensation; prediction and inference are possible through activation of appropriate schema.

scrapie: transmissible spongiform encephalopathy of sheep and goats; similar to Creutzfeldt-Jakob disease in humans; possibly related to the histopathologic changes associated with Alzheimer's disease.

secondary memory: long-term memory; theoretically a relatively permanent repository of information with unlimited capacity.

semantic knowledge: knowledge of the meaning properties and relations, referential properties and relations, and truth properties and relations expressed by language.

semantic memory: the highest-level cognitive modality, a hierarchically organized representational system; consisting of concepts, propositions, and schema; receives input from perceptual systems; system in which intermodality transfer of information occurs; the aspect of the mind wherein ideation and inferencing take place; it is the central processing unit of human knowledge and is particularly impaired in Alzheimer's disease.

semantic paraphasias: linguistic errors that are related in meaning to the intended word; for example, "pear" for "peach."

semantic priming: phenomenon in which a stimulus (e.g.,, a word, string of letters, category name) facilitates a target response (e.g., naming a word, deciding if a string of letters is a word, providing an example of a category) because the target is semantically related to the stimulus. For example, the word "dog" is processed faster after "cat" than after "pickle."

senile plaque: see neuritic plaque.

sensorineural hearing loss: loss due to a disorder of the cochlea or auditory nervous system.

sensory memory: conceptualized as a preattentive information registration system that is modality specific. See echoic and iconic memory.

skilled nursing care: a level of nursing home care and certification, stipulating 24-hour nursing care under the supervision of a physician.

somatostatin: peptide, decreased in Alzheimer's disease.

speaker reference: the speaker's intended meaning of an utterance; may be different from linguistic reference.

speech act theory: a theory about the ways linguistic utterances can be used.

stereotypies: frequent almost mechanical repetition of the same form of speech, or movement, or posture.

structural ambiguity: differences in meaning arising from the way in which words are grouped or chunked (e.g., he hit the man with the stick; he asked how old George was).

subcortical dementia: a controversial clinical classification of dementing diseases based on presumed subcortical preponderance of pathologic changes including Huntington's disease, multi-infarct dementia, normal pressure hydrocephalus, Parkinson's disease, and progressive supranuclear palsy.

substance P: peptide neurotransmitter found in the intestine, brain, and spinal cord; involved in the dilation of blood vessels and transmission of pain impulses.

substantia innominata: collection of nerve tissue including the nucleus basalis of Meynert, immediately ventral to the globus pallidus and ansa lenticularis and immediately caudal to the anterior perforated substance; area of neuropathologic change in Alzheimer's disease.

substantia nigra: one of the basal ganglia; composed of two zones, a dorsal zone of melanin (pigment)-containing cells, and a ventral zone lacking melanin. A hallmark neuropathologic finding in Parkinson's disease is depigmentation of the substantia nigra.

sylvian fissure: also known as the sulcus lateralis cerebri or lateral fissure; fissure running anterior to posterior; division between the temporal and frontal lobes of the brain.

syntactic knowledge: knowledge of the structure of a language; the rules for meaningfully ordering words and phrases.

tinnitus: a noice in the ears such as ringing, buzzing, roaring, clicking.

tissue hypoxia: a reduction in the oxygen supply to tissue.

Title XX: a portion of the 1974 Social Security Acts, providing federal block grants to states for reimbursement of health care costs, including monies dedicated to the elderly.

top-down activation: activation that proceeds from higher order mechanisms in semantic memory to lower order mechanisms.

transcortical motor aphasia: language impairment following a small, deep lesion within the left frontal subcortical matter or areas anterior or superior to Broca's area in the third frontal convolution; has similar features to those of Broca's aphasia, but with an exceptional ability to repeat.

transcortical sensory aphasia: language impairment secondary to focal brain lesions in area 37, the angular gyrus (area 39), and portions of area 22 of the dominant hemisphere; with a language profile similar to that of Wernicke's aphasia, but with an exceptional ability to repeat.

transient ischemic attack (TIA): temporary cessation of blood flow to brain tissue; due to trauma, thrombosis or embolism; results in temporary neurologic and/or neuropsychologic deficit.

tremor: involuntary oscillation of the musculature, due to asynchronous and antagonistic contraction of muscles.

trisomy-21: the presence of a third chromosome 21, resulting in Down syndrome.

vascular dementia: also multi-infarct dementia.

vasodilators: substances causing the dilation of blood vessels.

Wernicke's aphasia: initially described by Karl Wernicke in 1874; impairment in language and communication due to focal lesions in the posterior and superior left temporal gyrus, frequently extending into the second temporal gyrus and the parietal zone; typified by poor auditory and reading comprehension, poor repetition ability, fluent speech with semantic and phonemic paraphasias, and sometimes neologistic jargon.

Author Index

Subject Index

Note: Page numbers in *italics* refer to illustrations. Page numbers followed by /t/ refer to tables.